FOCUS ON HEALTH

W9-CIO-580

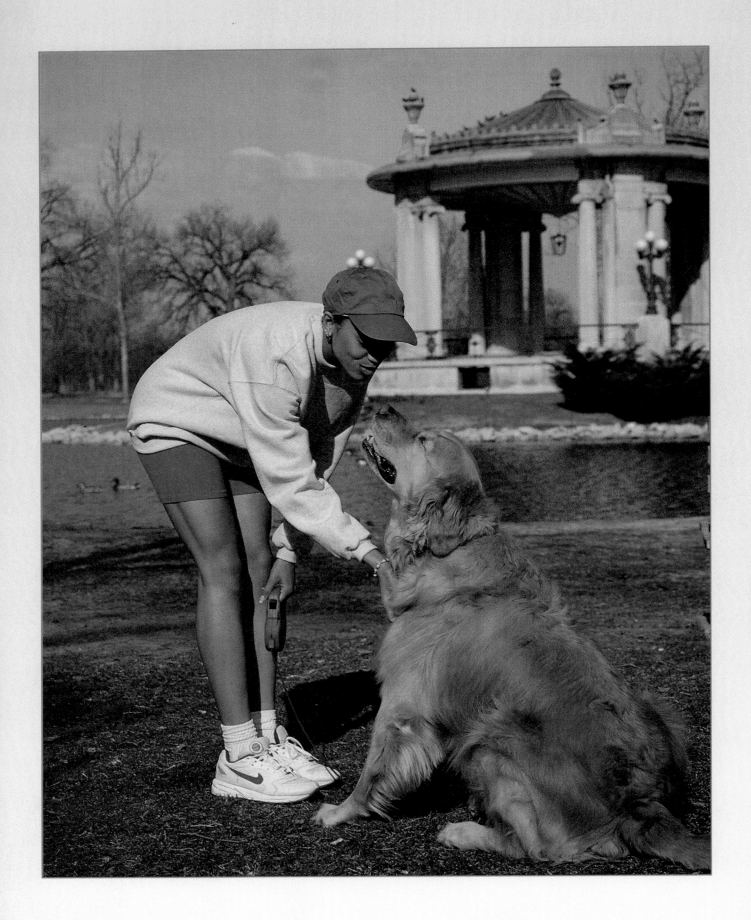

FOCUS ON HEALTH

Dale B. Hahn, Ph.D.
Georgetown College
Georgetown, Kentucky

Wayne A. Payne, Ed.D.
Ball State University
Muncie, Indiana

with 164 illustrations

WCB McGraw-Hill

Boston, Massachusetts   Burr Ridge, Illinois   Dubuque, Iowa
Madison, Wisconsin   New York, New York   San Francisco, California   St. Louis, Missouri

Third
Edition

WCB/McGraw-Hill

A Division of The McGraw-Hill Companies

Vice President and Publisher: James M. Smith
Senior Acquisitions Editor: Vicki Malinee
Developmental Editor: Melissa Martin
Project Manager: Carol Sullivan Weis
Production Editor: Rick Dudley
Designer: Sheilah Barrett
Manufacturing Supervisor: Karen Lewis
Cover Photo: Stewart D. Halperin

On the cover: A college student jogs through the park with her golden retriever. The companionship and affection a dog or cat provides can reduce stress and promote emotional wellness. Owning a large dog like this one can help protect our safety when we're outdoors alone and can make our homes more secure as well.

THIRD EDITION
Copyright © 1997 by Mosby-Year Book, Inc.

Previous editions copyrighted 1991, 1994

All rights reserved. No part of this publication may be reproduced, stored in a retrieval system, or transmitted, in any form or by any means, electronic, mechanical, photocopying, recording, or otherwise, without written permission of the publisher.

Permission to photocopy or reproduce solely for internal or personal use is permitted for libraries or other users registered with the Copyright Clearance Center, provided that the base fee of $4.00 per chapter plus $.10 per page is paid directly to the Copyright Clearance Center, 27 Congress Street, Salem, MA 01970. This consent does not extend to other kinds of copying, such as copying for general distribution, for advertising or promotional purposes, for creating new collected works, or for resale.

Printed in the United States of America
Composition by Black Dot
Printing/binding by Von Hoffmann Press, Inc.

International Standard Book Number 0-8151-4198-X

97 98 99 00 / 9 8 7 6 5 4 3 2

To all of our students, with the hope that the decisions they make will be healthy ones.

Preface

As a health educator, you already know that the personal health course is one of the most exciting courses a college student will take. Today's media-oriented college students are aware of the critical health issues of the 1990s. They hear about environmental issues, substance abuse, sexually transmitted diseases, fitness, and nutrition virtually every day. The value of the personal health course is its potential to expand students' knowledge of these and other health topics. Students will then be able to examine their attitudes toward health issues and modify their behavior to improve their health and perhaps even prevent or delay the onset of certain health conditions.

Focus on Health accomplishes this task with a carefully composed, well-documented manuscript written by two health educators who teach the personal health course to nearly 1000 students each year. We understand the teaching issues you face daily in the classroom and have written this text with your concerns in mind.

This book is written for college students in a wide variety of settings, from community colleges to large four-year universities. The content is carefully constructed to be meaningful to both traditional and nontraditional-age students. We have paid special attention to the increasing numbers of nontraditional students who have decided to pursue a college education. Points in the discussion often address the particular needs of these nontraditional students. *Focus on Health* continues to encourage students of all ages and backgrounds to achieve their goals.

NEW FEATURES OF THIS EDITION
Updated Content

As experienced health educators and authors, we know how important it is to provide students with the most current information available. Throughout each chapter we have included the very latest information and statistics, and the "As we go to press . . ." feature has allowed us to comment on breaking news right up to press time. In addition, we have introduced many timely topics and issues that are sure to pique students' interest and stimulate class discussion.

Occupational Dimension of Health

Two central themes, the multiple dimensions of health and the developmental tasks, are introduced in Chapter 1. We believe that a sixth dimension of health warrants inclusion in this edition: occupational health. An understanding of this aspect of total wellness is especially important for nontraditional students who must meet the demands of both school and work.

Healthy People 2000 Midcourse Reviews

Each chapter begins with an update of how far we've come as a nation in achieving the Healthy People 2000 objectives established in 1990. These national health care goals are explained and the reasons for progress or lack of improvement explored. Students will thus be motivated to evaluate their individual contributions to these trends and take proactive steps to modify their health habits and behavior.

Behavior Change

Chapter 1 includes an entirely new section on behavior change strategies, including determining areas for improvement, setting specific goals, making a personal contract, devising a plan of action, charting progress, preparing for obstacles, and rewarding achievements. Other suggestions for improving health-related behavior are presented throughout the book.

Integrated Presentation of Aging

Topics of interest to midlife and elderly adults no longer appear in the chapter on death and dying, thus sending a more positive message about aging. Instead, the material has been integrated into appropriate chapters according to subject. For example, Alzheimer's disease is now discussed in Chapter 11, Living with Cancer and Chronic Conditions. This reorganization allows both traditional and nontraditional students to learn about the physical and emotional changes that take place as we age.

Reorganized Discussion of Sexuality

The biological and psychosocial origins of sexuality, sexual behavior, and intimate relationships are now presented in a single, comprehensive chapter. This organization gives the student a better framework for studying these complex topics.

New Personal Safety Chapter

With good reason, students are more concerned than ever about issues related to violence and safety both on and off campus. This new chapter, Chapter 16, Protecting Your Safety, delves into critically important current issues such as homicide; domestic violence; hate crimes; sexual victimization; and recreational, residential, and motor vehicle safety.

Wellness and Disease Prevention

Throughout this new edition, you will notice that students are continually urged to be proactive in shaping their future health. For example, Chapter 5, Understanding Nutrition and Your Diet, explains the health benefits of following a semivegetarian or other low-fat diet. Chapter 10, Reducing Your Risk of Cardiovascular Disease, opens with a discussion of the "big four" risk factors for heart disease and emphasizes that prevention must begin early. Even the chapter titles themselves invite students to take control of their own health behavior.

Spirituality

A highly developed sense of spirituality is integral to wellness. Accordingly, we have included a "Focus On . . ." article in Chapter 2 that explores topics such as holistic healing, mind-body disciplines, and enhancement of spirituality through volunteering.

"Focus On . . ." Articles

New "Focus On . . ." articles examine current issues that students are hearing about in today's news, such as melatonin, telecommuting, smokers' rights, and even sex on the Internet. These often controversial health-related topics are a perfect starting point for class or group discussions. Because these essays are set at the end of each chapter, they can be covered or not at the instructor's option.

New Design and Revised Illustration Program

The fresh look, bold colors, and exciting graphics in this new edition will draw students in with every turn of the page. In addition, the illustration program has been substantially revised: photographs are sharp and appealing, new drawings are attractive and informative, and anatomical illustrations are accurately rendered and appropriately detailed. In addition, the anatomical illustrations in the cardiovascular disease and sexuality chapters have been enlarged for greater clarity.

"Exam Prep" Guide

A perforated exam preparation section is now included in the back of the book. The multiple-choice questions test students' retention of the material they have read. The critical thinking questions allow them to integrate the concepts introduced in the text with the information presented in class lectures and discussions.

Vegetarian Food Pyramid

Many students now follow or are considering a vegetarian diet. To help them understand how such a diet meets nutrient needs, we have printed a vegetarian food pyramid with the USDA Food Guide Pyramid inside the back cover of this textbook. For students who want to significantly reduce but not eliminate meat consumption, a new "Focus On . . ." article about the health benefits of following a semivegetarian diet is included in Chapter 5.

New or Expanded Topics

We are committed to making *Focus on Health* the most up-to-date health textbook available. Below is a sampling of topics that are either completely new to this edition or covered in greater depth than in the previous edition:

Chapter 1: Shaping Your Health
Occupational dimension of health
Behavior change strategies
Developmental tasks of midlife and elderly adults
Focus On . . . The diversity of today's college students

Chapter 2: Achieving Emotional Maturity
Taking a proactive approach to life
Emotional wellness of midlife and elderly adults
Focus On . . . Enhancing spirituality and wellness

Chapter 3: Managing Stress
Hardiness
Diaphragmatic breathing
Psychogenic and psychosomatic stress-induced illness
Focus On . . . Managing work-related stress

SUCCESSFUL FEATURES

Along with its new features, *Focus on Health* has many unique existing features that enhance student learning:

Two Central Themes

As mentioned earlier, two central themes—the multiple dimensions of health and the developmental tasks—are presented in Chapter 1. These give students a foundation for understanding their own health and achieving positive behavior change.

Flexibility of Chapter Organization

The third edition of *Focus on Health* has 18 chapters. The first stands alone as an introductory chapter that explains the focus of the book. The arrangement of the remaining chapters follows the recommendations of both the users of previous editions of the book and reviewers of this edition. Of course, professors can choose to cover the chapters in any sequence that suits the needs of their courses.

Health Reference Guide

The Health Reference Guide found at the back of the book lists many of the most commonly used health resources. In this edition, we have included many Internet addresses, as well as phone numbers and mailing addresses of various organizations and government agencies. The guide is perforated and laminated, making it durable enough for students to keep for later use.

Pedagogical Aids

In addition to the new pedagogical features listed previously, the teaching aids described below proved to be successful in the first two editions of this book and have been included in this new edition:

Star Boxes

In each chapter, special material in Star Boxes encourages students to delve into a particular topic or closely examine an important health issue.

Personal Assessment Inventories

Each chapter contains at least one Personal Assessment inventory, beginning with a comprehensive health inventory in Chapter 1. These self-assessment exercises serve three important functions: they capture students' attention, serve as a basis for introspec-

tion and behavior change, and provide suggestions for carrying the applications further.

Health Action Guides

These unique boxes provide step-by-step guidelines for achieving health behavior change. They allow students to apply their knowledge in practical and life-enhancing ways.

Definition Boxes

Key terms are set in boldface type and are defined in corresponding boxes. Pronunciation guides are provided where appropriate. Other important terms in the text are set in italics for emphasis. Both approaches facilitate student vocabulary comprehension.

Comprehensive Glossary

At the end of the text, all terms defined in boxes, as well as pertinent italicized terms, are merged into a comprehensive glossary.

Chapter Summaries

Each chapter concludes with a bulleted summary of key concepts and their significance or application. The student can then return to any topic in the chapter for clarification or study.

Review Questions

A set of questions appears at the end of each chapter to aid the student in review and analysis of chapter content.

Think About This . . .

These engaging questions encourage students to apply what they have learned in the chapter by analyzing their own health habits and finding appropriate solutions to the issues raised.

Suggested Readings

Because some students want to know more about a particular topic, a list of annotated readings is given at the end of each chapter. The suggested readings are readily available at bookstores or public libraries. This edition contains more than 45 new annotated readings.

Appendixes

Focus on Health includes four appendixes that are valuable resources for the student:

• **Commonly used over-the-counter products.** Popular categories of over-the-counter drugs are discussed in detail, with recommendations for consumers of these products. Newly available OTC products, such as naproxen, ketoprofen, minoxidil, and nicotine-containing gum, are included.

- **First aid.** This appendix outlines important general first-aid measures, such as what to do when someone is choking, bleeding, or in shock. It includes a special section on recognition and first-aid treatment of epileptic seizures.
- **Mental disorders.** Categories of mental disorders and therapeutic approaches are outlined in this appendix.
- **Body systems.** The systems of the human body have been clearly and accurately rendered in this appendix to make difficult anatomical concepts easier for students to understand.

ANCILLARIES

An extensive ancillary package is available to adopters to enhance the teaching-learning process. We have made a concerted effort to produce supplements of extraordinary utility and quality. This package has been carefully planned and developed to help instructors derive the greatest benefit from the text. We encourage instructors to examine them carefully. Beyond the following brief descriptions, additional information about these ancillaries is available from Mosby.

Instructor's Manual and Test Bank

Prepared by Virginia Lee Mermel, of Wellness Resources, the instructor's manual features chapter overviews, learning objectives, suggested lecture outlines with notes and recommended activities for teaching each chapter, Debating the Issues boxes, individual and community activities sections, suggestions for guest lectures, a list of current media resources, including software and on-line resources, and 60 full-page transparency masters of helpful illustrations and charts. In addition, the Personal Assessment inventories in the textbook and 50 others are combined into a single section of the instructor's manual. These assessments can be easily photocopied and given to each student as a single packet. The test bank, prepared by Dayna Brown, of Morehead State University, contains multiple-choice, true or false, matching, and critical thinking exam questions. It also includes questions to test students' knowledge of the new supplemental "Focus On . . ." boxes that appear at the end of each chapter in the text. The manual is perforated and three-hole punched for convenience of use.

Computerized Test Bank*

The test bank software provides a unique combination of user-friendly aids that enables the instructor to select, edit, delete, or add questions, as well as construct and print tests and answer keys. The computerized test bank package is available for IBM Windows and Macintosh computers.

Overhead Transparency Acetates*

Sixty key illustrations and graphics are available as transparency acetates. Attractively printed in full color, these useful tools facilitate learning and classroom discussion. They were chosen specifically to help the instructor explain complex concepts.

Personal Assessment Software*

For an additional charge, your students can receive 26 Personal Assessments on an IBM 3.5" or 5.25" diskette with the text. Using this software, students can automatically tally their responses and keep track of their performance.

Videodisc*

This ancillary includes many film clips on health issues facing students today. About 1 hour long, this visual presentation enhances classroom discussion. The videodisc is also available in videotape (VHS) format.

Mosby's Health Exchange*

This newsletter provides instructors with the latest information about "hot" health topics to supplement their Mosby health, fitness, sexuality, drugs, and wellness textbooks. Published twice a year, the newsletter is a useful resource for instructors. Each edition also includes a pullout center section containing information designed for student use.

VIEWSTUDY™ Presentation Software*

This CD-ROM, compatible with either Windows or Macintosh, contains key illustrations from Mosby's health, wellness, and fitness texts. Images are arranged by chapter, and a slide show tool allows selection of prearranged images. Illustrations can also be printed full size for use as transparency acetates and may be exported for use with other programs and applications, such as the computerized test bank.

Mosby's NUTRITRAC™ Software*

Compatible with either Windows or Macintosh, this nutrient-analysis software allows you and your

*Available to qualified adopters of the text.

students to analyze diets easily, using an icon-based interface and on-screen help features. Foods for breakfast, lunch, dinner, and snacks may be selected from more than 2250 items in the database. Records may be kept for any number of days. The program can provide intake analyses for individual foods, meals, days, or for an entire intake period. Intake analyses can compare nutrient values to RDA or RNI values and to the USDA Food Guide Pyramid, and can provide breakdowns of fat and calorie sources. Students may purchase NUTRITRAC™ with the text for a nominal fee.

ACKNOWLEDGMENTS

The publisher's reviewers made excellent comments and suggestions that were very useful to us in writing and revising this book. Their contributions are present in every chapter. We would like to express our sincere appreciation for both their critical and comparative readings.

For the third edition:

Dayna S. Brown
Morehead State University

Diane M. Hamilton
Georgia Southern University

Joe Herzstein
Trenton State College

Rebecca Rutt Leas
Clarion University

Dorinda Maynard
Eastern Kentucky University

Steven Navarro
Cerritos College

Mary Beth Tighe
The Ohio State University

For the second edition:

James D. Aguiar
Ithaca College

Carolyn M. Allred
Central Piedmont Community College

Joan Benson
University of Utah

Daniel E. Berney
California State University–Dominguez Hills

Ronnie Carda
Emporia State University

Barbara Funke
Georgia College

William C. Gross
Western Michigan University

Richard Hurley
Brigham Young University

Raeann Koerner Smith
Ventura College

L. Clark McCammon
Western Illinois University

Dan Neal
Southwestern Oregon Community College

David Quadagno
Florida State University

Leslie Rurey
Community Colleges of Spokane

Scott E. Scobell
West Virginia State College

Karen T. Sullivan
Marymount University

Joan Tudor
Chapman University

Stuart L. Whitney
University of Vermont

For the first edition:

Sandra L. Bonneau
Golden West College

Richard A. Kaye
Kingsborough Community College

Donald Haynes
University of Minnesota–Duluth

J. Dale Wagoner
Chabot College

SPECIAL ACKNOWLEDGMENTS

The third edition of *Focus on Health* is the ninth book we have written during the last decade. We could not have accomplished all of this without the help of many people. Among these are our faculty colleagues at Georgetown College and Ball State University, who continue to keep us abreast of new information in areas related to personal health. A special thanks goes out to all of you.

Additionally, we want to recognize our administrative colleagues. We are fortunate to have worked with administrators who maintain the vision that (a) textbooks represent important resources for today's college students, and (b) textbooks reflect faculty contributions that shed favorable light on a college community. We very much appreciate the support of Dr. Charles N. Boehms, Senior Vice President and Academic Dean of Georgetown College, and Dr. Ronald L. Johnstone, Dean of the College of Sciences and Humanities at Ball State University.

The list of dedicated people at Mosby is quite long. Many have played a direct part in influencing the direction of this writing project. Jim Smith, Vicki Malinee, Michelle Turenne, and Cathy Bailey are exceptional people who have championed this project for years. They understand clearly the demands authors face as they juggle family, teaching, and writing schedules. They do their best to provide a supportive environment for Mosby authors.

Another key player at Mosby is our newest developmental editor, Melissa Martin. This third edition of *Focus on Health* has been her special project for many months. It is difficult for us to realize how smooth her transition has been from the production side of publishing to the editorial side. She has been on top of every detail from the moment she took over this project. We appreciate her talent, effort, and humor very much.

We also wish to acknowledge the contributions of Virginia Lee Mermel and Dayna Brown. Over the years, we have learned the importance of providing professors with a comprehensive, well-written instructor's manual and test bank. Virginia Lee Mermel and Dayna Brown have developed an excellent instructor's manual and test bank that will benefit experienced instructors, as well as new ones.

One of the unique new features of this edition of *Focus on Health* is its "Focus On . . ." articles. Dawn L. Elmore-McCrary, of San Antonio College, and Thomas Neil McCrary combined their teaching experience and health expertise to develop, research, and write these outstanding essays. We are grateful for the considerable time and effort they devoted to making these articles up-to-date, exciting, and informative.

It is difficult for the authors to know the many people who work on the production end of a textbook project. Our principal connection with this part of Mosby has been our production editor, Rick Dudley. Rick made certain that every manuscript detail was clear and every production deadline met. In addition, the credit for the book's attractiveness goes to the designer, Sheilah Barrett.

Finally, we would like to thank our families for the continued support and love they have given us. Perhaps more than others, our families understand the effort and commitment it takes to write books. We truly appreciate their sacrifices.

Dale B. Hahn
Wayne A. Payne

Contents in Brief

Contents

Contents

Shaping Your Health

Healthy People 2000 Objectives

In 1990 a lengthy document titled *Healthy People 2000: National Health Promotion and Disease Prevention Objectives* formed the strategic plan for improving the health of the American public. Included in this plan were 300 health objectives in 22 priority areas. Some 47 of the 300 were identified as "sentinel' objectives—particularly significant goals that could quickly indicate the progress of health promotion efforts during the 1990s. In addition, three overall health goals were established: to increase the span of healthy life, to reduce health disparities among Americans, and to achieve access to preventive services for all Americans.

Progress toward achieving each of the 300 objectives, including the 47 sentinel objectives, and the three overall health goals is presented in a document titled *Healthy People 2000: Midcourse Review and 1995 Revisions.* Each chapter in *Focus on Health* will begin with a review of progress toward some of the health objectives that are related to the content of that chapter. Success in achieving the three overall health goals is assessed in the Star Box on p. 3.

This chapter focuses on two questions: "What is health?" and "How does health contribute to the process of living a satisfying life?" We help you answer these questions by providing a framework around which to view health, and we encourage you to study your own health as it relates to your growth and development throughout the stages of your life.

HEALTH CONCERNS OF THE LATE 1990s

As we move closer to the new century, health concerns such as heart disease, cancer, accidents, drug use, and mental health are important to us, even if we are not directly affected by them (Table 1-1). Environmental pollution, violence, health care costs, and acquired immunodeficiency syndrome (AIDS) and other sexually transmitted diseases are becoming increasingly significant. World hunger, population control, and the threat of worldwide ethnic violence represent major issues that will affect us, as well as the generations that follow.

The Star Box below lists the top five health issues facing college students in the 1990s. These health concerns are not unmanageable. By the turn of the century, we hope to see advancements in the way our society successfully tackles these problems. Fortunately, we as individuals can make choices in the way we live. At least on a personal level, we can decide to select a plan of healthful living that incorporates a sound diet, proper exercise, adequate rest, periodic medical checkups, and elimination (or moderation) of drug use, including tobacco and alcohol use. One goal of this textbook is to provide you with the information and motivation to help you select the lifestyle that will make you a happy and healthy person.

DEFINITIONS OF HEALTH-RELATED TERMS

A Traditional Definition of Health

One of the most widely recognized and frequently quoted definitions of health is that given by the Geneva-based World Health Organization[1]:

> Health is a state of complete physical, mental, and social well-being and not merely the absence of disease and infirmity.

This multifaceted view of health includes physical, mental, and social dimensions, indicating that health extends beyond the structure and function of your body to include feelings, values, and the ability to rea-

Table 1-1 Top 12 Causes of Death in the United States*	
Cause of Death	**Number of Cases**
1. Major cardiovascular diseases	939,180
2. Malignant neoplasms (cancers)	538,560
3. Chronic obstructive lung diseases	101,170
4. Accidents and adverse effects	88,370
5. Pneumonia and influenza	81,820
6. Diabetes mellitus	55,270
7. HIV infection	40,310
8. Suicide	30,570
9. Chronic liver disease and cirrhosis	25,660
10. Kidney diseases	24,690
11. Homicide	23,680
12. Septicemia (blood infections)	19,900
TOTAL (including all other causes)	2,286,000

*For the 12-month period ending December 1994.

Key Health Issues Facing College Students in the 1990s

At an annual meeting of the American College Health Association, a prominent group of health educators, medical professionals, and college residence hall staff professionals met to identify the most critical health issues facing college students in the 1990s.

The top five health issues of the 1990s (in order of their importance) were as follows:

- *Sexual health concerns*, including topics such as sexually transmitted diseases, relationship issues, unintended pregnancy, and sexual violence
- *Substance abuse*, including a wide range of issues related to the abuse of alcohol, tobacco, and other drugs, and dependency and codependency
- *Mental health concerns*, including stress management, fear of failure, coping skills, complex family relationships, and depression
- *Nutrition issues*, including healthful diets, weight management, chronic disease prevention, and eating disorders
- *Health care services*, including financing and delivering comprehensive, low-cost health services to students and their families

Does this list surprise you? Because of their importance to college students, we cover all of these health issues in this text, as well as numerous other important concerns for today's traditional and nontraditional students.

son. It also includes the nature of your interpersonal relationships. Furthermore, it can be inferred that health can exist in the presence of disease and infirmity; you do not have to be a "picture of health" to be productive and satisfied. Nevertheless, for all the definition's value, one question remains unanswered: "How does health contribute to the process of living a satisfying life?"

Holistic Health

One popular description of health expands the definition supplied by the World Health Organization. **Holistic health** extends the physical, mental, and social aspects of the definition to include intellectual, spiritual, and occupational dimensions. The holistically healthy person functions as a total person. Some experts say that holistically healthy people have reached a "high level of wellness."

Holistic health may be the broadest explanation of health. Through a holistic concept of health, we are better able to understand how a person who has a serious physical illness can also be considered quite healthy.

Health Promotion

The term **health promotion** is frequently linked to disease prevention.[2] Health promoters believe that if you accept scientific opinion regarding health and adopt specific health-enhancing practices, you will become healthy. On the basis of this view of health, if you have enhanced your health, you should live longer and have fewer health problems than the average person and feel better than an unhealthy person.

To promote the health of a person or a group, health professionals use a number of strategies (see the Star Box on p. 4). Health screenings (such as blood pressure or cholesterol measurements), health education activities (such as first aid, human immunodeficiency virus [HIV] education, or cardiopulmonary resuscitation [CPR] training), behavior change strategies (such as the use of specific eating plans or exercise programs), and health maintenance activities (such as the use of regular medical checkups) are examples of approaches used to keep people healthy and alive for many years.

Although these strategies are admirable, this interpretation presents health as an end in itself rather than a means to an end. Living a long time, not being sick, and doing only healthful things are important, but will they assure you of growing and developing to your fullest potential?

Wellness

Whereas *health promotion* is a term used by many in the health field, **wellness** may be the most popular health-related term of the late 1990s. High-level wellness suggests an optimistic way of looking at a person's health that extends beyond health measurements and life span. Wellness supports the concept that a person's health should not be judged primarily from a medical or disease standpoint but from the standpoint of reaching or achieving human potential. Wellness is a process for the continuous self-renewal needed for an exciting, creative, fulfilling life; it is a concept that extends beyond health promotion and disease prevention.

To achieve this human potential, wellness experts believe that individuals must take responsibility for their health behavior.[3] People must understand that they have more control over their health behavior than they might think. A wellness perspective encourages people to focus on the present and future and not on the past, especially when one's past includes negative health behavior. Wellness also discourages blaming others for one's own behavior.

Two wellness researchers, Brylinsky and Hoadley,[4] summarized the concept of wellness by writing:

> Wellness reflects a feeling, a conscious perception, or an awareness by the whole person that his/her components and processes are not only under control, but are also working harmoniously as a unit. Wellness also reflects a person's attitude and his/her unique response to living.

The college campus is an ideal place to view the concept of wellness in action. College administrators and even casual observers report that today's college

---

holistic health
Broadest view of the composition of health; views health in terms of its physical, emotional, social, intellectual, spiritual, and occupational makeup.

health promotion
A movement in which knowledge, practices, and values are transmitted to people for use in lengthening their lives, reducing the incidence of illness, and feeling better.

wellness
A broadly based term used to describe a highly developed level of health that encourages people to achieve their human potential.

Healthy People 2000 Midcourse Review

In this edition of *Focus on Health*, each chapter begins with a report on the progress our nation has made toward achieving the *Healthy People 2000* objectives established by the federal government in 1990. We highlight the progress made or lost during the first half of this decade in meeting many of these 300 key national health objectives.*

Three broad goals were established in the Healthy People 2000 report: (1) to increase the span of healthy life for each American, (2) to reduce health disparities among Americans, and (3) to achieve access to preventive health services for all Americans. Since 1990 the average life span for Americans has risen from 75 years to 76 years. However, the span of *healthy* life has actually declined despite the 1-year increase in longevity. An average of 11.4 years (about 15%) of an American's life is now considered unhealthy. We are living longer, but we are not necessarily healthier.

The second broad *Healthy People 2000* goal, to reduce differences "in health status and health outcomes between racial and ethnic minorities and the total population," does not seem likely to be met. Health status is often expressed as *years of potential life lost (YPLL)*, which is a measure of premature death calculated by subtracting the actual life span of each person in a particular population group from his or her life expectancy. The figure for all Americans is 8384 YPLL per 100,000 people, but for African-Americans it is 15,468 and for American Indians and Alaska Natives the figure is 11,875.

The third broad *Healthy People 2000* goal concerned improving access to preventive health services for all Americans. An important indicator of improved access is the percentage of Americans with health insurance coverage. The percentage of Americans under age 65 with private insurance coverage dropped from 77% in 1986 to 72% in 1992. In 1993, 39.7 million Americans had no health insurance.

Despite the lack of significant success in reaching these three broad goals, progress has been made in meeting many of the specific objectives set by *Healthy People 2000*. The nation has moved closer to fulfilling more than two thirds of the objectives for which there are adequate data. The challenge for health professionals is to continue to support programs that focus on disease prevention and improved access to health care for all.

*This information is from the 1996 U.S. Department of Health and Human Services publication *Healthy People 2000: Midcourse Review and 1995 Revisions*.

students seem to be embracing wellness. Students, faculty, and staff members realize the importance of health and are participating in activities designed to promote wellness, such as health screenings, nutrition awareness seminars, and fitness-focus weeks. Throughout this textbook, we encourage readers to develop the wellness lifestyle with which they feel most comfortable.

With the increased emphasis on wellness programs on many college campuses, it is not surprising to see the influence of wellness extending to many aspects of daily life, including schools and the workplace.[5,6] Commonly offered wellness programs cover smoking cessation, weight control, cholesterol screening, stress management, exercise, and nutrition. Many major corporations report that employee participation in wellness activities reduces health care costs (insurance premiums) and increases employee satisfaction and productivity.[7] Indeed, you will see wellness extending beyond your college campus.

Empowerment

Within the last few years, the term *empowerment* has been recognized and discussed within the health education literature.[8] In the context of health, empowerment refers to a process in which individuals or groups of people gain increasing measures of control over their health. To take control of health matters, people or groups must learn to "liberate themselves" from a variety of barriers that tend to restrict health enhancement, including the complicated and expensive health care system, limited access to health care or fitness facilities, the fear of discovering an illness or serious health condition, and the concern that one might be viewed as a "health nut."

When people empower themselves to overcome these barriers, they begin to take charge of their lives, regardless of the current forces that discourage positive health changes. Empowered people do not blame individuals or environmental realities for health conditions but focus on producing constructive change through dialogue and collaboration.

Empowerment programs have produced positive health consequences for individuals and groups that have been traditionally underserved by the health care system, such as the economically disadvantaged, the elderly, and minority populations. Have you seen empowerment programs working in your community? You probably have if you can identify programs where people have organized a grassroots campaign to prevent neighborhood violence, improve childhood nutrition, promote healthy lifestyles, or prevent drug use among youth. Only when people realize that they can "make a difference" will they become empowered. We believe that your personal health course can help you become empowered in your own life.

DEVELOPMENTAL TASKS FOR COLLEGE STUDENTS

Because *most* of today's undergraduate college students range between 18 and perhaps 40 years of age, we present five developmental tasks that reflect this broad student range (Figure 1-1). The first four tasks (involving identity, responsibility, independence, and social skills) are especially pertinent to the more traditional-age college student. The fifth task (concerning intimacy) is probably more important for students who have moved just beyond the **young adult years.** We hope that the gains you make with each of these tasks will help you move more successfully through your life.

However, keep in mind that many college students, regardless of their age, continue to make gains in all five developmental areas because each person's experience and development are unique. For example, **nontraditional students** remind us that their identity

young adult years
Segment of the life cycle from ages 18 to 24; a transitional period between adolescence and adulthood.

nontraditional students
Administrative term used by colleges and universities to refer to students who, for whatever reason, are pursuing undergraduate work at an age other than that associated with the traditional college years (18 to 24).

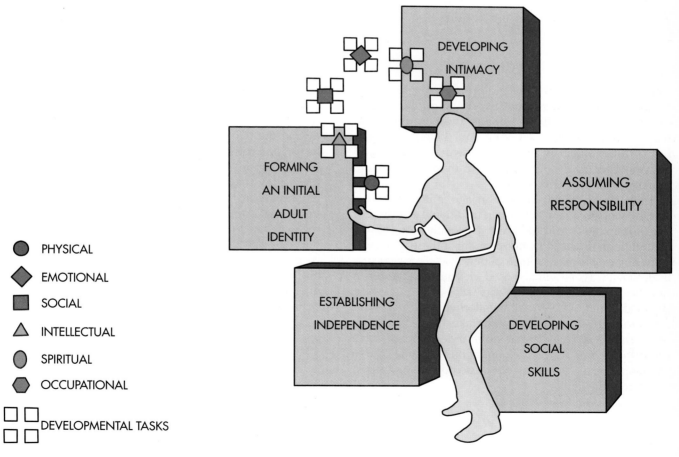

● PHYSICAL

◆ EMOTIONAL

■ SOCIAL

▲ INTELLECTUAL

◖ SPIRITUAL

⬡ OCCUPATIONAL

▢▢
▢▢ DEVELOPMENTAL TASKS

DEVELOPING INTIMACY

FORMING AN INITIAL ADULT IDENTITY

ASSUMING RESPONSIBILITY

ESTABLISHING INDEPENDENCE

DEVELOPING SOCIAL SKILLS

Figure 1-1   Mastery of the developmental tasks through a balanced involvement of the six dimensions of health will lead to your enjoying a more productive and satisfying life.

continues to change as they see themselves progressing through college. They realize that they are not the same people they were when they started back to school. Their identity keeps developing as they learn new concepts and meet new people.

Forming an Initial Adult Identity

For most of your youth, you were seen by adults within your neighborhood or community as someone's son or daughter. That stage has now nearly passed; both you and society are beginning to look at each other in new ways.

As an emerging adult, you probably wish to present a unique identity to society. Internally you are constructing a perception of yourself as the person you wish to be; externally you are forming the behavioral patterns that will project this identity to others.

The completion of this first developmental task is necessary so that you can have a productive and satisfying life. Through your experiences in achieving an adult identity, you will eventually be capable of answering the central question of young adulthood: "Who am I?" Interestingly, many nontraditional students are also asking this question as they progress through college.

Establishing Independence

In contemporary society the primary responsibility for socialization during childhood and adolescence is assigned to the family. For many years, your family was the primary contributor to your knowledge, values, and behavior. By this time, however, you should be demonstrating an interest in moving away from that dependent relationship.

Travel, peer relationships, marriage, military service, and, of course, college have been traditional avenues for disengagement from the family. Generally, your ability and willingness to follow one or more of these paths will help you to establish your independence. Your success in these endeavors will be based on your willingness to use the resources you have. You will need to draw on physical, emotional, social, intellectual, spiritual, and occupational strengths to undertake the new experiences that will bring about your independence. In a sense, your family laid the foundation for the resources and experiences you will now use to draw yourself away from the family.

Assuming Responsibility

The assumption of increasing levels of responsibility is a third developmental task in which you are

Social interaction can take place in many settings.

expected to progress. For adults, the opportunity to assume responsibility can come from a variety of sources. You may sometimes accept responsibility voluntarily, such as when you join a campus organization or establish a new friendship. Other responsibilities are placed on you when professors assign term papers, when dating partners exert pressure on you to conform to their expectations, or when employers require that you be consistently productive. In other situations, you may accept responsibility for doing a particular task not for yourself but for the benefit of someone else, such as when you donate a unit of blood during a campus blood drive.

As important and demanding as these areas of responsibility are, a more basic responsibility awaits the adult: that of maintaining and improving your health and the health of others. You will be challenged to be responsible for recognizing, improving, and then using the strengths that constitute your physical, emotional, social, intellectual, spiritual, and occupational makeup. At the same time, you will be equally responsible for recognizing, accepting, and working within your limitations. None of the specific areas of responsibility associated with school, employment, and parenting can be undertaken with maximum effectiveness unless you make a commitment to be responsible for your own health.

Developing Social Skills

A fourth developmental task is developing appropriate and dependable social skills. The college experience has traditionally prepared students very effectively in this regard, but the interactions in friendships, work relationships, or parenting may require that you make an effort to grow and develop beyond levels you might achieve from being a college student.

You will probably need to refine a variety of social skills, including communication, listening, and conflict management.

This need to interact socially will at times compromise your health. Examples might be the weekend party that prevents you from doing well on a Monday morning examination or the recreational or intramural activities that sometimes result in serious injury. Generally, however, social interaction contributes to your total health and is an important aid in helping you have a productive and satisfying life.

Developing Intimacy

This developmental task usually presents itself to people between young adulthood and midlife, when it appears important to establish one or more intimate relationships. Indeed, we are looking at intimacy in its broadest sense as a deeply close, sharing relationship. Intimacy may stem from a marriage relationship or other close friendship.

People vary in their number of intimate relationships, with some having many intimate friends, while others have only one or two deep relationships. The number does not matter. What matters is that each person has someone with whom to share intimate thoughts, feelings, and emotions.

After becoming familiar with these developmental tasks, you should see that there is considerable overlap in the accomplishment of each task. For example, your development and refinement of social skills can enhance your independence from your family. Your willingness to accept increasing responsibility may influence your ability to develop an intimate relationship with someone.

DEVELOPMENTAL TASKS OF MIDLIFE ADULTS

If you are a traditional-age student, have you wondered what it would be like to be 20 or 30 years older than you are now? What would you be doing, feeling, and thinking if you were the age of your parents? What are your parents thinking about and trying to accomplish as they move through their midlife years?

One thought that probably recurs all too often is the reality of their own eventual death. Their awareness that they will not live forever is a subtle but profoundly influential force that can cause them to be restless, to renew their religious faith, and to be more highly motivated to master the developmental tasks of midlife. This motivation and the awareness of the reality of death combine to produce the dynamic con-

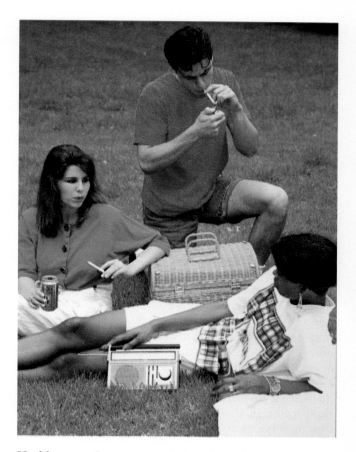

Healthy growth can occur during the college years . . . as can unhealthy growth.

cept of being at "the prime of life"—a time when there seems to be a great deal to accomplish and less time in which to accomplish it.

Achieving Generativity

In a very real sense, midlife people are asked to do something they have not been expected to do previously. As a part of their development as unique people, they are expected to "pay back" society for the support it has given them. Most people in midlife begin to realize that the collective society, through its institutions (families, schools, churches), has been generous in its support of their own growth and development and that it is time to replenish these resources. Younger and older people may have needs that middle-aged people can best meet. By meeting the needs of others, midlife people can fulfill their own needs to grow and develop. *Generativity* reflects this process of contributing to the collective good.[9] Generativity benefits both midlife people and society.

The process of repaying society for its support is structured around familiar types of activities. Developmentally speaking, midlife people are able to select the activities that best use their abilities to contribute to the good of society.[10]

The most traditional way in which midlife people repay society is through parenting. Children, with their potential for becoming valuable members of the next generation, need the support of people who recognize the contribution they can make. By supporting children, either directly through quality parenting or through institutions that function on behalf of children, middle-aged people repay society for the support they have themselves received. As they extend themselves outward on behalf of the next generation, they ensure their own growth and development. In similar fashion, their support of aging parents and institutions that serve the elderly provides another means to express generativity.

For people who possess artistic talent, generativity may be accomplished through the pleasure brought to others. Artists, craftsmen, and musicians have unique opportunities to speak directly to others through their talents. Volunteer work serves as another avenue for generativity. Most midlife people also express generativity through their jobs by providing quality products or services and thus contribute to the well-being of those who desire or need these goods and services.

Reassessing the Plans of Young Adulthood

It is also essential for midlife people to come to terms with the finality of their own deaths. Having done this, they often feel that it is time to think about their goals for adulthood they formulated 25 or more years previously. Their "dreams" must be revisited.[10] This reassessment constitutes a second developmental task of midlife adults.

By carefully reviewing the aspirations they had as young adults, middle-aged people can more clearly study their short- and long-term goals. Specifically, strengths and limitations that were unrecognizable when they were young adults are now more clearly seen. The inexperience of youth is replaced by the insights gained through experience. A commitment to quality often replaces the desire for quantity during the second half of the life cycle. Time is valued more highly because it is now seen in a more realistic perspective. The dream for the future is more sharply focused, and the successes and failures of the past are more fully understood as this developmental task of reassessing earlier plans of young adulthood is accomplished.

DEVELOPMENTAL TASKS OF ELDERLY ADULTS

In this section, we focus on the developmental tasks confronted by elderly people. Accepting the physical decline of aging, maintaining high levels of physical function, and establishing a sense of integrity are tasks of the elderly period.

Accepting the Decline of Aging

The general decline associated with the latter part of the life cycle is particularly serious between the seventh and eighth decades. Physically, emotionally, socially, intellectually, and occupationally, elderly people must accept at least some decline. For example, a person may no longer be physically able to drive a car, which could in turn limit participation in social activities. Even a spiritual loss may be encountered at those times when life seems less ordered or less humane. Clearly, a developmental task to be accomplished by the elderly is to accept the nature and extent of these losses.[11]

Maintaining a High Level of Physical Function

Because each segment of the life cycle should be approached with the fullest level of involvement possible, the second developmental task of the elderly is to maintain the highest level of physical function possible.

For areas of decline in which some measure of reversal is possible, the elderly are afforded an opportunity to seek **rehabilitation.** Whether through an individually designed program or through the aid of a skilled professional, the elderly can bring back some function to a previously high level.

The second approach, often used in combination with rehabilitation, is **remediation,** whereby an alternative to the area of loss is introduced. Examples of remediation include the use of hearing aids, audio cassettes, and prescription shoes. By using alternative resources, function can often be returned and may actually be improved.

rehabilitation
Return of function to a previous level.

remediation
Development of alternative forms of function to replace those that have been lost or were poorly developed.

For a growing number of older adults, rehabilitation and remediation are rarely necessary because of the high level of physical fitness that they enjoy. For these older people, physical fitness has been maintained through regular physical conditioning activities (see Chapter 4). For most, only minor modifications are necessary to enjoy injury-free involvement.

Establishing a Sense of Integrity

The third major developmental task that awaits the elderly is to establish a sense of *integrity,* or a sense of wholeness, concerning the journey that may be nearly complete.[9] The elderly must look back over their lives to see the value in what they were able to accomplish. They must address the simple but critical questions, "Would I do it over again?" "Am I satisfied with what I managed to accomplish?" "Can I accept the fact that others will have experiences to which I can never return?"

If the elderly can answer these questions positively, then they will feel a sense of wholeness, personal value, and worth. Having established this sense of integrity, they will believe that their lives have had meaning and fullness and that they have helped society.

Since they have already experienced so much, many elderly people have no fear of death, even though they may fear the process of dying. Their ability to come to terms with death thus reinforces their sense of integrity.

Like all of the other developmental tasks, this critical area of growth and development is a personal experience. The elderly must assume this last developmental task with the same sense of purpose they used for earlier tasks. When elderly people can feel this sense of integrity, their reasons for having lived will be fully understood.[12]

THE ROLE OF HEALTH

Having been introduced to the developmental tasks of college students, as well as those of midlife and elderly adults, you can better answer the question, "What is the *role of health* in my life?" The role of health is to assist you in mastering the developmental tasks that will make your life more satisfying and productive.

Health can be described meaningfully only in conjunction with your developmental tasks. If your health allows you to successfully complete your developmental tasks, then we would say that you have developed a high level of health.

For most of today's college students, the tasks we are identifying as those likely to be accomplished with high-level health are the five already presented. For midlife and elderly students, the continued refinement of these tasks and the mastery of additional tasks just presented will depend on their level of health.

THE COMPOSITION OF HEALTH

Your health is composed of six interacting, *dynamic* dimensions. By becoming familiar with these dimensions, you can more easily recognize what it is about your health that may or may not be helping you to master your developmental tasks. Fortunately, because your health is dynamic, you can modify aspects of its dimensions to make it a better tool to help you live a productive, satisfying life.

Your health is not static; it cannot be stored on a shelf or given to others. The health you had yesterday no longer exists. The health you aspire to have next week or next year is not guaranteed. However, scien-

HEALTH Action Guide

Cultural Diversity at Your Campus

To help you develop some understanding of the ethnically diverse culture at your college or university, try to find the answers to these basic questions:

- What are the minority population figures for the community in which your college is located? Try to include figures for African-Americans, Hispanics, Asians, and Native Americans.
- What are the minority population figures for your college or university?
- Do these figures surprise you?

The following is the resource center for the federal agency whose mission is to improve the health status of minority populations in the United States. To receive information or publications, call the 800 number listed below:

Office of Minority Health (OMH)
Information Resource Center
P.O. Box 37337
Washington, DC 20013-7337
(1-800-444-6472)

For more information about the diversity of today's college students, see the Focus Box on p. 20.

tific evidence suggests that what you do today will help determine the quality of your future health. We now briefly consider each of the six dimensions of health so that you can more clearly see how each forms a part of your total health.

Physical Dimension

A number of physiological and structural characteristics help you accomplish your developmental tasks, including your level of susceptibility to disease, body weight, visual ability, strength, coordination, level of endurance, and powers of recuperation. In certain situations the physical dimension of your health may be the most important. Perhaps this is why many authorities have for so long equated health with the design and operation of the body.

Emotional Dimension

Your emotional characteristics can also aid you as you grow and develop. The emotional dimension of health includes the degree to which you are able to cope with stress, remain flexible, and compromise to resolve conflict. This dimension may be the one that is most closely related to your feelings. How you feel about your family and friends, your life goals and ambitions, and your daily life situations is all tied to the emotional dimension of health.

Your growth and development can be associated with some vulnerability, which may lead to feelings of rejection and failure that could reduce your overall productivity and satisfaction. People who consistently try to improve their emotional health appear to lead lives of greater enjoyment than those who let feelings of vulnerability overwhelm them or block their creativity. Specific techniques for improving your emotional health are presented in Chapter 2.

Social Dimension

Social ability is the third dimension of total health. Whether you call it social graces, skills, or insights, you probably have many strengths in this area. Because most of your growth and development has occurred in the presence of others, you can appreciate how this dimension of your health may be a critically important factor in your life.

The social abilities of many nontraditional students may already be firmly established. Entering college may encourage them to develop new social skills that help them socialize with their traditional-age student colleagues. After being on campus for a while, non-traditional students often interact comfortably with tradi-

tional students in such diverse places as the library, the student center, and the bookstore, which enhances the social dimension of health for both types of students.

Intellectual Dimension

Your ability to process and act on information, clarify values and beliefs, and exercise your decision-making capacity ranks among the most important aspects of total health. Coping skills, flexibility, or the knack of saying the right thing at the right time may not serve you as well as does your ability to use information or understand a new idea. Certainly a refusal to grasp new information or to undertake an analysis of your beliefs could hinder the degree of growth and development that your college experience can provide.

Spiritual Dimension

The fifth dimension of health is the spiritual dimension.[13,14] Although you certainly could include your religious beliefs and practices in this category, we would extend it to include your relationship to other living things, the role of a spiritual direction in your life, the nature of human behavior, and your willingness to serve others.

Many of today's students appear to be searching for a deeper understanding of the meaning of life. Although you may not feel uneasy about the nature of your spiritual beliefs, many students do feel anxious about the spiritual side of their lives. In fact, one explanation for the renewed interest in the spiritual dimension of health probably stems from its value as a resource during periods of personal stress. The spiritual dimension of health is so significant that some health professionals believe it to be the actual "core of wellness."[13]

Cultivating the spiritual side of your health may help you discover how you "fit" into this universe. You can enhance your spiritual health in a variety of ways, many of which involve opening yourself to new experiences with nature, art, body movement, or music. Taking a walk in the woods, visiting an art museum, listening to classical music, talking with young children, writing poetry, caring for the environment, painting a picture, or pushing your body to its physical limits are just a few ways that you can develop spiritual health.

Occupational Dimension

The sixth dimension of health reflects the fact that employment satisfaction is directly related to many aspects of a person's health. When people feel good about their jobs, they tend to feel good about themselves and are more likely to have a healthier lifestyle. Usually, people have positive feelings about their employment situation if their jobs provide both external rewards (such as adequate salary and benefits) and internal rewards (such as positive social interactions and the opportunity for creative input).

As professors, we encourage our students to consider how closely their future occupations will be linked to their future health status. Fortunately, many colleges have career counseling offices, where students can talk with professionals about career opportunities. Sometimes during career counseling, students undertake a series of psychological tests to help in determining the kinds of jobs that could best fit their personality profiles. Students can also learn about job opportunities in their major areas of study by talking with professors and from volunteer work, student employment or internships, and summer job experiences.

It should also be noted that some health professionals are calling for the inclusion of additional dimensions of health. Although a case can be made for including environmental or consumer dimensions of health, we believe that too many dimensions can result in a watered-down view of health. Additional dimensions can probably fit under one of the six just discussed. For example, consumer health can be seen as a facet of social or intellectual health.

OUR DEFINITION OF HEALTH

By combining the role of health with the composition of health, we offer a new definition of health that we believe is unique to this book:

> Health is the blending of your physical, emotional, social, intellectual, spiritual, and occupational resources as they assist you in mastering the developmental tasks necessary for you to enjoy a satisfying and productive life.

Remember that this blending of your health resources is a never-ending process. Whether you are a traditional or nontraditional student, your ability to master the tasks that await you hinges on this unique combination of health dimensions.

CHARTING A PLAN FOR BEHAVIOR CHANGE

Students taking a personal health course usually decide to change their health behavior in one or more specific ways. We encourage our students to complete a "health behavior change project" as part of their course requirements. Sometimes, students know

LEARNING from ALL CULTURES

The Important Things in Life

What are the most important things in life for maintaining a happy and healthy existence? If any number of Americans responded to this question, the answers would vary. For some, success and happiness might mean a good job or a satisfying career, whereas for others, contentment with oneself, family, and friends might be the answer.

The same holds true for people of other cultures. There are common experiences, however, that people from different countries consider important to their well-being. Mexico, for example, is a country with a large gap between the rich and the poor; but for the great majority of Mexicans, celebrations or "fiestas" contribute greatly to their joy of living. Religious holidays and civil events are important occasions for fiestas and can be national or local celebrations. They are generally held outdoors and last from 1 to 3 days.[15]

Chile, like Mexico, is a country of the very rich and the very poor. Regardless of economic or social status, however, most Chileans derive pride and happiness from their families, and families typically are very close. Chileans generally are also extremely hospitable and enjoy interacting with strangers or visitors.[16]

Lebanese and other Middle Eastern people are also known for their hospitality and welcome visitors and foreigners into their homes for refreshment. In fact, much of their social life revolves around sharing refreshment, particularly Arabic coffee, with friends.[17]

Although all these countries face many challenges, their people still strive for happiness and continue to participate in things that bring them joy. What things in your life do you find most important for achieving happiness?

exactly which behavior they want to alter. They may have found this behavior while completing the Personal Assessment on p. 12.

Other students browse through various chapters in the textbook to see what topics are of special interest to them. It might be helpful for you to examine the personal assessments in each chapter. For example, if you are interested in behavior change related to alcohol use, you might look at p. 187 and complete the Personal Assessment entitled "How do you use alcoholic beverages?" If you are thinking about a behavior

Text continued on p. 15.

PERSONAL ASSESSMENT

A Personal Profile: Evaluating Your Health

Your health is influenced by behavior in a number of aspects of living. This personal health profile will help you assess this behavior. For each statement, circle the number of the response that best describes your behavior or how you think you will behave when confronted with a particular situation. At the end of each section, add the points received on the statements in that section and record your point total on the appropriate line. At the conclusion of the inventory you will be able to make a broad interpretation of the influence of your behavior on your personal health status.

Stress Management

	Rarely, if ever	Some of the time	Most of the time	Almost always
1. I seek out change and accept its presence with a sense of confidence and anticipation.	1	2	3	4
2. I participate regularly in a physical activity that allows me to expend nervous energy.	1	2	3	4
3. I turn to friends for advice and assistance during periods of disruption in my life.	1	2	3	4
4. I periodically reevaluate my experiences with stressful events in anticipation of future events of the same type.	1	2	3	4
5. I seek the counsel of professional advisors when stress becomes too difficult to manage.	1	2	3	4
6. I seek comfort and support from my faith when faced with a difficult period of adjustment.	1	2	3	4
				Points _____

Physical Fitness

1. I participate in vigorous activity for approximately 30 minutes four times per week.	1	2	3	4
2. I am active during the day and prefer a more vigorous approach to work and leisure activity.	1	2	3	4
3. I do exercises specifically designed to condition my muscles and joints.	1	2	3	4
4. I enter into vigorous activity only after I am warmed up, and I cool down after vigorous activity.	1	2	3	4
5. I select properly designed and well-maintained equipment and clothing for each activity.	1	2	3	4
6. I listen to my body regarding injury and fatigue, and I seek appropriate care when injured.	1	2	3	4
				Points _____

Social Relationships

1. I feel comfortable and confident when meeting people for the first time.	1	2	3	4
2. I establish social relationships with people of both genders with equal ease and enjoyment.	1	2	3	4
3. I participate in a wide variety of groups, including educational, recreational, religious, and occupational groups.	1	2	3	4
4. I find the roles of leader and subordinate to be equally acceptable.	1	2	3	4
5. I seek out opportunities to become proficient at a variety of social skills.	1	2	3	4
6. I am open and accessible to others in the development of intimate relationships.	1	2	3	4
				Points _____

	Rarely, if ever	Some of the time	Most of the time	Almost always

Spiritual Health

	Rarely, if ever	Some of the time	Most of the time	Almost always
1. I find myself searching for spiritual connections in my life.	1	2	3	4
2. I can identify ways I can improve the spiritual dimension of my health.	1	2	3	4

Points _____

Nutrition

	Rarely, if ever	Some of the time	Most of the time	Almost always
1. I select a wide variety of foods in an attempt to eat a balanced diet.	1	2	3	4
2. I select breads, cereals, fresh fruits, and vegetables in preference to pastries, candies, sodas, and fruits canned in heavy syrup.	1	2	3	4
3. I select such foods as peas, beans, and peanut butter as my primary sources of protein while limiting my consumption of red meat and high-fat dairy products.	1	2	3	4
4. I select foods prepared with unsaturated vegetable oils while reducing my consumption of red meats, organ meats, dairy products, and foods prepared with lard or butter.	1	2	3	4
5. I limit snacking, and I select nutritious foods when I do snack.	1	2	3	4
6. I attempt to balance my caloric intake with my activity level.	1	2	3	4

Points _____

Alcohol, Tobacco, and Drug Use

	Rarely, if ever	Some of the time	Most of the time	Almost always
1. I abstain from alcohol use, or I use alcohol infrequently and in very limited amounts.	1	2	3	4
2. I avoid riding with people who are consuming alcohol, and I drive defensively, remaining aware that other drivers may be using alcohol.	1	2	3	4
3. I avoid the use of tobacco products in all forms, including cigarettes, cigars, pipes, and smokeless tobacco products.	1	2	3	4
4. I limit my contact with others who are using tobacco, particularly when in confined spaces or when exposure would be for an extended period.	1	2	3	4
5. I take prescription drugs only in the manner prescribed, and I use over-the-counter drugs in accordance with directions.	1	2	3	4
6. I refrain from using illegal drugs.	1	2	3	4

Points _____

Safety

	Rarely, if ever	Some of the time	Most of the time	Almost always
1. I attempt to identify the sources of risk or potential danger in each new setting or activity.	1	2	3	4
2. I learn procedures and precautions before undertaking new recreational or occupational activities.	1	2	3	4
3. I select appropriate equipment for all activities and maintain equipment in good working order.	1	2	3	4
4. I curtail my participation in activities when I am not feeling well or am distracted by other demands.	1	2	3	4
5. I refrain from using alcohol or drugs when engaged in potentially dangerous recreational or occupational activities.	1	2	3	4
6. I repair or report dangerous conditions to individuals responsible for maintenance.	1	2	3	4

Points _____

Continued

Self-Care

	1	2	3	4
1. I maintain an accurate, updated personal health history.	Not at all	To a very limited degree	Almost completely	Completely
2. I routinely monitor my weight and blood pressure, as well as factors related to specific conditions applicable to my health.	Rarely, if ever	Some of the time	Most of the time	Almost always
3. I practice home dental health care, including brushing and flossing.	Rarely, if ever	Some of the time	Most of the time	Almost always
4. I maintain my immunization status and receive boosters when scheduled or required by specific conditions.	Not at all	To a very limited degree	Almost completely	Completely
5. I take prescription medication through the entire course of the prescribed period of use rather than stopping use when symptoms subside.	Rarely, if ever	Some of the time	Most of the time	Almost always
6. I consult a reliable home-medical reference book before beginning self-care.	Rarely, if ever	Some of the time	Most of the time	Almost always

Points _____

Answer When Applicable

	1	2	3	4
1. I routinely examine my testicles for the presence of small masses or other unusual signs.	Rarely, if ever	Some of the time	Most of the time	Almost always
2. I routinely examine my breasts for the presence of masses or other unusual signs.	Rarely, if ever	Some of the time	Most of the time	Almost always
3. I routinely receive a Pap smear test.	Rarely, if ever	Some of the time	Most of the time	Almost always
4. I use my birth control technique in the manner intended to maximize its effectiveness.	Rarely, if ever	Some of the time	Most of the time	Almost always

Points _____

Hereditary

	1	2	3	4
1. I can identify members of my family tree for the previous three generations.	Not at all	To a limited degree	Almost completely	Completely
2. I can identify the age at death and the cause of death for all family members to whom I am genetically related for the previous three generations.	Not for any	For a few but not for most	For most but not for all	For all
3. I receive medical consultation for conditions for which I may have a genetic predisposition (diabetes, hypertension, etc.).	Not at all	To a very limited degree	Relatively continuous consultation	Continuous consultation
4. I limit my exposure to radiation and to toxic environmental pollutants.	Rarely, if ever	Some of the time	Most of the time	Almost always
5. I will openly share information concerning inheritance abnormalities with potential mates.	Not likely	Perhaps	Very likely	Certainly
6. I will seek genetic counseling for known inherited conditions before having children.	Not likely	Perhaps	Very likely	Certainly

Points _____

Sleep, Rest, and Relaxation

	1	2	3	4
1. I plan my daily schedule to allow time for leisure activity.	Rarely, if ever	Some of the time	Most of the time	Almost always
2. I plan my daily schedule to allow time for contemplation, meditation, or prayer.	Rarely, if ever	Some of the time	Most of the time	Almost always
3. I receive between 7 and 8 hours of sleep daily.	Rarely, if ever	Some of the time	Most of the time	Almost always
4. I refrain from using sleep-inducing over-the-counter drugs.	Rarely, if ever	Some of the time	Most of the time	Almost always

5. I curtail activities when I need to recover from illnesses and injuries.

1	2	3	4
Rarely, if ever	Some of the time	Most of the time	Almost always

6. I attempt to leave the demands of work, school, or parenting outside of my leisure or relaxation time of the day.

1	2	3	4
Rarely, if ever	Some of the time	Most of the time	Almost always

Points _____

Health Consumerism

1. I am skeptical of practitioners and clinics who advertise or offer services at rates substantially lower than those charged by reputable providers.

1	2	3	4
Rarely, if ever	Some of the time	Most of the time	Almost always

2. I have the financial resources necessary to cover the costs associated with a major illness or hospitalization.

1	2	3	4
Not at all	To a limited degree	Almost completely	Completely

3. I am skeptical of claims that "guarantee" the effectiveness of a particular health-care service or product.

1	2	3	4
Rarely, if ever	Some of the time	Most of the time	Almost always

4. I accept information that is deemed valid by the established scientific community.

1	2	3	4
Rarely, if ever	Some of the time	Most of the time	Almost always

5. I pursue my rights in matters of misrepresentation or consumer dissatisfaction.

1	2	3	4
Rarely, if ever	Some of the time	Most of the time	Almost always

6. I seek additional opinions regarding diagnoses indicating a need for surgery or other costly therapies.

1	2	3	4
Rarely, if ever	Some of the time	Most of the time	Almost always

Points _____

YOUR TOTAL POINTS _____

Interpretation

213-264	Behavior is very supportive of high-level health.
164-212	Behavior is relatively supportive of high-level health.
115-163	Behavior is relatively destructive to high-level health.
66-114	Behavior is very destructive to high-level health.

To Carry This Further . . .

Were you surprised at your score? Remember that this assessment provides a brief look at your health behavior. It should help identify areas you may want to pay careful attention to as you read this book. We hope this assessment will serve as a positive motivator for you, regardless of your score. Remember that you can change your health behavior. This health textbook and your instructor can get you started in the right direction. Good luck.

---

change concerning weight management, you could take the Personal Assessment titled "Should you consider a weight loss program?" on p. 140.

Some of the health behaviors our students typically want to change are the following:

- To gain or lose weight
- To stop smoking
- To stop using smokeless tobacco
- To eliminate or reduce caffeine consumption
- To develop better sleeping patterns
- To reduce levels of stress
- To improve physical fitness
- To reduce alcohol consumption
- To eat more nutritiously
- To develop more friendships
- To enhance the spiritual dimension of health

To change your behavior, you must now attempt to complete the following 10 steps:

1. *Establish some baseline data about your behavior.* Baseline data is information about your current health and behavior that you can use later for comparison. This could take many forms, depending on your behavior. For example, you might weigh yourself for 3 consecutive days early in the morning. If you plan to stop smoking, keep track of your smoking patterns for a few days. If you are changing your diet, write down everything you eat for a 3- or 4-day period. We suggest keeping a journal and recording your activities and feelings related to the behavior.

2. *Summarize your baseline data.* Identify any patterns you see. Accept this information as an accurate indicator of your current health behavior. Use this textbook to find information about your behavior that could help you plan behavior-change strategies.

3. *Establish some specific goals.* Start with increments small enough to be within your grasp. For example, if you plan to lose weight, you might start out with a goal of 1 pound per week for the next 3 weeks. If you plan to stop smoking, you might start out by cutting down on your daily intake by five cigarettes. Think in terms of small, gradual progress toward your goals.

4. *Make a personal contract to accomplish your goals.* In this contract, you will want to indicate both starting and completion dates. Especially useful at this point are the Health Action Guides found in each chapter. These guides, such as the ones on p. 117 (Dietary Recommendations), p. 265 (Eat to Lower Your Cancer Risk), and p. 239 (Monitoring Your Cholesterol Level), will help you focus on specific activities to reach your goals. Identify any milestones along the way. Indicate the time, personal resources, and energy you will need to commit to this project.

5. *Devise a plan of action.* As you develop your strategy, try to control the environment in which you function so that you can replace old cues with new ones. For example, if you are trying to improve your sleep, you may wish to calm yourself before bed by reading rather than by listening to loud music or watching a television drama. If you are trying to improve your eating behavior, make a careful attempt to avoid walking by a place where donuts are available.

6. *Chart your progress in your diary or journal.* As you implement your behavior-change plan, keep a record of how you are doing. Making this chart visible also helps. For instance, posting an eating record on the refrigerator door is a good motivator for some people.

7. *Encourage your family and friends to help you.* Social support is important in any behavior-change attempt. Your friends may want to join you so that they can change their own behavior, and you can support each other. However, some friends or family members might be jealous of or misunderstand your efforts, and their behavior might discourage you. Avoid these people if at all possible . . . at least while your project is under way.

8. *Set up a reward system.* Rewards tend to motivate people and can serve to reinforce your positive changes. If you achieve success at a particular point in your plan, reward yourself with a special meal, new clothes, or a weekend trip. Pat yourself on the back occasionally for your efforts. Relish your success.

9. *Prepare for obstacles along the way.* No one who achieved anything of importance did it without a few setbacks along the way. For example, you might neglect your fitness plan during a long holiday weekend. Prepare yourself mentally for an occasional obstacle. The key is to try to get back on course as soon as possible after a setback. Work through your setbacks with a "forgive and forget" attitude.

10. *Revise your plan as necessary.* Try to remain somewhat flexible in your approach to behavior change. A strategy that works for a while might not work as well after a month or two, so be prepared to reevaluate your goals and try new techniques when necessary.

Summary

- The World Health Organization definition of health states that health is more than the absence of disease.
- Holistic health views health in its multiple dimensions.
- Health promotion, wellness, and empowerment reflect important movements in the health field.
- To move successfully through life, critical developmental tasks must be achieved. Chapter 1 focuses on five tasks that involve identity, independence, responsibility, social skills, and intimacy.
- One's health is composed of six dimensions: physical, emotional, social, intellectual, spiritual, and occupational.
- The authors define health in terms of the six dimensions' ability to help one successfully complete developmental tasks.
- Midlife adults have two key developmental tasks: achieving generativity and reassessing the plans of young adulthood.
- Developmental tasks of the elderly include accepting aging, maintaining physical function, and establishing a sense of integrity.

Review Questions

1. How does the World Health Organization's definition of health differ from the definition developed in this chapter?
2. Define holistic health, health promotion, wellness, and empowerment.
3. What were the three broad goals of the 1990 *Healthy People 2000* report?
4. What is a developmental task?
5. Identify the five developmental tasks of college students.
6. What is the difference between the *role* of health and the *composition* of health?
7. What is meant by "health is dynamic"?
8. Describe the six dimensions of health.
9. What developmental tasks exist for midlife and elderly adults?

Think About This . . .

- Does your lifestyle reflect a "wellness" approach to living?
- To what degree does your campus reflect a multicultural community?
- How closely related do you think the developmental tasks of independence and responsibility are? Can you have one without the other?
- Which of the six dimensions of health have you developed most fully? Least fully?

References

1. World Health Organization: Constitution of the World Health Organization, *Chronicle of the World Health Organization* 1:29-43, 1947.
2. Joint Committee on Health Education Terminology: Report of the 1990 Joint Committee on Health Education Terminology, *J Sch Health* 61(6):251-254, 1991.
3. Anspaugh DJ, Hamrick MH, Rosato FD: *Wellness: concepts and applications,* ed 2, St Louis, 1994, Mosby.
4. Brylinsky J, Hoadley M: A comparative analysis of wellness attitudes of "suicidal" and "at risk" college students, *Wellness Perspectives: Research, Theory, and Practice* 8(2):59-72, 1991.
5. DeGraw C: A community-based school health system: parameters for developing a comprehensive student health promotion program, *J Sch Health* 64(5):192-195, 1994.
6. Watts PR et al: A university worksite health promotion and wellness education program model, *Journal of Health Education* 23(2):87-94, 1992.
7. Anderson K: Cash rewards are made to faithful few, *USA Today,* 1B, May 27, 1992.
8. Fahlberg LL et al: Empowerment as an emerging approach in health education, *Journal of Health Education* 22(3):185-193, 1991.
9. Erikson E: *Childhood and society,* New York, 1963, WW Norton.
10. Levinson D: *The seasons of a man's life,* New York, 1978, Alfred A. Knopf.
11. Cavanaugh J: *Adult development and aging,* Belmont, Calif, 1990, Wadsworth.
12. Payne W, Hahn D: *Understanding your health,* ed 4, St Louis, 1995, Mosby.
13. Myers JE, Witmer M, Sweeney TJ: Spirituality: the core of wellness, *Wellness Connections* 4(2):1, 6-8, 1993.
14. Bensley RJ: Defining spiritual health: a review of the literature, *Journal of Health Education* 22(5):287-290, 1991.
15. Rummel J: *Mexico,* New York, 1990, Chelsea House.
16. Galvin IF: *Chile: land of poets and patriots,* Minneapolis, 1990, Dillon Press.
17. Cahill MJ: *Lebanon,* New York, 1987, Chelsea House.

Suggested Readings

Hoffman E: *Our health, our lives,* New York, 1995, Pocket Books.
Dr. Hoffman, a founding member of the Mt. Sinai School of Medicine's Women's Health Program, shows how medicine can function when it serves women's needs. Helps empower women to use the health care system to their advantage. Coverage of a wide range of health issues for women, including how to find a women-centered physician.

The good health fact book, Pleasantville, NY, 1992, The Reader's Digest Association.

This book is filled with current health facts written in an easy-to-read, question-and-answer format. Over 1000 health questions are answered. Illustrations are provided throughout. An appendix lists numerous health-related organizations.

Weil A: *Spontaneous healing,* New York, 1995, Alfred A. Knopf.
Written by a physician who is a leading voice in the practice of alternative medicine, including natural, noninvasive treatments. This book acknowledges that the body has an intrinsic healing system that mends the body and maintains well-being. Weil provides numerous case histories.

 AS WE GO TO PRESS . . .

The American Council of Education released a report that indicates a significant increase in minority enrollment in higher education. The 5% increase in 1994 doubled the 1993 increase in minority enrollment. Overall, 16% of the students enrolled in 4-year colleges are either Native American, Hispanic, or African-American.

ON...

The Diversity of Today's College Students

It's the fall of 1970, and you're about to meet Joe College, a student in a freshman health class at State University. Joe is an 18-year-old white man who graduated from City High School last summer in the top half of his class. He lives in State U's dormitory, and because his tuition is being paid by his parents, he is able to devote himself to his studies and college life on a full-time basis. When Joe looks around his health class, he sees some women and a few minorities and older students, but most of his fellow students are much like himself. In short, Joe College is a typical college student.

Flash forward to today. When you look around your health classroom, what kinds of students do you see? Undoubtedly, Joe College is still present in today's university; however, he no longer composes the overwhelming majority of the student body. The many changes in American society that have taken place over the past 25 years are reflected in today's colleges and universities. Nowadays, slightly more women than men are graduating from college. As more older people find that they need better skills and more training or a degree to keep their present jobs or to find new ones, the average age of college students has risen. Also, schools are focusing efforts to more actively recruit minority students. Finally, recent laws that affirm the rights of disabled Americans to have access to most public facilities have allowed disabled individuals the opportunity to attend college. As you look at your fellow students, you will probably notice that these changes are reflected in your health class and at your school in general. Because of these changes, schools must adapt to meet the educational needs of all their students.

Enrollment Statistics

College enrollment statistics cited in the *Chronicle of Higher Education* show that enrollment has increased dramatically for certain minority groups in the United States. The numbers of Asian students increased from 390,000 in 1984 to 724,000 in 1993, an increase of over 85%. Hispanic enrollment also increased by 84.9% over that same period. African-American enrollment increased by 31%, and Native American enrollment rose by 45.2%. White enrollment increased by only 8% from 1984 to 1993: enrollment of white men increased by only 1.4% during this span, whereas enrollment of white women increased by 14%.[1]

Even with the huge increases in enrollment within several groups, overall college enrollment only went up 16.9% from 1984 to 1993. This is because whites continue to make up the vast majority of college students, comprising 74.1% of all college students in 1993. Even so, the numbers show a gradual change in college demographics, since 80% of all college enrollees in 1984 were white.[1]

In 1993 a Census Bureau survey showed that over 40% of all students were 25 years of age or older.[1] This suggests that college campuses are no longer dominated by traditional-age students (age 18-24). The influx of older students, coupled with the strong increase in minority enrollment, has greatly increased the diversity on college campuses.

Causes Behind the Changes

So why are these changes occurring? Several factors seem to be affecting enrollment figures in the United States. Clearly the changing climate of the economy has affected enrollment. Corporate trends toward a more streamlined workforce and the gradual shift toward a service-oriented marketplace have caused many workers to seek training for new careers or to seek additional training for their current jobs. And although the nation's economy has been "growing" for the last several years, things do not always look so good to those outside of Wall Street. Many working people are finding that their wages are not enough to make ends meet, and many elderly people are finding that their Social Security benefits are not nearly enough to survive on. As a result, people who never thought they would see the inside of a classroom again are drawn back to school in hope of improving their careers.[2] Colleges have also become more accessible in recent years. The trend toward open admissions, especially at community colleges, has opened the doors of higher education to those who otherwise would be held back by low high school grades or low test scores. Colleges have attempted to meet the needs of these new students with remedial courses and special programs designed to prepare students whose academic records indicate that they are in need of extra help to meet academic standards.[3]

Social changes have also played an important role in the changing demographics on college campuses. The civil rights movement in the 1950s and 1960s was instrumental in making a college education available to minorities, and minority enrollment continues to increase as overall awareness of civil rights becomes more entrenched in society. Students with various physical disabilities are also finding it easier to obtain a college education. The Americans with Disabilities Act, signed into law in 1990, guarantees that people with disabilities will have access to employment, education, and public services. As a result, people with disabilities are able to pursue careers that were previously inaccessible, and many are heading to college to receive training for those careers.

As higher education has become more accessible, there has been an attitude change toward going to college. There is now a more prevalent feeling in society that everyone should go to college after high school. Population demographics as a whole may also have an effect on college demographics. Populations within minority groups have been increasing at a much higher rate than the white population in the United States, and this may in part account for the rise in minority enrollment.

Practical Implications of Diversity on Campus

With the rise of new populations on campuses, many practical changes have taken place at colleges and universities to reflect the needs and interests of students on today's campuses. San Antonio College, one of the largest community colleges in the United States, is a good example of the types of changes that are occurring nationwide. To meet the needs of students who are not prepared for college work, SAC has a large developmental education program designed to help students develop their skills in reading, writing, and mathematics. For working students, evening and weekend divisions offer courses in many disciplines to accommodate busy schedules. The college also houses the Student Support Services Project, an educational program sponsored by the United States Department of Education that serves the

needs of disabled and first-generation college students from low-income families.[4]

Changes are also reflected in SAC's course offerings, student organizations, and facilities. In addition to offering traditional courses in Western and American literature and history, the college also offers courses in African-American literature, Mexican literature, and world literature (including Third World works), and interdisciplinary studies courses that examine community issues, social issues, and the fine arts from a multicultural perspective. Student organizations include the Black Student Alliance, Chicanos in the Arts, and the Mexican American Engineering students, as well as more traditional student government organizations, major interest organizations, and honor societies. The campus learning center has large collections of multicultural literature and history books, and the library recently added a set of computers so that students can access the World Wide Web and use the Internet to make intercultural connections with other students from across the country and around the world.[4] All these changes were implemented (at least in part) to make the campus a more friendly and inviting environment for today's college students.

Changing Campuses and the Study of Health

Many changes have taken place on campus in recent years. Why mention them here in a health text? Because of the increasing diversity on college campuses, students studying health (and most other disciplines) should be made aware not only of issues that affect them personally but also of issues that affect others of different backgrounds as well. For example, many people are unaware of the fact that most pharmaceutical research is performed on men and then generalized to apply to women, a potentially dangerous practice given that women are at greater risk for adverse drug reactions.[5] Another good example of a cultural health issue is the use of alternative medical practitioners. Native Americans view health care as a holistic rather than symptom-based process, and they are more likely to respond to a "medicine man" who looks at both the physical and spiritual person than to a physician who examines only diseased body parts.[6] Similarly, some Mexican Americans will either rely on or supplement traditional health care with *curanderismo*, a medical system that combines Western health care practices with folklore, magic, herbalism, and religion.[7] Knowledge of these and other related cultural health care issues will allow college students to better understand all members of today's culturally diverse American society.

It is no longer possible to accept the traditional version of what health should be as the whole story. To get a complete picture of what health care issues are important today, we must understand health beliefs and health actions of the various segments of our culture.[8] Bringing cultural awareness into the health classroom can introduce students to concepts they might not otherwise be exposed to. During your college career, you will likely encounter students from a variety of backgrounds. They may be young or old, from a rich or poor family, from a rural or urban environment, or from an ethnic group different from yours. Just as your culture has its own unique health concerns, every other culture has its own set of health concerns as well, and you should be aware of them. *Focus on Health* will attempt to address the needs of students from different cultural backgrounds when appropriate.

For Discussion . . .
Consider the following items:

Prosthetics	Scurvy and rickets
Tay-Sachs disease	Cochlear implants
Sickle-cell anemia	Osteoporosis
Hemophilia	Cystic fibrosis
Alzheimer's disease	Breast cancer

For each item, determine which cultural group(s) are more likely to consider the item as a health concern (do a little research if needed). Can you think of other health concerns that are unique to certain cultures or groups? What are the particular health concerns of your culture?

References
1. The nation. *The chronicle of higher education,* Almanac Issue, 42(1), Sept 1, 1995.
2. Troyka LQ: Perspectives on legacies and literacy in the 1980s. In *A sourcebook for basic writing teachers,* New York, 1987, McGraw-Hill.
3. Mutnick D: *Writing in an alien world,* Portsmouth, NH, 1996, Boynton/Cook.
4. *San Antonio College Bulletin, 1995-1996,* San Antonio, Tex, 1995, San Antonio College.
5. Nechas E, Foley D: *Unequal treatment,* New York, 1994, Simon & Schuster.
6. Sorrell MS, Smith BA: Navajo beliefs: implications for health professionals, *Journal of Health Education* 24(6), 1991.
7. Stauber D: Curanderismo in the Mexican-American community, *Journal of Health Education* 25(6), 1994.
8. Airhihenbuwa CO: Culture, health education, and critical consciousness. *Journal of Health Education* 26(5), 1995.

PART 1

THE MIND

Achieving Emotional Maturity

Healthy People 2000 Objectives

In the area of emotional, mental, and cognitive disorders, an important objective of the Healthy People 2000 report was to reduce the prevalence of mental disorders within the general population. The Midcourse Review, however, does not address progress in reaching this objective. Perhaps in the short period of 5 years, it is difficult to assess the progress of such an ambitious quest.

Another important objective was to increase the use of community support services in the prevention and treatment of severe, persistent mental disorders. Data reported in the Midcourse Review clearly show that substantial gains have been made in the development of state-level clearinghouses to better identify existing resources. Unfortunately, adult patients of primary care providers, including family physicians, internal medicine specialists, and obstetricians and gynecologists, were unlikely to receive counseling or referral to these resources for treatment. For children, however, the picture is more encouraging. Most physicians routinely assess cognitive development, behavioral functioning, and child-parent interaction and refer their patients for appropriate care.

Emotionally healthy people have a high level of self-esteem and find social interaction to be comfortable and rewarding. Having stated that self-esteem is inseparable from emotional health, we must, however, caution that you cannot expect to feel personally fulfilled by everything. There will always be situations in which you must act against your own best interests so that others are best served. Additionally, self-esteem is not always enough to completely offset the health problems that can afflict us.

CHARACTERISTICS OF AN EMOTIONALLY WELL PERSON

We define an emotionally well person as one who is capable of using resources from each of the six dimensions of health mentioned in Chapter 1 to feel good about life and other people. A more specific yardstick for measuring emotional health comes from the National Mental Health Association. This group describes emotionally well people as having three fundamental characteristics[2]:

- They feel comfortable about themselves. They are not overwhelmed by their own feelings, and they can accept many of life's disappointments in stride. They experience the full range of human emotions (for example, fear, anger, love, jealousy, guilt, and joy) but are not overcome by them.
- They interact well with other people. They are comfortable with others and are able to give and receive love. They are concerned about others' well-being and have relationships that are satisfying and lasting.
- They are able to meet the demands of life. Emotionally healthy people respond appropriately to their problems, accept responsibility, plan ahead without fearing the future, and are able to establish reachable goals.

We do not wish to give the impression that emotionally well people are perfect. At times, emotionally healthy people experience stress, frustration, feelings of self-doubt, failure, and rejection. What distinguishes the emotionally well person is resilience—the ability to recapture a sense of emotional wellness within a reasonable period of time after encountering difficult situations.

EMOTIONAL AND PSYCHOLOGICAL WELLNESS

Is there a difference between emotional and psychological wellness? Many people believe that there is

little real difference between the terms. Rather, they both reflect the absence of emotional illness and psychopathology. However, some people believe that emotional health refers specifically to the feelings people experience in response to changes in their environment. These feelings, such as anger, jealousy, joy, disappointment, compassion, and sympathy, are familiar, healthy emotions. Responses to change vary from one person to the next and reflect each person's values. Emotionally healthy people feel good about their responses, whereas those who are less emotionally well feel negative about their responses.

In contrast to emotional health, some people think that psychological health refers more broadly to the development and functioning of a wide array of mental abilities, such as language, memory, perception, and awareness. For example, a person who believes he is being followed by government agents has faulty perception, so we would say that he is not psychologically healthy. Those who are psychologically healthy deal rationally with the world, have a fully functional personality, and resolve conflict nondestructively. Finally, the psychophysical (mind-body) interface of the psychologically healthy person is sound.

Normal Range of Emotions

Have you known people who seem to be "up" all the time? These people appear to be confident, happy, and full of good feelings 24 hours a day. Although some people may have these traits, they are truly the exceptions. For most people, emotions are more like a roller coaster ride. There are times when they feel good about themselves and others, and there are times when nothing seems to be going right. This is normal and healthy. Life has its ups and downs, and the concept of the "normal range of emotions" reflects this.

Self-Esteem

Perhaps the key to overall emotional wellness is self-esteem.[3] When people have positive self-esteem, they feel capable and are in control of social situations and their own thoughts and feelings. They are able to get along with others, cope in stressful situations, and make contributions when they work with others. Self-esteem may offset self-defeating or self-destructive behavior problems. For example, a young woman who is slightly overweight but has high self-esteem would be unlikely to go on an unhealthy crash diet in an effort to conform to the currently fashionable body image. As you will see when you complete the Personal Assessment on p. 26, people with high levels of

PERSONAL ASSESSMENT

How Does My Self-Concept Compare with My Idealized Self?

Below is a list of 15 personal attributes, each portrayed on a 9-point continuum. Mark with an X where you think you rank on each attribute. Try to be candid and accurate; these marks will collectively describe a portion of your sense of self-concept. When you are finished with

the above task, go back and circle where you *wish* you could be on each dimension. These marks describe your idealized self. Finally, in the spaces on the right, indicate the difference between your self-concept and your idealized self for each attribute.

Decisive					Indecisive				_____
9	8	7	6	5	4	3	2	1	

Anxious					Relaxed				_____
9	8	7	6	5	4	3	2	1	

Easily influenced					Independent thinker				_____
9	8	7	6	5	4	3	2	1	

Very intelligent					Less intelligent				_____
9	8	7	6	5	4	3	2	1	

In good physical shape					In poor physical shape				_____
9	8	7	6	5	4	3	2	1	

Undependable					Dependable				_____
9	8	7	6	5	4	3	2	1	

Deceitful					Honest				_____
9	8	7	6	5	4	3	2	1	

A leader					A follower				_____
9	8	7	6	5	4	3	2	1	

Unambitious					Ambitious				_____
9	8	7	6	5	4	3	2	1	

Self-confident					Insecure				_____
9	8	7	6	5	4	3	2	1	

Conservative					Adventurous				_____
9	8	7	6	5	4	3	2	1	

Extroverted					Introverted				_____
9	8	7	6	5	4	3	2	1	

Physically attractive					Physically unattractive				_____
9	8	7	6	5	4	3	2	1	

Lazy					Hardworking				_____
9	8	7	6	5	4	3	2	1	

Funny					Little sense of humor				_____
9	8	7	6	5	4	3	2	1	

To Carry This Further . . .

1. Overall, how would you describe the discrepancy between your self-concept and your self-ideal (large, moderate, small, large on a few dimensions)?

2. How do sizable gaps for any of your attributes affect your sense of self-esteem?

3. Do you think that any of the gaps exist because you have had others' ideals imposed on you or because you have thoughtlessly accepted others' ideals?

4. Identify several attributes that you realistically believe can be changed to narrow the gap between your self-concept and your self-ideal and, thus, foster a well-developed sense of self-esteem.

self-esteem find a comfortable balance between their idealized self and where they actually are.

For some people the lack of self-esteem is understandable. Growing up in a dysfunctional household, being overloaded with guilt in conjunction with religious upbringing, and failing in early undertakings can all damage feelings of self-worth.

The foundation of positive self-esteem can be

traced back to childhood. There are many ways in which interaction with young children imparts powerful messages about self-worth. Warm and supportive physical contact, verbal exchanges involving talking "with" rather than "to" children, and the gradual loosening of control so that more and more decisions become those of the child inform children that they are competent and valued. Children's emerging self-esteem, then, is strongly influenced by their parents' behavior. Children from less supportive or overly protective home environments will eventually seek positive feedback from other sources.

As important as parents and others, including the peer group, are to the development of self-esteem in children, people eventually become responsible for enhancing their own self-esteem. The extent to which people wish to nurture their own self-esteem varies. However, for those who want to take an active role in developing a more solid sense of self-worth, the Health Action Guide at right provides some assistance.

Hardiness

Working in conjunction with a sense of self-esteem to ensure emotional wellness is *hardiness*. As defined by Kobasa,[4] hardiness exists when a person consistently shows three important traits. First, a hardy person possesses a high level of *commitment* to something or someone and in doing so has the basis for a value orientation and a sense of purpose in life. The maintenance of this sense of commitment provides structure and direction even in the face of a wide variety of stressors (see Chapter 3). Second, a sense of *control* characterizes hardy people. By possessing the ability to orchestrate events in life, the hardy person reduces the chance of feeling helpless and vulnerable in the face of change imposed from outside. Third, the hardy person welcomes *challenge*. That is, he or she has the ability to take control of change and shape it in the direction of personal growth and fulfillment.

Hardiness may be more common among some types of people than others. Nevertheless, a high level of hardiness can be developed by focusing on signals from the body, assessing and responding to previous stressors, and engaging in activities that strengthen commitment, control, and challenge.

EMOTIONAL WELLNESS OF MIDLIFE AND ELDERLY ADULTS

An Optimistic View of Aging

It is not uncommon for our students to find the study of the aging process somewhat "uninteresting." However, for the nontraditional-age students, and eventually for the traditional-age students, aging is seen in a much more positive light. Older people report that they are generally happy and satisfied.

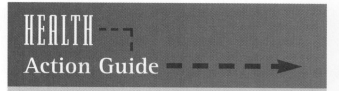

HEALTH ⌐¬ Action Guide ----►

Improving Your Self-Esteem

To improve your self-esteem, try to achieve success in these four areas:

- *Maintain satisfying relationships.* The best way to do this is to cultivate friendships or become affiliated with existing groups, such as social clubs, voluntary organizations, church groups, professional organizations, athletic groups, or any other group that you believe will help you feel a sense of "belonging."
- *Set and reach realistic goals.* Achieving their goals allows some people to feel personal power and control over themselves. In turn, this leads to improved self-confidence and further pride and motivation. The key is to make these goals realistic.
- *Realize your uniqueness.* The understanding and appreciation that you are indeed a unique and special person will enhance your self-esteem. Enjoy the satisfaction of a compliment when it is given to you. Take time out each day to think about your special strengths and abilities and how they differ from those possessed by others. Pat yourself on the back regularly, and remind yourself that you are a unique and special person.
- *Maintain contact with a mentor.* Look for certain key figures in your life who have been helpful to you and who have provided you with inspiration. These role models serve as mentors. The importance of making regular contact with your mentors should not be overlooked. ◄------

Many of our midlife (between 45 and 64 years of age) students report that they are starting a "new life." Intelligence, creativity, attractiveness, physical fitness, and sexual intimacy can continue in harmony with the aging process as long as people continue to participate in the activities that enhance these qualities.

The Joys of Midlife

Contrary to some stereotypical views, most midlife adults do not experience a multitude of problems that fill them with melancholy and despair. The lives of these midlife adults are characterized by positive elements. It is a myth that every midlife adult must have a midlife crisis. Most probably do not experience such an ordeal. Midlife adults may frequently find themselves more reflective than when they were young, but to label this behavior damaging is to fail to appreciate the value of careful self-examination. Perhaps midlife adults just have more to think about than they did when they were younger.

From our perspective, much of what midlifers think about is positive. Many see themselves as being in the prime of life. Certain potentially difficult aspects of life have been completed. Many have completed a formal education, become established in an occupation, gained financial security, and raised a family. Midlife adults can find great satisfaction with these accomplishments and can begin planning for future challenges.

By being relatively free from financial problems and no longer responsible for young children, midlife adults can pursue some of their own dreams. For example, it is not surprising to see midlife adults travel more than they did earlier in life. Many midlifers rededicate themselves to a fitness program or a hobby, such as reading or gardening. Some seem to love reliving their own college days vicariously through the lives of their college-aged children. For many midlifers, joyous moments also come with being grandparents. Can you think of other ways midlife adults experience deeply satisfying feelings?

The Midlife Crisis

For some adults, reaching midlife is a milestone that triggers a "midlife crisis," during which they reconsider the paths their lives have taken. They wonder whether they have made the right career and family decisions, and they reevaluate the meaning and value of their own lives. For some people, the midlife crisis can be a precarious period of reassessment because it coincides with a deep sense of vulnerability to time. The years seem to be slipping away, and they sense that personal growth should be occurring. If it is not, the alternatives seem to be limited. Dropping out of their current lives and starting over may seem like an attractive alternative to facing the future.

For most adults who have a midlife crisis, however, this period of questioning enhances emotional wellness because it prompts them to repeat the four-step process of emotional growth described on pp. 33-34.

Quality of Life for Elderly Adults

For the elderly, as for all adults, the quality of life is often judged on the basis of the status of several traits or conditions. We believe that life will be described as being "good" by older people who have not yet shown significant declines in the majority of areas listed below:

- *Health.* As long as the person feels well, has sufficient energy, and is not limited in terms of mobility, health is not a distracting factor to a good life.
- *Social status.* As long as the elderly person continues to participate in social activities that were enjoyed before retirement or the death of the spouse, social status remains unchanged and is not a negative factor in the quality of life.
- *Economic status.* As long as income is sufficient to maintain an acceptable lifestyle, provide the basic necessities, and form a cushion against unexpected major expenses, economic status is not a negative factor in a good life.
- *Marital status.* For most men, marital status remains unchanged. For women, widowhood can prove to be a significant factor detracting from the quality of life. If a support group can fill part of the void left by the spouse's death, the effect of a changed marital status can be minimized.
- *Living condition.* Only 5% of the elderly are living in nursing homes. As long as residential arrangements are unchanged, or, if changed, undertaken with minimal disruption, living conditions are not significant factors in defining the quality of life.
- *Educational level.* Educational level in general and an active interest in learning and experimenting in particular seem to foster positive experiences during aging. Limited education may inhibit some elderly people from learning more about the changing world around them.
- *Sexual intimacy.* Assuming the availability of a partner, sexual practices closely follow the patterns established during earlier periods of adulthood.[5] As long as both partners are satisfied, adjustment is not adversely influenced. Divergent expectations can cause difficulty for one or both partners.

AFFRONTS TO EMOTIONAL WELLNESS

In spite of their best efforts to be hardy and resilient, many people have a less than optimal level of emotional wellness. Depression is the most common and one of the most treatable of these dysfunctional emotional states. Loneliness, shyness, and, of course, thoughts of suicide are also challenges to high-level emotional wellness. Although this chapter focuses on emotional well-being rather than illness, an examination of these conditions is necessary because most of us at some time during our lives will either have emotional problems ourselves or know someone who is having difficulties.

Depression

Depression is an "emotional state characterized by exaggerated feelings of sadness, melancholy, dejection, worthlessness, emptiness, and hopelessness that are inappropriate and out of proportion to reality."[6] Some of the common symptoms of depression are listed in the accompanying Star Box. One key indicator of depression is the long-term presence of some of these symptoms. Everyone feels "down" or "blue" at times, but depression is characterized by a more chronic state of feeling "low."

In the United States, it is estimated that approximately 25% of the adult population will have some symptoms of major depression during their lifetime.[7] People with depression commonly have a number of compounding problems, including family problems and difficulty with social relationships. Depression is a common factor related to most suicides.[8]

Types of depression

According to mental-health experts, there are two main types of depression. When depression develops after a period of difficulty, such as a divorce or loss of a job, it is called *secondary* or *reactive depression*. However, when depression begins for no apparent reason, it is called *primary depression* and is caused by changes in brain chemistry. People with this type of depres-

sion are helped most by antidepressant drugs, whereas people with secondary depression often require counseling in addition to medication.

Through a variety of therapies, between 70% and 90% of depressed people can be helped. Types of therapy range from various "talking" strategies (including counseling) to the use of antidepressant drugs. Unlike the antianxiety or tranquilizer drugs that sedate the user, most antidepressant drugs prescribed today work by influencing neurotransmitters, chemicals released by the nervous system that help transmit impulses (see Chapter 7). Today, four main types of antidepressant medications are in use, including Prozac, the most frequently prescribed antidepressant.[9] When use is monitored carefully, many of today's antidepressant drugs produce few side effects.

Only a small percentage (about 33%) of depressed people ever seek help. This is unfortunate in light of the high rate of successful treatment. The Health Action Guide on p. 30 lists several resources available to help people with depression.

Loneliness

Many depressed people display signs of loneliness, although it is not always associated with depression. People are said to be lonely if they "desire close personal relationships but are unable to establish them."[10] It is possible to feel isolated and friendless even when you are around many people every day. In fact, loneliness is common among college students.

The difference between "being alone" and "feeling lonely" is important. Many people enjoy being alone occasionally to relax, to exercise, to read, to enjoy music, or just to think. These people can appreciate being alone, but they can also interact comfortably with others when they wish. However, when being alone or isolated is not enjoyable and seeking close relationships is very difficult, then feeling lonely can produce serious feelings of rejection.

One unfortunate aspect of loneliness is that it tends to continue in people year after year unless they take an active part in changing it. Chronically lonely people frequently cope with their loneliness by becoming consumed by their occupations or adopting habit-forming behavior that further makes them feel lonely.

Fortunately, there are successful techniques to help most lonely people. Counseling can help change how these people think about themselves when they interact with others. Another technique involves teaching people important social skills, such as starting a conversation, taking social risks, and introducing themselves. Through social skills training, people can also

Common Symptoms of Depression
Any of the following may be indications of possible depression:
- Persistent sad moods
- Feelings of hopelessness or pessimism
- Loss of interest or pleasure in ordinary activities, including sex
- Sleep and eating disorders
- Restlessness, irritability, or fatigue
- Difficulty concentrating, remembering, or making decisions
- Thoughts of death or suicide
- Persistent physical symptoms or pains that do not respond to treatment

HEALTH
Action Guide ➤

Resources for Help with Depression

If you or a friend had concerns about depression, would you know where to search for help? Regardless of where you are—large city, suburban community, or a rural area—a variety of resources are available.

- Seek help from your university health center, personal physician, or community health center.
- Try your university mental health counseling and treatment programs.
- Family and social service agencies can identify mental health specialists.
- Check the telephone book for private psychologists or psychiatric clinics.
- Talk with your professor.
- Contact one of the organizations listed below:

The Depression/Awareness, Recognition and Treatment Program (operated by the National Institute of Mental Health)
Room 15-C-05, 5600 Fishers Lane
Rockville, MD 20857
(301) 460-3062

The National Foundation for Depressive Illness
P.O. Box 2257
New York, NY 10016
(212) 268-4260

The National Mental Health Association
1021 Prince St.
Alexandria, VA 22314
(703)684-7722

---

learn how to talk comfortably on the telephone, give and receive compliments, and even enhance their appearance. If you need help in this area, contact your campus counseling center or health center.

Shyness

Is loneliness the result of an inability to interact comfortably with others, something brought about by shyness? If so, why are some people so shy? Some contend that shyness is a genetic component of temperament. Thus shy people do not want to be shy, they have not been conditioned to avoid contact with others, and they have not had unpleasant experiences with others; rather, they are genetically programmed to feel uncomfortable in settings involving other people. Accordingly, they cope by avoiding such situations. Even if shyness *is* a genetic trait, the social skills counseling and training suggested in the discussion of loneliness can help those who are shy.

Suicide

One of the tragedies of our times is the high incidence of suicide. In the last year for which statistics are available (1992), 32,000 people in the United States killed themselves.[11] Among young people (including college students), suicides follow accidents as the second leading cause of death.

What separates the potentially suicidal person from the nonsuicidal person is the degree of despair and depression the person feels and the ability to cope with it. Suicidal people tend to become overwhelmed with a range of destructive emotions, including anxiety, anger, loneliness, loss of self-esteem, and hopelessness. They may believe that death is the only solution to all of their problems.

In fact, college students who commit suicide to resolve academic failure, relationship difficulties, or unemployment leave problems for others that dwarf the original concerns.

Suicide prevention

Many communities now recognize the need to provide suicide prevention services or expand services that are already available. Most suicide prevention centers operate 24-hour hotlines and are staffed through volunteer agencies, mental health centers, public health departments, or hospitals. Staff members have extensive training in the counseling skills required to deal with suicidal people. Phone numbers for these services can be found in the telephone directory.

The Star Box on p. 31 lists the signs and symptoms we should watch for that could indicate that a person might be considering suicide. People need professional help when they show a clustering of these suicide warning signs for more than 2 weeks.

Warning Signs of Suicidal Behavior
- Change in appetite
- Change in sleep pattern
- Decreased concentration
- Decreased interest in activities that were a source of pleasure
- Sudden agitation or sudden slowing down in level of activity
- Social withdrawal
- Feelings of hopelessness, worthlessness, and self-reproach
- Inappropriate or excessive guilt
- Suicidal thoughts and/or talk
- Making a suicide plan
- Writing a suicide note
- Giving away prized possessions
- Recent humiliating life event
- Lack of social support

ENHANCING EMOTIONAL WELLNESS

Most people have the opportunity to function at an enhanced level of emotional well-being. This higher level of emotional health is often achieved by improving certain skills and abilities, including improving verbal and nonverbal communication, learning to use humor effectively, developing better conflict resolution skills, and taking a proactive approach to life. In this section, each of these facets of emotional well-being are explored.

Improving Communication

Communication can be viewed in terms of your role as sender or receiver of spoken language. In regard to sending messages, it may be possible to enhance effectiveness in *verbal* communication by implementing several specific types of behavior.[12] First, you should be willing to take time before speaking to understand what needs to be said. For example, does the audience need information, encouragement, humor, or something else? In addition, try to focus on the most important thoughts and ideas, since not every thought is central to effective communication. Effective speakers also talk with, rather than at, listeners to facilitate comfortable exchanges. Further, verbal exchanges should begin on a positive note so that you can establish and maintain a positive environment with listeners. Also, by seeking frequent feedback

from listeners through the use of "minimal encouragers," such as short questions, and by avoiding slanted language, spoken communication is more constructive. Lastly, you should recognize when other forms of communication, such as written notes, do a better job in transmitting information or ideas.

Effective verbal communication also requires that you function as a skilled listener. Certainly there are skills that can enhance listening abilities, such as the ability to listen attentively to hear everything that is being said. Also, listening selectively to filter out redundant ideas or information unrelated to the central theme allows you to pay greater attention to pertinent points. This technique is often used by adults when listening to young children or when information being shared by others is grossly inaccurate or exaggerated. A final measure can be used to be an effective listener: stopping the speaker from continuing the conversation by suggesting that he or she repeat or rephrase what was previously said. This technique ensures that you are hearing correctly the points the other person is trying to make rather than focusing only on your own responses.

Your ability to strengthen *nonverbal* communication skills may also enhance emotional well-being. For a variety of reasons, it may be necessary or desirable to communicate without speaking, a process that can be accomplished in many different ways.[5] One way is by using facial expressions. For example, a smile may open lines of communication that would have remained closed in the presence of a less friendly face. Eye contact, too, is an important component of positive nonverbal communication, although staring is undesirable. Effective eye contact can actually be practiced by studying facial expressions in the mirror.

Beyond facial expressions and mannerisms, other techniques for enhancing nonverbal communication exist. Touching comfortably, maintaining an appropriate distance from people, and wearing appropriate clothing aid in the silent exchange of information between people. In fact, the overall posture of the body may contribute to your ability to "hear" what others are attempting to communicate.

Using Humor Effectively

Possessing a sense of humor is an important component of high-level emotional health.[13] This means being able to see that life is not meant to be one long, boring exercise. Part of the reason for living is to have fun. You must not, therefore, take yourself or your life situations too seriously. In fact, as seen in the Learning from All Cultures box on p. 32, humor is an important component of life in all cultures.

LEARNING from ALL CULTURES

Humor

Humor is universal. In fact, there is no known culture in which humor is not present. People everywhere enjoy the funnier moments of everyday life. Humans all use the same elements of humor: incongruity, surprise, and familiar thinking patterns. Situations, however, differ from country to country, therefore making humor somewhat cultural.[14]

A nation's humor reflects its people's lives. Sexuality is a common topic for humor in Great Britain.[14] In the United States, sexual jokes are also popular, but in China and Israel, they are almost nonexistent. Israeli humor is described as aggressive humor, humor that

perhaps reflects the instability of its people's lives because of war and discrimination. This type of humor is evident in American society as we trade jokes about various groups of people, such as jokes about gays or women with blond hair. The French also are known to enjoy aggressive humor, by playfully making fun of others.[14]

A society's history, traditions, and language influence what its people find humorous. Imagine going through life without the ability to see, appreciate, and most importantly, laugh at the incongruities and surprises of our daily existence!

Recognizing the humor in daily situations and occasionally being able to laugh at yourself will make you feel better about yourself. People feel better when they build humor into their daily lives, and others enjoy being around them more. Some researchers have suggested that recovery from an injury or illness is enhanced when patients have a positive attitude that includes a sense of humor.

Improving Conflict Management Skills

In spite of our best efforts to avoid it, conflict regularly occurs when people interact. In fact, it is the presence of conflict, and the change that arises in the course of resolving it, that leads to growth. The ability to meet and resolve conflict reflects a mature state of emotional health. However, some forms of conflict resolution are more effective than others. In the discussion that follows, different approaches to conflict resolution are considered.[15]

Many people believe that a *hostile aggressive* approach to conflict resolution, in which the parties involved attempt to use force to win out, is the least emotionally mature approach to resolving differences. For example, attacking others for simply disagreeing with them shows both hostility and aggression. Regardless of whether the weapon of choice is a loud voice or a physical blow, the outcome of this approach is usually more and deeper conflict.

Although different in character from hostile aggres-

sion, the use of *submission* is also an unacceptable technique for resolving conflict. When one person involved in the conflict gives in, the disagreement may at first appear to have been resolved, but the accommodating party generally remains angry, with the conflict merely driven temporarily out of sight and likely to reappear later in a more intense form. Ask yourself, for example, "How long would I be willing to do only what others want, rather than what I would enjoy doing, before I became angry and resentful?"

A third and somewhat emotionally immature approach to conflict resolution is *withdrawal* by one or both parties. Simply walking out of a room to avoid further disagreement with others is an example of this conflict resolution approach. This regressive form of resolution may seem to calm the atmosphere but rarely leads to a true and constructive resolution of the conflict. However, withdrawal can be constructive if it provides time for one or both people to rethink the conflict situation and return to it later, using a more constructive approach.

One of the positive conflict resolution approaches is *persuasion*. In this approach, one or both parties to the conflict use words to explain their reasons for the position they are taking. Pointing out the advantages to pursuing one course of action versus another is an example of persuasion. In the face of a convincing presentation, it is hoped that the other party involved will become motivated to resolve the conflict, most likely by accepting the position being advanced. If all parties involved in the conflict are given an opportunity to "have the floor," this approach to conflict resolution can be considered more constructive than those described previously.

Perhaps the most mature conflict resolution technique is *dialogue*. In this approach, a verbal exchange of facts, opinions, and perceptions takes place to better understand the costs or benefits associated with each of the positions being advanced. The goal of this exchange is to reach an acceptable compromise that all parties involved will feel they had a share in formulating. Of course, this form of resolution frequently characterizes the lengthy negotiations that come before the signing of accords between nations. Often when this form of resolution is used, there are no losers in the traditional sense, but rather the compromise position agreed on allows all parties to contribute to a healthier relationship.

Taking a Proactive Approach to Life

Beyond the several approaches to high-level emotional health already discussed, the plan that follows is intended to give you even greater control of enhancing your feelings of self-esteem. A key to emotional health is the ability to control the outcomes of experiences and thus to learn about your own emotional resources.[16] Figure 2-1 shows a four-step process that continues throughout life: constructing perceptions of yourself, accepting these perceptions, undertaking new experiences, and reframing your perceptions based on new information. With some thought and practice, this process can be undertaken regularly by most people.

Constructing mental pictures

Actively taking charge of emotional growth begins when you construct a mental picture of what you are like. This mental picture or perception should be composed of the most recent and accurate information you have about yourself concerning the knowledge that is important to you, the values that you hold, and the activities in which you are competent.

To construct this mental picture, you will need to set aside a period of uninterrupted quiet time for reflection. Even in the midst of a busy schedule, most people can find several moments to complete a task that is important.

Before continuing to the second step in the plan for emotional development, it is important that you construct, in addition to a mental picture about *yourself,* similar mental pictures about yourself in relation to

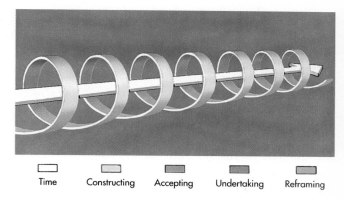

Time   Constructing   Accepting   Undertaking   Reframing

Figure 2-1   If you visualize the growth of the emotional dimension of health as a four-step process, you will see that continued emotional growth occurs in cycles throughout your life.

other people and *material objects,* including your residence and college or work environment, to gain a clearer picture of these relationships.

For example, Clara moved to a large city to become a jewelry designer after graduating from college with a degree in fine arts. Two years later, Clara's small business was thriving and she had been able to move to a spacious loft apartment in which one room served as her studio. Nevertheless, Clara felt that something was missing. She constructed a mental picture in which she saw herself as a resourceful, creative, independent person who was comfortable in her new surroundings. However, Clara realized that she wanted a partner with whom to share her success and her life.

Accepting mental pictures

The second step of the plan involves an *acceptance* of these perceptions. Acceptance implies a willingness to honor the truthfulness of the perceptions that you have formed about yourself and other people. For example, Clara should acknowledge her professional success and her artistic ability but must also accept that she has been unable to establish the long-term romantic relationship she desires.

As in the first step of the plan, the second stage requires time and commitment. Controlling emotional development is rarely a passive process. You must be willing to be *introspective* (inwardly reflective) about yourself and the world around you.

Undertaking new experiences

To mature emotionally, you must progress beyond the first two steps of the prescription and test the newly formed perceptions you have constructed. This *testing* is accomplished by *undertaking a new experience* or by reexperiencing something in a different way.

For example, I traveled to London with 31 students, and most of them took advantage of every opportunity out of class to meet new people, see new places, and have new experiences. No part of the United Kingdom (or Europe, for that matter) seemed to be beyond their reach. Over the course of our 15 weeks together, I could see them become more confident and self-assured as the result of being independent and self-directed in taking risks. In retrospect, I realize that no combination of reading assignments, guest lectures, and field trips could have produced the emotionally fulfilling maturation that was accomplished away from our university's London Centre.

New experiences do not necessarily require high levels of risk, foreign travel, or money. They may be no more "new" than deciding to move from the dorm into an apartment, to change from one shift at work to another, or to pursue new friendships. The experience itself is not the end that you should be seeking; rather, it is a means of collecting a new "pool" of information about yourself, others, and the objects that form your material world.

For instance, Clara volunteered to teach art therapy classes to chronically ill patients at a local hospital. This work was enjoyable and fulfilling for Clara, and she formed friendships with a few of the other hospital volunteers. Clara also met and began dating Marcel, a staff physical therapist.

Reframing mental pictures

When you have completed the first three steps in the plan for achieving emotional growth, the new information about yourself, others, and objects

Completing an internship in a career field that interests you could be a challenging new experience.

becomes the most current source of information available. Regardless of the type of new experience you have undertaken and its outcome, you are now in a position to modify the initial perceptions that were constructed during the first step of the plan. Once completed, you have new insights, knowledge, and perspectives.

Clara, whom we described previously, reframed her mental pictures in light of the changes that had taken place in her life. Her volunteer work gave her a new appreciation for art, and she discovered depths of caring in herself that she had not known existed. In addition, she now saw herself as part of a circle of friends and as a partner in a long-term relationship with Marcel. With her proactive approach to life, Clara had created challenges for herself from which she changed and grew.

The Star Box on p. 35 provides suggestions for fostering emotional growth and thus enhancing emotional well-being. Opportunities to participate in these activities exist on or near most college campuses.

REFLECTIONS OF EMOTIONAL WELLNESS

What characterizes people who have most fully developed their emotional wellness? In the discussion that follows, we suggest three areas in which emotional healthfulness can be evident to the observer. These include movement toward fulfilling the highest level of need as defined by Maslow, development of a mature level of faith, and expression of creativity in the context of a world that often restricts creative expression.

Maslow's Hierarchy of Needs

One of the most familiar constructs in the field of developmental psychology is Abraham Maslow's model of need fulfillment. Maslow views emotional growth in terms of inner needs and motivation. He lists motivational requirements in the following order: physiological needs, safety needs, belonging and love needs, esteem needs, and **self-actualization** needs (Figure 2-2).[17] Maslow distinguishes between the lower *deficiency needs* and the higher *being needs*. People do not seek the higher needs until the lower demands have been reasonably satisfied. Accordingly, people who are hungry, feel unsafe, or have few friends will be highly unlikely to have high self-esteem until their lower needs have been met.

Fostering Your Emotional Growth

Emotional growth requires both knowing about yourself and learning from new experiences. The activities listed below can be used in support of these requirements.

- Keep a daily journal. Writing down your thoughts and making note of experiences are effective tools in fostering greater self-understanding. Once written, the information that these accounts contain can be reprocessed for an even greater awareness of self.
- Join a support group. Sharing experiences and feelings in the presence of people who can "stand in your shoes" creates an environment that will support your efforts to grow as a more interesting and self-directed person. Additionally, being an active participant in a support group also functions as a "new experience" through which new insights into your sense of self-worth can be gained.
- Take an assertiveness course. Learning how to greet others, give and receive compliments, use "I" statements, express spontaneity, and state your feelings of disagreement are important tools in developing self-confidence. Very likely, an assertiveness course is or will be offered on your campus.
- Seek counseling. Nowhere is counseling generally more available and affordable than on a college campus. Clearly, much can be learned about your sense of self and the psychological factors that have shaped it. Furthermore, growth-enhancing skills can be formulated and tested in both individual and group counseling sessions. Contact the campus health center or the psychological services center for referral to an experienced psychologist or counselor.

What additional activities can you think of that would further your self-knowledge or serve as new experiences?

The healthiest and most effective people in society are those whose lives embody *being values* such as truth, beauty, goodness, faith, wholeness, and love. Maslow labels these as "Theory Z" people, or **transcenders.** Self-actualization, the highest level of self-development, is clearly evident in the personality of the transcender. Transcenders are described as follows[17]:

- Transcenders have more peak or creative experiences and naturally speak the language of being values.

- Transcenders are more responsive to beauty, are more holistic in their perceptions of humanity and the cosmos, adjust well to conflict situations, and work more wholeheartedly toward goals and purposes.
- Transcenders are innovators who are attracted to mystery and the unknown and see themselves as people who live according to transcendent values, such as unconditional acceptance, love, honesty, and forgiveness.
- Transcenders tend to fuse work and play. They are less attracted by the rewards of money and objects and more motivated by the satisfaction of being and service values.
- Transcenders are more likely to accept others with an unconditional positive regard, and they tend to be more oriented toward spiritual reality.

Most people will notice the similarity between transcenders and people with positive self-esteem. In following the Health Action Guide to improve self-esteem, you may also find yourself fulfilling Maslow's higher needs.

Spiritual or Faith Development

A fully developed sense of self-esteem most likely requires that you be knowledgeable and accepting of yourself as a person of **faith.** Certainly, many older adults have little difficulty sharing that they believe in something, such as the universal truths of beauty, honesty, and love, or someone greater than themselves and that this belief brings them great comfort and a sense of support. Many report that because of their personal level of faith, they do not fear death because they

---

self-actualization
The highest level of personality development; self-actualized people recognize their roles in life and use personal strengths to reach their fullest potential.

transcenders
Self-actualized people who have achieved a quality of being ordinarily associated with higher levels of spiritual growth.

faith
The purposes and meaning that underlie an individual's hopes and dreams.

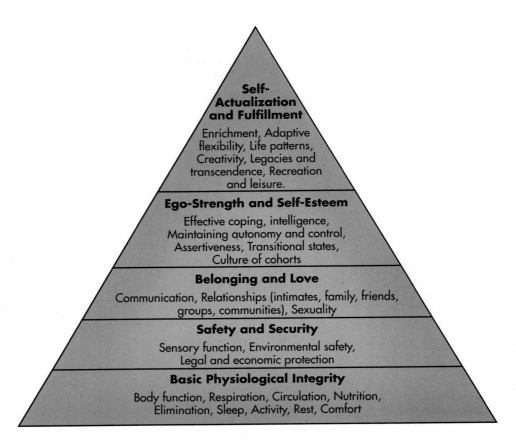

Figure 2-2   Maslow's hierarchy of needs.

know that their lives have had meaning within the context of their deeply held beliefs. Further, they would urge younger people to search for both the strength and direction in their lives that faith provides.[18]

As a resource in the spiritual dimension of health, the existence of faith provides a basis on which a belief system can mature and an expanding awareness of life's meaning can be fostered. In addition, the existence of faith gives meaning (or additional meaning) to your vocation and assists you in better understanding the consequences of your vocational efforts. For example, a college student might choose to major in education instead of marketing because he or she would find greater spiritual fulfillment in teaching than in business. Further, faith in something (or someone) influences many of the experiences that you will seek throughout life and tempers the emotional relationships that you have with these experiences.[19] The questions posed in the Star Box on p. 37 will help you consider how your faith affects your own life. The topic of spirituality is considered further in the Focus Box on p. 40.

In nearly all cultures, faith and its accompanying belief system provide individuals and groups with rituals and practices that foster a sense of community— "a community of faith." In turn, the community provides the authority and guidance that nurture the emotional stability, confidence, and sense of competence needed for living life fully.[18]

Creative Expression

Emotionally healthy individuals have a free and open approach to life. They think and act positively. They also assess people and situations realistically and constructively. When interacting with emotionally healthy people, others quickly notice their flexibility in solving problems. How did these people become so secure, competent, and constructive? Is it possible that most people will mature in this direction? What resources will you need to grow in a similar fashion?

Assuming that **creativity** is closely related to emotional health, these traits might help describe emotionally healthy people:

- Creative people are intuitive and open to new experiences. They are relatively free from fear

How Does My Faith Affect My Life?

James Fowler[14] describes the nature of faith as a fundamental, universal, but infinitely varied value response within the human experience. Faith can include religious practice but also can be quite distinct. Faith is the most fundamental category in the human quest for the meaning of life. It is a developing focus of the total person that gives purpose and meaning to thoughts.

By the time people reach college age, it is possible that the maturation of their faith has placed them into a series of uncomfortable situations. These include the need to take seriously the burden of responsibility for their own commitments, lifestyles, beliefs, and attitudes. Tension and anxiety can arise because the growth of faith requires them to make personal decisions. It demands objectivity and a certain amount of independence and requires finding a balance between personal aspirations and a developing sense of service to others. Finally, symbols and doctrines must be translated into personalized spiritual concepts that can then be validated on the basis of experience.

- In light of the potential for young adults to grow in their faith, what have been your own experiences?
- Would you consider yourself to be more or less "faithful" than your friends or other family members?
- What school-related experiences have affected most powerfully the spiritual dimension of your health?

Creative expression can occur in a variety of forms.

and are not disturbed by the unknown, the mysterious, or the puzzling.

- Creative people are less interested in detail than in meaning and implications. They tend to be more theoretical than practical in their orientation.
- Creative people are independent, self-accepting, and nonauthoritarian in their attitudes. They tend to resist group work and function best when allowed to work independently.
- Creative people are flexible. They do not use all-or-none thinking but recognize that there are many ways to interpret the same situation.
- Creative people have an internal set of values and are always working toward goals.

Some people may recognize many of these characteristics as being already well developed in their own personalities. Or they may not yet possess some of the traits listed, and these may now appear beyond their reach. Nevertheless, having a high level of health will increase their creativity by giving them the resources to face new challenges.

creativity
Innovative ability; insightful capacity to solve problems; ability to move beyond analytical or logical approaches to experiences.

Summary

- Emotionally well people feel comfortable about themselves and other people and are able to meet the demands of life.
- Emotional wellness refers specifically to one's feelings in response to change, whereas psychological wellness refers more broadly to the adequate development and proper functioning of mental abilities.
- Emotions are not always constant; people experience a normal range of emotions.
- A sense of self-esteem may be the essence of emotional and mental maturity.
- Hardiness reflects the existence of confidence and commitment and an ability to build on challenge.
- Depression can be recognized by the presence of characteristic symptoms.
- Loneliness results from the absence of adequate human contact.
- Shyness may be a basic component of temperament, yet social skills counseling can help shy people learn to interact more comfortably with others.
- Suicide represents an extreme and ineffective attempt to cope with life-centered problems.
- Effective verbal and nonverbal communication skills can be learned and will enhance emotional well-being.
- Humor can contribute to emotional health and well-being.
- Conflict management skills can include a variety of approaches, some of which are more effective than others.
- A four-step plan can be used to foster greater emotional growth and enhanced emotional wellness.
- The ability to meet basic human needs establishes a basis for pursuing higher emotional needs.
- People who possess a mature faith recognize the existence of guiding values in their lives and live within a community of faith.
- Creative people possess a positive outlook and take a unique approach to life and living.

Review Questions

1. What are the characteristics of an emotionally healthy person?
2. How is psychological health related to but different from emotional health?
3. What is meant by the "normal range of emotions"?
4. Define self-esteem. List strategies that can be used to improve self-esteem.
5. What are three characteristics of hardy people?
6. What is depression, and what are the behavioral patterns of depressed people? How do primary and secondary depression differ?
7. What is the important component missing in the lives of those who are lonely? What skills can be learned by lonely people that might be effective in easing their sense of loneliness?
8. On the basis of current understanding, what is the most likely origin of shyness?
9. What behavior characteristics indicate a suicidal tendency? How should someone who observes these traits in another person respond?
10. What are several characteristics of effective verbal communication?
11. What nonverbal cues encourage positive communication? What nonverbal cues detract from positive interpersonal communication?
12. What message is given to others by those who allow humor to be a part of their social interaction?
13. Which techniques are the more effective approaches to conflict management? Which are less effective?
14. Identify and explain the four components of the cyclic process that will help you enhance your emotional growth.
15. In what order are human needs encountered as one moves toward self-actualization?
16. What aspects of life are brought into focus as the spiritual dimension of health matures?
17. List several characteristics of creative people.

⚙ Think About This . . .

- How close do you come to meeting the characteristics of a mentally healthy person?
- Are you ready to undertake a new experience? What kind of experience will it be?

- Do you take yourself too seriously at times?
- Which traits of creativity have you developed?

References

1. McGinnis J, Lee P: Healthy People 2000 at mid decade, *JAMA* 73(14):1123-1129, 1995.
2. National Mental Health Association: *Mental health 1-2-3,* Alexandria, Va, 1992, The Association.
3. Robson P: Improving self-esteem, *Harvard Medical School Mental Health Letter* 6(12):3, 1990.
4. Kobasa S: Stressful life events, personality, and health: an inquiry into hardiness, *J Pers Soc Psychol* 37:1-11, 1979.
5. Haas A, Haas K: *Understanding sexuality,* ed 3, St Louis, 1993, Mosby.
6. *Mosby's medical, nursing, and allied health dictionary,* ed 4, St Louis, 1994, Mosby.
7. Johnson D, Weissman M, Klerman GL: Service utilization and social morbidity associated with depressive symptoms in the community, *JAMA* 267(11):1478, 1992.
8. Wells LA: *Psychiatric nursing,* St Louis, 1989, Warren H Green.
9. Ray O, Ksir C: *Drugs, society, & human behavior,* ed 7, St Louis, 1996, Mosby.
10. Baron RA, Byrne D: *Social psychology: understanding human interaction,* ed 6, Boston, 1991, Allyn & Bacon.
11. *Statistical abstract of the United States 1994,* ed 114, Washington, DC, 1994, US Department of Commerce, Bureau of the Census.
12. Masters W, Johnson V, Kolodny R: *Human sexuality,* ed 5, New York, 1995, HarperCollins.
13. Rose JF: Psychologic health of women: a phenomenologic study of women's inner strength, *Ad Nurs Sci* 12(2):56, 1990.
14. Ziv A, editor: *National styles of humor,* New York, 1988, Greenwood Press.
15. Tannen D: *That's not what I mean: how conversational style makes or breaks relationships,* New York, 1986, Ballantine.
16. Sprunger MJ: Personal communication, June 1995.
17. Maslow AH: *The farthest reaches of human nature,* Magnolia Mass, 1983, Peter Smith.
18. Hemenway JE, editor: *Assessing spiritual needs: a guide for care-givers,* Minneapolis, Minn, 1993, Augsburg Fortress.
19. Fowler J: *Faith development and pastoral care,* Philadelphia, 1987, Fortress Press.

Suggested Readings

Dowling C: *You mean I don't have to feel this way? New help for depression, anxiety, and addiction,* New York, 1992, Scribner.
This book supports a biological basis for many of the dysfunctions that occur today. Treatments appropriate for depression, eating disorders, and anxiety are discussed. The author believes that most people need professional assistance in dealing with their dysfunctional behavior.

Kinder M: *Going nowhere fast: step off life's treadmill and find peace of mind,* New York, 1990, Prentice Hall.
As a clinical psychologist, the author believes that our struggles to be "perfect" have put many of us on a dangerous treadmill that makes an enjoyable life virtually unattainable. Real peace of mind comes from our understanding of our inner selves. The author states that it is up to us to change ourselves.

Yapko MD: *Free yourself from depression,* Emmaus, Penn, 1992, Rodale Press.
The author, a psychologist and hypnotist, prescribes a variety of techniques for overcoming mild depressive symptoms. The book is specific in its direction, including the use of traditional therapies, medication, and self-help techniques. Information on the three principal causes of depression is also provided.

Fancher RT: *Cultures of healing: correcting the image of American mental health care,* New York, 1995, WH Freeman.
This is one of a series of recent books written by mental health professionals who are critical of the profession's use of *DSM (Diagnostic and statistical manual of mental disorders)* in labeling patients. The author sees misuse as a part of professional infighting regarding the effectiveness of various treatment approaches.

Kipfer BA: *14,000 things to be happy about,* New York, 1995, Workman.
This book is intended for reading on the "rainy days" oflife. The author presents in list format a wide array of frivolous things that bring happiness into her life, such as Coca-Cola commercials, cream cheese potatoes, green Jell-O, and, of course, puffed heart pendants.

Enhancing Spirituality and Wellness

Often our thoughts on the subject of health are confined to the scientific. Indeed, much of the study of health is involved with exploring topics in physical and emotional health from a practical point of view, with conclusions based on sound medical research. But are there other aspects to health and wellness that are not grounded in science? Some health care professionals are now beginning to embrace the concept that a person's spirituality may be an important factor in maintaining both emotional and physical health.[1,2]

Ways to Improve Spiritual Well-Being

The idea of "emotional wellness" may mean different things to different people. A person's emotional well-being can be affected by several components, including family, friends, finances, and occupation. For example, a person employed as a health care worker may gain a high degree of spiritual satisfaction from working. The same person may not be as spiritually fulfilled if he or she were a collections agent. Although a complete career change may not be possible in many cases, there are other things a person can do to increase spiritual well-being.

One simple way to achieve better spiritual health is to find a way to feel better about yourself. Helping others in need through volunteer work is one way to do that. Voluntarism is becoming more popular in the United States.[3] Besides the obvious benefits to the people being helped, the volunteer can also benefit. Charity work can boost self-confidence and make you feel good about what you are doing.[4] If you want to travel, some types of volunteer work can take you to other parts of the country (or even to other nations) and can help broaden your knowledge of other peoples. There are many opportunities close to home as well for those who cannot afford to travel or do not want to be away from home. Many community and neighborhood organizations offer opportunities for volunteer work,[3] and some businesses offer incentives for employees who perform community service.[4] If you cannot volunteer time, giving material goods or money can also help you feel better about your contribution to society. Providing toys, clothes, or used tools or furniture for those who need them can boost your sense of spiritual well-being.[5]

Teens and college students can also benefit by volunteering in a field related to their career interests.[3] Such work can improve skills, provide work experience, and increase the chances of obtaining a job in that field in the future. Such work also allows students to explore career fields they are interested in to determine which positions may be best for a future job. Families who volunteer as a unit can enjoy the benefits of helping others while spending quality time together.[5] Such work can bring families closer together. Children can learn about working with other people and gain an understanding about the community, and teaching kids early about the moral values associated with helping others may make them more likely to continue to volunteer as they grow older.[5]

If volunteer work doesn't interest you, other activities can also help improve your spiritual health. Taking time to do things you enjoy can make your outlook on life more positive. Take up a new hobby, spend more time with your family, listen to music, exercise, or do something that makes you happy. Although most recreational activities do not seem to fall under the classic definition spirituality, they can improve your emotional well-being by taking your mind off of stressful things in your life.

Religion and Mental Health

The traditional view of "spirituality" involves a person's religious or spiritual beliefs. Such beliefs can be very important in maintaining wellness. In recent years, churches and synagogues have experienced an increase in attendance, reflecting an upsurge in spiritual awareness in America. Money, education, and success might not have provided meaning to people's lives, so some are turning to religion to fill this void.[6] Congregating with people who have similar beliefs and values provides an outlet for sharing spiritual experiences and can make religion more meaningful. Many modern worshipers (especially those who are younger) tend to be very selective about where they attend, however. Often, people will try out several places of worship before settling on one they like. This suggests that people are looking for specific benefits from their place of worship, perhaps to make the experience more meaningful.

Spirituality may play a stronger role in people's health as they become older. Studies have shown that older people are in general more religious than younger people and that belief in God increases with age.[2] Some 50% of adults age 65 and older attend church on a regular basis.[2] Religion and the belief that there is something better than life on Earth may help older people cope with the various afflictions that come with the aging process. Spiritual beliefs may help people adapt to the stress that occurs as they grow older.[2] Spirituality may also help with mental disorders. Religion has been shown to fight the effects of depression. Several studies have suggested that there is an inverse relationship between religious coping and depression.[2] The better a person is able to use religion to cope with life's problems, the less likely he or she is to become depressed.

A person's spiritual well-being can be enhanced without embracing traditional Western religion. Mind-body disciplines, many of which are based in Far Eastern religions, have gained in popularity in the United States.[7] Mind-body disciplines such as yoga or t'ai chi require focused breathing in coordination with controlled body movements. Performing such activities calms the mind and boosts the spirit while toning and strengthening the muscles.[7] Meditation is a component of many of these disciplines, and it may be advantageous to combine meditation with exercise, since some people may not have the discipline to just sit and meditate.[7] Those who use mind-body disciplines regularly say that the exercise and meditation help them tap into unconscious issues and treat emotional or physical injuries.[7]

New age spirituality is also gaining a following. New age spirituality takes on many forms. Among the disciplines included in the new age category are yoga, meditation, and visualization. Other new age activities include the use of psychics, astrology, tarot cards, and crystals.[6] Most mainstream religious groups generally do not approve of such activities. They claim that many of the benefits touted by new age promoters, such as meditation, ordering of daily life, and group care of souls, are already present in traditional religion.[8] Nevertheless, new age publishing and retailing brings in $1 billion a year in sales, and $45 billion is spent yearly on self-development.[6]

The Changing Role of Spirituality in Health Care

If spirituality can play a positive role in emotional wellness, it follows that a person's physical health may benefit from spirituality also. The spiritual aspects of health and well-being have not been studied very extensively, but in recent years more people involved in medicine have been willing to embrace the idea that spirituality can have an effect on physical health. Traditionally, physicians have been unable or unwilling to pay attention to spiritual needs of patients, possibly because some doctors feared being labeled as "quacks" if they pushed the idea of holistic healing too much.[1] Others worried that patients might deny their illnesses.[1] Patients might concentrate solely on holistic methods for healing and ignore conventional medicine, therapy, and methods. And though statistics show that most Americans believe in a supreme being,[2] this may not be the case with certain

groups within the medical community. An American Psychiatric Association survey of psychiatrists showed that only 43% believed in God, and only 1.5% to 2.5% of published studies in four major psychiatric journals had a religious commitment.[2] But there is a growing belief among medical professionals that spirituality, in conjunction with conventional medicine, may help patients with the healing process.

There may be a connection between prayer and healing, and religion may help people cope with ailments. Spirituality has been cited as a positive force in the healing process, and religious beliefs may account for certain cases of spontaneous disease remission. Many patients ask for prayer as a component of their healing regimen, and more doctors of late have been willing to comply with their patients' wishes. The holistic health movement is increasing in popularity among physicians and patients alike.[1] There is some feeling in the medical community that physicians should consider and respect the religious and spiritual beliefs of patients. The American Psychological Association's *Diagnostic and Statistical Manual of Mental Disorders* now includes an entry for "Religious/Spiritual Problem," which may represent an acknowledgement from some medical professionals that faith can play a role in a person's health.[1]

There may be some advantages to looking at the person as a whole rather than as distinct parts. Although conventional exercise and medicine certainly help improve overall physical health, perhaps a spiritual component to healing should be considered as well. In some cases at least, physicians should be open to the idea that a patient's spirituality can be used as an important medical tool.

Thousands of volunteers used sandbags to shore up levees along the Mississippi River and its tributaries during the Great Flood of '93.

For Discussion . . .

In your personal experience, has your spirituality had an effect on your overall wellness? Does getting involved with a group project enhance your spirituality? Have you tried unorthodox methods of spirituality? Do you think that cases of "miracle cures" (spontaneous remission of disease) may be explained through religious or spiritual beliefs?

References

1. Martinez D: Rx: prayer—health care gets a dose of spirituality, *National Catholic Reporter* 30(24), 1994.
2. Marwick C: Should physicians prescribe prayer for health? *JAMA* 273(20), 1993.
3. Taibbi R: Teens who help, *Current Health 2* 21(3), 1994.
4. Caring in the community, *Management Today*, March 1995.
5. Friedman J: Family values, *MPLS-St. Paul Magazine* 21(12), 1993.
6. McDonald M: The new spirituality: mainstream N. America is on a massive search for meaning in life, *Maclean's* 107(41), Oct 10, 1994.
7. Hulet D: Mind over matter (return of spirituality), *Los Angeles Magazine*, 40(1), 1995.
8. Oder T C: Blinded by the 'lite': dying modernity is "into" spirituality, *Christianity Today* 38(10), 1994.

3

Managing Stress

Healthy People 2000 Objectives

An initial objective of the Healthy People 2000 report was to reduce the proportion of people with stress-related health conditions. At mid-decade, progress has unquestionably been made and is perhaps related to the fulfillment of a second objective: the development of worksite stress-management programs. The goal of increasing by 40% the number of employment sites (with 50 or more employees) at which stress management services are offered has almost been met.

Nevertheless, the mental health community has lost ground in its attempt to reduce the proportion of people who are experiencing stress but do not take steps to manage it. The reasons for this disappointing finding are unclear. Some of these people may be unable to practice the prevention strategies taught by the growing number of stress management programs, or they may not have access to such programs and thus lack coping skills.

Stress significantly influences the development of illnesses such as cancer, cardiovascular disease, and eating disorders. Being unable to control stress effectively is also linked to an increased incidence of violence. On the other hand, learning and practicing stress management skills promotes wellness. Our society must improve access to stress management services and find better ways to help people implement stress reduction techniques if we are to meet the Healthy People 2000 objectives in this area.

Change influences daily living. Each person, institution, and situation in a person's environment holds the potential for change, some of which may be seen as threatening. Being able to control or adjust to this change is often challenging, stimulating, and rewarding, which contributes to a sense of well-being.

When people handle change poorly, however, their responses result in stress that can be disruptive to their health and unpleasant to experience.

STRESS AND STRESSORS

Almost every day on a college campus, people can be heard commenting about how much **stress** they are under. Certainly, for both traditional and nontraditional college students, the demands of school, work, marriage, and parenting can produce feelings of distress that detract from wellness.

Although we have all experienced stress, we may have questions about what it is. Hans Selye, the originator of stress theory, described stress as "the nonspecific response of the body to any demand made on it."[1] Stress can be viewed as a physical and emotional response that occurs when people are exposed to change. The events that produce stress are called **stressors.** Stressors always come before stress. Stressors are the cause; stress is the effect.

Variation in Response to Stressors

Because individuals are unique, a stressor for one person might not be a stressor for another. For example, if the bookstore is out of a textbook or if a babysitter must be found because the local public schools are closed for a teachers' in-service day, some people are more *distressed* than others. This variation results from the unique information that each person applies in making decisions about the seriousness of the situation.[2]

Positive or negative stressors

Stressors produce the same generalized physical response whether an individual views the stressor as good or bad. Poor academic performance, loss of a friend, or being the only minority student on the dorm floor can cause stress, just as giving birth, receiving a promotion, or starting a passionate romance can be stressors. In each case, the effect on the body's physical systems is relatively similar.

Selye coined the word **eustress** for positive stress. Stressors that produce eustress can enhance longevity, productivity, and life satisfaction. Examples include the mild stress that helps you stay alert during a midterm examination, the anticipation felt on the first day of a new job, and the exhilarating stress you feel while exercising. In fact, some suggest that a personality type, type R (risk takers), may "require" the regular occurrence of high-risk activities.[3] Activities such as sky diving, roller coaster riding, and white-water rafting are undertaken frequently by those with type R personalities to generate an adrenaline rush (see p. 50) and thus a sense of well-being. These people in particular demonstrate a strong sense of confidence, self-effectiveness, courage, creativity, and optimism that they use to *plan to be stressed.*

Selye calls harmful, unpleasant stress **distress.** Distress that is not controlled can result in physical and emotional disruption, illness, and even death.[4] Examples of distress are chronic pain, lack of meaningful relationships, physical confrontation, and anxiety and depression. For some, when distress becomes overwhelming, thoughts of suicide may occur (see p. 30, Chapter 2).

Uncontrolled Stress Related to Disease States

If the effect of a stressor is not minimized or resolved, the human body becomes exhausted, producing emotional and physical breakdown. Depending on the strength of the stressor and the resistance of the person, this breakdown may occur quickly or over many years.

Clearly, the effects of unresolved stress can build up until the body begins to break down. This breakdown leads to stress-related diseases and disorders. Among the major diseases that have some origin in unresolved stress are hypertension, stroke, heart disease, kidney disease, depression, alcoholism, and gastrointestinal disorders (including ulcers, irritable bowel syndrome, and diverticulitis).[5] Other stress-

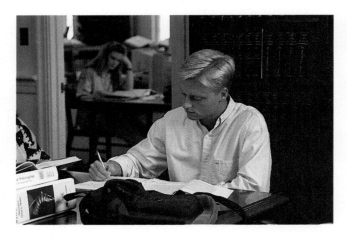

College life presents many stressors.

PERSONAL ASSESSMENT

Life Stressors

Which of the following events have you experienced in the past 12 months?

Life event	Point value
_____ Death of a close family member	100
_____ Jail term	80
_____ Final year or first year in college	63
_____ Pregnancy (yours or your partner's)	60
_____ Serious illness or injury	53
_____ Marriage	50
_____ Any interpersonal problems	45
_____ Financial difficulties	40
_____ Death of a close friend	40
_____ Arguments with your roommate (more than every other day)	40
_____ Major disagreements with your family	40
_____ Major change in personal habits	30
_____ Change in living environment	30
_____ Beginning or ending a job	30
_____ Problems with your boss or professor	25
_____ Outstanding personal achievement	25
_____ Failure in a course	25
_____ Final examinations	20
_____ Increased or decreased amount of dating	20
_____ Change in working conditions	20
_____ Change in your major	20
_____ Change in your sleeping habits	18
_____ Vacation of several days	15
_____ Change in eating habits	15
_____ Family reunion	15
_____ Change in recreational activities	15
_____ Minor illness or injury	15
_____ Minor violations of the law	11

SCORE: _____

Interpretation

Life events can function as stressors that influence the body through activation of the stress response. An accumulation of 150 or more points (see point ranges below) in a 1-year period may lead to increased physical illness during the coming year. Of course, you must remember that, for a given person, certain events may be more or less stressful than the point values indicated.

Less than 100: limited likelihood of stress-related illness

101 to 200: moderate likelihood of stress-related illness

201 or above: high likelihood of stress-related illness

To carry this further . . .

Having completed this Personal Assessment and evaluated your responses based on the interpretation, were you surprised by the number of stress points that you generated? Are there stressors listed that you have not encountered either in your own experiences or in those of your close friends?

related disorders are migraine headaches, allergies, asthma, hay fever, anxiety, insomnia, impotence, and menstrual irregularities. The dependency-related behaviors of cigarette smoking, overeating and undereating, and underactivity relate in part to unresolved stress. Even the immune system, which protects the body from infections and cancer, may be weakened by stress.[6] Completing the Personal Assessment above will help you determine your risk for stress-related illness.

COLLEGE–CENTERED STRESSORS

For some people who have not attempted college course work, the idea that college life could be stressful must seem strange. After all, even for nontraditional students, isn't college the good life?

stress
The physiological and psychological state of disruption caused by the presence of an unanticipated, disruptive, or stimulating event.

stressors
Factors or events, real or imagined, that elicit a state of stress.

eustress (**yoo** stress)
Stress that enhances the quality of life.

distress
Stress that diminishes the quality of life; commonly associated with disease, illness, and maladaptation.

PERSONAL ASSESSMENT

How Vulnerable Are You to Stress?

A wide variety of situations can function as stressors that influence us physically and psychologically. This assessment will help you to identify situations that could be stressful and to determine your overall vulnerability to stress. Use the following scoring system for each situation listed.

1 = Always (yes)
2 = Almost always
3 = Most of the time
4 = Some of the time
5 = Never (no)

Situation	Score
I get the appropriate amount of sleep my body needs to function.	
I exercise to the point of perspiring at least twice a week.	
I do not smoke, or I smoke less than half a pack of cigarettes a day.	
I regularly attend club or social activities.	
I have one or more friends to confide in about personal matters.	
I am able to vent my feelings when angry or worried.	
I am able to organize my time effectively.	
I drink fewer than three cups of coffee (or tea or cola drinks) a day.	
I take quiet time for myself during the day.	
I do not procrastinate; I get things done right away.	

Before a test, I go to bed at the same time I normally would.	
I live at home (with my family or spouse) while attending school.	
I try not to let other people's problems become my own.	
(If sexually active) I practice safe sex.	
The people closest to me are supportive of my goals.	
I have money to meet recreational expenses.	
I am attending college by choice.	
I rarely compare myself with my friends.	
I do not hold a job and go to school full time.	
My grade point average goal is set only for personal satisfaction.	
I do not plan to go on to higher levels of education.	

Scoring
Your Total Points _____ − 20 = _____ Final Score

Interpretation
30-49   Points = Vulnerable to stress
50-75   Points = Seriously vulnerable to stress
76-105   Points = Extremely vulnerable to stress

To carry this further . . .
Having completed this Personal Assessment and the interpretation based on your responses, is the "stress status" indicated by your score compatible with your feelings regarding your vulnerability to stress? Have you identified the specific types of behavior that need alteration to reduce your level of vulnerability to stress?

However, for those who study or teach on college campuses, these perceptions are hard to understand. They know all too well that the undergraduate experience is serious because of its role in preparation for life. For the part-time, nontraditional student who comes to campus for course work (often at night) and then returns to work, family, and community responsibilities, college classes can be especially stressful. Complete the Personal Assessment above to determine your level of vulnerability to stress.

In college and university settings, stressors could arise from a variety of areas, including the following:

- School policies that seem to make going to school too complicated, such as the inconvenient scheduling of classes and the restrictions on parking
- Expectations of faculty regarding various course requirements, such as attendance, out-of-class participation, and the type of examinations given by a particular instructor (see the Health Action Guide on p. 47)
- Difficulty in qualifying for loans or other forms of financial assistance, and, of course, the need to work to afford school
- Personal goals that become unachievable, including making an athletic team, earning a desired grade point average, or graduating with honors

HEALTH
Action Guide - - - - →

Coping With Test Anxiety

Examinations have been a major part of student life for decades and will likely continue to be so. Consequently, many students develop an incapacitating anxiety when preparing to take tests. Compare your current test preparation activities with the approach recommended by experts, described below.

- Find a location conducive to study.
- Set a formal schedule for your test preparation.
- Keep complete resources, including class notes, background reading material, and reference texts, available.
- Create learning aids to help you, such as review questions, illustrations, outlines, definitions of technical terms, and sample test items.
- Be your own best friend by going to class, taking notes, joining and contributing to an ongoing study group, asking questions in class, and making appointments to visit your professor to clarify material.
- Be kind to yourself by getting an adequate amount of sleep, eating balanced meals, exercising, taking time to be reflective, and staying sober.

On the basis of your comparisons, do you have any greater insight as to why you might be anxious about examinations? How do your study habits compare? Remember, most colleges and universities have counseling centers that can help you with study skills and test anxiety. ◄ - - - - -

- Uncertainties about previously held beliefs, including those related to religion, sexual abstinence, and politics
- Interpersonal relationships and decisions regarding interracial or interfaith dating, changing roommates, and, perhaps, being older than classmates
- Availability of a job or acceptance into graduate or professional school, and, or course, the rapid approach of "real world" responsibilities
- Family expectations concerning whether school is being taken seriously enough, friends will be made, or money will be used wisely

Education in a college or university setting is never passive. It nearly always demands active participation and effort and at times may demand more than you

Interpersonal relationships can be a source of stress.

believe you are capable of giving. Not surprisingly, it is frequently the source of many stressors.

Beyond the college setting, day-to-day living presents stressors that must be confronted and resolved. Although these stressors differ from those associated with college, these life-centered stressors hold the same potential for causing physical and emotional distress and challenges to well-being. Read the Focus Box on p. 60 for advice on coping with stress in the workplace.

GENERALIZED PHYSIOLOGICAL RESPONSE TO STRESSORS

Once under the influence of a stressor, people's bodies respond in remarkably similar, predictable ways. For example, on being asked to stand up in front of a group and talk, a person's heart rate increases, throat becomes dry, palms sweat, and he or she feels dizzy or lightheaded. The person may even become nauseated. Similar feelings would be felt if a person were told that she had lost her job or that her spouse wanted a divorce. It is clear that different stressors are able to elicit these common physical reactions.

Selye described the typical physical response to a stressor in his **general adaptation syndrome** model.

general adaptation syndrome
A sequenced physiological response to the presence of a stressor; the alarm, resistance, recovery, and exhaustion stages of the stress response.

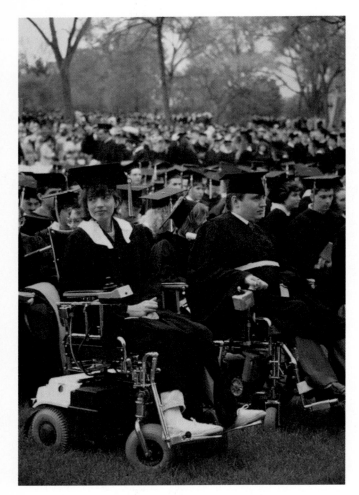

Graduation marks a transition from familiar stressors to new ones.

Selye stated that the human body moves through three stages when confronted by stressors, as explained below.

Alarm Reaction Stage

Once exposed to any event that is seen as threatening, the body immediately prepares for difficulty. The involuntary changes described in Figure 3-1 are controlled by hormonal and nervous system functions and quickly prepare the body for the **fight-or-flight response**.[7]

Resistance Stage

The second stage of response to a stressor, the resistance stage, reflects the body's attempt to reestablish internal balance, or a state of *homeostasis*. The high level of energy seen in the initial alarm stage cannot be maintained very long. The body therefore attempts to reduce the intensity of the initial response to a more manageable level. This is accomplished by reducing the production of adrenocorticotropic hormone (ACTH) (see p. xxx), thus allowing *specificity of adaptation* to occur. Specific organ systems become the focus of the body's re-sponse, such as the cardiovascular and digestive systems.[8]

Because of the ability to move from an alarm stage into a less damaging resistance stage, effective coping or a change in the status of the stressor will probably occur. In fact, as control over the stressful situation is gained, homeostasis is even more completely established and movement toward full recovery is seen. At the completion of the *recovery stage*, the body has returned to its prestressed state and there is minimal evidence of the stressor's existence.

Exhaustion Stage

Body adjustments required as a result of long-term exposure to a stressor often result in an overload. Specific organs and body systems that were called on during the resistance stage may not be able to resist a stressor indefinitely. Exhaustion results, and the stress-producing hormone levels again rise. In extreme or chronic cases, exhaustion can become so pronounced that death can occur.

THE STRESS RESPONSE

Why could something as familiar as a telephone ringing late at night cause a person to feel fear and near-panic? Why is it that the hands sweat, muscles tense, and the appetite leaves as you wait in the hallway outside the classroom in which your final examination is to be held? Is the "cotton-mouth" feeling described by athletes a valuable aid to performance? These answers are simple and based on the body's primitive interpretation of reality. The body is looking for energy because it believes that all change is threatening and can be confronted by running, fighting, scaring the "adversary" away, or engaging it in sexual activity (the flight, fight, fright, or folly response). For these responses, the body simply needs energy for physical activity. In the sections that follow, Figure 3-1 will be explained.

Stressors

For a state of stress to exist, a person must first be confronted by change, real or imagined. Any change

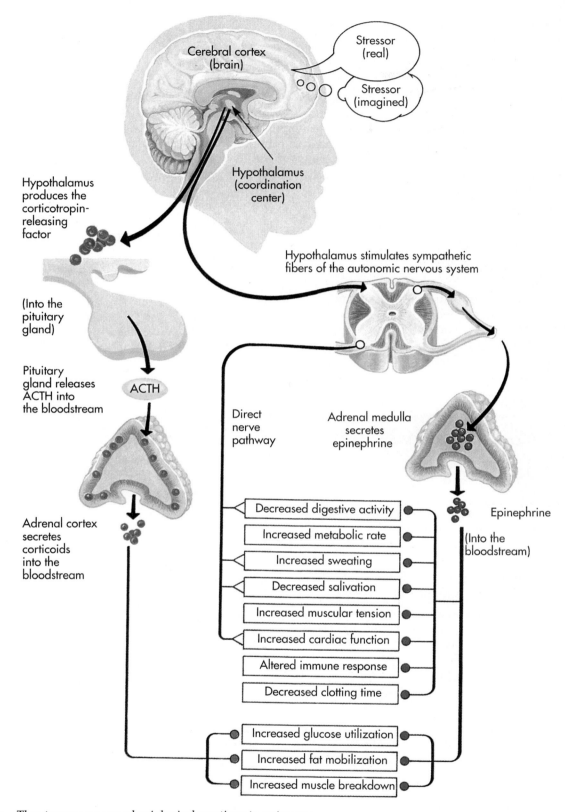

Figure 3-1   The stress response: physiological reactions to a stressor.

holds the potential for becoming a stressor and subsequently stimulating the stress response.

Sensory Modalities

Before a change event can be responded to as a stressor, however, it must first be sensed by the *central nervous system.* With the exception of stressors that are products of the imagination, a person must hear, smell, taste, feel, or see something changing so that they can be transformed into electrical impulses within the nervous system and thus capable of eliciting the stress response.

Cerebral Cortex

Events become stressors when, on entering the *cerebral cortex* of the brain, they are perceived as stressors. By a person's own determination, some, but not all, events are stressors. Remember the phone ringing late at night? Should that very same phone have rung 12 hours earlier (during the afternoon), its ringing would probably not have been interpreted as stressful.

Endocrine System Involvement

The body's response to the presence of a stressor involves not only the brain and nervous system but also the *endocrine system.* The process of interconnecting the nervous system and the endocrine system is the task of the **hypothalamus,** a structure located deep within the brain. The hypothalamus is situated immediately above the gland that plays the most important role in regulating the endocrine system, the **pituitary gland.**[9]

During periods of stress, communication between the hypothalamus and the pituitary gland is accomplished by the release from the hypothalamus of a chemical messenger into the blood flowing directly to the pituitary gland. This chemical stimulates the pituitary gland to produce its own powerful hormone, **adrenocorticotropic hormone (ACTH).** ACTH is then released into the bloodstream, ultimately reaching a pair of glands of the endocrine system called the **adrenal glands.**[10] ACTH stimulates the outer layer *(cortex)* of the adrenal glands to produce chemical substances called **corticoids.** Corticoids support the powerful hormone **epinephrine**

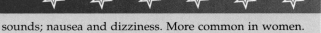

Headaches

An estimated 45 million Americans have frequent, bothersome headaches. If you have chronic headache symptoms or symptoms that are especially painful, you should seek medical help. Headaches can have many causes including stress. The three most common categories are described below:

Tension

Description
A dull, constricting pain centered in the hatband region. Pain may be on both sides of the head and extend down the neck to the shoulders. Produced by stress, eye strain, muscle tension, sinus congestion, TMJ dysfunction, nasal congestion, or caffeine withdrawal.

Treatment
Nonnarcotic pain relievers, muscle relaxants, relaxation exercises, massage.

Prevention
Preventive relaxation exercises, certain antidepressant medications.

Migraine

Description
Throbbing pain on one side of the head, usually preceded by visual disturbances. Sensitivity to lights and sounds; nausea and dizziness. More common in women. May be triggered by a number of causes. Can last from a few hours to 2 days.

Treatment
Rest in a quiet, dark place. Nonnarcotic pain relievers. Ergot compounds (prescription medications).

Prevention
Avoidance of certain foods, including red wines, other alcoholic beverages, ripened cheeses, chocolate, cured meats, and monosodium glutamate (MSG). In some cases, prescription medications are recommended.

Cluster

Description
Focused, intense pain near one eye, often producing a red and teary eye and a runny nose. Headaches occur daily for weeks or months. They mainly affect men and last up to 2 hours.

Treatment
Oxygen and/or ergot compounds during the headache.

Prevention
Avoidance of alcohol and nitrite-containing foods. Various prescription medications, including antidepressants, steroids, ergotlike compounds, or heart-regulating drugs.

(commonly known as **adrenaline**) in the production of energy.

The hypothalamus also activates the adrenal gland directly through a branch of the nervous system. This direct stimulation of the adrenal gland is responsible for the production of epinephrine. Epinephrine causes most of the changes that occur in the body to produce the rapid, short-term high energy levels required in the stress response.

Epinephrine-Influenced Responses

Once epinephrine has been released by the adrenal gland, many of the following tissue responses can be expected.

Decreased digestive activity

Because the body needs energy when a stressor must be avoided or an adversary must be defeated, it cannot wait for digestion to change food into glucose. Rather, the body must turn to the glucose already circulating in the bloodstream or in a storage form within tissue. As a consequence, the entire digestive system slows down. It is not surprising, then, that many people who are under chronic stress report gastric distress, constipation, hemorrhoids, or irritable bowel syndrome.

Increased metabolic rate

Epinephrine increases the **metabolic rate.** Glucose already within the system is rushed by blood circulation to the cells, where it is combined with oxygen (cellular respiration) for the release of energy.

Increased sweating

To control the elevated temperature generated by the accelerated energy production, the body sweats. The accumulated fluid forms on the skin surface, where it evaporates, thus lowering the body's temperature.

Decreased salivation

As a result of the overall shutdown of the digestive system, the production of saliva, which contains digestive enzymes, is also reduced. Thus people who are under the influence of any type of stressor may report a "cotton-mouth" sensation.

Increased muscular tension

Twitching and tautness of the arms and legs during times of stress reflect how close to the fully contracted state the body's skeletal muscles have become. By maintaining the muscles in this condition, the body is prepared for the fight-or-flight response. When mus-

cle tension is continued for extended periods, however, headaches (see the Star Box on p. 50), a stiff neck, and temporomandibular joint (TMJ) dysfunction can result.

Increased rate of cardiac and pulmonary function

During periods of stress, the heart and lungs shift into high gear. Epinephrine helps increase the rate of *cardiac* and *pulmonary* function. An overall upsurge in

---

fight-or-flight response
The reaction to a stressor by confrontation or avoidance (sometimes called the fight, fright, flight, or folly [or 4F] response).

hypothalamus (hype oh **thal** a muss)
The portion of the midbrain that connects the cerebral cortex and the pituitary gland.

pituitary gland (puh **too** it tary)
The "master gland" of the endocrine system; the wide variety of hormones produced by the pituitary are sent to structures throughout the body.

adrenocorticotropic hormone (ACTH) (uh **dreen** oh kore tick oh **trope** ick)
A hormone produced in the pituitary gland and transmitted to the cortex of the adrenal glands; stimulates production and release of corticoids.

adrenal glands
Paired triangular endocrine glands located on the top of each kidney; site of epinephrine and corticoid production.

corticoids (**kore** tick oids)
Hormones generated by the adrenal cortex; corticoids influence the body's control of glucose, protein, and fat metabolism.

epinephrine (epp in **eff** rin)
A powerful adrenal hormone whose presence in the bloodstream prepares the body for maximal energy production and skeletal muscle response.

adrenaline
The common name for epinephrine.

metabolic rate (met uh **bol** ick)
The rate or intensity at which the body produces energy.

heart output and blood pressure and the rate and depth of breathing ensure maximal oxygenation of tissue.

Altered immune system response

At the onset of the stress response, immune system cells are mobilized as if in anticipation of bodily injury. However, during periods of prolonged stress, elevated levels of adrenal hormones appear to have a destructive effect on important cells within the immune system.[11] Infectious illnesses contracted during or shortly after long periods of stress may be directly related to the suppression of these cells, which are part of the body's immune system.

Decreased clotting time

The body prepares for injury during the stress response. Blood clotting time decreases during stress. As a consequence, blood tends to clot more easily.

Stress–Related Disorders

In spite of the stress response's potential for degrading the body in search of energy for the fight-or-flight response, most encounters with stress leave little long-term signs of damage. On occasion, however, stress is the basis for conditions that involve changes in bodily function and, perhaps, actual tissue damage.

When the presence of change in our lives results in strong emotional feelings such as fear, anger, jealousy, disappointment, or unbridled excitement, we may begin to display symptoms suggesting altered *body function*. Conditions such as high blood pressure, spastic colon, chronic back pain, insomnia, and skin disruptions appear in conjunction with stressful situations and can therefore be called *psychogenic* conditions. These "mind-generated" changes in function (without tissue pathology) may not subside until the presence of stressors abates, or they may eventually serve as the basis of identifiable tissue change.

When stressors remain unabated for too long, conditions suggesting actual *tissue damage* may eventually appear. These *psychosomatic* illnesses, such as ulcerative colitis, body composition changes, and shifts in the type and number of immune system cells, are very familiar to physicians, as are, of course, the psychogenic conditions. Peptic ulcer was recently redefined as a bacterial induced erosion of the gastric mucosa rather than a purely psychosomatic condition resulting from increased acidity resulting from stress.

Influences of Corticoids and Epinephrine on Energy Release

Increased glucose use

Because glucose is the body's most basic source of energy, an early feature of the stress response is the release of glycogen (the storage form of glucose) from its deposit sites, particularly the liver.

Increased fat use

If a stressor is not eliminated promptly, the body's supply of glucose may become depleted. The body then turns to its two remaining energy reserves, fat deposits and muscle tissue. Fat breakdown will result in the production of metabolic waste products that will eventually cause the body to use its most protected energy deposits, muscle tissue.

Muscle tissue breakdown and use

If the stressor is unusually powerful, energy demands will continue to the point that muscle tissue becomes involved. Fortunately, most of today's stressors are resolved long before this occurs.

Although in the short term all of the responses shown in Figure 3-1 are valuable when confronting a stressor, long-term exposure to these breakdown processes has a destructive effect on physical health. During the resistance phase of the stress response, the body will shift the efforts of a prolonged "fight" to specific body systems. When this shift occurs, the **psychosomatic disorders** associated with chronic stress begin. These disorders are summarized in the Star Box at left, which includes a discussion of psychogenic and psychosomatic aspects of stress.

STRESS AND PSYCHOIMMUNOLOGY

In an earlier section of the chapter, the relationship of stress to both illness and the function of the immune system is briefly discussed (see p. 51). Additional information seems warranted in light of the growing interest in these topics within the scientific community.[12]

On the basis of clinical observation and laboratory studies, it is recognized that feelings associated with stress (depression and anxiety) and the disruption of social support systems relate to the weakening of the immune response and the development of some illnesses.[12] For example, a study involving self-assessment of stress levels and the occurrence of colds demonstrated that as stress levels increase, colds become more common.[13] In yet another study, immunizations were less effective in producing an immune response in students stressed by upcoming examinations than in those not scheduled to take examinations. What is not known, however, is which mechanisms certain stressors use in altering immune system function (nervous and endocrine systems versus nervous system only), whether studies done with immune cells removed from the body are reflective of what occurs in the body, and whether studies done with animals can be applied to humans.

In spite of these limitations, theoretical explanations for a strong relationship between stress and the absence of social support and immune system function can be made. Accordingly, a growing number of studies are under way to further clarify which pathways are involved in the stress–immune system interplay, and the use of social support therapy is becoming a component in the treatment of serious illness, such as breast cancer.

Personality Traits

Can personality play a role in making people more or less prone to stress? If so, what outlook on life is now considered to be the most stress-producing? The answer to the latter question has changed over the past two decades.

The initial, and still widely recognized, theory describing personality's role in fostering stress was that of type A and type B personalities, developed by cardiologists Friedman and Rosenman. In this model, time-dependence (hurry sickness) was related to high levels of stress and, eventually, to heart disease.

Today, the concept of time-dependence as being the most influential personality trait associated with high levels of stress has given way to concern over high levels of anger and cynicism. Anger is the intense feeling of rage and fury that accompanies unexpected change. For people who for whatever reasons seem to be always angry, the stress put on the body is detrimental to both physical and emotional health.[14] The term *angry heart* describes a condition frequently seen in people who have had a heart attack.

Closely akin to anger is cynicism, the second personality trait that fosters high levels of stress. This trait is associated with deeply held dislike and distrust of others and their ideas. Cynics have nothing good to say about others. They are, perhaps, profoundly angry about their relationships with others and can only express this feeling by being very critical. Regardless, cynicism, like anger, places the body under chronic stress and erodes the physical and emotional well-being of the cynic. Perhaps the only

effective treatment for chronically angry or cynical people is either a profoundly moving personal experience that truly changes their outlook on life, such as the birth of a child, or counseling to get in touch with the reasons underlying their negative outlook.

COPING: REACTING TO STRESSORS

It is in some ways more difficult than in the past to develop appropriate and effective coping skills. No longer is it socially acceptable to escape stressors through negative dependency behavior, withdrawal, or aggressiveness. The emphasis now is on lifestyle management techniques, such as time management (see the Health Action Guide on p. 54), that are not only effective but also supportive of overall health, social relationships, and the environment.

Stress Management Techniques

Experts in stress management have proposed several effective techniques for coping with stress. Each of these techniques is described in the material that follows, with specific instructions for use provided for some. You will not know whether a particular coping technique is effective for you until you study the technique and then use it for an adequate period of time.

Self-hypnosis

Techniques for increased awareness, mental relaxation, and enhanced self-directedness are taught by trained professionals to people capable of being hypnotized. These techniques, which can be learned in one lesson, are self-administered in daily sessions lasting 10 to 20 minutes each. Beware of unqualified practitioners, who frequently sell their services through newspaper advertisements. Professional organizations, such as psychological or psychiatric societies, can recommend qualified therapists.

The relaxation response

The "relaxation response" is a relaxation technique developed by Herbert Benson, M.D., through which one learns to quiet the body and mind. Relaxation technique centers on exhalation and allowing the body to relax while sitting in a comfortable position.

psychosomatic disorders (sye cho so **mat** ick) Physical illnesses of the body involving tissue change generated by the effects of stress.

HEALTH
Action Guide -------→

Time Management

Many college students think that the most significant problem about being a student is everything that can interfere with the academic side of school, including campus activities, athletics, work, marriage, parenting, and just having free time for relaxation. Therefore, too often perhaps, choices regarding time are made in ways that cause classroom work to be more stressful than it should be. Ultimately, however, it becomes an issue of priorities and the management of time so that academic demands can be met sufficiently.

Although there is no single best approach to managing time, most experts suggest that the following would be helpful:

1. Keep a log of how you use your time for 1 week. Make an entry about each half hour to see what you are doing.

2. Analyze your records, and eliminate those activities that unnecessarily take too much time.

3. Once the eliminations have been made, divide your time into blocks so that related activities can be scheduled together. There should be a block for each major area of responsibility applicable to you. Examples might include academics, employment, recreation, and social activities.

4. Schedule specific activities within each block of time. Attempt to conclude activities that you have started.

Reassess your time management activities occasionally, and make adjustments when necessary.[15]

◄------•

This technique can be learned in a single session but requires a commitment to making time to practice. Relatively effective for most people, the technique is described in Dr. Benson's book, *The Relaxation Response.*

Progressive muscular relaxation

Pioneered by the work of Edmund Johnson (author of *You Must Relax*), progressive muscle relaxation (PMR) is a procedure in which each of several muscle groups is systematically contracted and relaxed. By learning to recognize the difference between contracted and relaxed muscles, Johnson believed that people would be able to purposely place certain mus-

cles into a controlled state of stress-reducing relaxation.

PMR is based on the appropriate use of positioning, breathing, and concentration. The position of choice is lying on the floor, with the hands at the sides and palms facing upward. Once a comfortable position has been assumed, alternating periods of inhalation and exhalation are begun. As a person inhales, the muscles are contracted, whereas during exhalation, muscle groups are relaxed. Concentration is focused on the "feelings" of relaxation that accompany the release of tension during each exhalation. Once mastered, the basics of participation can be carried out in almost every setting, including a moving car, at work at one's desk, and in a college classroom. Depending on a person's levels of expertise, contractions last from a maximum of 100 seconds, through 50 seconds, to a minimum of 5 seconds. The face, jaw, neck, shoulders, upper chest, hands and forearms, abdomen, lower back, buttocks, thighs, calves, and

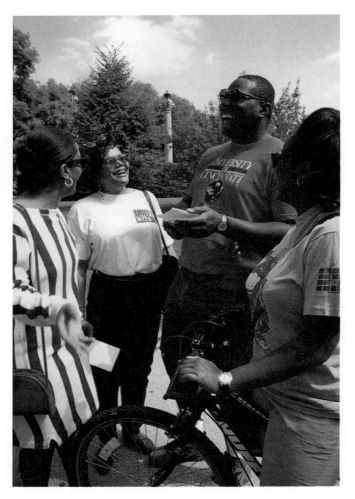

Periods of reduced stress are vital for mental health.

Reducing Stress

Many of us are looking for ways to reduce stress in our lives, whether we do it by exercising, reading self-help books, performing relaxation exercises, or seeing a therapist. Is peace of mind illusive, or is it achievable in today's society?

Stress is experienced by all people, regardless of culture. The Lebanese, for example, purchase "worry beads" and handle them for periods of time to help them deal with anger or anxiety. If one were to visit Lebanon, the clicking of beads might be a commonly heard sound.[17]

Perhaps we can learn from the Far Eastern cultures and their ways of dealing with stress. Eastern people seem to understand the concept of inner peace, and they work and practice to develop it. Many Japanese, through self-discipline and training, learn to block out outside disturbances and stressors. This practice is described as achieving tranquility.[18]

Tranquility does not come naturally to the Japanese. It is learned through very specific exercises. The exercises consist of three levels: stillness of the body, breathing, and the center of being. It is not known exactly how these exercises originated, but it has been suggested that they are derived from the practices of Buddhist monks and Shinto priests.[18]

For the Japanese, the idea of tranquility seems to be a way of life and a goal to achieve. Does one have to be from the Eastern culture to understand the concept of tranquility, or is it a practice that those of us from Western society can learn and internalize?

feet are tightened and then relaxed progressively. To the extent possible, each muscle group within the area is included.

Quieting

Quieting involves using a set of specific responses, such as striving for a positive mental state, an "inner smile," and a deep exhalation, with the tongue and the shoulders relaxed, immediately on sensing the onset of stress. This technique can be practiced at any time; it is easily learned and supplies immediate feelings of being "on top of stress." The technique can be learned by reading *QR: The Quieting Reflex,* by Charles Stroebel, M.D., Ph.D.

Yoga

An ancient exercise program for the mind and body, yoga can be learned from a qualified instructor in 1 to 3 months. Yoga is practiced daily in a quiet setting in sessions lasting 15 to 45 minutes. It can alter specific physiological functions, enhance flexibility, and free the mind from worry. Many good yoga books, classes, and videotapes are available.

Diaphragmatic breathing

A coping technique with elements of both relaxation and quieting is diaphragmatic breathing (Figure 3-2). Aspects of this practice are seen in the Lamaze approach to childbirth, yoga, and t'ai chi. Although no single explanation for its effectiveness can be given, when practiced regularly, diaphragmatic breathing produces relaxation that buffers the powerful stress response. A three-component approach to the practice of diaphragmatic breathing is described below:

1. **Assume a comfortable position.** Lie on the floor with arms by your sides, eyes closed, back straight. Begin breathing from the diaphragm, rather than by the normal method of lifting the chest.
2. **Concentrate.** The ability to concentrate is important in diaphragmatic breathing. This can be difficult but is most easily mastered by following the flow of air as it enters the body and flows deeply into the lower levels of the lungs, followed by the rising of the stomach as the air leaves the lungs. Each ventilation can be fragmented into four distinct steps: (1) take air into your lungs through the nose and mouth, (2) pause slightly before exhaling, (3) release the air to flow out via the path from which it entered, and (4) pause slightly after exhalation before repeating step 1.
3. **Visualize.** Diaphragmatic breathing promotes relaxation most fully when it is practiced in conjunction with visualization. What is visualized varies from person to person, but many feel that envisioning the air or even clouds entering the body with each breath, traveling down the path taken by the air, and leaving through the nostrils is very effective. Extending the image of the air flowing through the entire body (energy breathing) rather than only into the lungs is even more effective.

Once mastered, diaphragmatic breathing will quiet the body. Experienced users of this technique can temporarily lower their breathing rate from a typical rate of 14 to 18 breaths per minute to a few as four breaths per minute. In doing so, the entire nervous system is

1. Assume a Comfortable Position
Breathe from the diaphragm rather than by lifting the chest, as a person normally breathes.

2. Concentrate
Focus on the flow of air as it moves deeply into the lower levels of the lungs, followed by the rising of the stomach as the air leaves.

3. Visualize
Visualize the air flowing through the entire body, rather than only into the lungs.

Figure 3-2   Diaphragmatic breathing.

slowed, in direct opposition to its role in the stress response.

Transcendental meditation

Transcendental meditation (TM) allows the mind to transcend thought effortlessly when the person recites a mantra, or a personal word, twice daily for 20 minutes. TM is a seven-step program that is taught by trained professionals. TM centers are listed in the telephone directory under Transcendental Meditation.

Biofeedback

Biofeedback is a system for monitoring and subsequently controlling specific physiological functions, such as heart rate, respiratory rate, and body temperature. Training with an experienced instructor and appropriate monitoring instruments requires weekly sessions that last 1 hour or longer over a period of 12 or more weeks. When used with other tension reduction techniques, biofeedback provides concrete reinforcement of stress-reduction goals. For more infor-

mation, contact the Biofeedback Society of America, 4301 Owens Street, Wheat Ridge, CO 80033.

Exercise

A wide variety of movement activities are intended to reduce stress, expend energy, promote relaxation, provide enjoyment through social contact and, possibly, promote the formation of biological opiates. Running, jogging, lap swimming, walking, rope skipping, biking, stair climbing, and aerobic dancing workouts are all excellent ways to burn the energy produced by the stress response (see the Star Box on p. 57). Equipment needs, facilities, and required skills vary. Three to four sessions per week lasting a half hour per session are sufficient for most people. Health and fitness clubs offer exercise programs.

Health Practices and Stress

Beyond practicing the variety of stress reduction techniques and time management skills described in this chapter, one's health is important in the management of stress. There is little doubt that people who lead a wellness-oriented lifestyle have an advantage in dealing with stress. When people are rested, well conditioned, healthfully nourished, seen regularly by health care professionals, often in the company of friends, and secure in their beliefs, the demands imposed by change are more manageable. In fact, health, in combination with a realistic outlook on life such as that described in the next section, may be the basis on which all successful coping is built.

A Realistic Perspective on Stress and Life

Although we would like our lives to be stress-free, reality dictates otherwise. Therefore it is desirable that we approach life with a tough-minded optimism that provides a sense of hope and anticipation, as well as an understanding that life will never be without stress. The development of this realistic approach to today's fast-paced, demanding lifestyle may best be achieved by fostering many of the perspectives listed below[16]:

- **Do not be surprised by trouble.** Anticipate problems, and see yourself as a problem solver.
- **Search for solutions.** Act on a partial solution, even when a complete solution seems distant.
- **Take control of your own future.** Set out to accomplish all of your goals. Do not view yourself as a victim of circumstances.
- **Move away from negative thought patterns.** Do not extend or generalize difficulties from one area into another.
- **Rehearse success.** Do not disregard the possibility of failure. Rather, focus on the things that are necessary and possible to ensure success.
- **Accept the unchangeable.** The direction your life takes is only in part the result of your own doing. Cope as effectively as possible with the events over which you have no direct control.
- **Live each day well.** Combine activity, contemplation, and a sense of cheerfulness with the many things that must be done each day. Celebrate special occasions.
- **Act on your capacity for growth.** Undertake new experiences, and then extract from them new information about your interests and abilities.
- **Allow for renewal.** Make time for yourself, and take advantage of opportunities to pursue new and fulfilling relationships. Foster growth of your spiritual nature.
- **Tolerate mistakes.** Both you and others will make mistakes. Recognize that these can cause

Effective Coping: The Link Between Stress and Exercise

The energy produced by the stress response is most easily reduced through physical activity. In fact, coping by engaging in an exercise program during stressful situations closely resembles how our ancestors used the energy of their stress response—by fighting or fleeing.

The following list identifies physical activities that you can use to cope with stress during your lunch hour or before or after school or work. Describe your experience with each, including when, where, how long, and with whom you engaged in this activity. Then list the health benefits you received. For those activities you have not yet tried, describe what would be necessary to make them more attractive.

- *Walking (power, leisure):*

- *Jogging:*

- *Running (5 mph +):*

- *Aerobic Activities (stair stepping, dancing, rowing, aqua aerobics, etc.):*

- *Biking (12-15 mph +):*

- *Racquet Sports (squash, racquetball, tennis):*

- *Bowling:*

- *Weight Training (power, body building):*

- *Golf (with/without cart):*

- *Swimming:*

anger or frustration, and learn to avoid feelings of hostility.

With a realistic and positive outlook on life, you will need less coping time to live a satisfying and productive life. Change in all aspects of life is inevitable. In the presence of good health, change should be anticipated, nurtured, and then incorporated into the maturing sense of well-being.

Summary

- Stress is the physiological and emotional response to the presence of a stressor. Stressors are events that generate the stress response.
- Distress and eustress reflect similar physiological responses but different emotional interpretations.
- Uncontrolled stress can lead to a variety of illnesses. Since the effects of stress are cumulative, stress-related health problems can develop slowly.
- The college experience can generate stressors from several different areas, including finances, classroom requirements, and personal expectations.
- Day-to-day living is routinely the source of many types of stressors.
- The general adaptation syndrome consists of three distinct stages: alarm, resistance and reaction. Hopefully, exhaustion from excessive stress will not occur.
- An intricate interplay involving the brain, nervous system, and endocrine system results in a series of physiological changes that prepare the body to respond to stressors.
- The stress response mobilizes energy for the fight-or-flight response.
- Critical to the stress response are the senses, the cerebral cortex, the hypothalamus, the adrenal glands, the hormone ACTH, corticoids, and epinephrine.
- Stress influences the function of the immune system, resulting in susceptibility to illnesses.
- Chronic feelings of anger and cynicism can be central to feelings of stress.
- A variety of coping techniques can be easily learned and may prove to be beneficial in reducing stress.
- An optimistic outlook on life may protect some people from the potentially damaging effects of stressors. Further, a less stressful life enhances health and provides a greater sense of well-being.

Review Questions

1. What is the difference between stress and stressors?
2. How do distress and eustress differ? In what way are they similar?
3. What are several of the more familiar health conditions attributed to chronic unresolved stress? To what extent are the effects of stress cumulative?
4. In what way does the college experience contribute to the stress level of students? What life experience do typical Americans report as being most stressful?
5. In what predictable manner does the stress response unfold? What is the role of the endocrine system? How do the digestive and cardiovascular systems contribute to the fight-or-flight response?
6. What is psychoimmunology? To date, what has research found in regard to immune function and the occurrence of stress?
7. How has the popular type A/type B theory of time-dependence changed in regard to the cause of stress? In what manner do anger and cynicism contribute to stress? How do type R persons use the stress response?
8. What coping techniques have proved helpful when used on a regular basis? How are progressive muscular relaxation and diaphragmatic breathing practiced?
9. What traits characterize the optimistic lifestyle?

Think About This . . .

- Can you remember a stressful experience you recently had in which your body responses clearly followed the pattern of Selye's general adaptation syndrome? How long did you remain in each of the specific stages?
- If the body's response to stressors is similar for distress and eustress, how do we learn to distinguish between the two?
- Do you have a realistic perception about the potential stressful nature of life?
- Which dimension of your health (physical, emotional, social, occupational, intellectual, or spiritual) do you most frequently rely on when you are confronted with a stressful situation?
- If you believe that the enhancement of your stress management skills will be important to you in the future, which of the suggested approaches to coping with stress could you most comfortably develop? When can you start to develop these skills?

References

1. Selye H: *Stress without distress,* New York, 1975, New American Library.
2. Blonna R: *Stress management,* St Louis, 1996, Mosby.
3. Seaward BL: *Managing stress: principles and strategies for health and wellbeing,* Boston, 1994, Jones & Bartlett.
4. Julius M et al: Anger-coping types, blood pressure, and all causes of mortality: a follow-up in Tecumseh, Michigan (1971-1983), *Am J Epidemiol* 124:220-233, 1986.
5. McGinnis J: *Medicine for the layman: behavioral patterns and health,* US Department of Health and Human Services, NIH Pub No 85-2682, Washington, DC, 1986, US Government Printing Office.
6. Tyrrell DJ, Smith AP: Psychological stress and susceptibility to the common cold, *N Engl J Med* 325(9):606-613, 1991.
7. Girdano D, Everly G: *Controlling stress and tension: a holistic approach,* ed 4, Englewood Cliffs, NJ, 1992, Prentice Hall.
8. Swanton J: *The wellness book: the comprehensive guide to maintaining health and treating stress-related illness,* New York, 1991, Birch Lane Press.
9. Tate P, Seeley RR: *Understanding the human body,* St Louis, 1994, Mosby.
10. Thibodeau GA, Patton KT: *Human body in health and disease,* St Louis, 1992, Mosby.
11. O'Leary A: Stress, emotion, and human immune function, *Psychol Bull* 108(3):353-363, 1990.
12. Vitkovic L, Koslow SH, editors: *Neuroimmunology and mental health,* NIH Pub No 94-3274, US Department of Health and Human Services, Public Health Service, National Institutes of Health, National Institute of Mental Health, Rockville, MD, 1994, US Government Printing Office.
13. Cohen S et al: Psychological stress and susceptibility to the common cold, *N Engl J Med* 325:606-612, 1991.
14. Almada SJ et al: Neuroticism and cynicism and risk of death in middle-aged men: the Western Electric study, *Psychosom Med* 53(2):165-175, 1991.
15. Buchert W: A key to managing time: planning and discipline, *USA Today* 9A, April 16, 1990.
16. McGinnis L: *The power of optimism,* New York, 1990, Harper & Row.
17. Cahill MJ: *Lebanon,* New York, 1987, Chelsea House.
18. Durckheim K: *The Japanese cult of tranquility,* York Beach, Me, 1991, Samuel Weiser.

Suggested Readings

Davidson J: *Breathing space: living and working at a comfortable pace in a sped-up society,* New York, 1991, MasterMedia Limited.

Why are we moving so fast in today's world? According to the author, technological advances, such as the computer and the fax machine, have caused us to be pressed for time and thus in a leisure squeeze. Suggestions are given for making the most beneficial use of our remaining leisure time.

McGinnis A: *The power of optimism,* New York, 1990, Harper & Row.

People who are recognized for their optimism perceive life differently. Once adopted, their traits allow us to better understand the changes over which we have no control.

Dienstfrey H: *Where the mind meets the body,* New York, 1992, HarperCollins.

Describes a wide variety of topics related to the mind-body interface. Discusses type A behavior, relaxation, biofeedback, imagery, and hypnosis. Timely coverage in light of the government's recent decision to fund research into "alternative" health care.

Seligman M: *Learned optimism,* New York, 1990, Pocket Books.

Well written and easily understood, the author of this book contends that optimism and pessimism are both learned frames of reference regarding change. Accordingly, the former can be learned and the latter unlearned.

 ## AS WE GO TO PRESS . . .

While many living in the Midwest are experiencing an above average summer of precipitation, people living in the Southwestern United States are trying to cope with, perhaps, the worst drought in a century. The summer drought of 1996 follows an extremely dry winter and spring. Damage to farms and ranches is predicted to be in the billions of dollars. Many families are expected to face considerable financial difficulties and personal struggles as they cope with this environmental stressor.

Managing Work-Related Stress

When someone is introduced to you, the first bit of information you learn is the person's name. More often than not, the next part of the introduction will have some mention of that person's occupation, and at the very least you will have some idea about the person's job within the first few minutes of conversation. Americans often identify people with the jobs they perform, and much of our own self-identity is linked with our occupations. As a result, anything that threatens our jobs or our job performance is also a threat to our sense of personal worth.[1]

Job stress is becoming a part of everyday life. It affects society as a whole in a variety of ways, contributing to rising health care costs, increasing insurance rates, and decreasing national productivity.[2] If left unchecked, work-related stress can have profound effects on the physical and mental health of individuals as well.

Sources of Job Stress

Since we so often attach our jobs to our sense of self-worth, work-related stress can be an important problem in our daily lives. It is therefore important to identify things that can cause stress in the workplace (job stressors), and, when possible, deal with them in a healthy manner. Common job stressors include the following[1-3]:

- Conflicts with colleagues, supervisors, or workers under your supervision
- Changes in work routine
- Deadlines
- Too much (or too little) responsibility
- Lack of control over work methods and planning
- Long working hours
- Repetitive tasks
- Excessive or rhythmic noise
- Poor time management or organization
- Working with hazardous equipment or substances
- Threat of pay reduction or unemployment
- Lack of necessary resources

These are factors that nearly everyone has to deal with at one time or another in the workplace. These stressors may vary from job to job, and individuals react in different ways to these stimuli, but we are all usually affected in some way by job stressors.

Job Stress Among Older Workers

Although workers of any age can succumb to stress in the workplace, older workers in general are hit the hardest by job stress.[5] Technological advances tend to cause more stress for older workers, especially those who have been performing a similar routine for a long time and are suddenly forced to assimilate new technology into their daily work. Older workers are also prime targets for lay-offs. They have worked their way up the pay scale and in general are paid a higher wage than their younger counterparts. As a result, many older workers are leaving the workforce at an earlier age than they normally would because of increased stress.[5]

Stress in the Modern Workplace

Stress in the workplace has increased greatly over the last 15 years. Corporate mergers and buyouts have eliminated entire companies and thousands of jobs, new technology has caused a drastic increase in work pace, and the competitiveness of the modern economy has forced individual employees to take on much heavier workloads.[5]

Technology

Today's worker has to deal with stressors that are unique to the times we live in. The most obvious of these is the drastic increase in workplace technology. Increased mechanical efficiency leads to the need for fewer workers but requires employees to become more knowledgeable concerning the new machines they work with.[2,4] Personal computers and computer networks, although increasing workplace efficiency and speed, are themselves contributors to job stress. Increased work speed is a double-edged sword. Getting more work done within a specified time may mean more profit for a company, but it also leads to the expectation that more work will always be accomplished in less time. Computers drastically reduce the time needed to perform tasks, but the person running the computer may then be asked to perform more tasks within the workday, causing stress. Workers are also asked to know about the many uses of various computer software programs, which are constantly being changed and improved. The constant upgrading of computer programs requires that employees be reeducated continually to keep up. The increased productivity provided by the computer may lead to the elimination of many jobs, since one worker may now be able to do the work of two or more.

The computer itself may also contribute to physical problems. The monitor of the computer may cause eyestrain, headaches, fatigue, and muscle tension.[4] Constant work on a keyboard may place excess stress on fingers, hands, and wrists. This in turn may contribute to arthritic conditions or to the newly recognized affliction known as *carpal tunnel syndrome*. The simple act of sitting at the computer for extended periods with the body in a fixed position can put stress on the muscles and bones of the back, neck, and limbs.[3, 4]

Afflictions such as these, which are caused by repetitive motions, unusual body postures, or holding static joint positions over extended periods, are now referred to as repetitive strain injuries (RSIs). The risk of developing RSIs is increased during periods of emotional stress or while trying to beat a deadline.[6] RSIs can also develop because of improper placement of equipment (such as a keyboard) or by certain work practices.[6] Company production goals based on quotas, such as counting workers' keystrokes throughout the day, can force employees to work through needed break periods to meet the expected work output; this in turn can increase the risk of RSI development.

Downsizing

The current corporate trend of eliminating jobs to cut costs—"downsizing"—has contributed greatly to the problem of job stress. This practice affects not only rank-and-file workers but employees in management as well. Often cuts are made with little or no regard to an employee's years of service or experience (or because of this, to save money), so anyone on the payroll may be vulnerable. This lack of job security has been an important contributor to job stress over the last decade.

Although the current popularity of downsizing may be unprecedented, the effects of the fear of unemployment have been studied as early as the 1960s. For example, from 1965 to 1973 the workforce at Cape Canaveral was downsized from 65,000 employees to 32,000.[1] Aerospace workers, highly trained and highly paid, were being laid off in large numbers as the government cut back on the space program. With few skills that could be transferred to other jobs, many found themselves bagging groceries and taking tickets for a living.[1] The fear of being unemployed and the difficult transition after being laid off caused many physical and mental problems for Cape Canaveral workers and their families. Because of the heavy stress, these families suffered from anxiety and depression and led the nation in divorce rates, drinking, drug use, and sudden heart attack deaths.[1] Autopsies on these heart attack victims, some of whom were as young as 29, showed that no significant risk factors were present except for high levels of chemicals (such as epinephrine) that are released in response to stress.[1]

The situation that these aerospace workers were faced with is now happening in workplaces across the nation. Recent layoffs have occurred at many major corporations across the United States, and many of these are a direct result of corporate downsizing. AT&T, the telecommunications giant, is planning to lay off approximately 40,000 employees by the end of 1998, with up to 30,000 of those cuts coming in 1996.[7] Other major corporations, such as IBM, McDonnell-Douglas, and Apple Computer, have had layoffs in recent years as well.

Competition

Although there are more than enough jobs being created to replace those lost through downsizing, these new jobs offer lower pay, fewer benefits, and less desirable working conditions. As a result, competition for good jobs is growing stiffer.[8] A college education, which used to be a can't-miss ticket to a well-paying and rewarding job, is now merely a ticket to enter the fiercely competitive contest that is today's job market. Over 20% of adults hold at least a bachelor's degree, and over 40% of adults have some college experience. Over 14 million students are currently enrolled at institutions of higher education.[9] Workers whose jobs are cut are facing competition from new college graduates, who will often work for less money, as well as from others who have been laid off. New graduates, on the other hand, are competing with displaced workers, who usually have a wealth of work experience.

All of this uncertainty in the workplace has led many people to broaden their knowledge to become more competitive within their chosen field, or to change careers altogether. This has meant booming business for colleges and universities. Over 26% of all college students enrolled in the United States in the fall of 1993 were over the age of 30.[9] Many of these nontraditional students (and a great many traditional-age students) face the challenge of succeeding at school while trying to raise a family or hold down a job at the same time. Job stress is thus compounded with classroom stress. Even though the task seems daunting, more and more students are willing to try. It is not uncommon for students to attend classes either before or after working a full shift at a regular job.

Reducing Work-Related Stress

The changing climate of today's economy, marked by expanding technology, increasing demands on the individual, and decreasing job security, is taking its toll on the American worker. Since work-related stress appears to be increasing in nearly all professions, it is more important than ever to be able to recognize the physical signs of stress and to be able to reduce job stress when possible. Here are a few things you can do to reduce the effects of work-related stress[1-4]:

- Recognize when stress is getting to you. Be able to identify early warning signs that you may be under heavy stress. Emotional signs may include anxiety, lack of interest, and irritability. Mental fatigue, physical exhaustion, and frequent illness may be physical manifestations of stress as well. Not everyone reacts to stressful situations in the same way, so know yourself well enough to recognize when stressors are affecting you.
- Control your environment when you can. Not every work situation can be controlled, but controlling some situations can help reduce stress. Try not to schedule stressful work activities for the same time. Break larger jobs down into smaller parts. If it is safe to do so, rearrange your work area to keep things fresh.
- Know the things you cannot control and deal with them. Not even a CEO is under total control of his or her job. Becoming angry or obsessed over a situation you can't do anything about only increases your stress level. Developing a more flexible attitude toward situations on the job that are not flexible can be a very healthy thing to do.
- Take a break. Schedule some down time to keep yourself refreshed. If your breaks are scheduled for you, don't use them to get extra work done. Your physical and mental health can be helped immensely by taking advantage of your time off. When performing repetitive tasks, step away from the task whenever you can. If you work at a computer terminal, get up occasionally and move around.
- Get some exercise. Physical activity can be healthy for the mind and the body. Exercise can actually increase energy levels and increase physical resistance to stress.
- Make your workplace safe. Stress resulting from hazardous situations can be reduced by taking safety precautions when possible. If safety equipment is available, make use of it. Use a shade screen on your computer monitor if possible to reduce eyestrain and headaches. Staying safe on the job can prevent stressful situations that may occur because of an injury, such as missed work, decreased productivity, and physical pain.

If stress on the job seems to be greatly affecting you physically or mentally, it is important that you see your family doctor or a qualified mental health professional as soon as possible. Although everyone experiences some type of stress as a result of the workplace, this stress does not have to become an overwhelming factor in your life. Managing work-related stressors is an important skill that all employees of today must learn to master, so take some time to assess your problems and devise some strategies to deal with your stressful situations.

References

1. Eliot RS, Breo DL: *Is it worth dying for?* New York, 1984, Bantam Books.
2. Goliszek AG: *Breaking the stress habit*, Winston-Salem, NC, 1987, Carolina Press.

3. Gardell B: Efficiency and health hazards in mechanized work. In Quick et al, editors: *Work stress: health care systems in the workplace,* New York, 1987, Prager.

4. Haynes SG et al: The effect of high job demands and low control on the health of employed women. In Quick et al, editors: *Work stress: health care systems in the workplace,* New York, 1987, Prager.

5. Williams G: Flaming out on the job: How to recognize when it's all too much, *Modern Maturity,* 34(5), 1991.

6. Williamson E: Caught in the grip of RSI: a first-hand account, *Managing Office Technology,* 39(5), 1994.

7. "John Doe." American Telephone and Telegraph employee. Personal interview, January 29, 1996.

8. Church GJ: Are we better off? *Time,* 147(5), Jan 29, 1996.

9. The nation. *The Chronicle of Higher Education,* almanac issue, 42(1), Sept 1, 1995.

PART 2

THE BODY

Chapter

4

Becoming
Physically Fit

Healthy People 2000 Objectives

Many of the Healthy People 2000 objectives focused on getting Americans to increase their participation in activities that improve cardiorespiratory fitness. With an estimated 250,000 deaths per year in the United States attributable to the lack of physical activity, encouraging our sedentary society to become more active is clearly important.

The Midcourse Review concluded that progress toward achieving these objectives has been mixed. A somewhat higher percentage of adults now engage in moderate to vigorous physical activity. However, no progress has been made in reducing the percentage of adults who do not participate in leisure-time physical activity. The objective of increasing the number of worksite fitness programs has been fully achieved.

Unfortunately, the nation has lost ground in several areas. For example, since 1990 the percentage of students in grades 9 through 12 involved in physical education courses has decreased. The proportion of time that students are physically active during these class periods has also dropped.

When your day begins early in the morning, then you go to class or work or immerse yourself in family activities, and your day does not end until after midnight, you must be physically fit to keep up the pace. Even a highly motivated college student must have a conditioned, rested body to maintain such a schedule.

OK, let's simplify things a bit. The paragraph above reflects how college health professors might view the value of fitness—it helps people function well enough to cope with their hectic lifestyles. But what motivates students to value fitness? Quite simply, students say that overall body fitness helps them look and feel better.

Many college students want to look in the mirror and see the kind of body they see in the media: one with well-toned muscles, a trim waistline, and an absence of flabby tissue, especially on the arms and legs. Students become motivated to start fitness programs because they hope that they can build a better body for themselves. Through their efforts to do so, students usually start to feel better, both physically and mentally. They realize that change is possible, since they see it happening to their bodies with each passing week. "Go for it" and "just do it" then become more than just sports marketing phrases; they become reminders that the activities that lead to fitness are a meaningful part of their lives. Fitness actually becomes *fun*.

Fortunately, you do not have to be a top-notch athlete to receive the health benefits of physical activity. In fact, even a modest increase in your daily activity level can be rewarding (see the Health Action Guide at right). The health benefits of fitness can come from regular participation in moderate exercise, such as brisk walking or dancing.[1]

Your increase in physical activity will not only help you; it can help the nation to achieve its Healthy People 2000 Objectives. Further, although fitness will not guarantee you a longer life, it can help you enjoy the years that you have.

COMPONENTS OF PHYSICAL FITNESS

Physical fitness is achieved when "the organic systems of the body are healthy and function efficiently so as to resist disease, to enable the fit person to engage in vigorous tasks and leisure activities, and to handle situations of emergency."[2] In the following sections, we discuss cardiorespiratory endurance, muscular strength, muscular endurance, flexibility, and body composition.

Cardiorespiratory Endurance

If you were limited to improving only one area of your physical fitness, which would you choose—muscular strength, muscular endurance, or flexibility? Which would a dancer choose? Which would a marathon runner select? Which would an expert recommend?

We think the experts, who are exercise physiologists, would say that another fitness dimension is of even greater importance than those listed above. These research scientists regard improvement of your heart, lung, and blood vessel function as the key focal point of a physical fitness program. **Cardiorespiratory endurance** forms the foundation for whole-body fitness.

Cardiorespiratory endurance increases your capacity to sustain a given level of energy production for a

HEALTH Action Guide

Adding Activity to Your Day

If you find that you are not active during much of your day, why not try these suggestions?

- Get off the sofa during television commercials and walk around the house or in the yard.
- Whenever you can, take short, brisk walks. Brief extra walks around campus (for example, taking the long way to class) or your place of work can consume calories and place some beneficial exertion on your cardiorespiratory system.
- Instead of phoning people in your apartment or residence hall, walk to their rooms. Rather than phoning a colleague in an office building, you can walk to his or her office.
- When possible, use stairs instead of elevators.
- Instead of parking as close to a building as you can, park your car farther away to increase your walking distance.

cardiorespiratory endurance (**car** dee oh **ress** pur uh tory)
The ability of the heart, lungs, and blood vessels to process and transport oxygen required by muscle cells so that they can contract over a period of time.

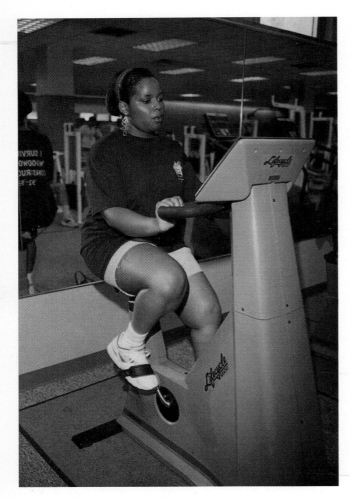

Cardiorespiratory endurance is produced by physical activity that requires continuous, repetitive movements.

prolonged period. Development of cardiorespiratory endurance helps your body to work longer and at greater levels of intensity.

Your body cannot always produce the energy it needs for long-term activity. Certain activities require performance at a level of intensity that will outstrip your cardiorespiratory system's ability to transport oxygen efficiently to contracting muscle fibers. When the oxygen demands of the muscles cannot be met, **oxygen debt** occurs. Any activity that continues beyond the point at which oxygen debt begins requires a form of energy production that does not depend on oxygen.

This oxygen-deprived form of energy production is called **anaerobic** (without oxygen) **energy production,** the type that fuels many intense, short-duration activities. For example, rope climbing, weight lifting for strength, and sprinting are short-duration activities that quickly cause muscle fatigue; they are generally considered anaerobic activities.

Activities that are not generally associated with anaerobic energy production (walking, distance jogging, and bicycle touring) become anaerobic activities when they are either increased in intensity or continued for an extended period.

If you usually work or play at low intensity but for a long duration, you have developed an ability to maintain **aerobic** (with oxygen) **energy production.** As long as your body can meet its energy demands in this oxygen-rich mode, it will not convert to anaerobic energy production. Thus fatigue will not be an important factor in determining whether you can continue to participate. Marathon runners, serious joggers, distance swimmers, bikers, and aerobic dancers can perform because of their highly developed aerobic fitness. The cardiorespiratory systems of these aerobically fit people take in, transport, and use oxygen in the most efficient manner possible.

Besides allowing you to participate in activities such as those mentioned, aerobic conditioning (cardiorespiratory endurance conditioning) may also provide certain structural and functional benefits that affect other dimensions of your life. These recognized benefits (see the Star Box on p. 69) have received considerable documented support. Some data, for example, strongly suggest that aerobic fitness can increase life expectancy[3] and reduce the risk of developing cancer of the colon, heart, uterus, cervix, and ovaries.[4]

Muscular Strength

Muscular strength is essential for your body to accomplish *work.* Your ability to maintain posture, walk, lift, push, and pull are familiar examples of the constant demands you make on your muscles to maintain or increase their level of *contraction.* The stronger you are, the greater your ability to contract muscles and maintain a level of contraction sufficient to complete tasks.

Muscular strength can best be improved by training activities that use the **overload principle.** By overloading, or gradually increasing the resistance (load, object, or weight) your muscles must move, you can increase your muscular strength. The following three types of training exercises are based on the overload principle.

In **isometric** (meaning "same measure") **exercises,** the resistance is so great that your contracting mus-

Structural and Functional Benefits of Cardiorespiratory (Aerobic) Fitness

Aerobic fitness can help you do the following:
- Complete and enjoy your daily activities
- Strengthen and increase the efficiency of your heart muscle
- Increase the proportion of high-density lipoproteins in your blood
- Increase the capillary network in your body
- Improve **collateral circulation**
- Control your weight
- Stimulate bone growth
- Cope with stressors
- Ward off infections
- Improve the efficiency of your other body systems
- Bolster your self-esteem
- Achieve self-directed fitness goals
- Reduce negative dependence behavior
- Sleep better
- Recover more quickly from common illnesses
- Meet people with similar interests
- Receive reduced insurance premiums

cles cannot move the resistant object at all. Thus your muscles contract against immovable objects, usually with increasingly greater efforts (Figure 4-1). Because of the difficulty of precisely evaluating the training effects, isometric exercises are not usually used as a primary means of developing muscular strength and can be dangerous for people with hypertension.

Progressive resistance exercises, also called *isotonic* or *same-tension* exercises, are currently the most popular type of strength-building exercises. Progressive resistance exercises include the use of traditional free weights (dumbbells and barbells), as well as Universal and Nautilus machines. People who perform progressive resistance exercises use various muscle groups to move (or lift) specific fixed resistances or weights. Although during a given repetitive exercise the weight resistance remains the same, the muscular contraction effort required varies according to the joint angles in the *range of motion*.[2] The greatest effort is required at the start and finish of the movement.

Isokinetic (meaning "same motion") **exercises** use mechanical devices that provide resistances that consistently overload muscles throughout the entire range of motion. The resistance will move only at a preset speed regardless of the force applied to it. For the exercise to be effective, a user must apply maximal force.[2] Isokinetic training requires elaborate, expensive equipment.

Thus the use of isokinetic equipment may be limited to certain athletic teams, diagnostic centers, or rehabilitation clinics. The most common isokinetic machines are Cybex, Orthotron, Mini-Gym, and Exergenie.

oxygen debt
The physical state that occurs when the body can no longer process and transport sufficient amounts of oxygen for continued muscle contraction.

anaerobic energy production
The body's means of energy production when the necessary amount of oxygen is not available.

aerobic energy production
The body's means of energy production when the respiratory and circulatory systems are able to process and transport a sufficient amount of oxygen to muscle cells.

collateral circulation
The ability of nearby blood vessels to enlarge and carry additional blood around a blocked blood vessel.

muscular strength
The ability to contract skeletal muscles to engage in work; the force that a muscle can exert.

overload principle
The principle whereby a person gradually increases the resistance load that must be moved or lifted; this principle also applies to other types of fitness training.

isometric exercises (eye so **met** rick)
Muscular strength training exercises in which the resistance is so great that the object cannot be moved.

progressive resistance exercises
Muscular strength training exercises in which traditional barbells and dumbbells with fixed resistances are used.

isokinetic exercises (**eye** so kin **et** ick)
Muscular strength training exercises in which machines are used to provide variable resistances throughout the full range of motion.

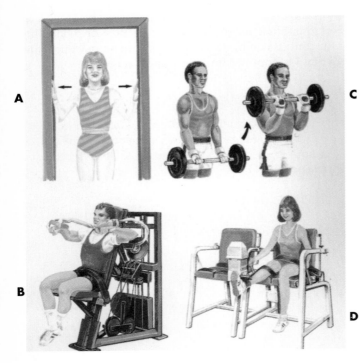

Figure 4-1 Three types of training exercises to improve muscular strength. **A,** Isometric exercise. **B** and **C,** Progressive resistance exercises. **D,** Isokinetic exercise. Exercise is important to the cardiorespiratory system at any age.

Which type of strength-building exercise (machines or free weights) is most effective? Take your choice, since all will help develop muscular strength. Some people prefer machines because they are simple to use, do not require stacking the weights, and are already balanced and less likely to drop and cause injury.

Other people prefer free weights because they encourage the user to work harder to maintain balance during the lift. In addition, free weights can be used in a greater variety of exercises than weight machines. Workouts with free weights are also associated with "tougher" images and sounds that some lifters prefer.

Muscular Endurance

Muscular endurance is a component of physical fitness associated with strength. When muscles contract and their individual muscle fibers shorten, energy is needed. Energy production requires that oxygen and nutrients be delivered by the circulatory system to the muscles. After these products are transformed into energy by individual muscle cells, the body must remove the potentially toxic waste by-products.

Amateur and professional athletes often wish to increase the endurance of specific muscle groups associated with their sports activities. This can be achieved by using exercises that gradually increase the number of repetitions of a given movement. However, muscular endurance is not the physiological equivalent of cardiorespiratory endurance. For example, a world-ranked distance runner with highly developed cardiorespiratory endurance and extensive muscular endurance of the legs may not have a corresponding level of muscular endurance of the abdominal muscles.

Flexibility

The ability of your joints to move through their natural range of motion is a measure of your **flexibility.** This fitness trait, like so many other aspects of structure and function, differs from point to point within your body and among different people. Not every joint in your body is equally flexible (by design), and over the course of time, use or disuse will alter the flexibility of a given joint. Certainly gender, age, genetically determined body build, and current level of physical fitness will affect your flexibility.

Inability to move easily during physical activity can be a constant reminder that aging and inactivity are the foes of flexibility. Failure to use joints regularly will quickly result in a loss of elasticity in the connective tissue and shortening of muscles associated with the joints. Benefits of flexibility include improved balance, posture, and athletic performance and reduced risk of low back pain.

As seen in young gymnasts, flexibility can be highly developed and maintained with a program of activity that includes regular stretching. Stretching also helps reduce the risk of injury. Athletic trainers generally prefer **static stretching** to **ballistic stretching** for people who wish to improve their range of motion. Guidelines for stretching are given in the Star Box on p. 71.

Body Composition

Body composition is the "makeup of the body in terms of muscle, bone, fat, and other elements."[2] Of particular interest to fitness experts are percentages of body fat and fat-free weight. Health experts are especially concerned about the large number of people in our society who are overweight and obese. Increasingly, cardiorespiratory fitness trainers are recognizing the importance of body composition and are including strength training exercises to help reduce

Static stretching can develop and maintain flexibility.

Guidelines for Static Stretching
Take the following precautions to reduce the possibility of injury during stretching:
- Warm up using a slow jog or fast walk before stretching.
- Stretch only to the point at which you feel tightness or resistance to your stretching. Stretching should not be painful.
- Be sure to continue normal breathing during a stretch. Do not hold your breath.
- Use caution when stretching muscles that surround painful joints. Pain is an indication that something is wrong—it should not be ignored.

body fat. (See Chapter 6 for further information about body composition, health effects of obesity, and weight management.)

AGING PHYSICALLY

With aging, physical decline will occur and the components of physical fitness become more difficult to maintain. From the fourth decade onward, a gradual decline in vigor and resistance eventually gives way to various types of illnesses. In the opinion of many authorities, people do not die of old age. Rather, old age worsens specific conditions responsible for death. However, physical decline can be slowed and the onset of illness delayed by staying physically active. The process of aging can be described on the basis of predictable occurrences[5]:

- *Change is gradual.* In aging, there are gradual changes in body structure or function that occur before specific health problems are identified.
- *Individual differences occur.* When two people of the same age are compared for the type and extent of change that has occurred with age, important differences can be noted. Even within the same person, different systems decline at differing rates and to varying extents.
- *Greatest change is noted in areas of complex function.* In physiological processes involving two or more major body systems, the most profound effects of physiological aging can be noted.

- *Homeostatic decline occurs with age.* Becoming older is associated with a growing difficulty in maintaining homeostasis (the dynamic balance among body systems). In the face of stressors the older adult's system takes longer to respond, does not respond with the same magnitude, and may take longer to return to baseline.

Like growth and development, aging is predictable yet unique for each person.

muscular endurance
The ability of a muscle or muscle group to function over time; supported by the respiratory and circulatory systems.

flexibility
The ability of joints to function through an intended range of motion.

static stretching
The slow lengthening of a muscle group to an extended stretch; followed by holding the extended position for a recommended period.

ballistic stretching
A "bouncing" form of stretching in which a muscle group is lengthened repetitively to produce multiple quick, forceful stretches.

Health Concerns of Midlife Adults

The period between 45 and 64 years of age brings with it a variety of subtle changes in the body's structure and function. When life is busy and the mind is active, these changes are generally not evident. Even when they become evident, they are not usually the source of profound concern. Your parents, older students in your class, and people with whom you will be working are, nevertheless, experiencing these changes[6]:

- Decrease in bone mass and density
- Increase in vertebral compression
- Degenerative changes in joint cartilage
- Increase in adipose tissue—loss of lean body mass
- Decrease in capacity to engage in physical work
- Decrease in visual acuity
- Decrease in basal energy requirements
- Decrease in fertility
- Decrease in sexual function

For some midlife adults these health concerns can be quite threatening, especially for those who view aging with apprehension and fear. Some middle-aged people reject these physical changes and convince themselves they are sick. Indeed, *hypochondriasis* is much more common among midlife people than among young people.

Osteoporosis

Osteoporosis is a condition frequently seen in late middle-aged women. However, it is not fully understood why white menopausal women are so susceptible to the increase in calcium loss that leads to fracture of the hip, wrist, and vertebral column. Well over 90% of all people with osteoporosis are white women.

The endocrine system plays a large role in the development of osteoporosis. At the time of menopause, a woman's ovaries begin a rapid decrease in the production of *estrogen,* one of two main hormones associated with the menstrual cycle. This lower level of estrogen may decrease the conversion of the precursors of vitamin D into the active form of vitamin D, the form necessary for absorbing calcium from the digestive tract. As a result, calcium may be drawn from the bones for use elsewhere in the body.

Additional explanations of osteoporosis focus on two other possibilities—*hyperparathyroidism* (another endocrine dysfunction) and the below-average degree of muscle development seen in osteoporotic women. In this latter explanation the reduced muscle mass is associated with decreased activity that in turn

deprives the body of the mechanical stimulation needed to facilitate bone growth.

Premenopausal women have the opportunity to build and maintain a healthy skeleton through an appropriate intake of calcium. Current recommendations are for an intake of 1200 mg of calcium per day. Three to four daily servings of low-fat dairy products should provide sufficient calcium. Adequate vitamin D must also be in the diet because it aids in the absorption of calcium.

Many women do not take in an adequate amount of calcium. Calcium supplements, again in combination with vitamin D, can be used to achieve recommended calcium levels. It is now known that calcium carbonate, a highly advertised form of calcium, is no more easily absorbed by the body than are other forms of calcium salts. Consumers of calcium supplements should compare brands to determine which, if any, they will buy.

In premenopausal women, calcium deposition in bone is facilitated by exercise, particularly exercise that involves movement of the extremities. Today, women are encouraged to consume at least the recommended servings from the milk group and engage in regular physical activity that involves the weight-bearing muscles of the legs, such as aerobics, jogging, or walking.

Postmenstrual women who are not elderly can markedly slow the resorption of calcium from their bones through the use of estrogen replacement therapy. When combined with a daily intake of 1500 mg of calcium, vitamin D, and regular exercise, estrogen therapy almost eliminates calcium loss. Of course, women will need to work closely with their physicians in monitoring the use of estrogen because of continuing concern over the role of estrogen replacement therapy and the development of breast cancer.

Osteoarthritis

Arthritis is an umbrella term for more than 100 forms of joint inflammation. The most common form is **osteoarthritis.** It is likely that as we age, all of us will develop osteoarthritis to some degree. Often called "wear and tear" arthritis, osteoarthritis occurs primarily in the weight-bearing joints of the knee, hip, and spine. In this form of arthritis, joint damage can occur to bone ends, cartilaginous cushions, and related structures as the years of constant friction and stress accumulate.

The object of current management of osteoarthritis (and other forms) is not to cure the disease but rather to reduce discomfort, limit joint destruction, and maximize joint mobility. Aspirin and nonsteroidal anti-inflammatory agents are the drugs most frequently used to treat osteoarthritis.

It is now believed that osteoarthritis develops most commonly in people with a genetic predisposition for excessive damage to the weight-bearing joints. Thus the condition seems to "run in families." Further, studies comparing the occurrence of osteoarthritis in those who exercise and those who do not demonstrate that regular movement activity may decrease the likelihood of developing this form of arthritis.

Health Concerns of Elderly Adults

In elderly people, it is frequently difficult to distinguish between changes caused by aging and those caused by disease. For virtually every body system, biomedical indexes for the old and young can overlap. In the respiratory system, for example, the oxygen uptake capacity of a man 70 years old may be no different from that of a man 55 years old who has a history of heavy cigarette smoking. Is the level in the elderly man to be considered an indicator of a disease, or should it be considered a reflection of normal old age? In dealing with the elderly, physicians frequently must make this kind of distinction.

In elderly people, as in midlife people, structural and physiological changes are routinely seen. In some cases, these are closely related to disease processes, but in most cases they reflect the gradual decline that is thought to be a result of the normal aging process. The most frequently seen changes include the following:

- Decrease in bone mass
- Changes in the structure of bone
- Decrease in muscle bulk and strength
- Decrease in oxygen uptake
- Loss of nonreproducing cells in the nervous system
- Decrease in hearing and vision abilities
- Decrease in all other sensory modalities, including the sense of body positioning
- Slower reaction time
- Gait and posture changes resulting from a weakening of the muscles of the trunk and legs

In addition to these changes, the most likely change seen in the elderly is the increased sensitivity of the body's homeostatic mechanism. Because of this sensitivity, a minor infection or superficial injury can be traumatic enough to decrease the body's ability to maintain its internal balance. An illness that would be easily controlled in a younger person could even prove fatal to a seemingly healthy 75-year-old person.

Continuing to follow a physical fitness plan throughout midlife and older adulthood is essential to minimizing age-related health problems. The plan should be modified as necessary to accommodate changes in physical functioning.

DEVELOPING A CARDIORESPIRATORY FITNESS PROGRAM

For people of all ages, cardiorespiratory conditioning can be achieved through many activities. As long as the activity you choose places sufficient demand on the heart and lungs, improved fitness is possible. In addition to the familiar activities of swimming, running, cycling, and aerobic dance, many people today are participating in brisk walking, rollerblading, cross-country skiing, swimnastics, skating, rowing, and even weight training (often combined with some form of aerobic activity). Regardless of age or physical limitations, you can select from a variety of enjoyable activities that will condition the cardiorespiratory system. Complete the Personal Assessment on pp. 74-75 to determine your level of fitness.

Many people think that any kind of physical activity will produce cardiorespiratory fitness. Golf, bowling, hunting, fishing, and archery are considered to be forms of exercise. However, these activities would generally fail to produce positive changes in your cardiorespiratory and overall muscular fitness; they may enhance your health, be enjoyable, and produce some fatigue after lengthy participation, but they do not meet the fitness standards recently established by the American College of Sports Medicine (ACSM), the nation's premier professional organization of exercise physiologists and sport physicians.[7]

The ACSM's most recent recommendations for achieving cardiorespiratory fitness were approved in 1990 and include five major areas: (1) mode of activity, (2) frequency of training, (3) intensity of training, (4)

osteoporosis
Loss of calcium from the bone, seen primarily in postmenopausal women.

osteoarthritis
Arthritis that develops with age; largely caused by weight bearing and deterioration of the joints.

PERSONAL ASSESSMENT

What Is Your Level of Fitness?

You can determine your level of fitness in 30 minutes or less by completing this short group of tests based on the National Fitness Test developed by the President's Council on Physical Fitness and Sports. If you are over 40 years old or have chronic medical disorders such as diabetes or obesity, check with your physician before taking this or any other fitness test. You will need another person to monitor your test and keep time.

Three-minute step test

Aerobic capacity. Equipment: 12-inch bench, crate, block, or step ladder; stopwatch. Procedure: face bench. Complete 24 full steps (both feet on the bench, both feet on the ground) per minute for 3 minutes. After finishing, sit down, have your partner find your pulse within 5 seconds, and take your pulse for 1 minute. Your score is your pulse rate for 1 full minute.

Scoring standards (heart rate for 1 minute)

Age	18-29		30-39		40-49		50-59		60+	
Gender	F	M	F	M	F	M	F	M	F	M
Excellent	<80	<75	<84	<78	<88	<80	<92	<85	<95	<90
Good	80-110	75-100	84-115	78-109	88-118	80-112	92-123	85-115	95-127	90-118
Average	>110	>100	>115	>109	>118	>112	>123	>115	>127	>118

Sit and reach

Hamstring flexibility. Equipment: yardstick; tape. Between your legs, tape the yardstick to the floor. Sit with legs straight and heels about 5 inches apart, heels even with the 15-inch mark on the yardstick. While in a sitting position, slowly stretch forward as far as possible. Your score is the number of inches reached.

Scoring standards (inches)

Age	18-29		30-39		40-49		50-59		60+	
Gender	F	M	F	M	F	M	F	M	F	M
Excellent	>22	>21	>22	>21	>21	>20	>20	>19	>20	>19
Good	17-22	13-21	17-22	13-21	15-21	13-20	14-20	12-19	14-20	12-19
Average	<17	<13	<17	<13	<15	<13	<14	<12	<14	<12

Arm hang

Upper body strength. Equipment: horizontal bar (high enough to prevent your feet from touching the floor); stopwatch. Procedure: hang with straight arms, palms facing forward. Start watch when subject is in position. Stop when subject lets go. Your score is the number of minutes and seconds spent hanging.

Scoring standards (heart rate for 1 minute)

Age	18-29		30-39		40-49		50-59		60+	
Gender	F	M	F	M	F	M	F	M	F	M
Excellent	>1:30	>2:00	>1:20	>1:50	>1:10	>1:35	>1:00	>1:20	>:50	>1:10
Good	:46-1:30	1:00-2:00	:40-1:20	:50-1:50	:30-1:10	:45-1:35	:30-1:00	:35-1:20	:21-:50	:30-1:10
Average	<:46	<1:00	<:40	<:50	<:30	<:45	<:30	<:35	<:21	<:30

Curl-ups

Abdominal and low back strength. Equipment: stopwatch. Procedure: Lie flat on upper back, knees bent, shoulders touching the floor, arms extended above your thighs or by your sides, palms down. Bend knees so that feet are flat and 12 inches from the buttocks. Curl up by lifting head and shoulders off the floor, sliding hands forward above your thighs or the floor. Curl down and repeat. Your score is the number of curl-ups in 1 minute.

Scoring standards (number in 1 minute)

Age	18-29		30-39		40-49		50-59		60+	
Gender	F	M	F	M	F	M	F	M	F	M
Excellent	>45	>50	>40	>45	>35	>40	>30	>35	>25	>30
Good	25-45	30-50	20-40	22-45	16-35	21-40	12-30	18-35	11-25	15-30
Average	<25	<30	<20	<22	<16	<21	<12	<18	<11	<15

Push-ups (men)

Upper body strength. Equipment: stopwatch. Assume a front-leaning position. Lower your body until chest touches the floor. Raise and repeat for 1 minute. Your score is the number of push-ups completed in 1 minute.

Scoring standards (number in 1 minute)

Age	18-29	30-39	40-49	50-59	60+
Excellent	>50	>45	>40	>35	>30
Good	25-50	22-45	19-40	15-35	10-30
Average	<25	<22	<19	<15	<10

Modified Push-ups (women)

Upper body strength. Equipment: stopwatch. Assume a front-leaning position with knees bent up, hands under shoulders. Lower your chest to the floor, raise, and repeat. Your score is the number of push-ups completed in 1 minute.

Scoring standards (number in 1 minute)

Age	18-29	30-39	40-49	50-59	60+
Excellent	>45	>40	>35	>30	>25
Good	17-45	12-40	8-35	6-30	5-25
Average	<17	<12	<8	<6	<5

To carry this further . . .

Note your areas of strengths and weaknesses. To improve your fitness, become involved in a fitness program that reflects the concepts discussed in this chapter. Talking with fitness experts on your campus might be a good first step. ☑

duration of training, and (5) resistance training. We summarize these recommendations. You may wish to compare your existing fitness program with these standards.

Mode of Activity

The ACSM recommends that the mode of activity be any continuous physical activity that uses large muscle groups and can be rhythmic and aerobic in nature. Among the activities that generally meet this requirement are continuous swimming, cycling, aerobics, basketball, cross-country skiing, rollerblading, step training (bench aerobics), hiking, walking, rowing, stair climbing, dancing, and running. Recently, water exercise (water or aqua aerobics) has become a popular fitness mode, since it is especially effective for pregnant women and elderly, injured, or disabled people.[8] (The Focus Box on p. 90 provides more information about exercise during pregnancy.)

Endurance games and activities, such as tennis, racquetball, and handball, are fine as long as you and your partner are skilled enough to keep the ball in play; walking after the ball will do very little for you. Riding a bicycle is a good activity if you keep pedaling. Coasting will do little to improve fitness. Softball and football are generally less than sufficient continuous activities—especially the way they are played by weekend athletes.

Regardless of which continuous activity you select, it should also be enjoyable. Running, for example, is not for everyone—despite what some accomplished runners say! Find an activity you enjoy. If you need others around you to have a good time, corral a group of friends to join you. Vary your activities to keep from becoming bored. You might cycle in the summer, run in the fall, swim in the winter, and play racquetball in the spring. To help you maintain your fitness program, see the suggestions in the Health Action Guide at right.

Frequency of Training

Frequency of training refers to the number of times per week a person should exercise. The ACSM recommends three to five times per week. For most people, participation in fitness activities more than five times each week does not significantly improve their level of conditioning. Likewise, an average of only two workouts each week does not seem to produce a measureable improvement in cardiorespiratory conditioning. Thus, although you may have a lot

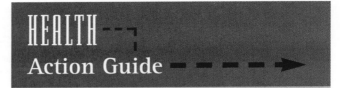

HEALTH
Action Guide

Tips to Help You Stick to Your Exercise Program

Sometimes it seems difficult to continue an exercise program. Here are a few tips to keep you going:
- Fit your program into your daily lifestyle
- Exercise with your friends
- Incorporate music into your activity
- Vary your activities frequently; crosstrain
- Reward yourself when you reach a fitness goal
- Avoid a complicated exercise program; keep it simple
- Measure your improvement by keeping a log or diary
- Take some time off to rest and recuperate
- Keep in mind how important physical activity is to your life and health

of fun cycling twice each week, do not expect to see a significant improvement in your cardiorespiratory fitness level.

Intensity of Training

How much effort should you put into an activity? Should you run quickly, jog slowly, or swim at a comfortable pace? Must a person sweat profusely to become fit? These questions all refer to **intensity** of effort.

The ACSM recommends that healthy adults exercise at an intensity level of between 60% and 90% of their maximum heart rate (calculated by subtracting your age from 220). This level of intensity is called the **target heart rate (THR).** This rate refers to the minimum number of times your heart needs to contract (beat) each minute to have a positive effect on your heart, lungs, and blood vessels. This improvement is called the *training effect.* Intensity of activity below the THR will be insufficient to make a significant improvement in your fitness level. Although intensity below the THR will still help you expend calories and thus lose weight, it will probably do little to make you more aerobically fit. On the other hand, intensity that is significantly above your THR will probably cause you to become so fatigued that you will be forced to stop the activity before the training effect can be achieved.

Choosing a particular THR between 60% and 90% of your maximum heart rate depends on your initial level of fitness. If you are already in relatively good physical shape, you might want to start exercising at 75% of your maximum heart rate. A well-conditioned person might select a higher THR for his or her intensity level, whereas a person with a low fitness level will still be able to achieve a training effect at the lower THR of 60% of maximum.

In the Star Box at right, the younger person would need to participate in a continuous activity for an extended period while working at a THR of 160 beats per minute. The older person would need to function at a THR of 117 beats per minute to achieve a positive training effect.

Determining your heart rate is not a complicated procedure. Find a location on your body where an artery passes near the surface of the skin. Pulse rates are difficult to determine by touching veins, which are more superficial than arteries. Two easily accessible sites for determining heart rate are the *carotid artery* (one on either side of the windpipe at the front of your neck) and the *radial artery* (on the inside of your wrist, just above the base of the thumb).

You should practice placing the front surface of your index and middle fingertips at either of these locations and feeling for a pulse. Once you have found a regular pulse, look at the second hand of a watch. Count the number of beats you feel in a 10-second period. Multiply this number by 6. This number is your heart rate. With a little practice, you can become very proficient at determining your heart rate.

Duration of Training

The ACSM recommends that the **duration** of training be between 20 and 60 minutes of continuous aerobic activity. Generally speaking, the duration can be on the shorter end of this range for athletic people whose activities use a high intensity of training (80% to 90% of maximum heart rate). Those who choose activities with a low range of intensity (60% to 70% of maximum heart rate) should maintain that activity for a longer time. Thus a fast jog and a moderate walk will require different lengths of time to accomplish the training effect. The fast jog might be maintained for 25 minutes, whereas the brisk walk should be kept up longer—perhaps for 50 minutes. Recently, however, some fitness experts have advocated a modified version of the ACSM's recommendations to accommodate less directed physical activity. See the Star Box on p. 78 for a more detailed discussion.

How to Calculate Your Target Heart Rate
The target heart rate (THR) is the recommended rate for increasing cardiorespiratory endurance. To maintain a training effect, you must sustain activity at your THR. To calculate your THR, subtract your age from 220 (the maximum heart rate) and multiply by .60 to .90. Here are two examples:

For a 20-year-old person who wants a THR of 80% of maximum
Maximum heart rate:
$220 - 20 = 200$
$200 \times .80 = 160$
THR = 160 beats per minute

For a 40-year-old person who wants a THR of 65% of maximum
Maximum heart rate:
$220 - 40 = 180$
$180 \times .65 = 117$
THR = 117 beats per minute

Muscular strength is an important component of physical fitness.

frequency
The number of times per week one should exercise to achieve a training effect.

intensity
The level of effort put into an activity.

target heart rate (THR)
The number of times per minute the heart must contract to produce a training effect.

duration
The length of time one needs to exercise at the THR to produce a training effect.

Resistance Training

Recognizing the important fact that overall body fitness includes muscular fitness, the ACSM now recommends resistance training in its current standards. The ACSM suggests participation in strength training of moderate intensity at least two times a week. This training should help develop and maintain a healthy body composition—one with an emphasis on lean body mass. The goal of resistance training is not to improve cardiorespiratory endurance but to improve overall muscle strength and tone. For the average person, resistance training with heavy weights is not recommended because it can induce a sudden and dangerous increase in blood pressure. See the Health Action Guide on p. 79 for safety precautions to observe during strength training.

The resistance training recommended by the ACSM includes one set of 8 to 12 repetitions of 8 to 10 different exercises. These exercises should be geared to the body's major muscle groups (that is, legs, arms, shoulders, trunk, and back) and should not focus on just one or two body areas. Isotonic (progressive resistance) or isokinetic exercises are recommended (see p. 69). For the average person, resistance training activities should be done at a moderate-to-slow speed, use the full range of motion, and not impair normal breathing. With just one set recommended for each exercise, resistance training is not very time consuming.

Warm-up, Workout, Cooldown

Each training session consists of three basic parts: the warm-up, the workout, and the cooldown.[2] The warm-up should last 10 to 15 minutes. During this period, you should begin slow, gradual, comfortable movements related to the upcoming activity, such as walking or slow jogging. All body segments and muscle groups should be exercised as you gradually increase your heart rate. Near the end of the warm-up period, the major muscle groups should be stretched. This preparation helps protect you from muscle strains and joint sprains.

The warm-up is a fine time to socialize. Furthermore, you can mentally prepare yourself for your activity or think about the beauty of the morning sky, the changing colors of the leaves, or the friends you will meet later in the day. Mental warm-ups can be as beneficial for you psychologically as physical warm-ups are physiologically.

The second part of the training session is the workout, the part of the session that involves improving muscular strength and endurance, cardiorespiratory

A Revised Approach to Fitness?

A number of health professionals have recently begun to urge the American public to consider the health benefits of less directed physical activity than that prescribed by the American College of Sports Medicine. These fitness experts believe that people shy away from physical activity because they are afraid that a fitness program requires too much effort and commitment.

One key aspect of this revised approach is the belief that the 20 to 60 minutes of daily physical activity does not have to be accomplished all at once. People can accumulate their minutes in segments over the course of the day. For example, raking leaves for 15 minutes, walking briskly for 10 minutes at lunch, and dancing for 10 minutes can produce health benefits if done on most days.

Opponents of this "kinder, gentler" approach to fitness are concerned that people who already exercise regularly may slack off and actually reduce their current fitness levels. Opponents also believe that, without a prescription for exercise, the public will fool itself into thinking it is much more active than it really is.

Which approach would be better for you? Do you wish to follow prescribed fitness guidelines, such as those given by the ACSM? Or do you believe that a lifestyle that incorporates short-term fitness activities throughout the day is a better approach for you?

endurance, and flexibility. Workouts can be tailor-made, but they should follow the ACSM guidelines discussed previously in this chapter.

The third important part of each fitness session, the cooldown, consists of a 5- to 10-minute session of relaxing exercises, such as slow jogging, walking, and stretching.[9] This activity allows your body to cool and return to a resting state. A cooldown period helps reduce muscle soreness.

Exercise for Older Adults

An exercise program designed for younger adults may be inappropriate for older people, particularly those over age 50. Special attention must be paid to matching the program to the interests and abilities of the participants. The goals of the program should include both social interaction and physical conditioning.

Older adults, especially those with a personal or family history of heart problems, should have a physical examination before starting a fitness program.

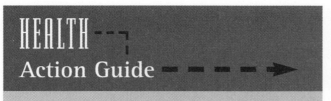

Safety Precautions for Strength Training

To avoid injury during strength training exercises, you should observe the following safety precautions:
- Warm up appropriately
- Use proper lifting techniques
- Always have a spotter if you are using free weights
- Do not hold your breath during a lift
- Avoid single lifts of very heavy weights
- Before using a machine (such as Nautilus, Universal, or Cybex), be certain you know how to use it correctly
- Seek advice for training programs from properly licensed or certified experts
- Work within your limitations; avoid "showing off"

This examination should include a stress cardiogram,[10] a blood pressure check, and an evaluation of joint functioning. Participants should learn how to monitor their own cardiorespiratory status during exercise.

Well-designed fitness programs for older adults will include activities that begin slowly, are monitored frequently, and are geared to the enjoyment of the participants. The professional staff coordinating the program should be familiar with the signs of distress (excessively elevated heart rate, nausea, breathing difficulty, pallor, and pain) and must be able to perform CPR. Warm-up and cooldown periods should be included. Activities to increase flexibility are beneficial in the beginning and ending segments of the program. Participants should wear comfortable clothing and appropriate shoes and should be mentally prepared to enjoy the activities.

A program designed for older adults will largely conform to the ACSM criteria specified previously in this chapter. However, except for certain very fit older adults (such as runners and triathletes), the THR should not exceed 120 beats per minute. Also, because of possible joint, muscular, or skeletal problems, certain activities may have to be done in a sitting position. Pain or discomfort should be reported immediately to the fitness instructor.

Fortunately, properly screened older adults will rarely have health emergencies during a well-monitored fitness program. Like their youthful counterparts, many older adults find fitness programs socially enjoyable, physically beneficial, and—occasionally—addictive.

Low Back Pain

A common occurrence among adults is the sudden onset of low back pain. Each year, 10 million adults develop this condition, which can be so uncomfortable that they miss work, lose sleep, and generally feel incapable of engaging in daily activities. Eighty percent of all adults who have this condition will experience these effects two to three times per year.

Although low back pain can reflect serious health problems, most low back pain is caused by mechanical (postural) problems. As unpleasant as low back pain is, the problem usually corrects itself within a week or two. The services of a physician, physical therapist, or chiropractor are not generally required after an initial visit.

By engaging in regular exercise, such as swimming, walking, and bicycling, and by paying attention to your back during bending, lifting, and sitting, you can minimize the occurrence of this uncomfortable and incapacitating condition.

FITNESS QUESTIONS AND ANSWERS

Along with the five necessary elements to include in your fitness program, you should consider many additional issues when you start a fitness program.

Should I See My Doctor Before I Get Started?

This issue has probably kept thousands of people from ever beginning a fitness program. The hassle and expense of getting a comprehensive physical examination is an excellent alibi for people who are not completely sold on the idea of exercise. A complete examination, including *blood analysis, stress test, cardiogram, serum lipid analysis,* and *body fat analysis,* is a valuable tool for developing some baseline physical data for your medical record.

Is this examination really necessary? Most exercise physiologists do not think so. The value of these measurements as safety predictors is questioned by many professionals. A good rule of thumb to follow is to

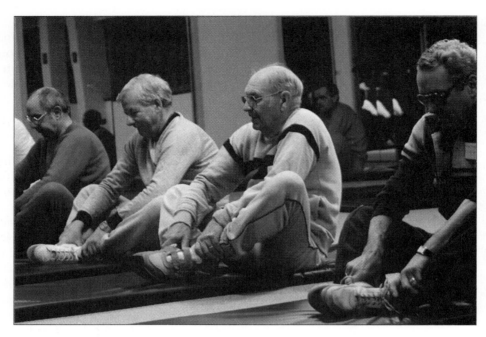

Exercise is important to maintain health at any age.

undergo a physical examination if (1) you have an existing medical condition (for example, diabetes, obesity, hypertension, heart abnormalities, or arthritis), (2) you are age 30 or over and have not pursued vigorous activity for at least 5 years, or (3) you smoke.

How Important Is Breast Support for Female Exercisers?

Because of the vigorous up-and-down and lateral breast movement that can occur with jumping and running activities, it is important that women wear bras that fully support their breasts. This is especially important for large-breasted women. A good support bra can reduce discomfort and distraction during physical activity. Also, adequate support reduces damage to the Cooper's ligaments. Damage to these ligaments can cause premature sagging of the breasts.

Another problem that female exercisers may face is a condition called *runner's nipples.* This is an abrasion caused by the constant friction from the jogger's shirt. A good bra prevents this, as well as a condition called *bicyclist's nipples,* in which the nipples become painful because of the combination of sweat evaporation and wind chill.[9]

Researchers believe that the characteristics of the ideal sports bra depend on a woman's weight and breast size, her physical activity, and what feels comfortable.

Sports bras should be made with (a) a material that is breathable, (b) minimal amounts of elastic, (c) no seams directly over the nipple area, (d) comfortable support under the breasts that prevents the bra from rising during activity, and (e) nonelastic straps that prevent the shoulder straps from slipping off during activity.

How Beneficial Is Aerobic Exercise?

One of the most popular fitness approaches is aerobic exercise, including aerobic dancing. Many organizations sponsor classes in this form of continuous dancing and movement. The rise in popularity of televised and videotaped aerobic exercise programs reflects the enthusiasm for this form of exercise. Because extravagant claims are often made about the value of these programs, the wise consumer should observe at least one session of the activity before enrolling. Discover for yourself whether the program meets the criteria outlined previously in this chapter: mode of activity, frequency, intensity, duration, and resistance training.

Street dancing is fast becoming one of the most popular aerobic exercises. Popularized by rap music, classic funk, and the growth of vigorous "street jam" dancing in music videos, street dancing is an excellent way of having fun and developing cardiorespiratory fitness. Have you experienced the exhilaration that results from an hour or two of dancing?

LEARNING from ALL CULTURES

Staying Fit

It is not uncommon in the United States for men and women to take time out of their day to go to an aerobics class, jog for several miles, or play a few games of racquetball. This practice is not unique to Americans. The people of Japan are also beginning to show a greater interest in fitness and sport, and commercialized sports facilities are rapidly developing. Japanese women, especially, are now participating in fitness activities. Many women who do not work outside the home participate in activities such as aerobic exercise, jazzercise, yoga, and Chinese martial arts; these activities are taught through programs at the sports centers.[14]

In China, commercialized sports centers do not exist, but there is an emphasis on physical fitness and sport. This emphasis comes from the government. For students in primary and secondary school, two physical education classes are required per week, each 50 minutes long. For adult workers, participation in exercise is also encouraged. In offices and factories, employees take 10-minute exercise breaks in the mornings and afternoons. Physical activities may include calisthenics and even eye exercises.[15]

Fitness seems to have gained popularity because many people recognize its benefits. However, one German visitor observed that many Americans get in their cars and drive to their fitness clubs, exercise, and then drive back to work or home. Merely walking to their destinations and forgetting the club seemed to make more sense to him!

Knowing how important fitness is to good health, think about your own daily routine. What kinds of exercise and activities do you participate in to enhance your fitness?

What Are Low-Impact Aerobic Activities?

Because long-term participation in some aerobic activities (for example, jogging, running, aerobic dancing, and rope skipping) may damage the hip, knee, and ankle joints, many fitness experts promote low-impact aerobic activities. Low-impact aerobic dancing, water aerobics, bench aerobics, and brisk walking are examples of this kind of fitness activity. Participants still conform to the principal components of a cardiorespiratory fitness program. THR levels are the same as in high-impact aerobic activities.

The main difference between low-impact and high-impact aerobic activities is the use of the legs. Low-impact aerobics do not require having both feet off the ground at the same time. Thus weight transfer does not occur with the forcefulness seen in traditional, high-impact aerobic activities. In addition, low-impact activities may include exaggerated arm movements and the use of hand or wrist weights. All of these variations are designed to increase the heart rate to the THR without damaging the joints of the lower extremities. Low-impact aerobics are excellent for people of all ages, and they may be especially beneficial to older adults.

In-line skating (rollerblading) is one of the fastest-growing participant fitness activities. This low-impact activity has cardiorespiratory and muscular benefits similar to those of running without the pounding effect that running can produce. Rollerblading requires important safety equipment: sturdy skates, knee and elbow pads, wrist supports, and a helmet.

What Is the Most Effective Means of Fluid Replacement During Exercise?

Despite all the advertising hype associated with commercial fluid replacement products, for an average person involved in typical fitness activities, water is still the best fluid replacement. The availability and cost are unbeatable. However, when activity is prolonged and intense, commercial sport drinks may be preferable to water because they contain electrolytes (which replace lost sodium and potassium) and carbohydrates (which replace depleted energy stores).[11] However, the carbohydrates in sports drinks are actually simple forms of sugar. Thus sports drinks tend to be high in calories just like regular soft drinks. Regardless of the drink you choose, exercise physiologists recommend that you drink fluids before and at frequent intervals throughout the activity.

What Effect Does Alcohol Have on Sport Performance?

It probably comes as no surprise that alcohol use is generally detrimental to sport performance. Alcohol consumption, especially excessive intake the evening before a performance, consistently decreases the level of performance. Many research studies have documented the negative effects of alcohol on activities involving speed, strength, power, and endurance.[12]

Lowered performance appears to be related to a variety of factors, including impaired judgment, reduced coordination, depressed heart function, liver interference, and dehydration. Understandably, sports federations within the International Olympic Committee have banned the use of alcohol in conjunction with sports competition.

Only in the sports of precision shooting (pistol shooting, riflery, and archery) have studies shown that low-level alcohol use may improve performance, by reducing the shooter's anxiety and permitting steady hand movements. However, alcohol use has also been banned from these sports.[12] Weapons and alcohol do not mix.

Why Has Bodybuilding Become So Popular?

It is true that the popularity of *bodybuilding* has increased significantly in recent years. There are many reasons for this growth. Bodybuilders often start lifting weights to get into better shape—to improve muscle tone. They may just want to look healthier and feel stronger. Once they realize that they can alter the shape of their bodies, they find that bodybuilding offers challenges that, through hard work, are attainable. Bodybuilders also report enjoying the physical sensations (the "pump") that result from a good workout. The results of their efforts are clearly visible and measurable. Some bodybuilders become involved in competitive events to test their advancements.

Perhaps we should dispel a few myths about bodybuilding. Are bodybuilders strong? The answer is emphatically—yes! Will muscle cells turn into fat cells if weightlifting programs are discontinued? *No,* muscle cells are physiologically incapable of turning into fat cells. Will women develop bulky muscles through weight training? *No,* they can improve muscle strength and tone, but unless they take steroids, their muscle mass cannot increase like men's muscle mass. Is bodybuilding socially acceptable? *Yes,* for many people. Just observe all the health clubs that cater to weightlifters and bodybuilders. Can strength training improve heart functioning? *Yes,* cardiovascular im-

Bodybuilding improves muscle tone and makes you look healthier and feel stronger.

provement has been seen among people who lift weights, especially those who use light weights repetitively.

Where Can I Find Out about Proper Equipment?

College students are generally in an excellent setting to locate people who have the resources to provide helpful information about sports equipment. Contacting physical education or health education faculty members who have an interest in your chosen activity might be a good start. Most colleges also have a number of clubs that specialize in fitness interests—cycling, hiking, and jogging clubs, for example. Attend one of their upcoming meetings.

Sporting goods and specialty stores (for runners, tennis and racquetball players, and cyclists) are convenient places to obtain information. Employees of these stores are usually knowledgable about sports and equipment (see the Star Box on pp. 85-86).

How Worthwhile Are Commercial Health and Fitness Clubs?

The health and fitness club business is booming. Fitness clubs offer activities ranging from free weights to weight machines to step walking to general aerobics. Some clubs have saunas and whirlpools and lots of frills. Others have course offerings that include wellness, smoking cessation, stress management, time management, dance, and yoga. The atmosphere at most clubs is friendly, and people are encouraged to have a good time while working out.

If your purpose in joining a fitness club is to improve your cardiorespiratory fitness, measure the program offered by the club against the ACSM standards. If your primary purpose in joining is to meet people and have fun, request a trial membership for a month or so to see whether you like the environment.

Before signing a contract at a health club or spa, do some careful questioning. Find out when the business was established, ask about the qualifications of the employees, contact some members for their observations, and request a thorough tour of the facilities. You might even consult your local Better Business Bureau for additional information. Finally, make certain that you read and understand every word of the contract.

What Is Crosstraining?

Crosstraining is the use of more than one aerobic activity to achieve cardiorespiratory fitness. For example, runners may use swimming, cycling, or rowing periodically to replace running in their training routines. Crosstraining allows certain muscle groups to rest and injuries to heal. Also, crosstraining provides a refreshing change of pace for the participant. You will probably enjoy your fitness program more if you vary the activities. Further, your enjoyment will make it more likely that the Healthy People 2000 Objectives can be reached.

What Are Steroids and Why Do Some Athletes Use Them?

Steroids are drugs that can be legally prescribed by physicians for a variety of health conditions, including certain forms of anemia, inadequate growth patterns, and chronic debilitating diseases. Steroids can also be prescribed to aid recovery from surgery or burns. **Anabolic steroids** are drugs that function like the male sex hormone *testosterone*.[13] They can be taken orally or by injection.

Anabolic steroids are used by athletes who hope to gain weight, muscular size and strength, power, endurance, and aggressiveness. Over the last few decades, many bodybuilders, weightlifters, track athletes, and football players have chosen to ignore the serious health risks posed by illegal steroid use.

The use of steroids is highly dangerous because of serious, life-threatening side effects and adverse reac-

tions. These effects include heart problems, certain forms of cancer, liver complications, and even psychological disturbances. The side effects on female steroid users are as dangerous as those on men. Figure 4-2 shows the adverse effects of steroid use.

Steroid users have developed a terminology of their own. Anabolic steroids are called "roids" or "juice." "Roid rage" is an aggressive, psychotic response to chronic steroid use. "Stacking" is a term that describes the use of multiple steroids at the same time.

Many organizations that control athletic competition (for example, the National Collegiate Athletic Association [NCAA], The Athletics Congress, the National Football League, and the International Olympic Committee) have banned steroids and are testing athletes for illegal use. The death of professional football player Lyle Alzado highlighted the serious threat posed by steroid use. Fortunately, athletes finally seem to be getting the message and are steering clear of steroids.

Are Today's Children Physically Fit?

Major research studies published during the last 10 years have indicated that U.S. children and teenagers lead very sedentary lives. Children ages 6 to 17 score extremely poorly in the areas of strength, flexibility, and cardiorespiratory endurance. In many cases, parents are in better shape than their children.

This information presents a challenge to educators and parents to emphasize the need for strenuous play activity. Television watching and parental inactivity were implicated as major reasons in these studies. For students reading this text who are parents or grandparents of young children, what can you do to encourage more physical activity and less sedentary activity?

How Does Sleep Contribute to Overall Fitness?

Although sleep may seem to be the opposite of exercise, it is an important adjunct to a well-planned exercise program (see the Star Box on p. 87). Sleep is so vital to health that people who are unable to sleep sufficiently (those with insomnia) or who are de-

> **anabolic steroids** (ann uh **bol** ick)
> Drugs that function like testosterone to produce increases in weight, strength, endurance, and aggressiveness.

Brain
Increased hostility can lead to tranquilizer use, hypertension, psychological dependence, and eating compulsions; increases aggression, which makes injuries more probable

Face
Facial hair growth, body hair growth, and baldness in women; acne in both men and women

Throat
Deepening of voice in women

Chest
Breast growth in men; breast cancer and decreased breast size in women

Heart
High blood pressure, clogging of arteries

Liver and prostate
Liver cancer in men and women; prostate cancer in men

Genitals
Sterility or atrophied testicles in men; menstrual irregularities, enlarged genitals in women

Arms, chest, and legs
Helps stimulate muscle growth, decreases recovery time needed between workouts

Figure 4-2   Adverse effects of steroids on various parts of the body.

Choosing an Athletic Shoe

Aerobic Shoes

When selecting shoes for aerobic dancing, J. Lynn Reese, president of J. Lynn & Co. Endurance Sports, Washington, DC, advises the following:

- Check the width of the shoe at the widest part of your foot. The bottom of the shoe should be as wide as the bottom of your foot; the uppers shouldn't go over the sides.
- Look for leather or nylon uppers. Leather is durable and gives good support, but it can stretch. Nylon won't stretch and gives support, but it's not as durable. Canvas generally doesn't offer much support.
- Look for rubber rather than polyurethane or black carbon rubber soles. Treads should be fairly flat in the forefoot. If you dance on carpet, you can go with less tread; if you dance on gym floors, you may need more grab.

Court Shoes

What's most important when choosing a tennis shoe? Jack Groppel, technical editor of *World Tennis* magazine and associate professor of bioengineering, University of Illinois, offers this list:

- Cushioning. Cushioning is especially important in the heel counter.
- Side support. Side support, also called *lateral* and *medial* support, is also important.
- Back-of-heel fit. Try on the shoe, and then put your little finger in behind the heel. It should fit snugly.
- Toe box (top front of shoe). Make sure the toe box isn't too tight or too loose.
- Traction. Keep in mind the surface you play on most often. Rubber gives better traction than synthetic materials, such as polyurethane, but is less durable.

When buying shoes for racquetball, Doug Richie, podiatrist, Seal Beach, California, advises the following:

- Choose side-to-side support over flexibility and cushioning.
- Choose a heavy shoe with lots of support.
- The tread should be relatively smooth—compatible with hardwood surfaces.
- Choose the brushed cotton jersey sock worn over terry liners.

Running Shoes

Need new running shoes? Here's advice from Jeff Galloway, former Olympic runner and founder and president of Phidippides International aerobic sports stores, headquartered in Atlanta.

- Take time to shop, and find a knowledgeable salesperson. Good advice is crucial.
- Check the wear pattern on your old shoes to see whether you have floppy or rigid feet. Floppy-footed runners wear out their soles on the outside and inside edges; rigid-footed runners wear out soles predominantly on the outside edges. Floppy-footed runners can sacrifice cushioning for support; rigid-footed runners can sacrifice support for cushioning.
- Know whether your feet are curved or straight and whether you have high arches or are flatfooted. The shoe should fit the shape of your foot.

Aerobic Shoes

Flexibility:
More at ball of foot than running shoes; less flexible than court shoes or running shoes; sole is firmer than running shoes

Uppers:
Most are leather or leather-reinforced nylon

Heel:
Little or no flare

Soles:
Rubber if you dance on wood floors; polyurethane for other surfaces

Cushioning:
More than court shoes; less than running shoes

Tread:
Should be fairly flat, especially on forefoot; may also have "dot" on the ball of the foot for pivoting

Continued

Court Shoes

Soles:
For tennis, flat; usually polyurethane—more durable for tennis courts; for racquetball, rounded (to allow for quicker side-to-side movement); usually rubber—less durable because wood courts are slicker and don't wear down shoes as fast

Flexibility:
Flexible at ball of foot

Cushioning:
Less than running shoes

Heel:
Not flared (flared heels reduce side-to-side support)

Tread:
Much flatter than running shoes; may have tread pattern designed around ball of foot where the foot pivots

Uppers:
Usually nylon mesh or nylon; leather; no canvas

Running Shoes

Heel:
Flare gives foot broader, more stable base

Soles:
Usually carbon-based for longer wear

Cushioning:
More than court shoes, especially at heel

Tread:
"Waffle" or other deep-cut tread for grip on many surfaces

prived of sleep experience deterioration in every dimension of their health. Fortunately, exercise is frequently associated with improvement in sleeping.

The value of sleep is apparent in a variety of positive changes in the body. Dreaming is thought to play an important role in supporting the emotional dimension of health. Problem-solving scenarios that occur during dreams seem to afford some carryover value in actual coping experiences. A variety of changes in physiological functioning, particularly a deceleration of the cardiovascular system, occur while you sleep. The feeling of being well rested is an expression of the mental and physiological rejuvenation you feel after a good night's sleep.

The amount of sleep needed varies among people. In fact, for any person, sleep needs vary according to activity level and overall state of health. As we age, the need for sleep appears to decrease from the 6 to 8 hours young adults require. Elderly people routinely sleep less than they did when they were younger. This decrease may be offset by the short naps older people often take during the day. For all people, however, periods of relaxation, daydreaming, and even an occasional afternoon nap promote electrical activity patterns that help regenerate the mind and body (see the Health Action Guide on p. 87).

What Exercise Danger Signs Should I Watch For?

The human body is an amazing piece of equipment. It functions well whether or not you are conscious of its processes. It also delivers clear signals when something goes wrong.

You should monitor any sign that seems abnormal during or after your exercise. "Listen to your body" is a good rule for self-awareness. The Star Box on p. 87 lists some common warning signs to monitor.

However, such occurrences are extremely unusual. Fear of developing these difficulties should not deter you from starting a fitness program. These risks are minimal—and the benefits far outweigh the risks.

Activities to Promote Sound Sleep

Can we work at being better sleepers? The answer is yes. There are many activities that when done at the appropriate time will aid you in your quest for sound sleep.

Activities for the Day

Schedule. Maintain a consistent schedule of daily activities; a disrupted day makes sleeping difficult.

Physical activity. Regular vigorous activity promotes sleep; exercising too near bedtime, however, can make you too energized to sleep soundly.

Eating. A large meal taken late in the evening interferes with sleeping; avoid heavy late-night snacks as well.

Alcohol use. A single drink in the evening may be relaxing, but too many drinks during the day can make sleeping difficult.

Central nervous system (CNS) stimulants. Coffee, tea, soft drinks with caffeine, and some medications can disrupt normal sleeping patterns.

Worry. Problems and concerns should be put behind you by the time you retire for the night; practice leaving your concerns at the office or in the classroom.

Rituals. A ritualistic "winding down" over the course of the evening promotes sleep; watching television, listening to music, and reading during the evening are excellent ways to prepare the body for sleep.

Activities for the End of the Day

Bathing. For many people, a warm bath immediately before retiring promotes sleep.

Yoga. The quiet, relaxing exercises of yoga promote sleep by slowing the body's activity level.

Snack or nightcap. A light snack of foods high in L-tryptophan (for example, eggs, tuna, and turkey) and a glass of milk will help you fall asleep.

Muscular relaxation. Alternating contraction and relaxation of the large muscles of the extremities aids the body in falling asleep.

Imaging. Quieting images can distract the mind, thus allowing you to fall asleep more easily.

Fantasies. Escaping into fantasies slows the mind and encourages the onset of sleep.

Breathing. Slow, deep breaths set a restful rhythm the body can "ride" into sleep.

Thinking. By envisioning yourself as sleeping soundly, you may actually fall asleep quicker.

HEALTH
Action Guide

The Power Nap

College students rarely get the amount of sleep they really need. This may be especially true for older students who are the parents of young children and students who are involved in many extracurricular activities, such as student government or athletics. College students should aim for 8 to 10 hours of sleep each night. If this amount of sleep cannot be achieved, students might want to consider the value of afternoon napping to make up the sleep debt. A short nap of about 20 or 30 minutes (a "power nap") can be quite refreshing and valuable to overall performance. Experts recommend that the nap remain short—never longer than an hour or two, since too much afternoon sleep might disrupt or delay one's nighttime sleep.

Exercise Danger Signs

- A delay of over 1 hour in your body's return to a fully relaxed, comfortable state after exercise.
- A change in sleep patterns.
- Any noticeable breathing difficulties or chest pains. Exercise at your THR should not initiate these problems. You should consult a physician.
- Persistent joint or muscle pain. Any lingering joint or muscle pain might signal a problem. Seek the help of an athletic trainer, a physical therapist, or your physician.
- Unusual changes in urine composition or output. Marked color change in your urine could signal possible kidney or bladder difficulties. Drink plenty of water before, during, and after you participate in your activity.
- Anything unusual that you notice after starting your fitness program. Examples are headaches, nosebleeds, fainting, numbness in an extremity, and hemorrhoids.

Summary

- Physical fitness allows one to avoid illness, perform routine activities, and respond to emergencies.
- The health benefits of exercise can be achieved through regular, moderate exercise.
- Fitness is composed of five components: cardiorespiratory endurance, muscular strength, muscular endurance, flexibility, and body composition.
- The American College of Sports Medicine's program for cardiorespiratory fitness has five components: mode of activity, frequency of training, intensity of training, duration of training, and resistance training.

- The *target heart rate* refers to the number of times per minute the heart must contract to produce a training effect.
- Training sessions should take place in three phases: warm-up, workout, and cooldown.
- Fitness experts are concerned about the lack of fitness in today's youth.
- Street dancing, step aerobics, and rollerblading are currently popular aerobic activities.
- College students who are interested in fitness should understand the important topics of steroid use, crosstraining, fluid replacement, bodybuilding, and proper sleep.

Review Questions

1. Identify the five components of fitness described in this chapter. How does each component relate to physical fitness?
2. What is the difference between anaerobic and aerobic energy production? What types of activities are associated with anaerobic energy production? With aerobic energy production?
3. List some of the benefits of aerobic fitness.
4. Describe the various methods used to promote muscular strength.
5. What does the principle of overload mean in regard to fitness training programs?

6. Identify the ACSM's five components of an effective cardiorespiratory fitness program. Explain the important aspects of each component.
7. Under what circumstances should you see a physician before starting a physical fitness program?
8. Identify and describe the three parts of a training session.
9. Describe some of the negative consequences of anabolic steroid use.
10. How can people improve their sleeping habits?

Think About This . . .

- What are your attitudes toward physical fitness? Do you participate in a regular physical fitness program? Why or why not?
- Does your present level of fitness allow you to effectively carry out the activities your schedule demands? Are there things that you would like to do but cannot because of your current level of fitness?
- Describe your level of fitness, taking into consideration cardiorespiratory endurance, strength, and flexibility.
- After determining your own THR, calculate the

THR for a parent or older friend. Talk to these people about starting their own fitness programs. Be ready to help with encouragement and accurate information. They may look to you as a role model for their own health.
- Design a physical fitness plan for yourself, taking into consideration all of the dimensions of body structure and function and the five components of an effective fitness program described in this chapter. What are the chances that you will continue this program after college?

References

1. Blair SN: Exercise and health, *Sports Science Exchange* 3(29):1-6, 1990.
2. Prentice WE: *Fitness for college and life,* ed 4, St Louis, 1994, Mosby.
3. Fit, fitter, fittest, *Harvard Medical School Health Letter* 15(4):2, 1990.
4. Simon HB: Can you run away from cancer? *Harvard Medical School Health Letter* 17(5):5-7, 1992.
5. Cavanaugh J: *Adult development and aging,* Belmont, Calif, 1990, Wadsworth.
6. Ferrini AF, Ferrini RL: *Health in later years,* ed 2, Madison, Wis, 1992, Brown & Benchmark.
7. American College of Sports Medicine: Position statement on the recommended quantity and quality of exercise for developing and maintaining fitness in healthy adults, *Med Sci Sports Exerc* 22(2):265-274, 1990.
8. White MD: *Water exercise,* Champaign, Ill, 1995, Human Kinetics.
9. Arnheim DD, Prentice WE: *Principles of athletic training,* ed 8, St Louis, 1993, Mosby.
10. What is an exercise stress test? *The Johns Hopkins Medical Letter: Health after 50,* 3(10):6-7, 1991.
11. Maughan RJ, Rehrer NJ: Gastric emptying during exercise, *Sports Science Exchange* 6(5):1-5, 1993.
12. Williams MH: Alcohol and sport performance, *Sports Science Exchange* 4(40):1-4, 1992.
13. Mishra R: Steroids and sports are a losing proposition, *FDA Consumer* 25(7):25-27, 1991.
14. Saeki T: Sport in Japan. In Wagner E, editor: *Sport in Asia and Africa: a comparative handbook,* New York, 1989, Greenwood Press.
15. Rizak G: Sport in the People's Republic of China. In Wagner E, editor: *Sport in Asia and Africa: a comparative handbook,* New York, 1989, Greenwood Press.

Suggested Readings

Burleigh WB: *Fitness lite: a guide for those who have never taken exercise seriously,* Santa Barbara, Calif, 1995, Capra Press.

A short, easy-to-read, humorous look at fitness. Disguised in the humor is a solid 16-week fitness program that incorporates important elements, including nutrition, weight management, and aerobic exercise. Fun to read.

Millman D: *The inner athlete: realizing your fullest potential,* Walpole, NH, 1994, Stillpoint.

Millman bridges the gap between physical conditioning and mental wellness. The author encourages focusing on the internal benefits of physical training, regardless of one's abilities. According to Millman, the mind is as important to overall success as are physical talent and effort.

Newby-Fraser P: *Peak fitness for women,* Champaign, Ill, 1995, Human Kinetics.

You might think a seven-time Ironman Triathlon champion would aim a fitness book at only swimming, cycling, and running. However, Newby-Fraser elaborates on strength training, nutrition, crosstraining, flexibility training, and competition for women. Sound information, excellent photos, and beneficial workout sheets are included.

Peterson JA, Bryant CX, Peterson SC: *Strength training for women,* Champaign, Ill, 1995, Human Kinetics.

This is a comprehensive yet easy-to-read guide to strength training for women. Free weights, weight machines, and non-equipment options are explored. Many illustrations and the pros and cons of various approaches are presented so that the user can tailor a program for herself.

Prentice WE: *Fitness for college and life,* ed 4, St Louis, 1994, Mosby.

This highly recommended, comprehensive textbook covers all aspects of fitness and wellness. The book provides particularly well-written coverage of strength training and stretching activities. The author's unique background as a scholar, athletic trainer, and physical therapist increases the credibility of the book.

Prentice WE: *Get Fit, Stay Fit,* St Louis, 1996, Mosby.

This text explains not only how to go about getting fit, but also why it is important to make fitness and exercise a part of your life. It includes specific techniques and guidelines so that you can tailor your fitness program to your individual needs.

White MD: *Water exercise,* Champaign, Ill, 1995, Human Kinetics.

Written by a licensed occupational and massage therapist, this book focuses on fitness development and injury rehabilitation through water activities. Nearly 80 exercises are discussed and illustrated. Step-by-step programs are presented from beginner to advanced levels.

Staying Fit During Pregnancy

Like many other attitudes, our thinking on fitness during pregnancy has changed in recent years. No longer is a pregnant woman treated as fragile. A woman needs to be quite careful when carrying a baby, but these days a doctor is more likely to advise against a sedentary lifestyle for a healthy pregnant woman. Exercise during pregnancy can increase a woman's muscle strength, making delivery of the baby easier and faster. Exercise can also help control her weight, making it easier to get back to normal weight after delivery. The baby may benefit from the mother's exercise program as well.

Importance of Exercise for Pregnant Women

Exercise in general is beneficial to the human body, and it is even more important for pregnant women to exercise regularly.[1] During pregnancy a woman's entire body undergoes many physical changes. Muscles are stretched, joints are loosened, and tissues are subjected to stress. If a woman is in good physiological condition, she is more likely to handle these changes with few complications.[2] The baby may also benefit: studies have shown that women who exercise during pregnancy tend to give birth to healthier babies.[1]

Types of Exercise

The types of exercises a woman should perform during pregnancy will vary with the individual and with the stage of pregnancy. General exercises that increase overall fitness and stamina should be practiced, as well as exercises that strengthen specific muscle groups. Muscles of the pelvic floor, for example, should be exercised regularly, since these muscles will be supporting most of the extra weight of the baby. The pelvic floor muscles are involved with control of the bladder and rectum and with controlling increases in pressure within the abdominal cavity resulting from pushing during labor.[2] General exercises for the pelvic floor muscles include Kegel exercises. These exercises involve the contraction of pelvic floor muscles, and they can be performed by squeezing and then relaxing the anal sphincter.[2] These exercises work on the sphincters (rings of muscle) that control the openings of the urethra and anus.

The abdominal muscles are responsible for supporting the load of the growing fetus in the front of the mother's body. They are also used for pushing during delivery. These muscles must be kept in good shape so they can adequately support the increased weight.[2] Muscles involved in maintaining good posture, such as the back and leg muscles, should also be exercised. Efficient breathing should be practiced as well.[2]

A variety of exercises are available, including walking, swimming, stretching, and strengthening exercises.[1] Yoga and t'ai chi are also good forms of exercise for pregnant women. The muscles of the pelvic floor, abdomen, and back are especially subject to stress and strain during pregnancy and delivery, so certain exercises can also be performed to strengthen these muscles.[2] Exercises can also be performed to speed up recovery after delivery. Such postpartum exercises can be started in some cases within 24 hours after delivery.[2] Exercises can even be started before conception if a pregnancy is anticipated.

Hydrotherapy is becoming a popular option for expectant mothers. Exercising in the water helps reduce stress on joints, since the buoyancy of water reduces body weight by up to 90% of what it is on land.[3] Water also provides more resistance than air, so muscles get a better workout. No special equipment is needed, but various props such as weights or fans can be used to increase resistance. Immersion in water has also been shown to decrease blood pressure, reduce heart rate, and reduce tissue swelling in pregnant women.[1,4] Exercising in water may also reduce the risk for pregnant women of getting overheated or tired.[3] The water must not be too warm, however, since water that is too hot (around 97° F or above) may damage the nervous system and brain of the fetus.[1]

Risks to the Fetus

Although exercise during pregnancy has definite advantages, there are some drawbacks that must be considered as well. Studies suggest that exercise can be harmful to the fetus in some cases. Women who undergo exercise for long periods may experience a prolonged increase in core body temperature (a condition called *hyperthermia*), which may in turn increase the body temperature of the fetus. It is thought that such increases in fetal temperature may in turn put the baby at risk for congenital malformations. It has been shown that fever-induced hyperthermia is related to congenital malformation in many mammals, and recent studies suggest that this may be true for humans as well.[4] If fever from illness can increase the expectant mother's core temperature enough to produce malformations in the fetus, then it is possible that an increase in the mother's core temperature resulting from prolonged exercise may have similar effects. Fortunately, exercise over short periods (15 minutes or less) is not likely to raise the mother's core temperature enough to cause problems.[4]

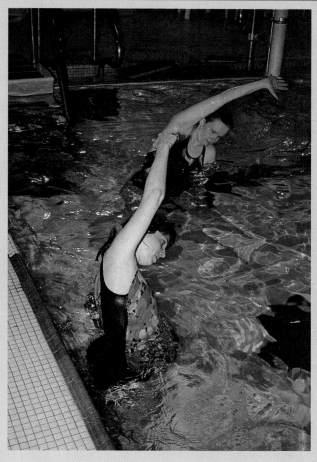

Water exercise is especially beneficial for pregnant women.

Exercising Safely

If the expectant mother exercised regularly before becoming pregnant, she may have to alter her exercise routine. Intense, high-impact workouts should be avoided in favor of moderate exercise, since very intense workouts may reduce blood flow to the fetus and deprive it of nutrients.[1] Sports that involve sudden stops, such as basketball or tennis, should be avoided,[5] and certain strenuous sports may eventually result in birth complications.[1] Exercises that involve lying on the back should not be performed after the first trimester of pregnancy, since they may reduce blood flow to the mother's heart and the heart of the fetus.[5] Exercises should be chosen that minimize the risk of injury to the fetus and the mother. Because of the changes in the mother's weight distribution during the course of pregnancy, she should be especially aware of balance during workouts. Exercises that may put her at a risk of losing balance and falling should be avoided, especially during the last trimester.[1]

Once safety factors have been accounted for, the healthy pregnant woman still has an array of options to choose from for her exercise routine. As with any workout program, she should consult her physician before beginning. Her obstetrician can tell her which exercises will be most beneficial and can also give tips to reduce potential injury to her and her baby. The obstetrician can give the expectant mother guidelines concerning safe levels of exertion and duration times of exercise as well.

For Discussion . . .

Do you think exercise during pregnancy is a good idea or not? Do the benefits outweigh the risks?

References

1. Marti J, Hine A: *The alternative health and medicine encyclopedia*, Gale, Cincinnati, 1995, Gale.
2. Noble E: *Essential exercises for the childbearing year*, ed 2, Boston, 1982, Houghton Mifflin.
3. Brody JE: For gentler aerobics, just add water, *The Saturday Evening Post* 263(6), Sept-Oct 1991.
4. Cefalo RC, Moos M-K: *Preconceptional health care: a practical guide*, ed 2, St Louis, 1995, Mosby.
5. Good news about exercise and pregnancy, *Parents*, 70(8), August 1995.

Understanding Nutrition and Your Diet

Healthy People 2000 Objectives

Nutrition and dietary practices are closely related to many aspects of wellness, including fitness, weight management, cardiovascular health, and the prevention of diseases such as cancer, osteoporosis, and diabetes mellitus. Accordingly, several important nutrition-related objectives were included in the Healthy People 2000 report.

One objective was to reduce the percentage of total calories from fat, especially saturated fat, in Americans' diets. We are now about one fourth of the way toward reaching the specific figure targeted in the report. A related objective was to stimulate the development, marketing, and consumer selection of fat-reduced foods in supermarkets and restaurants. In the area of processed foods sold in supermarkets and vending machines, this goal has actually been exceeded.

Consumer access to nutrition information, especially food labels, is essential to promoting more healthful eating. New labeling requirements introduced in the early 1990s have been helpful, but a more important factor is the consumer's willingness to act on this information. Some progress in this regard has been noted.

From the prenatal period throughout life, we must follow sound dietary practices to maintain high-level health. Food provides the body with the **nutrients** needed for production of energy, repair of damaged tissue, growth of new tissue, and regulation of physiological processes.

Physiologically, these nutrients—carbohydrates, fat, protein, vitamins, minerals, dietary fiber, and water—are essential in adequate quantity. In addition, the production, preparation, and serving of food enriches our lives in ways not directly related to its physiological value.

TYPES AND SOURCES OF NUTRIENTS

We discuss first the familiar nutrients: carbohydrates, fats, and proteins. These three nutrients provide our bodies with **calories.*** Calories are used quickly by our bodies in energy metabolism or are stored in the form of glycogen or adipose tissue, the tissue composed of fat cells designed to hold liquefied fat. Because the other nutrient groups are not sources of *energy* for the body, we discuss them later.

Carbohydrates

Carbohydrates are various combinations of sugar units, or saccharides. The body uses carbohydrates primarily for energy. Each gram of carbohydrate contains 4 calories. Since the average person requires approximately 2000 calories per day and about 60% of our calories come from carbohydrates, we obtain roughly 1200 calories per day from carbohydrates.[1]

Carbohydrates occur in three forms, depending on the number of saccharide (sugar) units that make up the molecule. Carbohydrates that contain only one saccharide unit are classified as monosaccharides (glucose, or blood sugar), those with two units are disaccharides (sucrose, or table sugar), and those with more than two units are polysaccharides (starches).

The average adult American now consumes about 125 pounds of sugar each year—usually in colas, candies, and pastries, which offer few additional nutritional benefits.[2] For years, excess sugar intake was blamed for a number of serious health problems, including obesity, mineral deficiencies, behavioral disorders, dental cavities, diabetes mellitus, and cardiovascular disease. However, with the exception of dental cavities, current scientific data fail to confirm that sugar per se directly causes any of these health problems. This said, however, the inability of some people to digest milk sugar (lactose) is well documented. Lactose-intolerant people lack an enzyme used in the digestion of this simple sugar. The brisk sales of enzyme supplements now available near dairy cases in supermarkets may, however, suggest that the problem is more widespread than experts believe. Regardless, today it is recommended that no more than 10% of our total calories come from simple sugars.

Much of the sugar we consume is hidden—that is, sugar is a principal product we may overlook in many food items. Foods such as ketchup, salad dressings, cured meat products, and canned vegetables and fruits frequently contain much hidden sugar. High-fructose corn syrup, often found in these items, is a very concentrated sugar solution.

Starches are complex carbohydrates composed of long chains of sugar units. However, these starches should not be confused with the adjective *starchy*. When people refer to starchy foods, they are usually referring to bland, bread-filled, or "heavy" foods. True starches are among the most important sources of dietary carbohydrates. Starches are found primarily in vegetables, fruits, and grains. Eating true starches is overall very nutritionally beneficial because most starch sources also contain much-needed vitamins, minerals, protein, and water.

Fats

Fats (lipids) are an important nutrient in our diets. Fats provide a concentrated form of energy (9 calories per gram) and help give our foods high *satiety value*.

---

*The term *calorie* is used here to mean kilocalorie (kcal), which is the accepted scientific expression of the energy value of a food.

nutrients
Elements in foods that are required for the energy, growth, and repair of tissues and regulation of body processes.

calories
Units of heat (energy); specifically, one calorie equals the amount of heat required to raise the temperature of 1 kilogram of water by 1° C.

carbohydrates
Chemical compounds composed of sugar units; the body's primary source of energy.

Eating patterns established in childhood can continue throughout life.

Fat also helps give food its pleasing taste, or *palatability*. Fats carry the fat-soluble vitamins A, D, E, and K. Without fat, these vitamins would quickly pass through the body. Fat insulates our bodies to help us retain heat.

Dietary sources of fat are often difficult to identify. The visible fats in our diet, such as butter, salad oils, and the layer of fat on some cuts of meat, represent only about 40% of the fat we consume. Most of the fat we eat is "hidden" in food. For example, the Star Box below illustrates how fat can be hidden in sweet snacks.

When shopping, we often notice that the fat content of some foods is reported in terms of a percentage of the product's weight. In selecting the type of milk we drink, for example, we see that milk ranges from skim milk (no fat) to ultralow-fat milk (½%) through low-fat milk (1% to 2%) to whole milk (3% to 4%). Most consumers do not know, however, how much of the product's calories come from fat.

Today, it is recommended that no more than 25% to 30% of our calories come from fat. Complete the Personal Assessment on pp. 95-96 to see whether you eat too many fatty foods. If so, the Health Action Guide on p. 97 offers tips for reducing the amount of fat in your diet. Children under 2 years of age, however, need adequate fat in their diets.[3] Check with your doctor before restricting the amount of fat in a young child's diet.

Every type of dietary fat is made up of a combination of three forms of fat: saturated, monounsaturated, and polyunsaturated, based on chemical composition. Consumers should pay attention to the amount of each type of fat in dietary fat because of the role that each form plays in heart disease (see Chapter 10). **Saturated fats,** including those found in animal sources and in vegetable oils to which hydrogen has

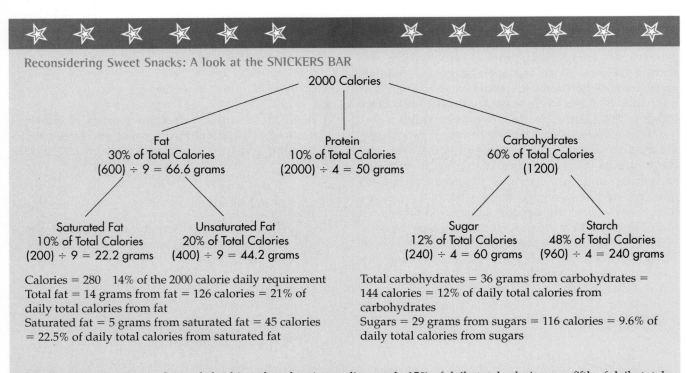

Reconsidering Sweet Snacks: A look at the SNICKERS BAR

2000 Calories

Fat	Protein	Carbohydrates
30% of Total Calories	10% of Total Calories	60% of Total Calories
(600) ÷ 9 = 66.6 grams	(2000) ÷ 4 = 50 grams	(1200)

Saturated Fat	Unsaturated Fat	Sugar	Starch
10% of Total Calories	20% of Total Calories	12% of Total Calories	48% of Total Calories
(200) ÷ 9 = 22.2 grams	(400) ÷ 9 = 44.2 grams	(240) ÷ 4 = 60 grams	(960) ÷ 4 = 240 grams

Calories = 280　14% of the 2000 calorie daily requirement
Total fat = 14 grams from fat = 126 calories = 21% of daily total calories from fat
Saturated fat = 5 grams from saturated fat = 45 calories = 22.5% of daily total calories from saturated fat

Total carbohydrates = 36 grams from carbohydrates = 144 calories = 12% of daily total calories from carbohydrates
Sugars = 29 grams from sugars = 116 calories = 9.6% of daily total calories from sugars

How nutritious can a single snack food item be when it supplies nearly 15% of daily total calories, one fifth of daily total calories from fat, and over one fifth of daily total calories from saturated fat? Using the technique used above, calculate the same values for the Quaker Chewy Granola Bar, and determine how it compares as a snack item with the Snickers bar.

PERSONAL ASSESSMENT

Do You Have Fatty Habits?

Fat has earned a bad reputation because of the health problems to which it contributes when we eat too much of it. The questionnaire below will help you think about the amounts and types of fat that you generally eat. For each general type of food or food habit, circle the response category that is most typical for you. If you never or almost never eat any items of a particular food type, just skip that type.

Food Type/Habit	High Fat	Medium Fat	Low Fat
Chicken	Fried with the skin	Baked, broiled, or barbecued with the skin	Baked, broiled, or barbecued without the skin
Fat present on meats	Usually eat	Sometimes eat	Never eat
Fat used in cooking	Butter, lard, bacon grease, chicken fat	Margarine, oil	Nonstick cooking spray or no fat used
Additions to rice, bread, potatoes, vegetables, etc.	Butter, lard, bacon grease, chicken fat, coconut oil, cream cheese	Margarine, oil, peanut butter	Butter-flavored granules or no fat used
Pizza toppings	Sausage, pepperoni, extra cheese, combination	Canadian bacon	Vegetable
Sandwich spreads	Mayonnaise or mayonnaise-type dressing	Light mayonnaise, oil and vinegar	Mustard, fat-free mayonnaise
Milk and milk products (e.g., yogurt)	Whole milk and whole-milk products	Low-fat milk and milk products	Skim milk and milk products
Sandwich side orders	Chips, potato salad, macaroni salad with creamy dressing	Coleslaw, pasta salad with clear dressing	Vegetable sticks, pretzels, pickle
Salad dressings	Blue cheese, ranch, Thousand Island, other creamy type	Oil and vinegar, clear-base dressing	Oil-free dressing, lemon juice, flavored vinegar
Typical meat portion eaten	6-8 ounces or more	4-5 ounces	2-3 ounces
Sandwich fillings	Beef or pork hot dogs, salami, bologna, pepperoni, cheese, tuna or chicken salad	Turkey hot dogs, 85% fat-free lunch meats, corned beef, peanut butter, hummus (chickpea paste)	95% fat-free lunch meats, roast turkey, roast beef, lean ham
Ground meats	Regular ground beef, sausage meat, ground meat, ground pork (about 30% fat)	Lean ground beef, ground chuck, turkey sausage meat (20%-25% fat)	Ground turkey, extra lean ground beef, ground round (about 15% fat)
Deep-fried foods (e.g., french fries, onion rings, fish or chicken patties, egg rolls, tempura)	Eat every day	Eat once a week	Eat once a month or never
Bread for sandwiches	Croissant	Biscuit	Whole wheat, French, tortilla, pita or pocket bread, bagel, sourdough, or English muffin

Continued

Food Type/Habit	High Fat	Medium Fat	Low Fat
Cheeses	Hard cheeses (e.g., cheddar, Swiss, provolone, Jack, American, processed)	Part skim mozzarella, part skim ricotta, low-fat cheeses	Nonfat cheeses, nonfat cottage cheese, no cheese
Frozen desserts	Premium or regular ice cream	Ice milk or low-fat frozen yogurt	Sherbet, Italian water ice, nonfat frozen yogurt, frozen fruit whip
Coffee lighteners	Cream, liquid or powdered creamer	Whole milk	Low-fat or skim milk
Snacks	Chips, pies, cheese and crackers, nuts, donuts, microwave popcorn, chocolate, granola bars	Muffins, toaster pastries, unbuttered commercial popcorn	Pretzels, vegetable sticks, fresh or dried fruit, air-popped popcorn, bread sticks, jelly beans, hard candy
Cookies	Chocolate coated, chocolate chip, peanut butter, filled sandwich type	Oatmeal	Ginger snaps, vanilla wafers, graham crackers, animal crackers, fruit newtons

SCORING: (_____ × 2)   +   (_____ × 1)   +   (_____ × 0)   =

Total Score _____

Once you have completed the questionnaire, count the number of circles in each column and calculate your score as follows: multiply the number of choices in the left-hand (high fat) column by 2 and multiply the number of choices in the middle by 1. Any number of choices in the right-hand column will equal 0.

Less than 10   =   Excellent fat habits
10 to 20   =   Good fat habits
20 to 30   =   Need to trim some fat
Over 30   =   Very high fat diet

If your score is 20 or above, try to substitute more foods from the middle (medium fat) column or, better still, the right (low fat) column for foods in the left-hand (high fat) column. ☑

been added (hydrogenated), becoming *trans-fatty acids,* need to be carefully limited in a modern healthy diet. Concern over the presence of trans-fatty acids (an altered form of normal vegetable oil molecule) is associated with changes to the cell membrane, including those cells lining the artery wall. This possibly prevents these vessel wall cells from freeing cholesterol from their surfaces.[4] The amount of trans-fatty acids in the diet can be reduced by using liquefied margarines rather than the solid stick forms. In addition, several products containing low-calorie fat substitutes are now on the market (see the Star Box on p. 97).

Tropical oils

Although all cooking oils (and fats such as butter, lard, margarine, and shortening) have the same number of calories by weight (9 calories per gram), some oils contain high percentages of saturated fats. All oils and fats contain varying percentages of saturated, monounsaturated, and polyunsaturated fats. However, the tropical oils—coconut, palm, and palm kernel—contain much higher percentages of saturated fats than do other cooking oils.[5] Coconut oil, for example, is 92% saturated fat (Figure 5-1). Tropical oils can still be found in some brands of snack foods, crackers, cookies, nondairy creamers, and breakfast cereals, although they have been removed from most national brands. Do you check for tropical oils on the ingredients labels of the foods you select?

Cholesterol

A high blood level of **cholesterol** has also been reported to be a risk factor for the development of cardiovascular disease (see Chapter 10). Cholesterol is necessary in all animal tissue and is manufactured by our bodies from carbohydrates and fats. Considerable evidence suggests that increased intake of saturated fats may increase serum (blood) cholesterol levels.[6] However, the relationship between intake of dietary cholesterol and serum cholesterol levels remains

HEALTH
Action Guide ----→

Tips for Reducing the Fat Content of Meals

A combination of the following practices can be used to reduce the fat content of meals. Can you suggest additional ways to reduce fat in your diet?

- Become familiar with today's food labels, and use the information provided to reduce the fat content of meals.
- Cut away and discard skin from meats such as chicken.
- When eating out, do not order foods with cream-based sauces, such as fettuccine alfredo.
- Trim fat from cuts of meat, including both the fat interspersed within the cut and that along the edges.
- Layer vegetables over baked potatoes to reduce the tendency to add butter, margarine, or sour cream.
- Request salad dressing and other condiments on the side so that you can control the amount you use.
- Eat more vegetables, fruits, and breads in place of meats and cheeses.
- Use jelly and apple butter in place of butter and margarine on toast, bread, and bagels. ◄-----•

Proteins

Proteins are found in every living cell; they are composed of chains of **amino acids.** Of the 20 naturally occurring amino acids, the body can synthesize

Low-Calorie Fat Substitutes

Newly developed products containing fat substitutes such as Simplesse, Simple Pleasures, Olestra, and Trailblazer are now or will soon be available. By combining high-protein sources such as egg whites and milk through a process called *microparticulation,* or by constructing new undigestible molecules, food technologists are able to restructure the configuration of protein to resemble that of fat. These new products contain no cholesterol and have 80% fewer calories than similar products made with fat. Because fat substitutes tend to be unstable when heated, they are being used in foods such as ice cream, salad dressing, cheese spreads, and yogurt. Whether significant health benefits can be derived from these products remains to be seen.

unclear.[7] Nevertheless, most doctors still recommend that people restrict their dietary intake of cholesterol to 300 mg or less per day, reduce total fat and saturated fat intake, and exercise regularly. High-cholesterol foods include whole milk, shellfish, animal fat, and egg yolks. Only foods of animal origin can contain cholesterol. Thus labels that appear on foods such as peanut butter and margarine trumpeting "cholesterol free" are overstating the obvious.

Low-fat foods

Reflecting our growing concern about the role of dietary fats in many health problems has been the explosion of fat-free, low-fat, or reduced-fat food items appearing in stores and restaurants. In 1994, for example, 1439 new foods of this type were introduced.[8] As favorable as this trend might be, however, it is important to remember that these food items may still be high in calories and, therefore, should not be consumed in large amounts just because of their lower-fat formulation.

saturated fats
Fats that are difficult for the body to use; they are in solid form at room temperature; primarily animal fats.

cholesterol
A primary form of fat found in the blood; lipid material manufactured within the body and derived from dietary sources.

proteins
Compounds composed of chains of amino acids; the primary components of muscle and connective tissue.

amino acids
The chief components of protein; can be manufactured by the body or obtained from dietary sources.

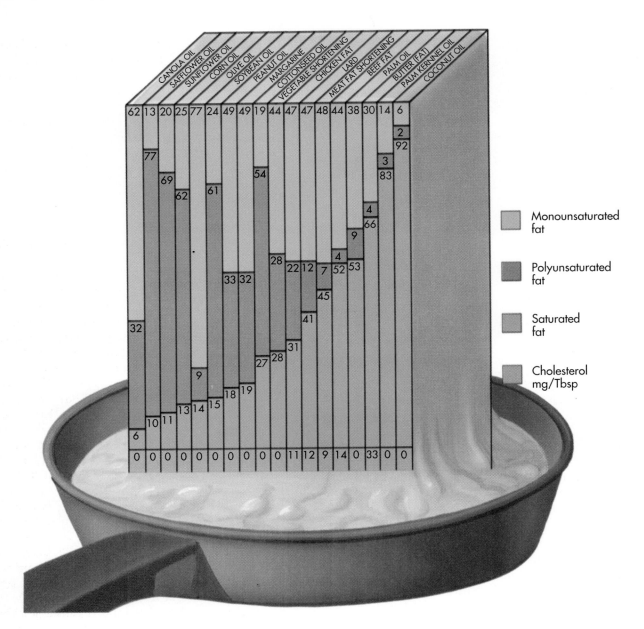

Figure 5-1 Comparison of dietary fats (fatty acid content normalized to 100%). Every fat shown above is a combination of three forms of fat: monounsaturated, polyunsaturated, and saturated.

all but nine *essential amino acids** from the foods we eat. A food that contains all nine essential amino acids is called a *complete protein* food. Sources of complete protein are animal products, including milk, meat, cheese, and eggs. A food source that does not contain all nine essential amino acids is called an *incomplete*

*Eight additional compounds are sometimes classified as amino acids; thus some nutritionists believe that there are more than 20 amino acids.

protein food. Vegetables, grains, and *legumes* (peas or beans—including chickpeas, butter beans, soybean curd [tofu], and peanuts) are principal sources of incomplete protein. For some people, including vegan vegetarians (see pp. 117-120 and the Focus Box on p. 125), people with limited access to animal-based food sources, or those who have significantly limited their meat, egg, and dairy product consumption, it is important to understand how essential amino acids can be obtained from incomplete protein sources. This requires the careful selection of plant foods in combi-

LEARNING from ALL CULTURES

A Variety of Diets

Do you eat to live or live to eat? Maybe it depends on what day it is! We do know that to stay healthy we need to eat a variety of good foods.

What we eat reflects our culture. In the United States, we have "American" food, such as hamburgers and corn on the cob. Because of the variety of ethnic groups in this country, we also enjoy many foods from other cultures. In fact, it would be difficult to identify the staple foods of the American diet.

People in other countries often consume those particular foods that are most widely available. Corn, for example, is the main ingredient in food for most Mexicans, and it is eaten in a variety of forms. Beans, or *frijoles*, are another staple food found in the Mexican diet. There are many varieties, and they are commonly eaten with rice and hot peppers. The diet is basically a healthy one, but there is not enough food to feed all the people, especially the poorest peasants.

Seafood is enjoyed by many Canadians. Fishing is an important industry for northern Canadian natives. Some Native Canadian groups have a long history of commercial fishing. Salmon and cod have been caught and sold by the Inuit of Labrador for many years, and fish were sold to the Gold Rush miners by Native Canadians from the Yukon. Fisheries run by Native Canadians are operational today, through government assistance, and provide fish to northern and southern parts of the country.

Can you identify food choices in your own diet that are commonly found in other cultures, such as Asian cuisine?

nations that will provide all of the essential amino acids. The list below shows many usable combinations that include legumes and grains:

- Sunflower seeds/green peas
- Navy beans/barley
- Green peas/corn
- Red beans/rice
- Sesame seeds/soybeans
- Black-eyed peas/rice and peanuts
- Green peas/rice
- Corn/pinto beans

When even one essential amino acid is missing from the diet, deficiency can develop.

Protein primarily promotes growth and maintenance of body tissue. However, when caloric intake falls, protein will be broken down and converted into glucose. This loss of protein can impede growth and repair of tissue. Protein also is a primary component of enzyme and hormone structure, helps maintain the *acid-base balance* of our bodies, and is a source of energy (4 calories per gram consumed). Nutritionists recommend that 12% to 15% of our caloric intake be from protein, particularly that of plant origin.

Vitamins

Vitamins are organic compounds that are required in small amounts for normal growth, reproduction, and maintenance of health. Vitamins differ from carbohydrates, fats, and proteins in that they do not provide calories or serve as structural elements for our bodies. Vitamins are *coenzymes*. By facilitating the action of **enzymes,** vitamins help initiate a wide variety of body responses, including energy production, use of minerals, and growth of healthy tissue.

Vitamins can be classified as *water soluble* (capable of being dissolved in water) or *fat soluble* (capable of being dissolved in fat or lipid tissue). Water-soluble vitamins include the B-complex vitamins and vitamin C. Most of the excess of these water-soluble vitamins will be eliminated from the body in the urine. The fat-soluble vitamins are vitamins A, D, E, and K. Excessive intake of these vitamins causes them to be stored in the body in the adipose (fat) tissue. It is therefore possible to consume and retain too many of these vitamins, particularly vitamins A and D. Because excess fat-soluble vitamins are stored in the body's fat, organs that contain fat, such as the liver, are primary storage sites. (See Tables 5-1 and 5-2 for general properties of fat-soluble and water-soluble vitamins.)

Because water-soluble vitamins dissolve quickly in water, you should be careful not to lose them during the preparation of fresh fruits and vegetables. One precaution is not to overcook fresh vegetables. The longer vegetables are steamed or boiled, the more

vitamins
Organic compounds that facilitate the action of enzymes.

enzymes
Organic substances that control the rate of physiological reactions but are not themselves altered in the process.

Table 5-1   The Fat-Soluble Vitamins, Their Functions, Deficiency Conditions, and Food Sources

Vitamin	Major functions	Deficiency symptoms	People most at risk	Dietary sources	RDA	Toxicity symptoms
Vitamin A (retinoids) and provitamin A (carotenoids)	1. Vision, light, and color 2. Promotes growth 3. Prevents drying of skin and eyes 4. Promotes resistance to bacterial infection	1. Night blindness 2. Xerophthalmia 3. Poor growth 4. Dry skin (keratinization)	People in poverty, especially preschool children (still very rare)	Vitamin A Liver Fortified milk Provitamin A Sweet potatoes Spinach Greens Carrots Cantaloupe Apricots Broccoli	Women: 800 RE (4000 IU) Men: 1000 RE (5000 IU)	Fetal malformations, hair loss, skin changes, pain in bones
Vitamin D (cholecalciferol and ergocalciferol)	1. Facilitates absorption of calcium and phosphorus 2. Maintains optimum calcification of bone	1. Rickets 2. Osteomalacia	Breastfed infants, elderly shut-ins	Vitamin D-fortified milk Fish oils Tuna fish Salmon	5-10 micrograms (200-400 IU)	Growth retardation, kidney damage, calcium deposits in soft tissue
Vitamin E (tocopherols, tocotrienols)	1. Antioxidant: prevents breakdown of vitamin A and unsaturated fatty acids	1. Hemolysis of red blood cells 2. Nerve destruction	People with poor fat absorption (still very rare)	Vegetable oils Some greens Some fruits	Women: 8 α-tocopherol equivalents Men: 10 α-tocopherol equivalents	Muscle weakness, headaches, fatigue, nausea, inhibition of vitamin K metabolism
Vitamin K (phylloquinone and menaquinone)	1. Helps form prothrombin and other factors for blood clotting	1. Hemorrhage	People taking antibiotics for months at a time	Green vegetables Liver	60-80 micrograms	Anemia and jaundice

RE, Retinol equivalents; IU, international units.

water-soluble vitamins will be lost. You may wish to drink (or use in cooking) any water in which vegetables were boiled or steamed.

To ensure an adequate vitamin intake, eat a variety of foods. Unless there are special circumstances, such as pregnancy, lactation, infancy, or an existing health problem, nearly everyone who eats a reasonably well-rounded diet consumes enough vitamins to prevent deficiencies.

In spite of the availability of vitamin-rich foods, not all people eat a balanced diet based on a variety of foods. Recent studies suggest that a somewhat higher intake of vitamins A, C, and E for adults might reduce the risk of developing cancer, atherosclerosis, and

depressed levels of HDL cholesterol (see Chapter 10).[9,10] In addition, consumption of an adequate amount of folic acid before and during pregnancy has been shown to reduce the incidence of birth defects.[11] To date, most of these findings have not been translated into specific recommendations, but they are drawing increased interest from both the scientific community and the general public.[12] It is the antioxidation properties of vitamins A, C, and E that most keenly interest health experts. At the same time that many health experts are reconsidering recommendations concerning additional consumption of vitamins, the Food and Drug Administration (FDA) has set forth new restrictions on the labeling of *food supplements,* banning unsubstantiated claims

Table 5-2   The Water-Soluble Vitamins, Their Functions, Deficiency Conditions, and Food Sources

Name	Major functions	Deficiency symptoms	People most at risk	Dietary sources	RDA or ESADDI	Toxicity
Thiamin	Coenzyme involved with enzymes in carbohydrate metabolism; nerve function	Beriberi, nervous tingling, poor coordination, edema, heart changes, weakness	People with alcoholism, people in poverty	Sunflower seeds, pork, whole and enriched grains, dried beans, peas, brewer's yeast	1.1-1.5 milligrams	None possible from food
Riboflavin	Coenzyme involved in energy metabolism	Inflammation of mouth and tongue, cracks at corners of the mouth, eye disorders	Possibly people on certain medications if no dairy products consumed	Milk, mushrooms, spinach, liver, enriched grains	1.2-1.7 milligrams	None reported
Niacin	Coenzyme involved in energy metabolism, fat synthesis, fat breakdown	Pellagra, diarrhea, dermatitis, dementia	People in severe poverty where corn is dominant food, people with alcoholism	Mushrooms, bran, tuna, salmon, chicken, beef, liver, peanuts, enriched grains	15-19 milligrams	Flushing of skin at >100 milligrams
Pantothenic acid	Coenzyme involved in energy metabolism, fat synthesis, fat breakdown	Using an antagonist causes tingling in hands, fatigue, headache, nausea	People with alcoholism	Mushrooms, liver, broccoli, eggs; most foods have some	4-7 milligrams	None
Biotin	Coenzyme involved in glucose production, fat synthesis	Dermatitis, tongue soreness, anemia, depression	People with alcoholism	Cheese, egg yolks, cauliflower, peanut butter, liver	30-100 micrograms	Unknown
Vitamin B$_6$, pyridoxine, and other forms	Coenzyme involved in protein metabolism, neurotransmitter synthesis, hemoglobin synthesis, many other functions	Headache, anemia, convulsions, nausea, vomiting, flaky skin, sore tongue	Adolescent and adult women, people on certain medications, people with alcoholism	Animal protein foods, spinach, broccoli, bananas, salmon, sunflower seeds	1.8-2 milligrams	Nerve destruction at doses >100 milligrams

Continued

Table 5-2, cont'd.

Name	Major functions	Deficiency symptoms	People most at risk	Dietary sources	RDA or ESADDI	Toxicity
Folate (folic acid)	Coenzyme involved in DNA synthesis	Megaloblastic anemia, inflammation of tongue, diarrhea, poor growth, mental disorders	People with alcoholism, pregnant women, people taking certain medications	Green leafy vegetables, orange juice, organ meats, sprouts, sunflower seeds	180-200 microgram	None, nonprescription vitamin dosage is controlled by FDA
Vitamin B$_{12}$ (cobalamins)	Coenzyme involved in folate metabolism, nerve function	Macrocytic anemia, poor nerve function	Elderly because of poor absorption, vegans	Animal foods, especially organ meats, oysters, clams (B$_{12}$ not naturally in plant foods)	2 micrograms	None
Vitamin C (ascorbic acid)	Collagen synthesis, hormone synthesis, neurotransmitter synthesis	Scurvy: poor wound healing, pinpoint hemorrhages, bleeding gums, edema	People with alcoholism, elderly men living alone	Citrus fruits, strawberries, broccoli, greens	60 milligrams	Doses >1-2 grams cause diarrhea and can alter some diagnostic tests

for the cure or prevention of disease.[13] Not surprisingly, the manufacturers of these products attempted to curtail this action by strongly suggesting to consumers that the FDA planned to take vitamins off the over-the-counter (OTC) market and make them available by prescription only. Today, the sale of food supplements (vitamins, minerals, and amino acids) is a huge industry in this country, with 75 million Americans using *dietary aids* at an annual cost of more than $1.5 billion.

Minerals

Nearly 5% of the body is composed of inorganic materials, the *minerals*. Minerals function primarily as structural elements (in teeth, muscles, hemoglobin, and hormones). They are also critical in the regulation of body processes, including muscle contraction, heart function, blood clotting, protein synthesis, and red blood cell formation. Approximately 21 minerals have been recognized as essential for human health.

Major minerals are those that are seen in relatively high amounts in our body tissues. Examples of major

minerals are calcium, phosphorus, sulfur, sodium, potassium, and magnesium. Examples of **trace elements,** minerals seen in relatively small amounts in body tissues, include zinc, iron, copper, selenium, and iodine. Trace elements are required only in small quantities; nevertheless, they are essential for good health. (See Tables 5-3 and 5-4 for lists of minerals and their functions.) As with vitamins, the safest, most appropriate way to prevent a mineral deficiency is to eat a balanced diet.

Water

Water may well be our most essential nutrient, since without water most of us would die from **dehydration** effects in less than a week. We could survive for weeks or even years without some of the essential minerals and vitamins, but not without water. More than half our body weight comes from water. Water provides the medium for nutrient and waste transport, controls body temperature, and plays a key role in nearly all of our body's biochemical reactions.

Table 5-3   Key Trace Minerals

Mineral	Major functions	Deficiency symptoms	People most at risk	RDA or ESADDI	Nutrient–dense dietary sources	Results of toxicity
Iron	Part of hemoglobin and other key compounds used in respiration; used for immune function	Low serum iron levels, small, pale red blood cells, low blood hemoglobin values	Infants, preschool children, adolescents, women in childbearing years	Men: 10 milligrams Women: 15 milligrams	Meats, spinach, seafood, broccoli, peas, bran, enriched breads	Toxicity is seen in children who consume 200-400 milligrams in iron pills and in people with hemochromatosis; in this latter case, people over-absorb iron
Zinc	Over 200 enzymes need zinc, including enzymes involved in growth, immunity, alcohol metabolism, sexual development, and reproduction	Skin rash, diarrhea, decreased appetite and sense of taste, hair loss, poor growth and development, poor wound healing	Vegetarians, women in general, the elderly	Men: 15 milligrams Women: 12 milligrams	Seafood, meats, greens, whole grains	Reduces iron and copper absorption; can cause diarrhea, cramps, and depressed immune function
Selenium	Part of antioxidant system	Muscle pain, muscle weakness, heart disease	Unknown	55-70 micrograms	Meats, eggs, fish, seafood, whole grains	Nausea, vomiting, hair loss, weakness, liver disease
Iodide	Part of thyroid hormone	Goiter, poor growth in infancy when mother is deficient in pregnancy	None in America, since salt is usually fortified	150 micrograms	Iodized salt, white bread, saltwater fish, dairy products	Inhibition of function of the thyroid gland
Copper	Aids in iron metabolism; works with many enzymes, such as those involved in protein metabolism and hormone synthesis	Anemia, low white blood cell count, poor growth	Infants recovering from malnutrition, people who use overzealous supplementation of zinc	1.5-3 milligrams	Liver, cocoa, beans, nuts, whole grains, dried fruits	Vomiting, nervous system disorders

Continued

Table 5-3, cont'd

Mineral	Major functions	Deficiency symptoms	People most at risk	RDA or ESADDI	Nutrient-dense dietary sources	Results of toxicity
Fluoride	Increases resistance of tooth enamel to dental caries	Increased risk of dental caries	Areas where water is not fluoridated and dental treatments do not make up for this lack of fluoride	1.5-4 milligrams	Fluoridated water, toothpaste, dental treatments, tea, seaweed	Stomach upset, mottling (staining) of teeth during development
Chromium	Enhances blood glucose control	High blood glucose levels after eating	People on total parenteral nutrition and perhaps elderly people with non–insulin-dependent diabetes mellitus	50-200 micrograms	Egg yolks, whole grains, pork	Caused by industrial contamination, not dietary excess
Manganese	Aids action of some enzymes, such as those involved in carbohydrate metabolism	None in humans	Unknown	2-5 milligrams	Nuts, rice, oats, beans	Unknown in humans
Molybdenum	Aids action of some enzymes	None in humans	Unknown	75-250 micrograms	Beans, grains, nuts	Unknown in humans

Most people seldom think about the importance of an adequate intake of water and fluids. Adults require about six to ten glasses a day, depending on their activity level and environment. People who drink beverages that tend to dehydrate the body (tea, coffee, and alcohol) should increase their water consumption. Of course, we also obtain needed fluids from fruits, vegetables, fruit and vegetable juices, milk, and noncaffeinated soft drinks. The latter are important sources of fluids because Americans tend to consume more of these beverages than they do water.

Fiber

Although not considered a nutrient by definition, **fiber** is an important component of sound nutrition. Fiber consists of plant material that is not digested but rather moves through the digestive tract and out of

the body. Cereal, fruits, and vegetables all provide us with dietary fiber.

Fiber can be classified into two large groups on the basis of water solubility. *Insoluble* fibers are those that can absorb water from the intestinal tract. By absorbing water, the insoluble fibers give the stool bulk and decrease the time it takes the stool to move through the digestive tract. In contrast, *soluble* fiber turns to a "gel" within the intestinal tract and in so doing binds to liver bile, to which cholesterol is attached. Thus the soluble fibers may be valuable in removing cholesterol, which lowers blood cholesterol levels.[14] Also, since foods high in soluble fiber are generally low in sugar and saturated fats, fiber may indirectly contribute to keeping the blood sugar level low and reducing the risk of colon cancer associated with diets high in saturated fat.[15]

In recent years, attention has been directed toward

Table 5-4   Water and the Major Minerals

Name	Major functions	Deficiency symptoms	People most at risk	RDA or minimum requirement	Nutrient–dense dietary sources	Results of toxicity
Water	Medium for chemical reactions, removal of waste products, perspiration to cool the body	Thirst, muscle weakness, poor endurance	Infants with a fever, elderly in nursing homes	1 milliliter per calorie burned*	As such and in foods	Probably occurs only in mental disorders: headache, blurred vision, convulsions
Sodium	A major ion of the extracellular fluid; nerve impulse transmission	Muscle cramps	People who severely restrict sodium to lower blood pressure (250-500 milligrams/day)	500 milligrams	Table salt, processed foods	High blood pressure in susceptible individuals
Potassium	A major ion of intracellular fluid; nerve impulse transmission	Irregular heartbeat, loss of appetite, muscle cramps	People who use potassium-wasting diuretics or have poor diets, as seen in poverty and with alcoholism	2000 milligrams	Spinach, squash, bananas, orange juice, other vegetables and fruits, milk	Slowing of the heartbeat; seen in kidney failure
Chloride	A major ion of the extracellular fluid; acid production in stomach; nerve transmission	Convulsions in infants	No one, probably, when infant formula manufacturers control product quality adequately	700 milligrams	Table salt, some vegetables	High blood pressure in susceptible people when combined with sodium
Calcium	Bone and tooth strength; blood clotting; nerve impulse transmission; muscle contractions; cell regulation	Poor intake increases the risk for osteoporosis	Women in general, especially those who constantly restrict their energy intake and consume few dairy products	800 milligrams (older than 24 years old)	Dairy products, canned fish, leafy vegetables, tofu, fortified orange juice	Very high intakes may cause kidney stones in susceptible people

Continued

*An approximation; best to keep urine volume greater than 1 liter (4 cups) per day.

Table 5-4, cont'd.

Name	Major functions	Deficiency symptoms	People most at risk	RDA or minimum requirement	Nutrient–dense dietary sources	Results of toxicity
Phosphorus	Bone and tooth strength; part of various metabolic compounds; major ion of intracellular fluid	Probably none; poor bone maintenance possible	Elderly consuming very nutrient-poor diets, possibly total vegetarians and those with alcoholism	800 milligrams (older than 24 years)	Dairy products, processed foods, fish, soft drinks	Hampers bone health in people with kidney failure; poor bone mineralization if calcium intakes are low
Magnesium	Bone strength; enzyme function; nerve and heart function	Weakness, muscle pain, poor heart function	People on thiazide diuretics, women in general	Men: 350 milligrams Women: 280 milligrams	Wheat bran, green vegetables, nuts, chocolate	Causes weakness in people with kidney failure
Sulfur	Part of vitamins and amino acids; drug detoxification; acid-base balance	None	People who do not meet their protein needs	None	Protein food	None likely

Table 5-5A   Adult Recommended Dietary Allowances,[1] Revised 1989

Category	Age (years)	Weight[2] (kg)	(lb)	Height[2] (cm)	(in)	Protein (g)	Vitamin A (µg RE)[3]	Vitamin D (µg)[4]	Vitamin E (µg α-TE)[5]	Vitamin K (µg)
Males	15-18	66	145	176	69	59	1000	10	10	65
	19-24	72	160	177	70	58	1000	10	10	70
	25-50	79	174	176	70	63	1000	5	10	80
	51+	77	170	173	68	63	1000	5	10	80
Females	15-18	55	120	163	64	44	800	10	8	55
	19-24	58	128	164	65	46	800	10	8	60
	25-50	63	138	163	64	50	800	5	8	65
	51+	65	143	160	63	50	800	5	8	65
Pregnant						60	800	10	10	65
Lactating	1st 6 Months					65	1300	10	12	65
	2nd 6 Months					62	1200	10	11	65

[1]The allowances, expressed as average daily intakes over time, are intended to provide for individual variations among most normal people as they live in the United States under usual environmental stresses. Diets should be based on a variety of common foods to provide other nutrients for which human requirements have been less well defined. See text for detailed discussion of allowances and of nutrients not tabulated.

[2]Weights and heights of reference adults are actual medians for the U.S. population of the designated age, as reported by NHANES II. The use of these figures does not imply that the height-to-weight ratios are ideal.

three forms of soluble fiber—oat bran, psyllium (from the weed plantain), and rice bran—because of their ability to lower blood cholesterol levels. Psyllium can be obtained by using laxatives, such as Metamucil, Konsyl, Fiberall fiber wafers, and Perdiem Fiber.

Although earlier studies were contradictory regarding the effectiveness of soluble fiber in lowering cholesterol levels, today it appears that oat bran can lower cholesterol levels by five to six points in people whose initial cholesterol levels are moderately high.[16] To accomplish this reduction, a daily consumption of oat bran equal to a large bowl of cold oat bran cereal or three or more packs of instant oatmeal would be necessary. Of course, oatmeal can be eaten as a cooked cereal or used in other foods, such as hamburgers, pancakes, or meat loaf.

THE FOOD GROUPS

As is so frequently heard, the most effective way to take in adequate amounts of nutrients is to eat a **balanced diet,** that is, to eat a diet that includes a wide variety of foods from different food groups (Table 5-5, *A* to *C*). Over the past several decades, various methods of grouping foods have identified five, seven, four, and now (again) five food groups from which selections are to be made. Today, the United States Department of Agriculture (USDA) Food Guide Pyramid outlines five groups for which recommendations

have been established and an additional group (fats, oils, and sweets) for which no specific recommendations exist (Figure 5-2). Table 5-6 summarizes the major nutrients each food group supplies. To determine whether you are eating a healthful diet balanced with choices from each food group, complete the Personal Assessment on p. 110.

Fruits

Two to four daily servings from the fruit group are recommended for an adult. The important functions

trace elements
Minerals present in very small amounts in the body; micronutrient elements.

dehydration
The abnormal depletion of fluids from the body; severe dehydration can be fatal.

fiber
Plant material that cannot be digested; found in cereal, fruits, and vegetables.

balanced diet
A diet featuring food selections from each of the five basic food groups.

Water-soluble vitamins							Minerals						
Vitamin C (mg)	Thiamin (mg)	Riboflavin (mg)	Niacin (mg NE)[6]	Vitamin B$_6$ (mg)	Folate (µg)	Vitamin B$_{12}$ (µg)	Calcium (mg)	Phosphorus (mg)	Magnesium (mg)	Iron (mg)	Zinc (mg)	Iodide (µg)	Selenium (µg)
60	1.5	1.8	20	2.0	200	2.0	1200	1200	400	12	15	150	50
60	1.5	1.7	19	2.0	200	2.0	1200	1200	350	10	15	150	70
60	1.5	1.7	19	2.0	200	2.0	800	800	350	10	15	150	70
60	1.2	1.4	15	2.0	200	2.0	800	800	350	10	15	150	70
60	1.1	1.3	15	1.5	180	2.0	1200	1200	300	15	12	150	50
60	1.1	1.3	15	1.6	180	2.0	1200	1200	280	15	12	150	55
60	1.1	1.3	15	1.6	180	2.0	800	800	280	15	12	150	55
60	1.0	1.2	13	1.6	180	2.0	800	800	280	10	12	150	55
70	1.5	1.6	17	2.2	400	2.2	1200	1200	320	30	15	175	65
95	1.6	1.8	20	2.1	280	2.6	1200	1200	355	15	19	200	75
95	1.6	1.7	20	2.1	260	2.6	1200	1200	340	15	16	200	75

[3]Retinol equivalents. 1 retinol = 1 µg retinol or 6 µg ß-carotene.
[4]As cholecalciferol. 10 µg cholecalciferol = 400 IU of vitamin D.
[5]α-Tocopherol equivalents. 1 mg d-α tocopherol = 1 α-TE.
[6]1 NE (niacin equivalent) is equal to 1 mg of niacin or 60 mg of dietary tryptophan.

Table 5-5B   Estimated Safe and Adequate Daily Dietary Intakes (ESADDIs) of Selected Vitamins and Minerals for Adults*

Vitamins		Trace elements†				
Biotin (µg)	Pantothenic acid (mg)	Copper (mg)	Manganese (mg)	Fluoride (mg)	Chromium (mg)	Molybdenum (µg)
30-100	4-7	1.5-3.0	2.0-5.0	1.5-4.0	50-200	75-250

*Because there is less information on which to base allowances, these figures are not given in the main table of RDAs and are provided here in the form of ranges of recommended intakes.
†Because the toxic levels for many trace elements may be only several times the usual intake, the upper levels for the trace elements given in this table should not be habitually exceeded.

Table 5-5C   Estimated Minimum Sodium, Chloride, and Potassium Requirements of Healthy People*

Age	Weight (kg)*	Sodium (mg)*†	Chloride (mg)*†	Potassium (mg)‡
10-18	50.0	500	750	2000
>18§	70.0	500	750	2000

*No allowance has been included for large, prolonged losses from the skin through sweat.
†There is no evidence that higher intakes confer any health benefit.
‡Desirable intakes of potassium considerably exceed these values (~3500 mg for adults).
§No allowance included for growth. Values for those below 18 years assume a growth rate at the 50th percentile reported by the National Center for Health Statistics and averaged for men and women.

Figure 5-2   The USDA Food Guide Pyramid.

Table 5-6	Guide to Daily Food Choices		
Food group	**Serving**	**Major contributions**	**Foods and serving size***
Milk, yogurt, and cheese	2 (adult†) 3 (children, teens, young adults, and pregnant or lactating women)	Calcium Riboflavin Protein Potassium Zinc	1 cup milk 1½ oz cheese 2 oz processed cheese 1 cup yogurt 2 cups cottage cheese 1 cup custard/pudding 1½ cups ice cream
Meat, poultry, fish, dry beans, eggs, and nuts	2-3	Protein Niacin Iron Vitamin B_6 Zinc Thiamin Vitamin B_{12}‡	2-3 oz cooked meat, poultry, fish 1-1½ cups cooked dry beans 4 T peanut butter 2 eggs ½-1 cup nuts
Fruits	2-4	Vitamin C Fiber	¼ cup dried fruit ½ cup cooked fruit ¾ cup juice 1 whole piece fruit 1 melon wedge
Vegetables	3-5	Vitamin A Vitamin C Folate Magnesium Fiber	½ cup raw or cooked vegetables 1 cup raw leafy vegetables
Bread, cereals, rice, and pasta	6-11	Starch Thiamin Riboflavin§ Iron Niacin Folate Magnesium ‖ Fiber ‖ Zinc ‖	1 slice of bread 1 oz ready-to-eat cereal ½-¾ cup cooked cereal, rice, or pasta
Fats, oils, and sweets		Foods from this group should not replace any from the other groups. Amounts consumed should be determined by individual energy needs.	

This is a practical way to turn the RDA into food choices. You can get all essential nutrients by eating a balanced variety of foods each day from the food groups listed here. Eat a variety of foods in each food group, and adjust serving sizes appropriately to reach and maintain desirable weight.

*May be reduced for children's servings.   ‡Only in animal food choices.   §If enriched.
†≥25 years of age.   ‖Whole grains especially.

of this group are to provide vitamin A, vitamin C, complex carbohydrates, and fiber in our diets. At least one serving high in vitamin C should be eaten daily.

Vegetables

Three to five servings from the vegetable group are recommended for an adult. As with the fruit group, the important functions of this group are to provide vitamin A, vitamin C, complex carbohydrates, and fiber. Foods included in this group are dark green, yellow, and orange vegetables, canned or cooked vegetables, and tossed salads. **Cruciferous vegetables,** such as broccoli, cabbage, brussels sprouts, and cauliflower, may be especially important in the prevention of certain forms of cancer.[17]

PERSONAL ASSESSMENT

Seven-Day Diet Study

A primary requirement for good nutrition is a balanced diet. A variety of food selections from each food group forms the basis of this diet.

For a 7-day period, assign yourself the points indicated when each dietary requirement is met. Record your points in the appropriate column for each day. Total your daily and weekly points. Negative points for junk food consumption should be subtracted from your daily and weekly totals.

Food	Points	Maximum Score	M	T	W	T	F	S	S
Milk and milk products		30							
One cup of milk or equivalent	10								
Second cup of milk	10								
Third cup of milk	10								
Protein-rich foods		25							
One serving of egg, meat, fish, poultry, cheese, dried beans, or peas	15								
One or two additional servings of egg, meat, fish, poultry, or cheese	10 each								
Fruits and vegetables		30							
One serving of green or yellow vegetables	10								
One serving of citrus fruit, tomato, or cabbage	10								
Two or more servings of other fruits and vegetables, including potatoes	5 each								
Breads and cereals		15							
Four or more servings of whole-grain or enriched cereals or breads	5 each								
Junk foods (or negative point value foods)									
Sweet rolls	−5								
Fruit pies	−5								
Potato chips, corn chips, or cheese curls	−5								
Candy	−5								
Nondiet sodas	−5								
		100							

Point Record

Weekly point total	———	
Negative point total	———	
Adjusted weekly point total	———	

Interpretation

600-700	Excellent dietary practices
450-599	Adequate dietary practices
300-449	Marginal dietary practices
Below 300	Poor dietary practices

Milk, Yogurt, and Cheese

This group contributes two primary nutritional benefits: high-quality protein and calcium (required for bone and tooth development). Foods included in this group are whole milk, low-fat milk, yogurt, cheese, and ice cream. The adult recommendation is 2 to 3 cups of milk or two to three equivalent servings from this group each day. Premenopausal women should consume three to four daily servings from this group to provide maximal protection from osteoporosis.

Because of the general concern about saturated fat, cholesterol, and additional calories, low-fat milk products are recommended in place of high-fat milk products. The Star Box below depicts the differences in calories (per cup), fat content (in grams) and cholesterol content (in milligrams) among various types of dairy products, including whole, 2%, 1%, and skim milk. Low-fat and high-fat dairy products provide similar nutritional benefits.

Meat, Poultry, Fish, Dry Beans, Eggs, and Nuts

Our need for daily selections from the protein-rich group is based on our daily need for protein, iron, and the B vitamins. Meats include all red meat (beef, pork, and game), fish, and poultry. Meat substitutes include eggs, cheese, dried peas and beans (legumes), and peanut butter. Eggs can also be used as meat substitutes; however, using only the separated egg whites provides excellent protein without the accompanying fat, including cholesterol. The current recommendation for adults is 4 ounces total per day, preferably in two to three servings.

The fat content of meat varies considerably. Some forms of meat yield only 1% fat, whereas others may be as high as 40% fat. Poultry and fish are usually significantly lower in overall fat than red meat. Interestingly, the higher the grade of red meat, the more fat will be marbled throughout the muscle fiber and thus the higher will be its caloric value.

Bread, Cereal, Rice, and Pasta

The nutritional benefit from this group lies in its contribution of B-complex vitamins and energy (in the form of calories) to our diets. Some nutritionists believe that the use of foods from this group also promotes protein intake, since many foods in this group are prepared with foods in other groups as complete-protein foods: macaroni and cheese, cereal and milk, and bread and meat sandwiches. Six to eleven servings daily from this group is recommended. Several daily servings of any **enriched** or whole-grain bread or cereal is recommended.

Fats, Oils, and Sweets

Where do such items as butter, candy, colas, cookies, corn chips, and pastries fit into this food group pattern? They are included under the label "fats, oils, and sweets." Most of the items mentioned contribute relatively little to healthful nutrition other than providing additional calories (generally from table sugar) and large amounts of salt and fat. This concern about sugar and high total calories must also be extended to the popular new cookies, crackers, and desserts that are "fat free" or "low fat." It is not surprising that many of these items are referred to collectively as *junk foods*.

FAST FOODS

Fast foods are convenience foods usually prepared in walk-in or drive-through restaurants. In contrast to that of junk foods, the nutritional value of fast foods can vary considerably (see the Star Box on pp. 112-113). As you can see in the "Calories from fat (%)" column, **fat density** is a serious limitation of fast foods. In

---

Skimming Off Fat, Calories, and Cholesterol
Below is a comparison of calories, fat, and cholesterol in 1 cup of several types of milk:
- **Whole.** 150 calories, 8 grams of total fat, 5 grams of saturated fat, 33 mg cholesterol
- **2%.** 120 calories, 5 grams of total fat, 3 grams of saturated fat, 18 mg cholesterol
- **1%.** 100 calories, 2.5 grams of total fat, 1.5 grams of saturated fat, 10 mg cholesterol
- **Skim.** 80 calories, 0 fat, 0 saturated fat, 4 mg cholesterol

---

cruciferous vegetables (crew **sif** er us)
Vegetables that have flowers with four leaves in the pattern of a cross.

enrichment
The process of returning to foods some of the nutritional elements (B vitamins and iron) removed during processing.

fat density
The percentage of a food's total calories that are derived from fat; above 30% is considered to be a high fat density.

Facts about Fast Foods

Will you stop at a fast-food restaurant today? Consider these points before you do: (1) Will this be an extra meal, or have I planned for it as a part of my food intake for the day? (2) Can fast foods be part of a balanced diet? (3)

Do I realize how fat-dense this meal will be? If you answer yes to these questions, then you are practicing responsible, healthful nutrition planning.

Food	Calories	Protein (g)	Carbohydrate (g)	Fat (g)	Calories from Fat (%)	Cholesterol (mg)	Sodium (mg)
Hamburgers							
McDonald's hamburger	263	12.4	28.3	11.3	38.6	29.1	506
Dairy Queen single hamburger w/cheese	410	24	33	20	43.9	50	790
Hardee's ¼ pound cheeseburger	506	28	41	26	46.2	61	1950
Wendy's double hamburger, white bun	560	41	24	34	54.6	125	575
McDonald's Big Mac	570	24.6	39.2	35	55.2	83	979
Burger King Whopper sandwich	640	27	42	41	57.6	94	842
Jack in the Box Jumbo Jack	485	26	38	26	48.2	64	905
Chicken							
Arby's chicken breast sandwich	592	28	56	27	41.0	57	1340
Burger King chicken sandwich	688	26	56	40	52.3	82	1423
Dairy Queen chicken sandwich	670	29	46	41	55.0	75	870
Church's Crispy Nuggets (one; regular)	55	3	4	3	49.0	—	125
Kentucky Fried Chicken Nuggets (one)	46	2.82	2.2	2.9	56.7	11.9	140
Fish							
Church's Southern fried catfish	67	4	4	4	53.7	—	151
Long John Silver's Fish & More	978	34	82	58	53.3	88	2124
McDonald's Filet-O-Fish	435	14.7	35.9	25.7	53.1	45.2	799
Others							
Hardee's hot dog	346	11	26	22	57.2	42	744
Jack in the Box taco	191	8	16	11	51.8	21	406
Arby's roast beef sandwich (regular)	350	22	32	15	38.5	39	590
Hardee's roast beef sandwich	377	21	36	17	40.5	57	1030
French fries							
Arby's french fries	211	2	33	8	34.1	6	30
McDonald's french fries (regular)	220	3	26.1	11.5	47.0	8.6	109
Wendy's french fries (regular)	280	40	35	14	45.0	15	95
Shakes							
Dairy Queen	710	14	120	19	24.0	50	260
McDonald's							
Vanilla	352	9.3	59.6	8.4	21.4	30.6	201
Chocolate	383	9.9	65.5	9	21.1	29.7	300
Strawberry	362	9	62.1	8.7	22.3	32.2	207

Facts about Fast Foods—cont'd.

Soft Drinks

Coca-Cola Classic	144	—	38	—	—	—	14
Coca-Cola	154	—	40	—	—	—	6
Diet Coke	0.9	—	0.3	—	—	—	16
Sprite	142	—	36	—	—	—	45
Tab	1	—	1	—	—	—	30
Diet Sprite	3	—	0	—	—	—	9

Fast foods can be a part of a balanced diet, especially since many companies are reformulating their products to provide better nutrition. However, you should remember that fast foods do have limitations, including their low calcium content, low vitamin A and vitamin C levels, and high calorie content. Plan carefully for your fast food intake, remembering to eat a wide variety of all foods from each of the five basic food groups.

comparison with the recommended standard (25% to 30% of total calories from fat), 40% to 50% of the calories in fast foods come from fats. The conversion by many fast-food restaurants from animal fat to vegetable oil for frying (to reduce cholesterol levels) did not lower the fat density of these food items. One fast-food meal supplies over one half the amount of fat needed in a day. In addition, fast foods are often high in sugar and salt, which contribute to tooth decay and increase the risk for high blood pressure, respectively.

On the positive side, fast-food restaurants have broadened their menus to include whole-wheat breads and rolls, salad bars, lower-fat meats, and low-fat milk products. Many of the larger fast-food restaurants provide nutritional information for consumers on request. The Health Action Guide on p. 114 offers advice for choosing healthful foods when you're eating out.

PHYTOCHEMICALS

In recent years a large group of physiologically active components thought to be able to deactivate carcinogens or function as antioxidants have been identified in a variety of fruits and vegetables. Among these are the carotenoids (from green vegetables), polyphenols (from onions and garlic), indoles (from cruciferous vegetables), and the allyl sulfides (from garlic, chives, and onions). These *phytochemicals* may play an important role in reducing the risk of cancer in people who consume a large quantity of foods (vegetarian or semivegetarian diets) from these two food groups.[18] So important are these several distinct classes of chemicals that they have been called "as essential as vitamins."[19] Whether the recommended minimum number of servings from the fruit and vegetable groups will be increased based on this new information remains to be seen.

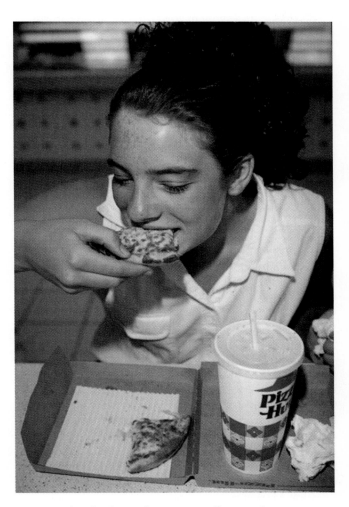

Pizza is a fast food popular among college students.

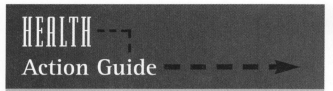

Eating Healthfully Away from Home

Today, more than ever before, people eat more meals away from home. Many of these are fast-food meals characterized by high fat density and excessive use of sweeteners. It is possible, however, to eat nutritiously while eating on the run if you follow these suggestions:

- Choose nutritious foods, such as salads, baked potatoes, and whole-grain breads, instead of french fries.
- At a salad bar, choose the plain vegetables; avoid mayonnaise-based salads, and limit your use of cheese, croutons, and salad dressings.
- Order a plain hamburger without condiments; when you add your own, you control the amounts.
- Add lettuce and tomato to hamburgers to add vitamins, not calories.
- Order plain chicken; it has fewer calories than beef.
- Avoid breaded and fried foods.
- Choose skim milk, low-fat milk, juice, or water, not soda or shakes.
- For dessert, bring a piece of fresh fruit with you.
- Eat a small, nonfat, low-calorie snack at 10 AM and another at 2 PM. This kind of "grazing" can be healthier than gulping down one big, fat-filled meal at noon.

FOOD ADDITIVES

The nostalgia some people have for the "good old days" certainly extends to our current food supply. Today many people believe that the food they consume is unhealthy because of the 2800 generally recognized as safe (GRAS) **food additives** that can be put into food during production, processing, and preparation.[20] But should these additives be banned?

Today's food manufacturers add chemical compounds to the food supply for several reasons that they believe we the consumers support: (1) to maintain the nutritional value of the food; (2) to maintain the food's freshness by preventing changes in its color, flavor, and texture; (3) to contribute to the processing of the food by controlling its texture, acidity, and thickness; and (4) to make the food more appealing to the consumer by enhancing its flavor and standardizing its color. Market research indicates that consumers will continue to accept these alterations regardless of what we might say about our desire that they not be made.

Proposed Definitions for Nutrient Content Claims
- *Free:* an amount that is "nutritionally trivial" and unlikely to have a physiological consequence
- *Calorie Free:* fewer than 5 calories per serving
- *Sugar Free:* less than 0.5 grams of sugar per serving
- *Sodium Free* and *Salt Free:* less than 5 milligrams of sodium per serving
- *Fat Free:* less than 0.5 grams of fat per serving, provided that it has no added fat or oil ingredient
- *Low Fat:* 3 grams or less of fat per serving per 100 grams of the food
- *Low in Saturated Fat:* may be used to describe a food that contains 1 gram or less of saturated fat per serving and not more than 15% of calories from saturated fat
- *Cholesterol Free:* less than 2 milligrams of cholesterol per serving and 2 grams or less of saturated fat per serving
- *Low in Cholesterol:* 20 milligrams or less of cholesterol per serving and per 100 grams of food, and 2 grams or less of saturated fat per serving

Apparently we recognize that living in urban areas, working outside the home, and having foods available at all times during the year are worth the price of additives being a part of our once "natural" food supply.

FOOD LABELS

Since 1973, food manufacturers have been required by the FDA to provide nutritional information (labels) on products to which one or more additional nutrients have been added or for which some nutritional claim has been made. Despite the presence of these labels, there was concern about whether the public could understand the labels as they appeared and whether additional information was required. Accordingly, the FDA, in consultation with individual states and public interest groups, developed new labeling regulations. Revised labels began appearing on food packages in May 1993. The newly adopted label is shown in Figure 5-3. Specific types of information contained on the new label are highlighted. Additionally, newly developed definitions for nutrition-related terms are shown in the Star Box above.

Proposals for the labeling of raw foods, including fresh produce, meat, and seafood, are now being studied. Concern for consumer protection stems from recent disclosures regarding inadequate meat inspection, undercooking of hamburgers, and the risk of contaminated seafood. Currently, single-ingredient meat, fish, and poultry products are not required to have a

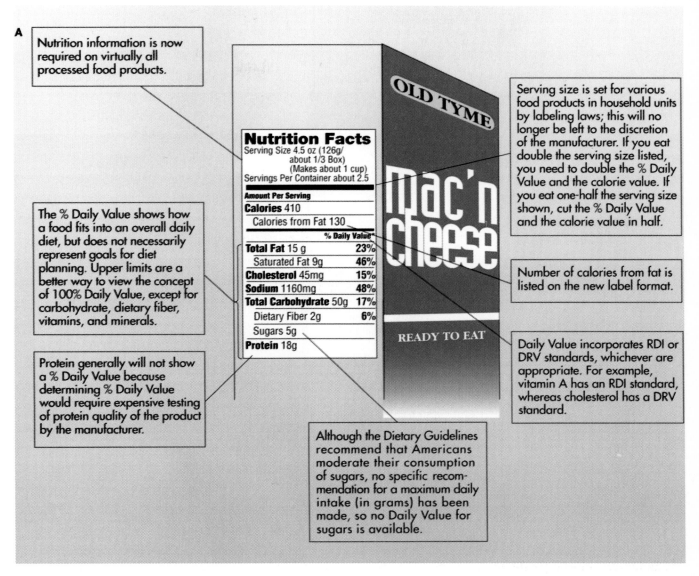

A

Nutrition information is now required on virtually all processed food products.

The % Daily Value shows how a food fits into an overall daily diet, but does not necessarily represent goals for diet planning. Upper limits are a better way to view the concept of 100% Daily Value, except for carbohydrate, dietary fiber, vitamins, and minerals.

Protein generally will not show a % Daily Value because determining % Daily Value would require expensive testing of protein quality of the product by the manufacturer.

Nutrition Facts
Serving Size 4.5 oz (126g/
about 1/3 Box)
(Makes about 1 cup)
Servings Per Container about 2.5

Amount Per Serving

Calories 410

Calories from Fat 130

% Daily Value*

Total Fat 15 g   23%

Saturated Fat 9g   46%

Cholesterol 45mg   15%

Sodium 1160mg   48%

Total Carbohydrate 50g   17%

Dietary Fiber 2g   6%

Sugars 5g

Protein 18g

Serving size is set for various food products in household units by labeling laws; this will no longer be left to the discretion of the manufacturer. If you eat double the serving size listed, you need to double the % Daily Value and the calorie value. If you eat one-half the serving size shown, cut the % Daily Value and the calorie value in half.

Number of calories from fat is listed on the new label format.

Daily Value incorporates RDI or DRV standards, whichever are appropriate. For example, vitamin A has an RDI standard, whereas cholesterol has a DRV standard.

Although the Dietary Guidelines recommend that Americans moderate their consumption of sugars, no specific recommendation for a maximum daily intake (in grams) has been made, so no Daily Value for sugars is available.

OLD TYME
mac'n cheese
READY TO EAT

Figure 5-3   The Nutrition Facts panel on a current food label. **A,** Top of panel. **B,** Bottom of panel.   *Continued*

label. In most areas of the country, however, the standard food label is being applied. Combination meat, fish, and poultry products, such as hot dogs, fish sticks, and chicken patties, must be labeled. Produce, such as vegetables and fruit, is not required to be labeled. (Food Labeling Education Information Center, USDA, May 9, 1996 [personal communication].)

GUIDELINES FOR DIETARY HEALTH

Although dietary guidelines of one type or another have been issued on many occasions, the Dietary Guidelines for Americans are the most current and

widely disseminated guidelines. The newest version appeared in 1995 as the fourth edition of *Nutrition and Your Health: Dietary Guidelines for Americans.*[21] As presently constructed, these guidelines are directed to healthy Americans 2 years of age and older and to the health professional who can influence public dietary practices. Information contained within these guidelines came from a variety of sources, including the

food additives
Chemical compounds intentionally added to our food supply to change some aspect of the food, such as its color or texture.

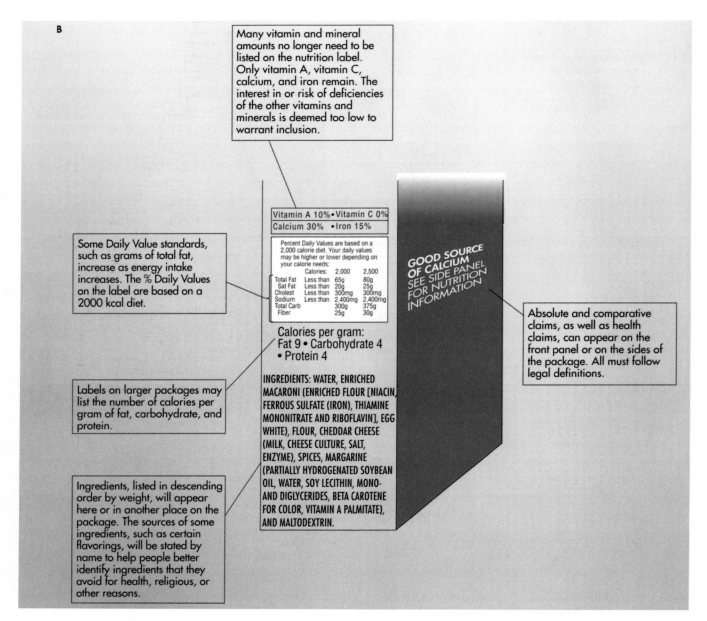

Figure 5-3   *cont'd.* For legend see previous page.

Surgeon General's Report on Nutrition and Health. The most recent dietary guidelines are shown in Figure 5-4 and in the Star Box on p. 117.

Table 5-7 shows how healthful dietary changes can lead to reduced chances of developing certain major diseases. Notice that a reduction in fat and better control of caloric intake are important factors in reducing the likelihood of chronic illness.

Whether the newest Dietary Guidelines for Americans will be more fully implemented than their predecessors remains to be seen. Regardless, almost all Americans could move much closer to meeting these guidelines. The Health Action Guide on p. 117 presents recommendations for making healthful food choices.

NONTRADITIONAL DIETARY PRACTICES

It is not uncommon during the college years to follow some kind of nontraditional diet. Vegetarian diets, weight-reduction diets, and overreliance on fast foods represent some of these nontraditional diet approaches. Most nutritionists believe that these diets

Dietary Recommendations

Issues for Most People

Your nutritional health could probably be improved by implementing the practices described below.

- **Fats and cholesterol:** Reduce consumption of fat (especially saturated fat) and cholesterol. Choose foods relatively low in fat and cholesterol, such as vegetables, fruits, whole-grain foods, fish, poultry, lean meat, and low-fat dairy products. Use food preparation methods that add little or no fat.
- **Energy and weight control:** Achieve and maintain a desirable body weight. To do so, choose a dietary pattern in which energy (caloric) intake is consistent with energy expenditure. To reduce energy intake, limit consumption of foods relatively high in calories, fat, and sugar and minimize alcohol consumption. Increase energy expenditure through regular and sustained physical activity.
- **Complex carbohydrates and fiber:** Increase consumption of whole-grain foods and cereal products, vegetables (including dried beans and peas), and fruits.
- **Sodium:** Reduce sodium intake by choosing foods relatively low in sodium and limiting the amount of salt added in food preparation and at the table.
- **Alcohol:** To reduce the risk of chronic disease, drink alcohol only in moderation (no more than two drinks

a day), if at all. Avoid drinking any alcohol before or while driving, operating machinery, taking medications, or engaging in any other activity requiring judgment. Avoid drinking alcohol while pregnant.

Issues for Some People

The following recommendations are for people with special nutritional needs:

- **Fluoride:** Community water systems should contain fluoride at optimal levels for prevention of tooth decay. If such water is not available, use other appropriate sources of fluoride.
- **Sugars:** Those who are particularly vulnerable to dental caries (cavities), especially children, should limit their consumption and frequency of use of foods high in sugar.
- **Calcium:** Adolescent girls and adult women should increase consumption of foods high in calcium, including low-fat dairy products.
- **Iron:** Children, adolescents, and women of childbearing age should consume foods that are good sources of iron, such as lean red meat, fish, certain beans, and iron-enriched cereals and whole-grain products. This issue is of special concern for low-income families, since iron-rich foods, particularly lean meat, may be too expensive to consume on a regular basis.

need not be discontinued or avoided, but that they should be undertaken with care and insight because of potential nutritional limitations.

Dietary Guidelines for Americans—1995

- Eat a variety of foods.
- Balance the food you eat with physical activity—maintain or improve your weight.
- Choose a diet with plenty of grain products, vegetables, and fruits.
- Choose a diet low in fat, saturated fat, and cholesterol.
- Choose a diet moderate in sugars.
- Choose a diet moderate in salt and sodium.
- If you drink alcoholic beverages, do so in moderation.

Vegetarian Diets

A *vegetarian diet* relies on plant sources for all or most of the nutrients needed by the body. Vegetarian diets encompass a continuum from diets that allow some animal sources of nutrients to those that not only exclude animal sources but also are restrictive in terms of the plant sources of nutrients permitted. We briefly describe three types of vegetarian diets, beginning with the least restrictive.

Ovolactovegetarian diet

Depending on the particular pattern of consuming eggs *(ovo)* and milk *(lacto)* or using one but not the other, **ovolactovegetarianism** can be an extremely sound approach to healthful eating during the adult years. Ovolactovegetarian diets provide the body with the essential amino acids and limit the high intake of fats seen in more conventional diets. The exclusion of meat as a protein source lowers the total

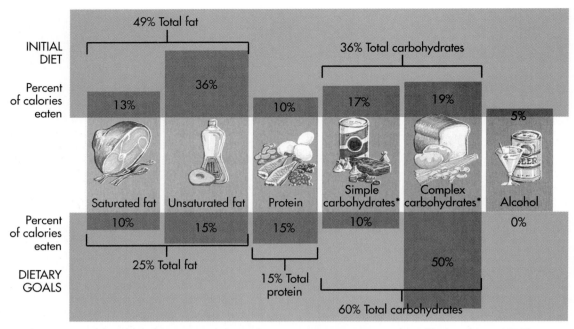

INITIAL DIET

49% Total fat

36% Total carbohydrates

Percent of calories eaten

13%   36%   10%   17%   19%   5%

Saturated fat   Unsaturated fat   Protein   Simple carbohydrates*   Complex carbohydrates*   Alcohol

Percent of calories eaten

10%   15%   15%   10%   0%

DIETARY GOALS

25% Total fat

15% Total protein

50%

60% Total carbohydrates

*Estimates based on Senate Select Subcommittee on Nutrition and Health data (circa 1970).
**Some versions of the Dietary Goals use ranges rather than specific values:
Fats   25%-30%
Protein   12%-15%
Carbohydrate   58%-60%

Figure 5-4   Where do your calories come from? This figure compares the present sources of calories in the U.S. diet with the sources that are currently recommended by nutritionists. How close are you to obtaining your calories from these sources in the recommended percentages? Some experts express each goal as a range: 25% to 30% of calories should come from fat, 12% to 15% from protein, and 58% to 60% from carbohydrates.

fat intake, and the consumption of milk or eggs allows an adequate amount of saturated fat to remain in the diet. The consistent use of vegetable products as the primary source of nutrients complies with the current dietary recommendations for an increase in overall carbohydrates, complex carbohydrates, and fiber.

Lactovegetarian diet

People who include dairy products in their diet but no other animal products, including eggs, are *lactovegetarians*. As with the ovolactovegetarian diet, there is little risk associated with this dietary pattern.

| Table 5-7   Recommended Dietary Changes to Reduce the Risk of Diseases and Their Complications |
Change in Diet:	Reduce Fats	Control Calories	Increase Starch* and Fiber	Reduce Sodium	Control Alcohol
Reduce risk of:					
Heart disease	√	√		√	
Cancer	√	√	√		√
Stroke	√	√		√	√
Diabetes	√	√	√		
Gastrointestinal disease†	√	√	√		√

*Starch refers to complex carbohydrates provided by fruits, vegetables, and whole grain products.
†Primarily gallbladder disease (fat), diverticular disease (fiber), and cirrhosis (alcohol).

HEALTH Action Guide ----→

Making Healthful Food Choices

It is very likely that you can improve your dietary health and reduce the risk of developing heart disease and cancer by implementing the following practices.

Eat More High-Fiber Foods
- Choose dried beans, peas, and lentils more often.
- Eat whole-grain breads, cereals, and crackers.
- Eat more vegetables—raw and cooked.
- Eat whole fruit in place of drinking fruit juice.
- Try other high-fiber foods, such as oat bran, barley, brown rice, or wild rice.

Eat Less Sugar
- Avoid regular soft drinks. One 12-ounce can has nine teaspoons of sugar!
- Avoid eating table sugar, honey, syrup, jam, jelly, candy, sweet rolls, fruit canned in syrup, regular gelatin desserts, cake with icing, pie, or other sweets.
- Choose fresh fruit or fruit canned in natural juice or water.
- If desired, use sweeteners that don't have any calories, such as saccharin or aspartame, instead of sugar.

Use Less Salt
- Reduce the amount of salt you use in cooking.
- Try not to salt your food at the table.
- Eat fewer high-salt foods, such as canned soups, ham, sauerkraut, hot dogs, pickles, and foods that taste salty.
- Eat fewer convenience and fast foods.

Eat Less Fat
- Eat smaller servings of meat. Eat fish and poultry more often. Choose lean cuts of red meat.
- Prepare all meats by roasting, baking, or broiling. Trim off all fat. Be careful of added sauces or gravy. Remove skin from poultry.
- Avoid fried foods. Avoid adding fat when cooking.
- Eat fewer high-fat foods, such as cold cuts, bacon, sausage, hot dogs, butter, margarine, nuts, salad dressing, lard, and solid shortening.
- Drink skim or low-fat milk.
- Eat less ice cream, cheese, sour cream, cream, whole milk, and other high-fat dairy products. ◄------

Vegan vegetarian diet

A **vegan vegetarian diet** is one in which not only meat but also other animal products, including milk, cheese, and eggs, are not part of the diet. When compared with the ovolactovegetarian diet, the vegan diet requires greater nutritional understanding to avoid malnourishment.

When plants are the body's only source of nutrients, some difficulties can arise. The novice vegan will need to be particularly alert for these difficulties. One potential difficulty is obtaining all the essential amino acids. Since a single plant source does not contain all the essential amino acids, the vegan must learn to consistently use a complementary diet. By carefully combining various grains, seeds, and legumes, amino acid deficiency can be prevented. This diet probably should not be used by children, pregnant women, and **lactating** mothers.

In addition to the potential difficulty with amino acid deficiency, the vegan could have some difficulty in maintaining the necessary intake of vitamin B_{12}.

Vegans often have trouble maintaining adequate intakes of iron, zinc, and calcium. In addition, vitamin D deficiencies can occur.

Because of its nutritional limitations, many nutritionists do not recommend the vegan vegetarian diet. This diet should be followed only for reasons related to ecological, philosophical, or animal rights beliefs, since the total exclusion of animal products seems

ovolactovegetarian diet (oh voe **lack** toe vegetarian)
A diet that excludes all meat but does include the consumption of eggs and dairy products.

vegan vegetarian diet (**vay** gan *or* **vee** gan)
A vegetarian diet that excludes all animal products, including eggs and dairy products.

lactating
Breastfeeding, nursing.

to accomplish little from a nutritional point of view that cannot be accomplished through ovolactovege-tarianism. Clearly, the ovolactovegetarian diet is much less likely to lead to malnutrition than is the vegan diet. Many people have now adopted semiveg-etarian diets, in which meat consumption is signifi-cantly reduced but not eliminated. We take a closer look at this type of diet in the article on pp. 125-126.

High-Risk Dietary Practices

Whereas the health benefits and relatively low risks make vegetarian diets attractive, the diets that follow can pose serious health risks.

Macrobiotic diet

At the extreme end of the vegetarian continuum is the **macrobiotic diet.** One form of this diet is the Zen macrobiotic diet. Characterized by an almost total dependence on brown rice as the source of nutrients, this diet moves the individual through progressive stages, each of which gradually removes "undesir-able" foods until little remains other than brown rice. So potentially harmful is this limited approach to nutrition (with deficiencies in vitamin C, calcium, and high-quality protein) that dietitians warn against its use.

Unbalanced and fad diets

A second area of concern about collegiate dietary practices is following **unbalanced diets** to achieve or maintain weight loss. An unbalanced diet might con-sist of a *single food* (like pizza) or food selections from just one or two of the five main food groups. Whether grapefruit, bananas, avocados, or any other "special foods" are used, the point is the same: a diet lacking variety and balance generally cannot provide all of the essential nutrients.

NUTRIENT DENSITY

For many college students, the consideration of nutrient density may prompt certain dietary adjust-ments. The *nutrient density* of a food item relates to its ability to supply proportionally more of the RDA for select vitamins and minerals than it does daily calorie requirements. Foods with a high nutrient den-sity are better choices than those that supply only *empty calories* (Figure 5-5). For example, a bag of potato chips or a bottle of beer has a much lower nutrient density than either a serving of lightly steamed mixed vegetables or a 3-oz. serving of

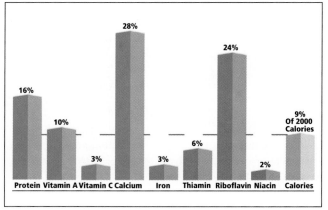

Nutrient density of chocolate milk

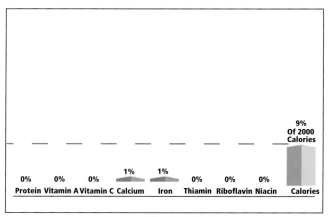

Nutrient density of soda

Figure 5-5   A comparison of the nutrient density of choco-late milk with that of soda. **A,** The bars that represent pro-tein, vitamin A, calcium, and riboflavin are all taller than the calorie bar, showing that chocolate milk is nutrient dense for these nutrients. **B,** All of the nutrient bars are shorter than the calorie bar, illustrating that soda has a low nutrient density relative to the number of calories it sup-plies.

broiled skinless chicken breast. Choosing to eat foods with high nutrient density is especially important for people who are trying to limit caloric intake.

NUTRITION AND THE OLDER ADULT

Nutritional needs change as adults age. Age-related changes to the structure and function of the body are primarily responsible for altered nutritional requirements. These age-related changes can involve the teeth, salivary glands, taste buds, oral muscles, gastric acid production, and peristaltic action. In addition, chronic constipation resulting from changes in gastrointestinal tract function can decrease interest in eating.

The progressive lowering of the body's basal metabolism is another factor that will eventually influence the dietary patterns of older adults. As energy requirements fall, the body gradually senses the need for less food. Because of this decreased need for calories, nutrient density—the nutritional value of food relative to calories supplied—is an important consideration for the elderly.

In addition to the physiological factors that influence dietary patterns among the elderly, psychosocial factors alter the role of food in the lives of many older adults. Social isolation, depression, chronic alcohol consumption, loss of income, transportation limitations, and housing are lifestyle factors that can alter the ease and enjoyment associated with the preparation and consumption of food.[22] Consequently, a person's food intake might decrease.

INTERNATIONAL NUTRITIONAL CONCERNS

Whereas nutritional concerns in this country are centered on overnutrition, including fat density and excessive caloric intake, the main concern in many areas of the world is the limited quantity and quality of food. Reasons for these problems are many, including the limitations imposed by weather, the availability of arable land, religious practices, political unrest, war, social infrastructure, and material and technical shortages. Underlying nearly all of these factors, however, is unabated population growth.

In an attempt to increase the availability of food to countries whose demand for food outweighs their ability to produce it, a number of steps have been suggested, including the following:

- Increase the yield of land currently under cultivation.
- Increase the amount of land under cultivation.
- Increase animal production on land not suitable for cultivation.
- Use water (seas, lakes, and ponds) more efficiently for the production of food.
- Develop unconventional foods through the application of technology.
- Improve nutritional practices through education.

Little progress is being made despite impressive technological breakthroughs in agriculture and food technology (such as "miracle" rice, disease-resistant high-yield corn, and soybean-enhanced infant foods), the efforts of governmental programs, and the support of the Food and Agricultural Organization of the United Nations and the USDA. Particularly in Third World countries, where fertility rates are two to four times higher than those of the United States, annual food production would have to increase between 2.7% and 3.9%. If population growth and food production are not altered in these countries, basic needs will continue to be unmet.

LEARNING from ALL CULTURES

A Comparison of Dietary Practices

Dietary practices differ among various areas of the world. This simple concept is clearly demonstrated when comparing dietary patterns in China with those in the West. These differing patterns then influence the prevalence of health problems. Notice in the data presented below that the average cholesterol difference could be explained on the basis of dietary practices. It is likely that the limited consumption of meat and the heavy consumption of vegetables gives China an advantage in "heart health."

Dietary Intake	China	West
Total protein	64.1 g	91.0 g
Plant protein	60.0 g	27.0 g
Complex carbohydrates	371.0 g	120.0 g
Fat as a percent of total calories	14.5%	38.8%
Cholesterol	127 mg/100 mg	212 mg/100 mg

macrobiotic diet (mack row bye **ott** ick)
A vegetarian diet composed almost entirely of brown rice.

unbalanced diet
A diet lacking adequate representation from each of the five basic food groups.

Summary

- Carbohydrates, fat, and protein supply the body with calories.
- Carbohydrates differ on the basis of their molecular makeup, with sugars being the least complex and starches the most complex.
- Fat plays important roles in nutritional health beyond serving as the body's primary means of storage of excess calories.
- Saturated fats, including trans-fatty acids, should be carefully limited because of their association with chronic diseases.
- Dietary intake of cholesterol should be limited through careful monitoring of food choices.
- Protein supplies the body with amino acids needed to construct its own protein.
- When few foods of animal origin are consumed, incomplete protein sources must be carefully balanced to provide complete protein in the diet.
- Vitamins serve as catalysts for body responses and are found in water-soluble and fat-soluble forms.
- The use of vitamin supplements is desirable for some people, but extensive use of food supplements can be dangerous.
- Minerals are incorporated into various tissues of the body and participate in regulatory functions within the body.
- An adequate amount of water and other fluids is required by the body daily and is obtained from a variety of food sources, including beverages.
- Fiber is undigestible plant material and has two forms, water-soluble and water-insoluble.

- Foods are currently classified into six groups, although recommendations regarding the needed number of daily servings have been given for only five of them.
- Fat-free or low-fat foods can be more calorie dense than anticipated.
- Fast foods should play only a limited role in daily food intake because of their high fat density and their high levels of sugar and sodium.
- Phytochemicals, capable of protecting the body from carcinogens or free radicals, are now being identified in many types of vegetables.
- Food additives enhance the overall quality and convenient use of our food supply.
- New food labels provide considerably more information for the consumer than did labels used previously.
- Current dietary recommendations focus on the role of fat, saturated fat, starch, and sodium in health and disease.
- Ovolactovegetarianism, lactovegetarianism, vegan vegetarianism, and macrobiotic diets are different forms of vegetarianism. Semivegetarianism is similar in some important ways to other forms of vegetarianism.
- Nutrient density plays an important role in the management of caloric intake for people of all ages, particularly older adults.
- A variety of factors contribute to malnourishment in many areas of the world.

Review Questions

1. Which nutrients supply the body with calories?
2. How do sugars differ structurally from starches?
3. What roles does fat play in nutritional health besides serving as the body's primary means of storage for excess calories? What is the basis of our current concern about saturated fats, cholesterol, and trans-fatty acids?
4. What is the principal role of protein in the body? How can complete protein be obtained by people who eat few or no animal products?
5. Which vitamins are water soluble and which are fat soluble? What is the current perception regarding the need for vitamin supplementation? Which vitamins are regarded as antioxidants?
6. What functions do minerals have in the body? What is a trace element?
7. What are the two principal forms of fiber, and how does each of them contribute to health?
8. How many glasses of water daily are currently recommended?
9. What method of grouping foods is now used?
10. What are the current dietary recommendations regarding fat, saturated fat, starch, and sodium intake?
11. How can fat-free or low-fat foods be both low in nutritional density and high in caloric density?
12. What are phytochemicals? What are their principal dietary sources?

13. What information can be obtained from our current food labels?
14. If additives were eliminated from our food, what lifestyle adjustments would the public be forced to make?
15. What are an ovolactovegetarian diet and semivegetarianism, and how do they differ from a vegan diet and a macrobiotic diet?
16. What is nutrient density, and how does it relate to the aging process?

 ## Think About This . . .

- Is it more economical to buy a generic brand of cereal and take a generic multivitamin than to buy a highly supplemented but more expensive brand-name cereal?
- What nutrients are missing from your diet?
- Do your roles in parenting, employment, school, or home management compromise your ability to eat healthfully?
- Analyze your diet in terms of the recommendations made by *Nutrition and Your Health: Dietary Guidelines for Americans.*

- Consider your own dietary practices and those of your friends. Are sound nutritional guidelines being followed?
- Would you say that you live to eat or eat to live?
- What are the most immediate changes that need to be made in your diet?
- In your opinion, what is the role of diet in both the cause and prevention of chronic disease? Are we currently too concerned about the role of food in preventing disease and enhancing health?

References

1. Guthrie H: *Introductory nutrition,* ed 7, St Louis, 1989, Mosby.
2. Wardlaw G, Insel P, Seyler M: *Contemporary nutrition: issues and insights,* ed 2, St Louis, 1994, Mosby.
3. US Department of Health and Human Services: *Report on the expert panel on population strategies for blood cholesterol reduction,* NIH Pub No 9-3046, Washington, DC, 1990, US Government Printing Office.
4. Willet WC, Ascherio A: Transfatty acids: are the effects only marginal? *Am J Public Health* 84:722, 1994.
5. Wardlaw G, Insel P: *Perspectives in nutrition,* ed 3, St Louis, 1996, Mosby.
6. United States Department of Health and Human Services: *The Surgeon General's report on nutrition and health,* DHHS Pub No 88-50210. Washington, DC, 1988. US Government Printing Office.
7. Addis P: Coronary heart disease: an update with emphasis on dietary lipid oxidation products, *Food & Nutrition News* 62(2):7-14, 1990.
8. Carey AR, Stacey J: Low-fat saturating market, *USA Today,* p 1B, June 7, 1995.
9. Rimm EB et al: Vitamin E consumption and the risk of coronary heart disease in men, *N Engl J Med* 328(20):1450-1456, 1993.
10. Leary WE: Vitamins cut cancer in China study, *The New York Times,* Sept 15, 1993.
11. Czeizel AE, Dudas I: Prevention of the first occurrence of neural-tube defects by periconceptional vitamin supplementation. *N Engl J Med* 327(26): 1832-1835, 1992.
12. Food and Nutrition Board, Commission on Life Science, National Research Council: *Diet and health: implications for reducing chronic disease risk/Committee on Diet and Health,* Washington, DC, 1989, National Academy Press.
13. Food labeling: Health claims and label statements: antioxidant vitamins and cancer, *Federal Register* 58(3):2622-2660, Washington, DC, January 6, 1993, US Government Printing Office.
14. Neiman DC, Butterworth DE, Nieman CN: *Nutrition,* Dubuque, Iowa, 1990, Wm C Brown.
15. Fiber: essential to a healthy diet, *Worldview* 3(3):1-5, 1991.
16. Ripsin CM et al: Oat products and lipid lowering: a metaanalysis, *JAMA* 267(24):3317-3325, 1992.
17. American Cancer Society: *Cancer facts and figures—1995,* Atlanta, 1995, The Association.
18. Phytochemicals in disease prevention, *Nutri-News,* St Louis, Mosby, January 1995.
19. Schardt D: Phytochemicals: plants against cancer, *Nutrition Action Health Letter,* April 1994.
20. Office of the Federal Register National Archives and Research Administration: *Code of federal regulations: food and drugs,* 21(Parts 170 to 199):417-420, 1991.
21. US Department of Agriculture, US Department of Health and Human Services: *Nutrition and your health: dietary guidelines for Americans,* ed 4, Home & Garden Bulletin no 232, Washington, DC, 1995, US Government Printing Office.
22. Worthington-Roberts BD, Williams SR: *Nutrition throughout the life cycle,* ed 3, St Louis, 1995, Mosby.

Suggested Readings

Carper J: *The food pharmacy guide to good eating,* New York, 1991, Bantam Books.

Recommendations for health and a longer life through healthful eating are central to this book. The author provides 22 guidelines that should all be followed in selecting and preparing food, as well as recipes for low-fat, low-cholesterol, and low-sodium meals. Disease prevention and health promotion are stressed.

Connor SJ, Connor WE: *The new American diet system,* New York, 1991, Simon & Schuster.

This is a book of tested recipes intended to move Americans in the direction of lower-fat (low–saturated fat) diets. Some recipes are new, and others are modifications of recipes familiar to most Americans.

Copper KH: *Dr. Kenneth H. Cooper's anti-oxidant revolution,* New York, Thomas Nelson, 1994.

A widely recognized name in the fields of aerobic activity, physical fitness, and preventive medicine, Kenneth Cooper throws his full support behind the use of antioxidant vitamins in the prevention of disease. Cooper explains the role of free radicals in altering the structure and function of the body and provides a recipe for an "antioxidant cocktail," intended to reduce free radical formation.

Heslin J, Natow A: *The fast-food nutrition counter,* New York, Pocket Books, 1994.

This handy little book details the contribution to good nutrition (or lack of it) by over 5000 fast-food items. The authors provide helpful hints regarding what to look for that makes a particular fast-food item better or worse than another. For example, breading as a "grease sponge" is shown to make even chicken a less than nutritionally sound choice.

Jacobson MK: *What are we feeding our kids?* New York, Workman, 1994.

Developing sound nutritional habits in children is a difficult task in the face of fast food and other faulty eating practices that can be learned outside and inside the family. The author encourages parents to set a healthy example by following sound nutrition practices and presents lists of foods that should and should not be found in the home.

Following a Semivegetarian Diet

People become vegetarians for many reasons. Some shun meat and animal products for ethical reasons. Others may choose vegetarianism for health reasons. Often it seems that vegetarians are placed in opposition to those who eat meat, and that the two lifestyles are not compatible. In recent years, however, some people are choosing a "middle ground" between the two eating styles. These so-called "semivegetarians" are increasing their intake of vegetables and cutting back greatly on meat consumption but not necessarily eliminating meat entirely.

There are several types of vegetarians. *Vegans* are the most restrictive with their diets, eating only fruits, grains, and vegetables.[1] *Lactovegetarians* consume milk products along with fruits, vegetables, and grains, and *lactoovovegetarians* include both eggs and milk products in their diets.[1] *Semivegetarians* add occasional servings of fish and poultry to the lactoovovegetarian diet,[1] and some even eat red meat on occasion.[2,3]

Benefits of Vegetarianism

Semivegetarianism is the most popular option among the 12 million Americans who consider themselves to be vegetarians.[3] Whereas most vegetarians seem to embrace this lifestyle for health reasons,[3] some people become vegetarians for ethical reasons. These people cite the inhumane conditions in which factory farm animals are raised and processed as reasons to boycott the eating of animal products.[4] The convictions of these people suggest that they are more likely to be vegans, lactovegetarians, or lactoovovegetarians than semivegetarians.

The health benefits of vegetarianism are many. Six of the ten leading causes of death in the United States are linked to red meat consumption.[5] Cutting meat consumption can decrease the risk of heart attacks,[3] and eating more vegetables in place of meat may decrease the risk of some types of cancer.[1,6] In addition, animals raised in factory farms are often given antibiotics to keep them healthy until they get to market; however, constant exposure to antibiotics may cause some bacteria to become resistant, and these bacteria may therefore be present in meat at the store.[7] A vegetarian diet can also aid in weight loss and prevention of obesity.[1]

There are risks associated with following a purely vegetarian diet, however. Protein in plants is generally of lower quality than protein found in animal products,[1] so those on a vegetarian diet must be careful to eat a variety of plant foods to get all of the essential amino acids. Eliminating meat altogether may also lead to a deficiency of vitamin B_{12}, which can lead to brain and nerve damage.[1] Eating foods (such as cereals) fortified with this vitamin or taking vitamin supplements can ward off B_{12} deficiency.[1] Vitamin D, which is needed for bone and tooth development, may be lacking in vegetarian diets.[1] Vegans must make sure they get enough vitamin D by eating fortified foods or getting enough sunlight exposure to promote vitamin D production in the body. Vegetarians should eat plant foods high in iron to prevent deficiency, and calcium supplements may also be necessary, since vegan diets may make calcium difficult to absorb.[1]

Is Semivegetarianism Really Vegetarian?

There is some controversy over whether the semivegetarian diet truly qualifies as "vegetarian." Many people on a strict vegetarian diet do not consider the semivegetarian diet to be vegetarian. To them, any consumption of meat products is considered a compromise to vegetarian principles.[4] Likewise, there are debates over the appropriate use of dairy products and eggs among the various vegetarian groups. Some semivegetarians even acknowledge that they are not "real" vegetarians.[8]

The use of the term "semivegetarian" may not be acceptable to some vegetarians, but there is little doubt that the semivegetarian diet is much healthier than the typical meat-laden Western diet. Interest in the semivegetarian diet came about as a result of recommendations from several groups in the 1980s. The American Cancer Society, the American Heart Association, and the National Academy of Scientists all recommended dietary changes that were closely related to the typical semivegetarian diet.[7] The health benefits of such a diet are well documented. The debate over whether semivegetarians should be categorized as vegetarians seems to revolve around ethical questions concerning treatment of animals. Many vegans especially denounce the eating of any meat or animal products, since animals must be exploited to obtain these foods,[4] and they are thus morally opposed to semivegetarianism. Cutting back, however, may at least cause a decrease in demand for meat and animal products, and some semivegetarians may see this as a moral justification for their dietary changes. Although the semivegetarian diet may not effectively address the ethical questions raised by animal rights activists, it has become an acceptable way of eating for many people who are looking for a way to eat more healthfully.

Becoming Semivegetarian

The semivegetarian diet may be desirable to some people because the limited consumption of meat products may help ward off some nutrient deficiencies,[3] and such a diet can be healthier than that of the typical American. A person who wishes to adopt the semivegetarian diet should not make the change overnight.[2] A sudden elimination of most meat and other animal products can be too drastic of a change to adhere to, so it is best to cut back on them gradually. Such a change should also be discussed first with a doctor, since dietary alterations can cause difficulty for people who are pregnant, nursing, or have health problems.[3]

A gradual cutback in meat consumption can be accomplished by keeping track of how much meat you consume per day. Reduce meat consumption slowly until you have tapered off to about 4 ounces a day.[9] Meat can be used as a condiment (such as chicken strips on a salad) instead of as a main course, and fish can be substituted for red meat.[9] Try new vegetarian foods at each meal, and keep track of your likes and dislikes.[2] Adding more fruit to your meals can increase the variety of your diet as well.[2]

Arlene Spark, a nutrition expert from New York Medical College, has developed a vegetarian food pyramid to help non–meat eaters and semivegetarians to follow a healthful diet (see the inside back cover of this textbook). This pyramid is similar to the USDA Food Guide Pyramid (see Figure 5-2), but it replaces the meat, poultry, fish, dry beans, eggs, and nuts group with a meat/fish substitutes group. It also includes special recommendations for vegans. The pyramid advises vegetarians of all types to eat 6 to 11 servings of grains or starchy vegetables, at least 3 servings of other vegetables, 2 to 4 servings of fruit, and 2 to 4 servings of milk or milk substitutes per day.[10] Legumes can be used as a substitute for

meats for obtaining iron, calcium, protein, and zinc, but keep in mind that vitamin B_{12} is not found in plant foods.[9] Semivegetarians can obtain some B_{12} from the limited meats they consume, but should be careful not to decrease B_{12} intake too much. Also, the occasional fast-food meal is not forbidden. Fast food can provide a change of pace,[2] and many healthy fast-food meals are available.[5]

Children can also be involved in the change of diet (but consult your pediatrician first to be safe). Making dietary changes a "family affair" can make the adjustment easier. Getting kids involved in meal planning, cooking, and label reading can make things more interesting for them.[5] Dietary changes can be a difficult adjustment for kids, however, so don't hold them to the same restrictions as the adults.[2] This may help parents and children avoid arguments over meals and can make meals more enjoyable for the kids.

A semivegetarian diet may be an acceptable alternative for people who want to cut back significantly on meat consumption but who do not want to give up meat altogther. Reducing the amount of meat in the diet can have definite health benefits. Check with your doctor to see if such a diet could have advantages for you.

For Discussion . . .

Is semivegetarianism more ethically sound than the typical Western diet, or is there no difference between eating meat occasionally and eating it often? Should semivegetarians be considered vegetarians? Is the ethical treatment of animals a consideration for you in the food choices you make? Is health a concern for you in your diet?

References

1. *Macmillan health encyclopedia, Vol 4*, New York, 1993, Macmillan.
2. Monroe C, Fuller K: Hooked on good health, *Better Homes and Gardens* 73(3), March 1995.
3. Springer I: Are you ready to go vegetarian? *Cosmopolitan* 219(4), October 1995.
4. Singer P: *Animal liberation*, New York, 1975, Avon.
5. Dinwiddie-Boyd E: Raising vegetarians, *Essence* 23(1), May 1992.
6. Eat your vegetables, *Harvard Health Letter* 20(1), Nov 1994.
7. Null G: *The vegetarian handbook*, New York, 1987, St Martin's Press.
8. Lee K: *The occasional vegetarian*, New York, 1995, Warner.
9. Nash J: The transition diet: from meat eater to vegetarian, *Essence* 25(9), Jan 1995.
10. Vegetarian pyramid, *Better Homes and Gardens*, October 1994.

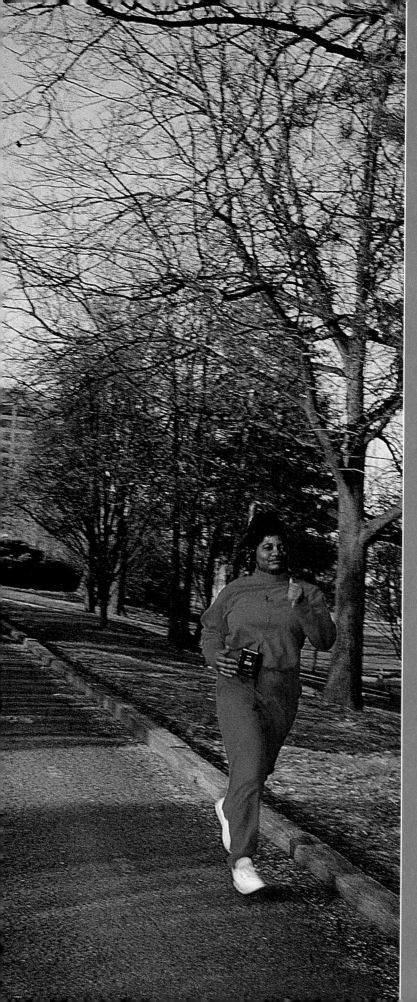

6

Maintaining a Healthy Weight

Healthy People 2000 Objectives

In the area of weight management, the Healthy People 2000 Midcourse Review indicates almost no progress. For all adults between ages 18 and 74, obesity has increased by over 100%. Particularly distressing has been the lack of success in controlling weight among those under age 18. This failure may be partly due to the decline in the number of physical activity programs in schools. In people over age 18, men have been less successful than women in preventing the development of obesity, with a nearly 200% movement away from the stated objective.

These disappointing findings are especially puzzling in light of the progress made in some areas of weight management. For example, many worksite physical fitness programs have been established since the late 1980s. Worksite nutrition programs are also more common now, and many of these programs include weight management components. Further, there has been a small increase in the percentage of adults who report exercising moderately or vigorously almost daily.

You are probably aware that obesity is a serious health concern. Still, most people are above their healthy weight, and a large percentage of adults (25% to 30%) are classified as obese.[1] In a society that has an abundance of high-quality food and a wide variety of labor-saving devices, being overweight is almost the rule rather than the exception.

When the body is supplied with more energy than it can use, a predictable response is seen—the storage of excess energy (or a **positive caloric balance**) in the form of fat. This continuous buildup of fat can eventually result in obesity. The prevailing feeling has been that in terms of medical risk, being only mildly overweight is not dangerous. Today, however, some information suggests otherwise. In fact, in a large study of thousands of nurses, it was found that being average to slightly below average weight relates positively with lower levels of premature death.[2] A recent, smaller study, however, suggests a relatively low risk for slight to moderate obesity.

Regardless of whether slight to moderate overweight is unhealthy, few experts question the real dangers to health and wellness from extreme obesity.[3] Among the health problems caused by or complicated by excess body fat are increased surgical risk, hypertension, various forms of heart disease, stroke, type II diabetes mellitus, several forms of cancer, deterioration of joints, complications during pregnancy, gallbladder disease, and an overall increased risk of mortality (see the Star Box at right).

BODY IMAGE AND SELF-CONCEPT

In spite of some disagreement among professionals, for our image-conscious general population there is little debate about overweight being a problem. All too often, the media tell people that being overweight is undesirable, particularly when it interferes with their ability to conform to certain ideal body images (such as being tall, thin, and "cut" with muscular definition). To cite a case in point, the average actress and model is thinner than 95% of the female population and weighs 23% less than the average woman. Today's lean but muscular version of perfection is a very demanding standard for both women and men to meet.

In light of this challenge, people may become dissatisfied and concerned about their inability to resemble these ideals. The scope of this dissatisfaction is evident in a study of over 800 women, which revealed that nearly half were unhappy with their weight, muscle tone, hips, thighs, buttocks, and legs (men may not be very different in this regard).[4] Not surpris-

Health Risks of Obesity
Each of the diseases listed below is followed by the percentage of cases that are caused by obesity:

Colon cancer   10%
Breast cancer   11%
Hypertension   33%
Heart disease   70%
Diabetes (type II, non–insulin-dependent)   90%

As these statistics show, being obese greatly increases your risk of many serious and even life-threatening diseases.

ingly, when this dissatisfaction exists, people can begin to question their own attractiveness, and eventually, for some, their self-concept changes and self-esteem declines. Only growing older lessens, but does not eliminate, this dissatisfaction.

In comparison with being overweight, there has traditionally been little media attention paid to being underweight (see pp. 147-148). However, the body image problems experienced by some extremely thin people can be equally distressing.

OVERWEIGHT AND OBESITY DEFINED

How can we tell the difference between overweight and obesity? Nutritionists have traditionally said that obesity is present when fat accumulation produces a body weight that is more than 20% above an ideal or **desirable weight.** People are said to be overweight if their weight is between 1% and 19% above their desirable weight. As weight increases above the 20% level, the label *obese* is routinely applied. Of course, an exception to this relationship between overweight and obesity is excessive weight caused by extreme muscularity, such as that seen in many football players.

The term *obesity* requires further refinement. When people are between 20% and 40% above desirable weight, their obesity is described as *mild* (about 90% of all obese people), whereas excessive weight in the range of 41% to 99% above desirable weight is defined as *moderate obesity* (9%) and weight of 100% or more above desirable weight is defined as *severe, gross,* or *morbid obesity* (< 1%).

Being most familiar with the weight guidelines

used in the past, most clinicians and the general public continue to use standard height-weight tables to determine the extent to which scale weight exceeds desirable weight and thus the existence of mild, moderate, or severe obesity. At this time, however, other, more precise techniques are available that can be used to determine body composition. In the following section, several of those techniques, including waist-to-hip ratio (*healthy body weight*), body mass index, hydrostatic weighing, skin fold measurements, and electrical impedance, are described.

DETERMINING WEIGHT AND BODY COMPOSITION

As mentioned previously, a variety of techniques can be used to determine the existence of overweight and obesity. Some techniques are common and routinely used by the general public, whereas others are expensive and of limited availability.

Height-Weight Tables

Over the last 40 years a number of height and weight tables have been developed to assist people in determining the relationship between their weight and desirable standards. Criticisms of one kind or another have been made against nearly every version of these tables, including the absence of consideration of variables such as gender, age, frame size, and body composition. Further, some versions were thought to be too rigorous in establishing cutoff points for desirable or ideal weight, and others were deemed too generous in allowing people to weigh too much. Accordingly, these tables are being gradually replaced by other assessment techniques. Regardless, height and weight tables remain available. Table 6-1 shows the most widely used of these tables.[5,6]

Healthy Body Weight

You can determine your **healthy body weight** by using the weight guidelines (Table 6-2) that are found in the *Dietary Guidelines for Americans*.[5] This assessment involves converting two body measurements, the waist and the hip circumferences, into a waist-to-hip ratio (WHR) that can then be applied to weight ranges for people of particular ages and heights. Among people who have an acceptable WHR, female "healthy weight" is near the lower end of each weight range, whereas male "healthy weight" is at the higher end of each weight range.

Table 6-1   1983 Metropolitan Life Insurance Height and Weight Table

Height	Small Frame	Medium Frame	Large Frame
		Weight in pounds	
Men*			
5'2"	128-134	131-141	138-150
5'3"	130-136	133-143	140-153
5'4"	132-138	135-145	142-156
5'5"	134-140	137-148	144-160
5'6"	136-142	139-151	146-164
5'7"	138-145	142-154	149-168
5'8"	140-148	145-157	152-172
5'9"	142-151	148-160	155-176
5'10"	144-154	151-163	158-180
5'11"	146-157	154-166	161-184
6'0"	149-160	157-170	164-188
6'1"	152-164	160-174	168-192
6'2"	155-168	164-178	172-197
6'3"	158-172	167-182	176-202
6'4"	162-176	171-187	181-207
Women†			
4'10"	102-111	109-121	118-131
4'11"	103-113	111-123	120-134
5'0"	104-115	113-126	122-137
5'1"	106-118	115-129	125-140
5'2"	108-121	118-132	128-143
5'3"	111-124	121-135	131-147
5'4"	114-127	124-138	134-151
5'5"	117-130	127-141	137-155
5'6"	120-133	130-144	140-159
5'7"	123-136	133-147	143-163
5'8"	126-139	136-150	146-167
5'9"	129-142	139-153	149-170
5'10"	132-145	142-156	152-173
5'11"	135-148	145-159	155-176
6'0"	138-151	148-162	158-179

*Weights at ages 25 to 59, based on lowest mortality. Weight in pounds according to frame (in indoor clothing weighing 5 lb, shoes with 1" heels).

†Weights at ages 25 to 59, based on lowest mortality. Weight in pounds according to frame (in indoor clothing weighing 3 lb, shoes with 1" heels).

positive caloric balance
Caloric intake greater than caloric expenditure.

desirable weight
The weight range deemed appropriate for people of a specific gender, age, and frame size.

healthy body weight
Body weight within a weight range appropriate for a person with an acceptable weight-to-height ratio.

Table 6-2   Healthy Weight: Recommended Guidelines

Height without shoes	Weight without clothes	
	19–34 years	35 years and over
5'	97-128	108-138
5'1"	101-132	111-143
5'2"	104-137	115-148
5'3"	107-141	119-152
5'4"	111-146	122-157
5'5"	114-150	126-162
5'6"	118-155	130-167
5'7"	121-160	134-172
5'8"	125-164	138-178
5'9"	129-169	142-183
5'10"	132-174	146-188
5'11"	136-179	151-194
6'	140-184	155-199
6'1"	144-189	159-205
6'2"	148-195	164-210
6'3"	152-200	168-216
6'4"	156-205	173-222
6'5"	160-211	177-228
6'6"	164-216	182-234

To use these new weight ranges, the following procedure must be performed:

1. Measure around your waist near your navel while you stand relaxed, not pulling in your stomach.
2. Measure around your hips, over the buttocks where hips are the largest.
3. Divide the waist measurement by the hip measurement.

For example, a woman with a 25-inch waist and 36-inch hips has a WHR of .69, which is well within the healthful range. Women with a WHR of less than .85 generally have a body weight that falls within the healthy range for their age and height; men with a WHR of less than 1.00 will also probably fall within the range that is considered healthy for their age and height. Any person whose WHR is equal to or greater than the recommended ratio should attempt to lose weight. Weight loss should occur no faster than ½ to 1 pound per week.

This new system was developed because of the growing concern over the relationship between the amount of fat that is around the waist (the spare tire) and the development of several serious health problems. In addition to an unacceptably high WHR, a bulging stomach or high blood pressure indicates a need to lose weight. Certainly people who exhibit all three of these signs are most in need of weight loss.

Body Mass Index

Another procedure for assessing healthy body weight is the **body mass index (BMI)**. The BMI indicates the relationship of body weight (expressed in kilograms) to height (expressed in meters) for both men and women.[7] The BMI does not reflect body composition (fat versus lean tissue) or consider the degree of fat accumulated within the central body cavity, nor is it adjusted for age. It is, nevertheless, widely used in determining obesity. A BMI greater than 27.8 for men or 27.3 for women indicates obesity.

An alternative method of determining the BMI is to use a **nomogram** such as that in Figure 6-1. Like the BMI, the nomogram requires information about both weight and height.

Once the BMI has been obtained, its relationship to a desirable BMI can be determined using Table 6-3.

Electrical Impedance

Electrical impedance is a relatively new method used to determine body composition. This computerized assessment procedure measures the electrical impedance (resistance) to a weak electrical flow directed through the body. Electrodes are attached to the arm and leg. Because adipose tissue resists the passage of the electrical current more than muscle tissue does, electrical impedance can be used to accurately calculate the percentage of body fat. Fortunately, electrical impedance measurements are painless. Additional techniques in which highly accurate but expensive technology is used to determine body composition, including *computerized axial tomography (CAT) scans, magnetic resonance imaging (MRI), infrared light transmission,* and *neutron activation,* may become common ways of measuring body composition in the future.

Skinfold Measurements

Skinfold measurements are a relatively precise and inexpensive indicator of body composition. In this assessment procedure, constant-pressure **calipers** are used to measure the thickness of the layer of fat beneath the skin's surface, the *subcutaneous fat layer.* Skinfold measurements of subcutaneous fat are taken at key places on the body (Figure 6-2). Through the use of specific formulas, skinfold measurements can be used to calculate the percentage of body fat. Additionally, the percent body fat value can be used in determining desirable weight.

Young adult men normally have a body fat percentage of 10% to 15%. The normal range for young adult women is 20% to 25%.[8] When a man's body fat percentage is higher than 20% and a woman's body

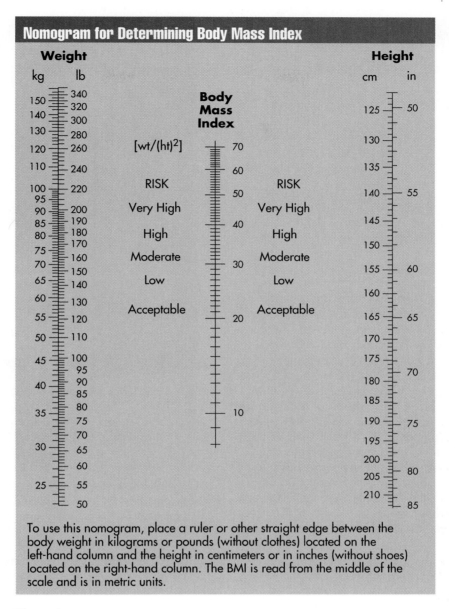

Nomogram for Determining Body Mass Index

Weight

kg   lb

Body Mass Index

$[wt/(ht)^2]$

RISK

Very High

High

Moderate

Low

Acceptable

RISK

Very High

High

Moderate

Low

Acceptable

Height

cm   in

To use this nomogram, place a ruler or other straight edge between the body weight in kilograms or pounds (without clothes) located on the left-hand column and the height in centimeters or in inches (without shoes) located on the right-hand column. The BMI is read from the middle of the scale and is in metric units.

Figure 6-1

fat percentage is above 30%, they are considered to be obese. The higher percentage of fat typically found in women is related to preparation for pregnancy and breastfeeding.

Hydrostatic Weighing

Hydrostatic (underwater) *weighing* is yet another precise method for determining the relative amounts of fat and lean body mass that make up body weight. A person's percentage of body fat is determined by comparing the underwater weight with the body weight out of water. The need for expensive facilities (a tank or pool) and experienced technicians make the

body mass index (BMI)
A numerical expression of body weight based on height and weight.

nomogram
Graphic means for finding an unknown value.

electrical impedance
Method to test for the percentage of body fat using resistance to the flow of electrical current.

calipers
A device used to measure the thickness of a skinfold, from which percent body fat can be calculated.

Table 6–3 Desirable Body Mass Index in Relation to Age	
Age Group (years)	BMI (kg/m^2)
19–24	19–24
25–34	20–25
35–44	21–26
45–54	22–27
55–65	23–28
>65	24–29

availability and cost of this procedure limited to small-scale application, usually at a large research university or teaching hospital.

Appearance

Despite the many ways to determine obesity, the simplest method may be to look in the mirror. The old saying "mirrors don't lie" speaks for itself. For most people, this method is fairly accurate and certainly inexpensive. Unless a person is very muscular or has retained an excessive amount of water, the reflection in the mirror should be a good indicator of whether one's weight is appropriate. Although this simple method does not allow a person to pinpoint a body fat percentage, the person should be able to visually determine whether he or she is excessively fat.

For some overweight and obese people, however, it can be difficult to be objective. They may not accurately judge their bodies. Their imagined (or desired) **body image** and their actual image are markedly different. For these people, disappointment and frustration are likely.

ORIGINS OF OBESITY

Experts continue to investigate the origins of obesity. Many theories focus on factors within the individual and from the environment. If the definitive cause of obesity is ever identified, it will probably have a complex basis that includes strong genetic and **neurophysiological** factors. However, until such a discovery is made, it is safe to assume that no two obese people will have gained their excess weight in exactly the same way or for the same reasons.

Genetic Basis for Obesity

Based on studies involving identical and nonidentical twins, some raised together and others separately, researchers have concluded that both environment and genetics influence obesity. In some cases an

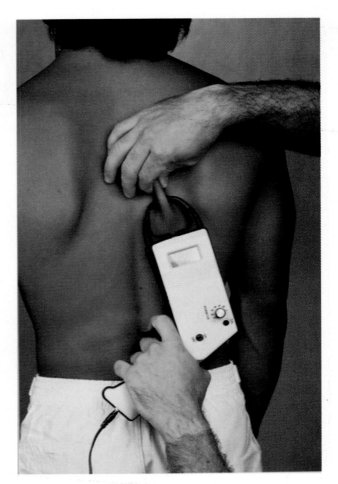

Figure 6-2 Subscapular body fat determination using skinfold calipers. Skinfold measurements are used in equations that calculate body fat density and percent body fat.

inherited tendency toward excessive weight appears to be almost solely responsible for the amount and distribution of body fat, whereas in other cases the role of genetics is clearly limited.

In recent months the role of a genetic contribution has been clarified somewhat by the discovery of "fat" genes in mice and, subsequently, an "obese" gene in humans.[9,10] Speculation regarding the influence of these (or additional) genes centers on flawed genetic receipt of a protein that normally signals the body to terminate food consumption.[11] Research, in fact, found this protein, *leptin,* in low levels in overweight mice. Researchers suspected that leptin would be found in lower levels in obese humans compared with those of average weight. Their results demonstrated, however, that obese humans actually have higher levels of leptin than those of average weight.[12]

In addition, a genetic basis for an altered form of metabolism in people whose adipose tissue tends to accumulate in the midline may now be known. The "spare tire," associated unhealthy body weight, severe obesity, and type II diabetes mellitus (see p. 266), is now thought to reflect an abnormal β_3-adrenergic gene.[13]

Appetite Center

Building on this new information about the neurophysiological basis of obesity, researchers have identified centers for the control of eating within the hypothalamus of the CNS. These centers, the *feeding center* for hunger and the *satiety center* for fullness, tell the body when it should begin consuming food and when food consumption should stop. These centers are thought to monitor continuously a variety of factors regarding food intake, including olfactory and visual cues, the body's stores of glucose, amino acids and free fatty acids, the degree of stomach distention, and information regarding basal metabolic rate and gastrointestinal hormone level.[14] The ability of several drugs to influence, at least temporarily, either hunger or **satiety,** including the amphetamines, fenfluramine, and the antidepressant Prozac, support the important role of the CNS in controlling food consumption. A protein that controls satiety in rats, GLP-1, was identified in 1996. If this protein functions in humans in the same manner, a highly effective weight management medication could follow.

Set Point Theory

Traditional theory has suggested that the energy expenditure and energy storage centers of the body possess a genetically programmed awareness of the body's most physiologically desirable weight. To "honor" this so-called **set point** for desirable weight, the body adjusts its baseline use of energy, the basal metabolic rate (see pp. 137-138), upward or downward to accommodate an excessive intake of calories or an inadequate intake of calories, as the case may be. Thus by burning more energy or storing more energy, the body maintains its "best" weight through the process of **adaptive thermogenesis.**

Using the set point theory to explain the difficulty of losing weight, it has been suggested that in the case of a person with a genetically conditioned tendency to store excessive energy (to gain weight easily), the body prevents planned weight loss from occurring easily by adjusting the set point to a lower level. In addition, according to the set point theory, to prevent further episodes of "starvation" from occurring, a new, higher set point is established and lost weight is regained to a level above that of the initial set point. Every time the dieter again attempts to lose weight, he or she will **yo-yo** between weight loss and subsequent weight gain.

Today, a body of evidence suggests that the yo-yo dieting model, explained on the basis of set point readjustment, may not be accurate. Perhaps the weight gain that follows a period of dieting occurs merely because of the tendency for most people to gain fat and weight as they age. Perhaps, however, it is a reflection of the difficulty of losing weight only through caloric restriction, without increasing caloric expenditure.[15]

Related somewhat to set point and adaptive thermogenesis is the renewed interest in whether the small stores of brown fat (most fat is white fat) found in humans are involved in weight control. Located in small amounts in the upper back between the shoulder blades, this fat has the physiological ability to expend calories solely as heat without generating the high-energy units that are capable of being stored in fat cells.[16] Perhaps in people who have little difficulty controlling weight, brown fat is more successful in producing heat rather than material suitable for storage in fat cells.

Although considered dangerous by health experts, some have experimented with the use of an enzyme, 2,4 Dinitrophenol (DNP), that is capable of "uncoupling" high-energy units in a manner similar to that done naturally by brown fat, thus preventing energy storage and weight gain.

---

body image
A person's subjective perception of how his or her body appears.

neurophysiological
Pertaining to nervous system functioning; processes through which the body senses and responds to its internal and external environments.

satiety (suh **tie** uh tee)
A state in which there is no longer a desire to eat; fullness.

set point
A genetically programmed range of body weight beyond which a person finds it difficult to gain or lose additional weight.

adaptive thermogenesis
Physiological response of the body to adjust its metabolic rate to the presence of food.

yo-yo syndrome
The repeated weight loss followed by weight gain experienced by many dieters.

Body Type

An inheritance basis for obesity could involve the interplay of *somatotype* (body build) and other unique energy processing characteristics passed on from parents to their children.

The classic work of Sheldon is credited with establishing the now-familiar body types: *ectomorph, mesomorph,* and *endomorph.* In the case of the ectomorphic body type, a tall slender body seems to virtually protect individuals from difficulty with excessive weight. Ectomorphs usually have difficulty maintaining normal weight for their height.

The somewhat shorter, more heavily muscled, athletic body of the mesomorph represents a genetic middle ground in inherited body types. During childhood, adolescence, and adulthood, as long as activity levels are maintained, mesomorphic people will appear to be "solid" without appearing to be obese. For well-conditioned mesomorphs, scale weight may suggest obesity, but the excessive weight is more likely the result of heavy muscularity. Mesomorphs have their greatest difficulty with obesity during adulthood when eating patterns fail to adjust to a decline in physical activity.

Endomorphs have body types that tend to be round and soft. Many endomorphs have excessively large abdomens and report having had weight problems since childhood.

Sheldon was interested in the personality traits and temperament of people with each body type. The relationship of body type to inheritance, body weight, and weight management cannot, however, go unnoticed. Sheldon's work simply gives us labels with which to discuss our observations.

Infant and Adult Feeding Patterns

Obesity can be categorized according to the way in which feeding patterns seem to produce it. Two general feeding patterns are related to two forms of obesity: hypercellular obesity and hypertrophic obesity.

The first of these patterns involves infant feeding. Many researchers believe that the number of fat cells a person has will be initially determined during the first 2 years of life. Babies who are overfed will develop a greater number of fat cells than babies who receive a balanced diet of appropriate, infant-sized portions. Overfed babies, especially those with a family history of obesity, will tend to develop **hypercellular obesity.** When these children reach adulthood, they will have more fat cells.

Late childhood and adolescence are also times during which excessive weight gain may result in the formation of addition fat cells. For adults, substantial weight gain can also stimulate an increase in the number of fat cells and thus move them toward hypercellular obesity.

A second type of obesity that has its origins in an eating pattern is called **hypertrophic obesity.** This form of obesity is related to a long-term positive caloric balance during adulthood. Over a period of years, existing fat cells increase in size to accommodate excess food intake.

Hypertrophic obesity is generally associated with excessive fat around the waist and is thought to contribute to conditions such as diabetes mellitus (type II, non–insulin-dependent diabetes), high levels of fat in the blood, high blood pressure, and heart disease. In our society, hypertrophic obesity shows itself during middle age—a time when our physical activity generally declines while our food intake remains the same.

Endocrine Influence

For a number of years, people believed that obesity was the result of "glandular" problems. Often the thyroid gland was said to be underactive, thus preventing the person from "burning up" food. Today, it is known that only a few obese people have an endocrine dysfunction of the type that would cause obesity.

Pregnancy

During a normal pregnancy, approximately 75,000 additional calories are required to support the development of the fetus and the formation of *maternal supportive tissues* and to fuel the mother's basal metabolic rate. In addition, the woman will develop approximately 9 extra pounds of fat tissue, which will be used as an energy source during breastfeeding. In total, the typical woman gives birth having gained approximately 28 pounds over her prepregnancy weight.[17]

After the birth of the baby, the mother will ideally have a weight gain of only 2 to 3 pounds over her prepregnancy weight. This small amount of additional weight will normally be lost by the end of the sixth to eighth month after birth. Of course, in the absence of the sound diet and exercise components stressed in the prenatal period, weight gain could be considerably greater.

Decreasing Basal Metabolic Rate

The body's requirement for energy to maintain basic physiological processes falls steadily with age. This change reflects the loss of muscle tissue with age in both men and women. Although on a short-term basis little adjustment needs to be made to maintain

LEARNING *from* ALL CULTURES

Satisfying Our Appetites

All people satisfy hunger by eating, but because of cultural differences, when and how our appetites are satisfied vary. All people usually eat at least one meal in a 24-hour period. Some African tribes and other developing societies are accustomed to eating only one meal per day, as a result of occasional or continual food shortages. Other substances are known to be used by some of these societies to suppress hunger, such as coca leaves (which contain cocaine), peyote (a hallucinogen derived from a cactus), tobacco, coffee, and tea.[18] Appetite suppressants in the form of diet aids in the United States serve the same purpose but for different reasons.

Typically in North America, three meals a day is the custom, although skipping regular meals and snacking are common. The British usually eat four times a day, whereas continental European people may eat five or six times. Of course, these practices vary according to changing lifestyles.[18]

For most, eating is a pleasurable experience, but not just for the sake of nourishment. Business deals are made over lunch, agreements between countries are discussed over a meal, relationships are begun during a romantic dinner, and events are celebrated by the sharing of food.

Think about your own eating habits. Why and when do you eat? How do your eating habits reflect your culture and lifestyle?

weight, weight gain can become a problem over time if adjustments are not made. A gradual decrease in food intake or an effort to exercise more can be effective in preventing the gradual onset of obesity.

Family Dietary Practices

Food preferences and eating practices are among the many areas of instruction for which the family assumes responsibility. In some families the lessons are taught as though they were outlined from a nutrition textbook, whereas for others the lessons taught are destined to lead to a lifetime of malnourishment, including obesity. For example, between-meal snacking involving highly sugared or high-fat foods, large serving sizes, multiple servings, and high-calorie meals are poor lessons taught by some families.

Inactivity

When weight management experts are asked to identify the single most important reason there is so much obesity in today's society, they are almost certain to point to inactivity. People of all ages tend to do less and therefore burn fewer calories than did their ancestors only a few generations ago. Automation in the workplace, labor-saving devices in the home, the inactivity associated with watching television, and a general dislike of sweating are a few of the reasons that account for this inactivity.

CALORIC BALANCE

As previously mentioned, any calories consumed in excess of those that are used by the body are converted to fat. We gain weight when our energy input is greater than our energy output. On the other hand, we lose weight when our energy output is greater than our energy input (Figure 6-3). Weight remains constant when caloric input and output are identical. In such situations, our bodies are said to be in *caloric balance.*

ENERGY NEEDS OF THE BODY

What are our energy needs? How many calories should we consume (or burn) to achieve a healthy weight? Although there are some ballpark estimates for college-aged men (2500 to 3300 calories daily) and women (approximately 2500 calories daily), we all

hypercellular obesity
A form of obesity seen in people who possess an abnormally large number of fat cells.

hypertrophic obesity (high per **troh** fick)
A form of obesity in which fat cells are enlarged but not excessive in number.

vary in our specific energy needs.[19] These needs are based on three factors: (1) activity requirements, (2) basal metabolic rate, and (3) the thermic effect of food.

We often ignore opportunities to become more active.

Activity Requirements

Each person's caloric *activity requirements* vary directly according to the amount of daily physical work completed. For example, sedentary office workers will require a smaller daily caloric intake than will construction workers, lumberjacks, or farm workers.

Physical activity that occurs outside the workplace also increases caloric needs. Sedentary office workers may be quite active in their recreational pursuits. Active employees may spend their off hours lounging in front of the television. You must closely examine the total amount of work or activity an individual engages in to accurately estimate that person's caloric requirements. Physical activity uses 20% to 40% of caloric intake. See Table 6-4 for a breakdown of caloric expenditures for various recreational pursuits.

Basal Metabolism

Of the three factors that determine energy needs, basal metabolism uses the highest proportion (50%

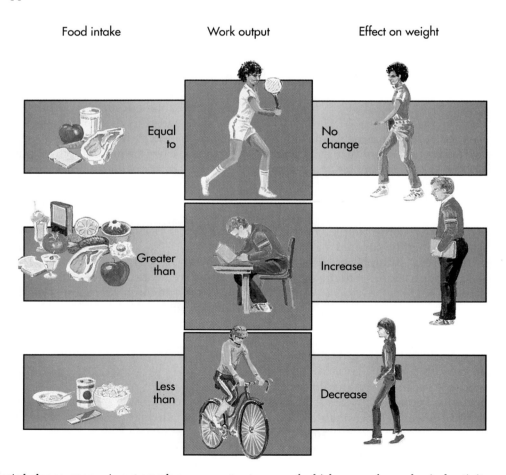

Figure 6-3   Caloric balance: energy input equals energy output, some of which comes from physical activity.

to 70%) of the total calories required by each person. Expressed as a **basal metabolic rate (BMR),** basal metabolism reflects the minimum amount of energy the body requires to carry on all vital functions, such as blood circulation and glandular activity. Even when a person is totally relaxed or sleeping, these vital body functions continue to expend calories.

Basal metabolism changes as people age. For both males and females, the BMR is relatively high at birth and continues to increase until the age of 2. Except for a slight rise at puberty, their BMR will then gradually decline throughout life.[16] If people

fail to recognize that their BMR decreases as they grow older (2% per decade), they might also fail to adjust their food intake and activity level accordingly. Thus they will gradually put on unwanted pounds as they move through the life cycle. Use the formula given in the Star Box on p. 138 to determine your BMR.

Thermic Effect of Food

Formerly called the *specific dynamic action* of food, or *dietary thermogenesis*, the thermic effect of food represents the energy our bodies require for the diges-

---

Table 6-4   Calories Expended During Physical Activity

To determine the number of calories you have spent in an hour of activity, simply multiply the *calories per hour per pound* column by your weight (in pounds). For example, after an hour of archery, a 120-pound person will have expended 209 calories; a 160-pound person, 278 calories; and a 220-pound person, 383 calories.

Activity	Calories/hour/pound	Activity	Calories/hour/pound
Archery	1.74	Marching (rapid)	3.84
Basketball	3.78	Painting (outside)	2.10
Baseball	1.86	Playing music (sitting)	1.08
Boxing (sparring)	3.78	Racquetball	3.90
Canoeing (leisure)	1.20	Running (cross-country)	4.44
Climbing hills (no load)	3.30	Running	
Cleaning	1.62	11 min 30 sec per mile	3.66
Cooking	1.20	9 min per mile	5.28
Cycling		8 min per mile	5.64
5.5 mph	1.74	7 min per mile	6.24
9.4 mph	2.70	6 min per mile	6.84
Racing	4.62	5 min 30 sec per mile	7.86
Dance (modern)	2.28	Scrubbing floors	3.00
Eating (sitting)	0.60	Sailing	1.20
Field hockey	3.66	Skiing	
Fishing	1.68	Cross-country	4.43
Football	3.60	Snow, downhill	3.84
Gardening		Water	3.12
Digging	3.42	Skating (moderate)	2.28
Mowing	3.06	Soccer	3.54
Raking	1.44	Squash	5.76
Golf	2.34	Swimming	
Gymnastics	1.80	Backstroke	4.62
Handball	3.78	Breaststroke	4.44
Hiking	2.52	Free, fast	4.26
Horseback riding		Free, slow	3.48
Galloping	3.72	Butterfly	4.68
Trotting	3.00	Table tennis	1.86
Walking	1.14	Tennis	3.00
Ice hockey	5.70	Volleyball	1.32
Jogging	4.15	Walking (normal pace)	2.16
Judo	5.34	Weight training	1.90
Knitting (sewing)	0.60	Wrestling	5.10
Lacrosse	5.70	Writing (sitting)	0.78

tion, absorption, and transportation of food. This energy breaks the electrochemical bonds that hold complex food molecules together, resulting in smaller nutrient units that can be distributed throughout the body. This energy need is in addition to activity needs and basal metabolic needs. The thermic effect of food is estimated to represent about 10% of total energy needs.[20] Some nutritionists now consider the thermic effect of food merely a component of overall basal metabolism.

Lifetime Weight Control

Obesity and frequent fluctuation in weight are thought to be associated with higher levels of morbidity and mortality. Therefore the maintenance of weight and body composition at or near optimum levels is highly desirable. Although people may believe that this is a difficult goal to achieve, it is not unrealistic when begun early in life and from a starting point at or near optimum levels. The following are some keys to success:

- *Exercise:* Caloric expenditure through regular exercise, including cardiovascular exercise and strength training, is a key to maintaining optimum weight and body composition (see Chapter 4).
- *Dietary modification:* Meals planned around foods low in total fat and saturated fat and high in complex carbohydrates also play an important role in maintaining optimum weight and body composition (see Chapter 5).
- *Lifestyle support:* Not only must people be committed to a lifestyle featuring regular physical activity and careful food choices, they must also build a support system that will encourage them in these endeavors. People should inform family, friends, classmates, and co-workers about their intent to rely on them for support and encouragement.
- *Problem solving:* People should reevaluate their current approaches to dealing with stressors. They must replace any reliance on food as a coping mechanism with nonfood options, such as exercise or talking with friends or family members.
- *Redefinition of health:* People must develop the ability to think about health and wellness in a manner that recognizes the importance of proactivity (see Chapter 2) and involvement, rather than simply focusing on not becoming sick or incapacitated.

Assuming that a person has an acceptable weight and body composition at this time, the lifestyle choices just suggested will make a significant contribution to avoiding a weight problem during the adult years.

WEIGHT MANAGEMENT TECHNIQUES

For those who are already overweight, the need to reduce weight to attain their optimum weight and

Calculating Basal Metabolic Rate

The basal metabolic rate (BMR) reflects the amount of energy in calories (C) that your body requires to sustain basic functions. The formula below can be used to calculate your approximate basal metabolic rate.

$$\text{BMR per day} = 1\,C \times \frac{\text{body weight (lb)}}{2.2} \times 24$$

EXAMPLE: 150-lb person

$$\text{BMR per day} = 1\,C \times \frac{150}{2.2} \times 24$$

$$= 1\,C \times 68.2 \times 24$$

$$= 1636.8\,C$$

This person would need approximately 1637 calories to sustain the body at rest for an entire day. Activity of any kind, of course, elevates the requirement for calories.

NOTE: A woman's BMR would be approximately 5% lower than that of a man of the same age.

A daily surplus of 10 calories yields 10 unwanted pounds in 10 years.

body composition will require intervention that may be different from the total lifestyle approach just described. However, on reaching a more healthful weight and body composition, maintenance of that status will depend on adopting the lifestyle changes described above.

Weight loss occurs when the amount of energy taken into the body is less than that demanded by the body for physiological maintenance and voluntary activity. A number of approaches to weight loss can be pursued. Complete the Personal Assessment on p. 139 to determine whether you are a candidate for weight loss.

Dietary Alterations

A diet that reduces caloric intake is the most common approach to what seems to be a national obsession with weight loss. The choice of foods included in the diet and the amount of food that can be consumed are the two factors that distinguish the wide range of diets currently available. Unfortunately, dieting alone usually does not result in long-term weight loss. In fact, whether managing their diets by themselves or following the advice of one of the widely recognized weight loss programs, most dieters regain at least two thirds of the weight they lost within 2 years after their initial loss.[21] The Health Action Guide on p. 141, left, provides suggestions for changing your eating patterns to increase your chances for long-term success.

Balanced diets supported by portion control

For nutritional health, a logical approach to weight loss and subsequent weight maintenance is to establish a nutritionally sound balanced diet (low in fat, especially saturated fat, and high in complex carbohydrates) that controls portions. This approach is best undertaken with nutritionists and physicians who are knowledgeable about diet management. After a study of a person's day-to-day energy needs, they can establish a diet designed to produce a gradual loss. A working understanding of portion size can be achieved using diet scales or through a nutrition education program in which realistic models of food servings are used. A balanced diet, portion control approach to weight loss is a nutritionally sound program with which there is some probability of success.

Fad diets

People use a variety of fad diets in an attempt to lose weight within a short time. These popular diets are often promoted in best-selling books written by people who claim to be nutrition "experts" (see the Health Action Guide on p. 141, right). With few

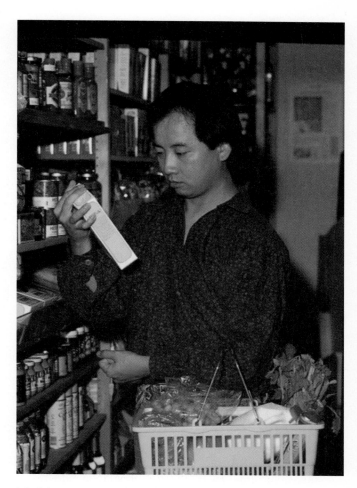

Modifying your eating behavior requires making thoughtful food choices.

exceptions, these approaches are both ineffective and potentially unhealthful. In addition, some require far greater expense than would be associated with weight loss or management techniques using portion control and regular physical activity. The pros and cons of a variety of popular diet plans are presented in Table 6-5.

Low-calorie or low-fat foods and controlled serving sizes

Recently a variety of familiar foods have been developed in a reduced-calorie form. By lowering the carbohydrate content with the use of nonnutritive sweeteners, reducing the portion size, or reducing the

basal metabolic rate (BMR) (**bay** sal)
The amount of energy (in calories) your body requires to maintain basic functions.

PERSONAL ASSESSMENT

Should You Consider a Weight Loss Program?

Before undertaking a program, it is important to look at your past experiences and feelings about weight loss. Perhaps in doing so, you might decide that you would do better with other alternatives besides dieting.

Answer each of the following items with a "True" or "False" as it applies to you.

_____ 1. I am frustrated about my inability to stick to a diet.

_____ 2. I have less self-control than most dieters.

_____ 3. Most of the times I try to lose weight, I lose control and go off my diet.

_____ 4. When I try to develop a habit of regular exercise, something always interferes and I stop.

_____ 5. Exercise seems to be an ordeal to me.

_____ 6. I often feel tired during the day.

_____ 7. My weight has gone up and down several times when I go on and off diets.

_____ 8. My body seems to be getting thicker in the middle over the years.

_____ 9. My weight seems to be increasing over the years.

_____ 10. I find myself thinking about food more than I should.

_____ 11. I find myself thinking about my weight all through the day.

_____ 12. I feel there is probably no hope for my weight problem.

_____ 13. Sometimes I lose control and really binge on food.

_____ 14. I use food to make myself feel better when I am angry, nervous, or depressed.

_____ 15. Some people reject me as a friend because I am too heavy.

_____ 16. My social life is limited because of my weight.

_____ 17. My sex life is limited because of my weight.

_____ 18. Other people think I am unattractive because of my weight.

_____ 19. I put a lot of effort into choosing clothes that tend to cover up my weight problem.

To Carry This Further . . .

For those items that you answered as true, consider these recommendations:

Items 1, 2, and 3: Rather than going on a diet, why not try to reduce your fat intake by avoiding fried food and foods with added fat. Eat more low-fat foods, and make certain that your dairy products are low-fat and your meats are lean.

Items 4, 5, and 6: You need a gradual but regular exercise program. Check around your community, and identify a reputable program that has a proven success rate in helping others who have had a weight problem.

Items 7, 8, and 9: These items indicate the development of a weight problem that could truly be damaging your health. These are reasons for being serious about weight loss that go beyond appearance.

Items 10, 11, 12, 13, and 14: You may be into "living to eat" rather than "eating to live." Now is the time to give serious thought on what is important in your life, other than appearance-related needs.

Items 15, 16, and 17: Work at forming new relationships. Seek out people who are capable of looking beyond your physical appearance for those attributes that they will find to be attractive in you.

Items 18 and 19: As for 15 to 17, assess your current relationships. Put your efforts into relationships with people who seem capable of looking "into" you, rather than only "at" you. ☑

---

fat content of the original formulations, manufacturers have produced "lite" versions of many food products. For example, numerous frozen entrees, such as Healthy Choice Oriental Beef with Vegetables (290 calories), Weight Watchers Lasagna Florentine (210 calories), and Healthy Choice Fettucine with Turkey and Vegetables (350 calories), are attractively low in calories. An additional aid to selecting lower-calorie and lower-fat foods is the newly required food label, described in Chapter 5.

Controlled fasting

In cases of extreme obesity, physicians place some patients on a complete fast in a hospital setting. The patient is maintained on only water, electrolytes, and vitamins. Weight loss is profound because the body is quickly forced to begin **catabolizing** its fat and muscle tissues. Sodium loss, a negative nitrogen balance, and potassium loss are particular concerns.

Today, some people regularly practice unsupervised, short periods of modified fasting. Solid foods

HEALTH Action Guide

Changing Your Eating Patterns

Following the tips listed below will help you achieve your weight loss goals:

- Keep a log of the times, settings, reasons, and feelings associated with your eating.
- Set realistic long-term goals (for example, loss of a pound per week instead of 5 lb per week).
- Do not completely deprive yourself of enjoyable foods (occasionally reward yourself with a small treat).
- Realize that the sacrifices you are making are what *you* feel are important for *your* health and happiness.
- Eat slowly. It takes about 20 minutes for your brain to recognize satiety signals from your body.
- Put more physical activity into your daily routine (taking stairs instead of elevators or parking in the distant part of a parking lot, for example).
- Reward yourself when you reach your goals (with new clothes, sporting equipment, a vacation trip).
- Share your commitment to weight loss with your family and friends so that they can support your efforts.
- Keep careful records of daily food consumption and weight change.
- Be prepared to deal with occasional plateaus and setbacks in your quest for weight loss.
- Remember that low-fat, low–saturated fat, and high–complex carbohydrate meals in combination with regular physical activity is the basis on which these strategies are applied.

HEALTH Action Guide

Choosing A Diet Book

- Make sure the program described in the book incorporates a balanced diet, an exercise program, and behavior modification.
- Beware of inflexible plans, such as those that require you to eat certain foods on certain days.
- Avoid plans that allow fewer than 1200 calories a day, the minimum needed to get essential nutrients.
- Make sure the recommended rate of weight loss does not exceed 2 lb per week.
- Steer clear of books that promote vitamins, pills, shots, gimmicks, gadgets, or brand-name diet foods.
- Read reviews to see if the book received approval from a reputable nutrition expert, institution, or journal.
- Check the author's credentials. He or she should have a degree in nutrition from an accredited university or should use reliable sources for the information.
- Make sure the book is based on up-to-date scientific research.
- Beware of diets that promise fast, easy, or effortless weight loss or "a new secret formula."
- Choose a plan that teaches how to keep the weight off once you've lost it.

are removed from the diet for a number of days. Fruit juice, water, supplements, and vitamins are used to minimize the risks described in association with total fasting. However, too frequent unsupervised short-term fasting can be dangerous and is not generally recommended.

Self-help weight reduction programs

In virtually every area of the country, at least one version of the popular commercial weight reduction programs, such as TOPS (Take Off Pounds Sensibly), Jenny Craig, and Nutri-Systems Weight Loss Centers, can be found. Popularized by Weight Watchers, these programs generally feature a format consisting of (1) a

well-balanced diet emphasizing portion control and low-fat, low–saturated fat, and high–complex carbohydrate foods, (2) realistic weight loss goals to be attained over a reasonable period of time, (3) encouragement from supportive leaders and fellow group members, (4) emphasis on regular physical activity, and (5) a weight management program (follow-up program). The Star Box on p. 144 presents some guidelines for choosing a commercial weight loss program.

Although in theory these programs offer an opportunity to lose weight for people who cannot or will not

catabolism
The metabolic process of breaking down tissue for the purpose of converting it into energy.

Table 6-5   Advantages and Disadvantages of Selected Diets

Type of diet	Advantages	Disadvantages	Examples
Limited food choice diets	Reduce the number of food choices made by the users Limited opportunity to make mistakes Almost certainly low in calories after the first few days	Deficient in many nutrients, depending on the foods allowed Monotonous—difficult to adhere to Eating out and eating socially are difficult Do not retrain dieters in acceptable eating habits Low long-term success rates No scientific basis for these diets	Banana and milk diet Grapefruit and cottage cheese diet Kempner rice diet Lecithin, vinegar, kelp, and vitamin B_6 diet Beverly Hills Diet Fit for Life
Restricted-calorie, balanced food plans	Sufficiently low in calories to permit steady weight loss Nutritionally balanced Palatable Include readily available foods Reasonable in cost Can be adapted from family meals Permit eating out and social eating Promote a new set of eating habits	Do not appeal to people who want a "unique" diet Do not produce immediate and large weight losses	Weight Watchers Diet Prudent Diet (American Heart Association) The I Love New York Diet UCLA Diet Time-Calorie Displacement (TCD) Fit or Fat Target Diet Take Off Pounds Sensibly (TOPS) Overeaters Anonymous
Fasting starvation diet	Rapid initial loss	Nutrient deficient Danger of ketosis >60% loss is muscle <40% loss is fat Low long-term success rate	ZIP Diet
High-carbohydrate diet	Emphasizes grains, fruits, and vegetables High in bulk Low in cholesterol	Limits milk, meat Nutritionally very inadequate for calcium, iron, and protein	Beverly Hills Diet Quick Weight Loss Diet Pritikin Diet Carbohydrate Cravers

participate in an activity program, their effectiveness is very limited. In fact, the limited success of these programs and the difficulty that working women have in attending meetings has resulted in falling enrollment and the development of home-based programs,[22] such as those developed by hospital-based wellness programs, many YMCAs and YWCAs, and even Weight Watchers. Further, these programs are costly when compared with self-directed approaches, especially when the program markets its own food products.

Physical Intervention

A second approach to weight loss involves techniques and products designed to alter basic eating patterns. These techniques range from those that are

Type of diet	Advantages	Disadvantages	Examples
High-protein, low-carbohydrate diets Usually include all the meat, fish, poultry, and eggs you can eat Occasionally permit milk and cheese in limited amounts Prohibit fruits, vegetables, and any bread or cereal products	Rapid initial weight loss because of diuretic effect Very little hunger	Too low in carbohydrates Deficient in many nutrients— vitamin C, vitamin A (unless eggs are included), calcium, and several trace elements High in saturated fat, choles- terol, and total fat Extreme diets of this type could cause death Impossible to adhere to these diets long enough to lose any appreciable amount of weight Dangerous for people with kid- ney disease Weight lost, which is largely water, is rapidly regained Expensive Unpalatable after first few days Difficult for dieter to eat out	Dr. Stillman's Quick Weight Loss Diet Calories Don't Count by Dr. Taller Dr. Atkin's Diet Revolution Scarsdale Diet Air Force Diet
Low-calorie, high-protein supplement diets Usually a premea- sured powder to be reconstituted with water or a prepared liquid formula	Rapid initial weight loss Easy to prepare—already mea- sured Palatable for first few days Usually fortified to provide rec- ommended amount of micronutrients Must be labeled if >50% protein	Usually prescribed at danger- ously low calorie intake of 300 to 500 Cal Overpriced Low in fiber and bulk—consti- pating in short amount of time	Metracal Diet Cambridge Diet Liquid Protein Diet Last Chance Diet Oxford Diet
High-fiber, low-calorie diets	High satiety value Provide bulk	Irritating to the lower colon Decreases absorption of trace elements, especially iron Nutritionally deficient Low in protein	Pritikin Diet F Diet Zen Macrobiotic Diet
Protein-sparing modified fats <50% protein: 400 Cal	Safe under supervision High-quality protein Minimize loss of lean body mass	Decreases BMR Monotonous Expensive	Optifast Medifast
Premeasured food plans	Provide prescribed portion sizes—little chance of too small or too large a portion Total food programs Some provide adequate calories (1200) Nutritionally balanced or sup- plemented	Expensive Do not retrain dieters in accept- able eating habits Preclude eating out or social eating Often low in bulk Monotonous Low long-term success rates	Nutri-System Carnation Plan

Choosing a Reputable Weight Loss Program

When checking out commercial weight loss programs, keep the following criteria in mind. Steer clear of any program that:

- Is not led by qualified specialists, including a registered dietitian
- Promises or encourages quick weight loss
- Does not require a preenrollment physical examination
- Does not warn clients of the risk of developing health problems related to weight loss, such as ketosis and diabetes-related complications
- Claims that an unusually high percentage of its clients are successful in achieving and maintaining weight loss
- Requires you to buy its products, such as foods or nutritional supplements
- Does not encourage lifestyle changes, including an exercise program
- Does not provide follow-up support after you reach your weight loss goal

self-selected and self-applied to those that must be administered within an institutional setting by highly trained professionals.

Hunger- and satiety-influencing products

One of the fondest wishes of overweight people is to lose the desire to eat or to feel that they have had enough to eat. Today some OTC and prescription medications are being used or developed in an attempt to achieve these outcomes.

At this time, several nonprescription appetite suppressants containing **phenylpropanolamine (PPA)** are being sold in supermarkets. Controversy concerning the safety of this active ingredient may alter its future availability. The drug is clearly dangerous for some people. People with high blood pres-sure, thyroid problems, diabetes, depression, or glaucoma should not use PPA. In addition, it can interact with other medications to produce dangerous side effects.

In regard to prescription-based approaches the drug *fenfluramine,* in combination with a second agent, *phentermine,* has shown some promise in lessening the desire for food. Specifically, this combination of agents alters the activity of the neurotransmitter serotonin. However, considerable concern exists over its unsupervised or long-term use. Also, the antidepressant drug Prozac is sometimes used to reduce appetite even though the agent has not been approved by the FDA for that purpose. Prozac is a very effective antidepressant, but its effectiveness in reducing appetite may be limited over time.

Although far from being approved by the FDA for general use, three interesting new pharmaceutical agents for reducing excessive weight and body fat have been identified. The first of these is *Orlistat,* a drug that reduces the percentage of fat that can be absorbed from the digestive tract. The second pharmaceutical agent is a topically applied cream, *aminophylline,* that appears to stimulate fat cell metabolism in the area to which the cream has been applied. However, critics suggest that only localized dehydration has occurred. The third approach to altering body composition is the use of testosterone patches in men. When absorbed through the skin, testosterone may reduce some adipose tissue layering around the major abdominal organs.

As for drugs to "cure" obesity, hope springs eternal, and some believe the recently approved drug dexflenfluramine (Redux) might be that cure. Like fenfluramine, it influences neurotransmitter activity, producing feelings of satiety. When used with dietary modification, exercise, and group support, it could be a helpful tool for achieving and maintaining moderate weight loss. Some concern exists over the drug's use and both neurological problems and pulmonary hypertensive disease. Experts, however, remain cautious in predicting that a major discovery will be made soon in this approach to our national weight problem.

Surgical Measures

When weight loss is imperative and a person is morbidly obese, surgical intervention may be considered. A *gastric resection* is a major operation in which a portion of the small intestine is bypassed in an attempt to decrease the body's ability to absorb nutrients. Although the procedure can produce a major loss of body weight, it is associated with many unpleasant side effects (including diarrhea and liver damage) and various nutritional deficiencies.

Gastroplasty (stomach stapling) is a surgical procedure that involves sealing off about half of the stomach with surgical staples. Once the procedure has been completed, the reduced capacity of the stomach decreases the amount of food that can be processed at any one time. As a result, patients feel full more quickly after eating a small meal. This procedure is reversible but carries the risks associated with surgery and the costs of a major surgical procedure.

Liposuction

Another form of surgical weight loss management is *liposuction,* or *lipoplasty.* During this expensive procedure, a physician inserts a small tube through the skin and vacuum aspiration sucks away fat cells. This procedure is generally used for stubborn, localized pockets of fat and is usually appropriate for people under the age of 40.

Liposuction is more a cosmetic procedure than a general approach to weight loss. Along with unrealistic expectations, the risks of infection, pain and discomfort, bruising, swelling, discoloration, abscesses, and unattractive changes in body contours are possible outcomes of liposuction. Therefore people considering this procedure should carefully investigate all aspects of it, including the training and experience of the surgeon, to determine whether it is appropriate.

EATING DISORDERS

Perhaps it is not surprising that some people have medically identifiable, potentially serious difficulties with body image, body weight, and food selection. Among these disorders are two that are frequently seen among college students, anorexia nervosa and bulimia. In addition, compulsive exercising, compulsive eating, and disorders involving various combinations of anorexic and bulimic practices are also found in college populations. We have included these topics in the chapter on weight management because most eating disorders begin with dieting. However, most eating disorders also involve inappropriate food choices, as well as deep emotional needs. Those issues are discussed in Chapters 2 and 5.

Anorexia Nervosa

A young woman, competitive and perfectionistic by nature, determines that her weight (and appearance) is unacceptable. She begins to disregard her appetite, and her food consumption virtually ceases.

The young woman in this description may be seen by her friends or roommates as active and intelligent and simply dieting and exercising with an unusual degree of commitment. Eventually, however, they observe that her food consumption has nearly stopped. Her weight loss has continued beyond the point that is pleasing—at least to others. Nevertheless, her activity level remains high. When questioned about her weight loss, she says that she still needs to lose more weight.

This person is suffering from a medical condition called **anorexia nervosa** (see the Star Box on p. 146). This self-induced starvation is life-threatening in 5% to 20% of cases. The stunning amount of weight that some anorexic people lose—up to 50% of their body weight—eventually leads to failure of the heart, lungs, and kidneys.

As weight loss–oriented as this condition seems, experts believe that the anorexic person is attempting to meet a much deeper need for control. Specifically, in a family setting in which much is expected of the individual but little opportunity for self-directed behavior is provided, control over the body becomes a need-fulfilling tool. Eventually, however, a normal body image is lost and the condition progresses in the manner described above. Fortunately, psychological intervention in combination with medical and dietary support can return the anorexic person to a more life-sustaining pattern of eating. Thus the anorexic person needs to seek professional help. Your obligation when you observe this condition in a friend is to secure immediate assistance for this person.

Bulimia Nervosa

Bulimia is an eating disorder in which people gorge themselves with food. When people practice a pattern of massive eating followed by **purging,** they are said to suffer from *bulimarexia,* or *bulimia nervosa* (see the Star Box on p. 146). Most often, however, the term *bulimia* is used to describe this binge-purge pattern. As with anorexic people, most people with bulimia are young women.

People with bulimia lose or maintain weight not because they stop eating but because they eat and then purge their digestive system by vomiting, using laxatives, or taking syrup of ipecac, a dangerous drug used to stimulate vomiting after an accidental poisoning. People with bulimia may gorge themselves with food (up to 10,000 calories in a sitting) and then disappear, only to return later seemingly unaffected by

anorexia nervosa
A disorder of emotional origin in which appetite and hunger are suppressed and marked weight loss occurs.

bulimia
A disorder of emotional origin in which binge eating patterns are established; usually accompanied by purging.

purging
Using vomiting or laxatives to remove undigested food from the body.

phenylpropanolamine (PPA)
The active chemical compound found in most over-the-counter diet products.

Recognizing Anorexia Nervosa and Bulimia

The American Psychological Association uses the following diagnostic criteria to identify anorexia nervosa and bulimia:

Anorexia

- 15% or more below desirable weight
- Fear of weight gain
- Altered body image
- Three or more missed menstrual periods

Bulimia

- Binge eating two or more times a week for 3 months
- A lack of control over bingeing
- Purging
- Concern about body image

Characteristic symptoms include the following. However, it is unlikely that all the symptoms will be evident in any one individual.

Anorexia

- Looks thin and keeps getting thinner
- Skips meals, cuts food into small pieces, moves food around plate to appear to have eaten

- Loss of menstrual periods
- Wears "layered look" in an attempt to disguise weight loss
- Loss of hair from the head
- Growth of fine hair on face, arms, and chest
- Extreme sensitivity to cold

Bulimia

- Bathroom use immediately after eating
- Inconspicuous eating
- Excessive time (and money) spent food shopping
- Shopping for food at several stores rather than one store
- Menstrual irregularities
- Excessive constipation
- Swollen and/or infected salivary glands, sore throat
- Bursting blood vessels in the eyes
- Damaged teeth and gums
- Dehydration and kidney dysfunction

the amount of food they ate. In all likelihood, they have quickly and quietly regurgitated the food. In the mid-1980s, medical experts estimated that as many as 19% of 18- to 22-year-old women developed all the principal symptoms of bulimia. However, when all of the criteria mentioned in the Star Box are applied rather than simply reporting "experience" with bulimia-associated behavior, the percentage drops to less than 2%.

In addition to the binge-purge disorder, people who binge but do not purge also suffer from an eating disorder. Whether called *bulimia*, "eating disorder not otherwise specified," or *binge-eating disorder*, this practice also requires intervention and effective treatment.

Compulsive Exercise and Compulsive Eating

The compulsive nature of some people's exercising or eating patterns suggests a slightly different version of the two principal eating disorders. More than likely, a wide array of causes can account for both of these behavior patterns. In the case of compulsive exercise, a desire for control may exist, as in anorexia nervosa, whereas with compulsive eating the role of food in reducing feelings of insecurity and stress may

explain the inability to resist food whenever it is present. Again, dieting may be the starting point for both of these behavior patterns. As in the more classic eating disorders, family members and friends should not fail to identify and respond to these conditions.

Treatment for Eating Disorders

The treatment of eating disorders is complex and demanding. The initial physical care for a person with anorexia most often begins with hospitalization to stabilize the physical deterioration associated with starvation. Stomach tubes and intravenous feedings are sometimes necessary, particularly when the patient will not (or cannot) eat. In addition, drug therapy to decrease hyperactivity and stimulate appetite is often used. Behavior modification, including eating contracts, is used, as is psychotherapy in both individual and group formats. Nutritional and family counseling complete the therapy.[23]

Treatment for bulimia involves individual, family, and nutritional counseling. Unlike treatment for anorexia, however, bulimia treatment does not as frequently involve hospitalization. The Star Box on p. 147 lists resources for people with eating disorders.

Resources for Anorexia and Bulimia Treatment

Local Resources
- College or university health centers
- College or university counseling centers
- Comprehensive mental health centers
- Crisis intervention centers
- Mental health associations

Organizations and Self-Help Groups
American Anorexia/Bulimia Association, Inc.
418 East 76th Street, New York, NY 10021
(212) 501-8351

Anorexia Nervosa and Associated Disorders, Inc.
P.O. Box 7, Highland Park, IL 60035
(708) 831-3438

Anorexia Nervosa and Related Eating Disorders, Inc.
P.O. Box 5102, Eugene, OR 97405
(503) 344-1144

This nonprofit organization, which collects information about eating and exercise disorders, distributes information through booklets and a monthly newsletter. Staff lead workshops, self-help groups, and training programs for professionals. They also provide speakers.

Bulimia Anorexia Nervosa Association
Windsor, Ont (Canada)
(519) 253-7421 or 7545

National Eating Disorders Association (NEDO) at Laureatte Psychiatric Hospital,
P.O. Box 470207, Tulsa, OK 74147
(918) 481-4092
This organization publishes a quarterly newsletter appropriate for professional and personal use.

UNDERNUTRITION

For some young adults, the lack of adequate body weight is a serious concern. Particularly for those who have inherited an ectomorphic body build (tall, narrow shoulders and hips, tendency to thinness), attempts to gain weight are routinely undertaken, often with limited success. If these people are to be successful in gaining weight, they must discover an effective way to take in more calories than they burn (see the Health Action Guide below and the article on pp. 151-152).

Nutritionists believe that the healthiest way to gain weight is to increase the intake of calorie-dense food.

HEALTH Action Guide

Weight Management Tips

Tips for Weight Loss
- You probably didn't gain your excessive weight eating alone. Seek the encouragement and support of family and friends in your weight loss efforts.
- Eat only at the table. Leave the table immediately after finishing your meal. By all means never take your meal with you into other rooms of the house.
- Stop eating after one serving. A second helping contributes more fat and calories than your diet can afford.
- If you must snack between meals, choose small, nutritious, low-fat snacks.
- Stay away from the kitchen. An innocent look into the refrigerator will almost certainly lead to a taste, a snack, or even a meal.

Tips for Weight Gain
- Make certain that there is no medical reason for your thinness.
- Have your current dietary practices evaluated so that appropriate modifications can be made.
- Begin a moderate exercise program to enhance your physical fitness.
- Incorporate the following recommendations into your dietary practice:
  - Substitute juice, soup, or hot chocolate for coffee.
  - Eat a healthy breakfast.
  - Learn appropriate portion sizes.
  - Replace junk foods with more healthy foods.

These foods are characterized by high fat density resulting from high levels of vegetable fats (polyunsaturated fats). Particularly good foods in this regard are dried fruits, bananas, nuts, granola, and cheeses made from low-fat milk. It is important, however, to consume these foods later in a meal so that the onset of satiety that quickly follows eating fat-rich foods does not occur.

A second component of weight gain for those who are underweight is the curtailment of excessive physical activity. By carefully reducing their activity level, they can prevent the "burning up" of calories and thus use them for development of body fat. Of course, activity should not be restricted to the point that cardiovascular conditioning declines or enjoyable activities are no longer available.

For those who cannot gain weight in spite of having tried the above approaches, a medical evaluation could supply an explanation for being underweight. If no medical explanation can be found, the person must begin to accept the reality of his or her unique body type. The article on pp. 151-152 explores further the problems of being underweight.

Summary

- Overweight and obesity are the most common forms of malnutrition in the United States.
- Obesity results from an abnormal accumulation of fat.
- Little question exists regarding the health implications of moderate to severe obesity, but the seriousness of mildly obese or overweight is questioned by some.
- Body image and self-concept can be adversely influenced by obesity.
- Obesity and overweight can be defined in a variety of ways and determined using any of several methods.
- Maintaining a healthy body weight is desirable because central body cavity obesity relates to a variety of serious health problems.
- Theories regarding the cause of obesity focus on factors from within the individual and from the environment.
- Many complex theories exist regarding the role of inheritance, set point, body type, feeding patterns, pregnancy, aging, inactivity, and family eating patterns.
- Caloric balance influences weight gain, loss, and maintenance.
- The body's energy needs arise from three areas: BMR, activity, and the thermic effect of food.
- Weight loss can be attempted through dieting, which is the restriction of food intake.
- Drugs, behavior modification, and other techniques, including surgery, can be used to achieve weight loss.
- A combination approach involving low-fat, low–saturated fat, high–complex carbohydrate food, portion-controlled dieting, and exercise may be the most effective way to lose weight.
- Although many people can lose some weight through dieting, very few who do are able to maintain that weight loss.
- The weight loss industry is facing declining participation as people become more aware of information regarding limited success rates.
- Serious eating disorders usually begin with dieting but are often sustained in an attempt to meet deeper needs.
- Underweight is a condition of concern to many that may be resolved through the use of calorie-dense and nutrient-dense foods.

Review Questions

1. Why are obesity and overweight considered to be forms of malnutrition and potentially serious health problems?
2. How are obesity and overweight defined? Why is it possible to be overweight without being over-fat? What is the set point?
3. In what ways can obesity be determined? What is desirable weight? What is body mass index? What is waist-to-hip ratio? Why is central body cavity obesity of concern to physicians?
4. Describe the role that each of the following could play in causing obesity: heredity, set point, body type, infant feeding patterns, pregnancy, aging, inactivity, and family eating patterns.

5. What is caloric balance? What are the body's three areas of energy needs? How does aging influence caloric balance? What role exists for exercise in both weight loss and long-term weight maintenance?

6. What is the role of surgery, fasting, and fad diets? What advances are being made in the development of drugs that are effective in weight management?

7. How effective is dieting in terms of both immediate success and later weight maintenance? Why has participation in some commercial weight loss programs fallen in recent years?

8. What two techniques are used in a combination approach to weight loss? How should this program be structured to ensure the highest level of success?

9. What are the two principal eating disorders within the college community? In what ways do they differ? What is *binge-eating disorder*? What are compulsive exercise and compulsive eating? How are eating disorders treated?

 ## Think About This . . .

- What methods have you used to determine whether you are underweight, overweight, or obese?
- What are your attitudes toward people with weight control problems? Why do you feel this way?
- Do you believe that being underweight is as psychologically traumatic as being overweight?
- If you have ever attempted to lose weight, what methods have you used? Were any of these methods potentially dangerous?

- Regardless of your weight, which of your personality traits do others find positive? How can you present these attributes to others?
- If you have a weight problem, do you agree or disagree that you have a responsibility to yourself and to other people to reduce your weight?
- What do you see as your responsibility in dealing with a friend or family member who is displaying signs of an eating disorder?

References

1. Morgan K, Morgan S, Quitno N, editors: *Health care state rankings 1995: health care in the 50 United States,* Lawrence, Kan, Morgan Quitno Press, 1995.
2. Manson J et al: Body weight and mortality among women, *N Engl J Med* 333(11):677-685, 1995.
3. Crowley LV: *Introduction to human disease,* ed 3, Boston, 1992, Jones & Bartlett.
4. Cash T, Henry P: Women's body images: the results of a national survey in the U.S.A., *Sex Role: A Journal of Research,* 33(1-2):19-29, 1995.
5. United State Department of Agriculture/United States Department of Health and Human Services: *Nutrition and your health: dietary guidelines for Americans,* 1990, Home and garden bulletin 232.
6. Chart your upper limit, *USA Today,* p 1D October 4, 1995.
7. Bray GA: Obesity: a blueprint for progress, *Contemporary Nutrition* 12(7):1-2, 1987.
8. Prentice WE: *Fitness for college and life,* ed 4, St Louis, 1994, Mosby.
9. The obsession with obesity, *Nature Genetics* 11(1):1-2, 1995 (editorial).
10. Clement K et al: Genetic variation in the B_3-adrenergic receptor and an increased capacity to gain weight in patients with morbid obesity, *N Engl J Med* 333(6):352-354, 1995.
11. Halaas J et al: Weight-reducing effects on the plasma protein encoded by the obese gene, *Science* 269(5223):543-546, 1995.
12. Considine R et al: Serum immunoreactrive-leptin concentrations in normal-weight and obese humans, *N Engl J Med* 334(5):292-295, 1966.
13. Widen E et al: Association of a polymorphism in the ß$_3$-adrenergic-receptor gene with features of the insulin resistance syndrome in Finns, *N Engl J Med* 333(6)348-351, 1995.
14. Moffett D, Moffett S, Schauf C: *Human physiology: foundations and frontiers,* ed 2, St Louis, 1993, Mosby.
15. National Task Force on the Prevention and Treatment of Obesity: Weight cycling, *JAMA* 272(15):1196-1202, 1994.
16. Ganong WF: *Review of medical physiology,* ed 7, Norwalk, Conn, 1995, Appleton & Lange.
17. Schauberger CW, Rooney BL, Brimer LM: Factors that

influence weight loss in the puerperium, *Obstet Gynecol* 79(3):424-429, 1992.

18. Fieldhouse P: *Food and nutrition: customs and culture,* London, 1986, Cromm Helm.
19. Food and Nutrition Board: *Recommended dietary allowances,* Washington, DC, 1989, National Academy of Sciences, National Research Council.
20. Wardlaw GM, Insel PM, Seyler MF: *Contemporary nutrition,* ed 2, St Louis, 1994, Mosby.
21. Losing weight: what works and what doesn't work, *Consumer Report* 58(6):347-352, 1993.
22. Neuborne E: Weight-loss programs going hungry, *USA Today,* p 1B, July 28, 1994.
23. Schlundt D, Johnson W: *Eating disorders: assessment and training,* New York, 1990, Allyn & Bacon.

Suggested Readings

Hess MA, Hunt AE, Stone BM: *A healthy start: a worry-free guide to feeding young children,* New York, 1991, Henry Holt.

This guide describes how to feed young children in a way that fosters health and decreases the likelihood of obesity. Recipes for nutritious food that children will like are provided, as well as information about food fads and snacking.

Kleinman RE, Jellinek MS: *Let them eat cake! The case against controlling what your children eat,* New York, 1994, Villard Books.

Picky eaters are made, not born. Rather than forcing children to eat food that they have little interest in eating, this book suggests that parents help children make choices regarding good foods and lead by example. Food and mealtime should be pleasurable, social, and enjoyable.

LeShan L: *Meditating to attain a health body weight,* New York, 1994, Doubleday.

For people interested in a unique approach to weight loss, this book introduces meditation as a tool worth mastering. Through the use of one or both of the techniques described, meditation assists readers in gaining control over their use of food.

Freedman LC: *Bodylove: learning to like our looks and ourselves,* New York, 1989, Harper & Row.

Widely recommended by clinicians who deal with eating disorders, this book assists the reader in recognizing the positive nature of many different body configurations. The natural "inner" body becomes the basis of happiness and self-esteem regardless of its external counterpart.

Gaining Weight Healthfully

"I can't believe how thin you are! It must be so great to eat whatever you want. I wish I had your problem. Of course, it wouldn't hurt you to put on a few pounds. You sure would look healthier!"

"Hey, stick! Do you have anorexia or what? Don't you ever eat?"

These excerpts from real-life exchanges are just two examples of how cruel people can be to the underweight. Some observers think that naturally thin people must have an eating disorder because of their appearance; others are envious because they wish they could indulge in high-fat foods without a second thought. Even in a society where thin is in, being too thin can be just as emotionally and physically devastating as being too heavy. Our society has little understanding or sympathy for people who can eat all they want and never gain a pound.

Causes of Being Underweight
A person is considered to be underweight when he or she is 10% to 15% or more under the ideal weight as indicated on a standard height and weight chart.[1,2] Such a condition can be caused by heredity, poor eating habits, or disease.[2,3] Hereditary causes of being underweight center on high metabolism. Being underweight can be caused by a tendency to burn more calories than are taken in.[3] Many researchers believe that people have a natural "set point" for their metabolic rate[4] that determines how quickly and efficiently calories are used in the body. Metabolism also may prevent people from reaching unrealistic goals with regard to weight gain.[4]

Poor eating habits may also play a role in being underweight. The same concept applies to eating as to metabolism; not consuming enough calories can lead to a person burning more calories than are taken in.[3] High-calorie foods may be lacking in the diets of some underweight people. Other underweight people may include high-calorie foods in their diets but simply do not consume enough total calories to gain weight.[3] Weight control disorders resulting from anorexia, bulimia, or other diseases should be treated by a doctor and are not considered here.

Effects of Being Underweight
Being underweight can cause a variety of physical problems. Women who are underweight are at increased risk of amenorrhea, a reproductive system disorder characterized by a complete absence of menstrual flow.[5] Underweight people tend to have lower bone mass than people of normal weight, which may place underweight people at risk for bone fractures and osteoporosis.[6-8] Being female, over 65, and underweight can increase the risk for hip fractures.[6] Being too thin can also shorten the life expectancy for men and women.[1,7]

The dangers of being underweight are gradually being discovered. Some studies have shown that being underweight may be as dangerous as being overweight. Government weight guidelines now include data showing that being too thin is as dangerous as being too heavy, and people who are obese by government standards are living longer than those who are underweight.[7]

Being underweight can cause psychological problems in addition to physical problems. Anna, a young woman who spent her youth, teenage years, and early twenties as an underweight person, recalls what life was like for her during that time. "It was like a never-ending nightmare. I hated to go to school because the kids made fun of me all the time. They called me names like 'concentration camp victim' and 'twig.' Many nights I would cry myself to sleep because I hated the way I looked so much. I tried everything I could think of to gain weight: eating as much high-calorie food as I could, using commercial weight-gain products, even not exercising in hopes that I'd get fatter. Nothing worked. When I graduated from high school, I was five feet eight inches tall and still weighed 98 lbs. So many people had told me that I was ugly that I believed it must be true. I spent 6 years in therapy trying to get my self-esteem back. Thank God I finally began to gain weight when I graduated from college. I'm actually a little overweight now. If I had to choose between being this way or being the way I was, there's no question in my mind that I'd choose to be like I am now. People say and do things to underweight people that they'd never dream of saying or doing to people who are overweight."[9]

Gaining Weight Safely
If you are underweight, gaining weight safely is not just a matter of continuously gorging on food. Gaining fat pounds will increase a person's actual weight but will not make him or her any healthier. Diet and exercise plans are available for those who wish to gain weight safely. You should first consult a physician to determine the cause of being underweight. If it has been determined that the underweight condition is not due to disease, a combination of diet and exercise can be prescribed to gain lean body mass. Such a weight-gain plan should include a diet that is high in complex carbohy-

drates and low in fat. About 60% of the caloric intake should consist of complex carbohydrates,[10] which can be obtained from foods such as pastas. Fat intake should be low (about 10% of total caloric intake), since gaining weight in the form of fat is not healthy.[4,10] Protein should make up about 30% of the caloric intake, but protein supplements are not recommended,[4,10] since their use could damage the kidneys.

An underweight person must exercise to gain muscle mass. The exercise program should be a combination of weight training and endurance training.[4,10] About 80% of the exercise program should consist of weight training, with the other 20% consisting of endurance exercises such as aerobics.[10] Fairly heavy weights should be used with fewer repetitions to gain lean body mass,[10] since more repetitions with lighter weights will not increase lean body mass as effectively. Stretching and calisthenics can be incorporated into the weight training as well.[4] Weight training can help underweight people (and women in particular) gain upper body strength that may be lacking.[4] Exercise is also important because it improves cardiovascular fitness and may deter osteoporosis.[4]

The important thing to remember about such changes in diet and lifestyle is that they must be continued on a long-term basis. It may take 6 to 12 months to see results,[4] and if the program is halted, any weight gained may be lost again.[10] A person must maintain a lifetime commitment to gaining the weight and keeping it on. As always, consult your physician before starting any exercise or diet program.

For Discussion . . .
Why might being underweight be just as dangerous as being overweight? Is it easier to chastise underweight people than overweight people? What are the similarities and differences between people who are thin resulting from metabolism and those who are thin resulting from disease (such as anorexia)?

References
1. Weight control, *Grolier wellness encyclopedia, vol 15*, Guilford, Conn, 1992, Dushkin.
2. Nutrition and fitness ("Underweight"), *Macmillan health encyclopedia, vol 4*, New York, 1993, Macmillan.
3. Nutrition and fitness ("weight gain strategy"), *Macmillan health encyclopedia, vol 4*, New York, 1993, Macmillan.
4. Blackburn GL: Gaining weight without "getting fat," *Prevention* 40(10), 1988.
5. Amenhorrea: What your body is trying to tell you, *Cosmopolitan* 25(4), 1993.
6. Cooper C, Barker JP: Risk factors for hip fracture, *N Engl J Med* 332(2), 1995.
7. Good news for heavyweights, *USA Today Magazine*, 122(2585), Feb 1994.
8. Who is at risk? *USA Today Magazine*, 122(2585), Feb 1994.
9. "Anna," Personal interview, 1996.
10. Bishop D, MD, Personal interview, 1996.
11. Schrieber B: Living and learning, *Shape* 14(12), Aug 1995.

PART 3

ADDICTIVE SUBSTANCES

Choosing a Drug-Free Lifestyle

Healthy People 2000 Objectives

Achieving the Healthy People 2000 objectives in the area of drug abuse is critically important for the nation. Substance abuse is directly responsible for 120,000 deaths each year in the United States, 100,000 of which are related to alcohol abuse and 20,000 to other drug use. In addition, substance abuse harms the emotional health of individuals, destroys families, and devastates communities.

No headway has been made in preventing drug-related deaths or in reducing the number of drug-related hospital emergency room visits, probably because there is a group of hard-core drug users whom it is difficult to reach with anti-drug abuse messages. In addition, there has been no progress in raising the age of first use of cigarettes, alcohol, or marijuana by children.

However, the number of adolescents and young adults who report having used alcohol, marijuana, or cocaine during the past month seems to be declining. This is especially true of cocaine use in the 12-to-17 and 18-to-25 age-groups. Cocaine use among people in these groups has dropped dramatically, and the Healthy People 2000 objectives have been met for this category.

The use of psychoactive drugs can be tremendously disruptive in many people's lives, from tragic deaths to the loss of employment opportunities (most Fortune 500 companies use preemployment drug testing) to the deterioration of personal relationships. Perhaps realizing this, college students have generally moved away from using the most dangerous illegal drugs.[1]

Since the early 1980s, college students' illegal drug use has consistently dropped. However, a 1993 major survey of college students' drug use reported that this decline may have bottomed out (Figure 7-1).[2] For the first time in years, there was a slight increase in the percentage of students who reported using an illegal drug within the past year: in 1991, 29.2% of college students used an illegal drug, but in 1992, 30.6% of college students used an illegal drug. Overall, drug use remained steady or actually dropped in all drug categories except hallucinogens and marijuana.

It is safe to say that in the late 1990s, drug use remains a significant problem for both college students and the general population. Alcohol is the most important problem drug for most college students (see Chapter 8), but other drugs pose risks for certain students. Some of these drugs are specified in the Healthy People 2000 objectives. Additionally, many nontraditional students see the destructive effects of drug use on their neighborhoods and worry about their children being exploited by those who deal drugs.

ADDICTIVE BEHAVIOR

This chapter explores the health consequences of drug use, misuse, and abuse. Before talking about specific drugs, however, drug use should be put in the broader context of addictive behavior. Experts in human behavior view drug use and abuse as just one of the many forms of addictive behavior. Addictive behavior includes addictions to shopping, eating, gambling, sex, television, video games, and work, as well as addictions to alcohol or other drugs.

The Process of Addiction

The process of developing an addiction has been a much-studied topic. There seem to be three common aspects of addictive behavior.

Exposure

An addiction can begin after a person is exposed to a drug (such as alcohol) or a behavior (such as gambling) that he or she finds pleasurable. Perhaps this drug or behavior temporarily replaces an unpleasant feeling or sensation. This initial pleasure gradually (or in some cases quickly) becomes a focal point in the person's life.

Compulsion

Increasingly more energy, time, and money are spent pursuing the drug use or behavior. At this point

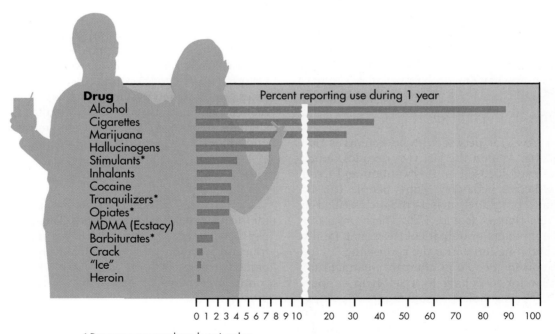

Drug	Percent reporting use during 1 year
Alcohol	
Cigarettes	
Marijuana	
Hallucinogens	
Stimulants*	
Inhalants	
Cocaine	
Tranquilizers*	
Opiates*	
MDMA (Ecstacy)	
Barbiturates*	
Crack	
"Ice"	
Heroin	

0 1 2 3 4 5 6 7 8 9 10   20   30   40   50   60   70   80   90   100

* Drug use was not under a doctor's orders.

Figure 7-1   Alcohol, cigarettes, marijuana, and hallucinogens are the four most common substances used by college students.

in the addictive process, the person can be said to have a compulsion for the drug or behavior. Frequently, repeated exposure to the drug or behavior continues despite negative consequences, such as the gradual loss of family and friends, unpleasant physical symptoms after taking the drug, and problems at work.

During the compulsion phase of the addictive behavior, a person's "normal" life is likely to degenerate while she or he searches for increased pleasures from the drug or the behavior. An addicted person's family life, circle of friends, work, or study patterns become less important than the search for more and better "highs." The development of tolerance and withdrawal are distinct possibilities. (These terms are discussed later in the chapter.)

Why some people develop compulsions and others do not is difficult to pinpoint, but addiction might be influenced by genetic makeup, family dynamics, physiological processes, personality type, peer groups, and available resources for help.

Loss of control

Over time, the search for highs changes to a search to avoid the effects of withdrawal from the drug or behavior. Addicted people lose their ability to control their behavior. Despite overwhelming negative consequences (for example, deterioration of health, alienation of family and friends, or loss of all financial resources), addicted people continue to behave in ways that make their lives worse. The person addicted to alcohol continues to drink heavily, the person addicted to shopping continues to run up heavy debts, and the person addicted to food continues to eat indiscriminately. This behavior reflects a loss of control over one's life. Frequently, a person has addictions to more than one drug or behavior.

Intervention and Treatment

The good news for people with addictions is that help is available. Within the last two decades, much attention has been focused on intervention and treatment for addictive behavior. Many people can be helped through programs such as those described at the end of this chapter (see p. 170). These programs often include inpatient or outpatient treatment, family counseling, and long-term aftercare counseling.

It is common for people in aftercare treatment for addictive behavior to belong to a self-help support group, such as Alcoholics Anonymous, Gamblers Anonymous, or Sex Addicts Anonymous. These groups are often listed in the phone book or in the classified section of the newspaper.

DRUG TERMINOLOGY

Before discussing drug actions or drug behavior, you must first be familiar with some basic terminology. Much of this terminology originates from the field of *pharmacology*, or the study of the interaction of chemical agents with living material.

What does the word *drug* mean? Each of us may have different ideas about what a drug is. Although a number of definitions are available, we will consider a drug to be "any substance, other than food, that by its chemical or physical nature alters structure or function in the living organism."[3] Included in this broad definition is a variety of psychoactive drugs, medicines, and substances that many people do not usually consider to be drugs.

Psychoactive drugs alter the user's feelings, behavior, perceptions, or moods. Psychoactive drugs include stimulants, depressants, hallucinogens, opiates, and inhalants. *Medicines* function to heal unhealthy tissue. Medicines are also used to ease pain, prevent illness, and diagnose health conditions. Although some psychoactive drugs are used for medical reasons, as in the case of tranquilizers and some narcotics, the most commonly prescribed medicines are antibiotics, sulfa drugs, diuretics, oral contraceptives, and antihypertensive drugs. Legal substances not usually considered to be drugs (but which certainly are drugs) include caffeine, tobacco, alcohol, aspirin, and other over-the-counter (OTC) preparations. These common substances are used so frequently in our society that they are rarely perceived as true drugs.

For organizational reasons, this chapter primarily deals with psychoactive drugs. Alcohol is covered in Chapter 8. The effects of tobacco are delineated in Chapter 9. Prescription and OTC drugs and medicines are discussed at length in Chapter 15. Environmental pollutants are covered in Chapter 17. Anabolic steroids, drugs used primarily for increasing muscle growth, are discussed in Chapter 4.

Dependence

Psychoactive drugs have a strong potential for the development of **dependence.** When users take a psychoactive drug, the patterns of nervous system function are altered. If these altered functions provide perceived benefits for the user, drug use may continue, perhaps at increasingly larger dosages. If persistent use continues, the user can develop a dependence on the drug. Pharmacologists have identified two types of dependences—physical and psychological.

A person can be said to have developed a *physical dependence* when the body cells have become reliant on a drug. Continued use of the drug is then required because body tissues have adapted to its presence.[4] The person's body needs the drug to maintain homeostasis, or dynamic balance. If the drug is not taken or is suddenly withdrawn, the user develops a characteristic **withdrawal illness.** The symptoms of withdrawal reflect the attempt by the body's cells to regain normality without the drug. Withdrawal symptoms are always unpleasant (ranging from mild to severe irritability, depression, nervousness, digestive difficulties, and abdominal pain) and can be life threatening, as in the case of abrupt withdrawal from barbiturates or alcohol. In this chapter the term *addiction* is used interchangeably with physical dependence.

Continued use of most drugs can lead to **tolerance.** Tolerance is an acquired reaction to a drug in which continued intake of the same dose has diminishing effects.[4] The user needs larger doses of the drug to receive previously felt sensations. The continued use of depressants, including alcohol, and opiates can cause users to quickly develop a tolerance to the drug.

For example, college seniors who have engaged in 4 years of beer drinking usually recognize that their bodies have developed a degree of tolerance. Many such students can vividly recall the initial and subsequent sensations they felt after drinking. For example, five beers consumed during a freshman social gathering might well have resulted in inebriation, but if these same students continued to drink beer regularly for 4 years, five beers would probably fail to produce the response they experienced as freshmen. Perhaps seven or eight beers would be needed to produce such a response. Clearly, they have developed a tolerance to alcohol.

Furthermore, tolerance developed for one drug may carry over to another drug within the same general category. This phenomenon is known as **cross-tolerance.** The heavy abuser of alcohol, for example, might require a larger dose of a preoperative sedative to become relaxed before surgery than the average person. The tolerance to alcohol "crosses over" to the other depressant drug.

A person who possesses a strong desire to continue using a particular drug is said to have developed *psychological dependence* (see the Star Box on p. 158, top). People who are psychologically dependent on a drug believe that they need to consume the drug to maintain a sense of well-being. They crave the drug for emotional reasons in spite of having persistent or recurrent physical, social, psychological, or occupational problems that are caused or worsened by the drug use. Abrupt withdrawal from a drug by such a person

would not trigger the fully expressed withdrawal illness, although some unpleasant symptoms of withdrawal might be felt. The term *habituation* is often used interchangeably with psychological dependence.

Drugs whose continued use can quickly lead to both physical and psychological dependence are the depressants (barbiturates, tranquilizers, and alcohol), narcotics (the opiates, which are derivatives of the Oriental poppy: heroin, morphine, and codeine), and synthetic narcotics (Demerol and methadone). Drugs whose continued use can lead to various degrees of psychological dependence and occasionally to significant (but not life-threatening) physical dependence in some users are the stimulants (amphetamines, caffeine, and cocaine), hallucinogens (LSD, peyote, mescaline, and marijuana), and inhalants (glues, gases, and petroleum products).

Drug Misuse and Abuse

So far in this chapter we have used the term *use* (or *user*) in association with the taking of psychoactive drugs. At this point, however, it is important to define *use* and to introduce the terms *misuse* and *abuse.*[3] By doing so, we can more accurately describe the ways in which drugs are used.

The term *use* is all-encompassing and describes drug-taking in the most general way. For example,

psychoactive drug
Any substance capable of altering feelings, moods, or perceptions.

dependence
General term that refers to the need to continue using a drug for psychological and/or physical reasons.

withdrawal illness
Uncomfortable, perhaps toxic response of the body as it attempts to maintain homeostasis in the absence of a drug; also called *abstinence syndrome.*

tolerance
An acquired reaction to a drug; continued intake of the same dose has diminished results.

cross-tolerance
Transfer of tolerance from one drug to another within the same general category.

Why People Use Drugs
- To medicate themselves
- To get high (a buzz)
- To be cool
- To ease pain
- To experiment
- Peer pressure
- Family problems
- To calm nerves
- To get down
- To escape
- To commit suicide
- Because it feels good
- Because they are addicted
- To work better
- To be alert
- Because they are bored
- To hurt themselves
- To hurt someone else
- To get in a good mood
- For a dare
- Fear of stopping

Americans use drugs of many types. The term *use* can also refer more narrowly to misuse and abuse. We most often use the word in this latter regard.

The term **misuse** refers to the inappropriate use of legal drugs intended to be medications. Misuse may occur when a patient misunderstands the directions for use of a prescription or OTC drug or when a patient shares a prescription with a friend or family member for whom the drug was not prescribed. Misuse also occurs when a patient takes the prescription or OTC drug for a purpose or condition other than that for which it was intended or at a dosage other than that recommended.

The term **abuse** applies to any use of an illegal drug or any use of a legal drug when it is detrimental to health and well-being. The costs of drug abuse to the individual are extensive and include absenteeism and underachievement, loss of job, marital instability, loss of self-esteem, serious illnesses, and even death. Complete the Personal Assessment below to determine whether you or someone you know may be abusing drugs.

PERSONAL ASSESSMENT

Recognizing Drug Abuse

To assess whether you or someone you know may be abusing drugs circle **Y** for yes and **N** for no.

1. A sudden increase in or loss of appetite or sudden weight loss or gain   Y   N
2. Moodiness, depression, irritability, or withdrawal   Y   N
3. Disorientation, lack of concentration, or forgetfulness   Y   N
4. Frequent use of eye drops or inappropriate wearing of sunglasses   Y   N
5. Disruption or change in sleep patterns or a lack of energy   Y   N
6. Borrowing money more and more, working excessive hours, selling personal items, or stealing or shoplifting   Y   N
7. Persistent and frequent nosebleeds, sniffles, coughs, and other signs of upper respiratory infection   Y   N
8. Change in speech patterns or vocabulary or a deterioration in academic performance   Y   N
9. Feeling ill at ease with family members and other adults   Y   N
10. Neglect of personal appearance   Y   N

Interpretation:
A yes response to more than three questions indicates that there may be drug dependence, and professional help should be obtained.

To Carry This Further . . .
See the Star Box on p. 171 and the Health Reference Guide at the back of this text for information about national groups and hot lines for drug use. They will help you find additional information about drug dependence and how to combat it.

EFFECTS OF DRUGS ON THE CENTRAL NERVOUS SYSTEM

To better understand the disruption caused by the actions of psychoactive drugs, a general knowledge of the normal functioning of the nervous system's basic unit, the **neuron,** is required.

First, stimuli from the internal or external environment are received by the appropriate sensory receptor, perhaps an organ such as an eye or an ear. Once sensed, these stimuli are converted into electrical impulses. These impulses are then directed along the neuron's **dendrite,** through the cell body, and along the **axon** toward the *synaptic junction* near an adjacent neuron. On arrival at the **synapse,** the electrical impulses stimulate the production and release of chemical messengers called *neurotransmitters.*[5] These neurotransmitters transmit the electrical impulses from one neuron to the dendrites of adjoining neurons. Thus neurons function in a coordinated fashion to send information to the brain for interpretation and to relay appropriate response commands outward to the tissues of the body.

The role of neurotransmitters is critically important to the relay of information within the system. A substance that has the ability to alter some aspect of transmitter function has the potential to seriously disrupt the otherwise normally functioning system. Psychoactive drugs are capable of exerting these disruptive influences on the neurotransmitters. Drugs "work" by changing the way neurotrans-mitters work, often by blocking the production of a neurotransmitter or forcing the continued release of a neurotransmitter (see the Star Box on p. 160).

DRUG CLASSIFICATIONS

Drugs can be categorized according to the nature of their physiological effects. Most psychoactive drugs fall into one of six general categories: stimulants, depressants, hallucinogens, cannabis, narcotics, and inhalants (Table 7-1).

Stimulants

In general, **stimulants** excite or increase the activity of the CNS. Also called "uppers," stimulants alert the CNS by increasing heart rate, blood pressure, and the rate of brain function. Users feel uplifted and less fatigued. Examples of stimulant drugs include caffeine, amphetamines, and cocaine. Most stimulants produce psychological dependence and tolerance relatively quickly, but they are unlikely to produce significant physical dependence when judged by life-threatening withdrawal symptoms. The important

exception is cocaine, which seems to be capable of producing psychological dependence and withdrawal so powerful that continued use of the drug is inevitable in some users.

Caffeine

Caffeine, the tasteless drug found in chocolate, some soft drinks, coffee, tea, some aspirin products, and OTC "stay-awake" pills, is a relatively harmless stimulant when consumed in moderate amounts (Table 7-2). Many coffee drinkers believe that they cannot start the day successfully without the benefit of a cup or two of coffee in the morning.

Pregnant women are advised to consume caffeine sparingly.[6] For the average healthy adult, moderate consumption of caffeine is unlikely to pose any serious health threat. However, excessive consumption (equivalent to 10 or more cups of coffee daily) could lead to anxiety, diarrhea, restlessness, delayed onset of sleep or frequent awakening, headache, and heart palpitations.

Amphetamines

Amphetamines produce increased activity and mood elevation in almost all users. The amphetamines include several closely related compounds:

---

misuse
Inappropriate use of legal drugs intended to be medications.

abuse
Any use of a legal or illegal drug in a way that is detrimental to health.

neuron (**noor** on)
A nerve cell.

dendrite (**den** drite)
The portion of a neuron that receives electrical stimuli from adjacent neurons; neurons typically have several such branches or extensions.

axon
The portion of a neuron that conducts electrical impulses to the dendrites of adjacent neurons; neurons typically have one axon.

synapse (**sinn** aps)
The location at which an electrical impulse from one neuron is transmitted to an adjacent neuron; also referred to as a *synaptic junction.*

stimulants
Psychoactive drugs that stimulate the function of the central nervous system.

Effect of Drugs on the Central Nervous System

This illustration depicts the disruption caused by the action of psychoactive drugs on the central nervous system.[1] Neurotransmitters are chemical messengers that transfer electrical impulses across the synapses between nerve cells.[2] Psychoactive drugs interrupt this process, thus disrupting the coordinated functioning of the nervous system.

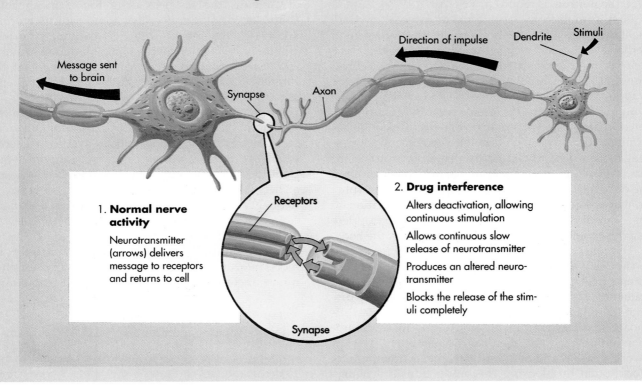

Message sent to brain

Direction of impulse

Dendrite

Stimuli

Synapse

Axon

Receptors

Synapse

1. Normal nerve activity

Neurotransmitter (arrows) delivers message to receptors and returns to cell

2. Drug interference

Alters deactivation, allowing continuous stimulation

Allows continuous slow release of neurotransmitter

Produces an altered neurotransmitter

Blocks the release of the stimuli completely

Table 7-1   Psychoactive Drug Categories

Drugs	Trade or Common Names	Medical Uses	Possible Effects
Stimulants			
Cocaine*	Coke, flake, snow, crack	Local anesthetic	Increased alertness, excitation, euphoria, increased pulse rate and blood pressure, insomnia, loss of appetite
Amphetamines	Biphetamine, Delcobese, Desoxyn, Dexedrine, mediatric, methamphetamine (ice)	Hyperactivity, narcolepsy, weight control	
Phendimetrazine	Prelu-2		
Methylphenidate	Ritalin, Methidate		
Other stimulants	Adipex, Bacarate, Cylert, Didrex, Ionamin, Plegine, PreSate, Sanorex, Tenuate, Tepanil, Voranil		
Depressants			
Chloral hydrate	Noctec, Somnos	Hypnotic	Slurred speech, disorientation, drunken behavior without odor of alcohol
Barbiturates	Amobarbital, Butisol, phenobarbital, phenoxbarbital, secobarbital, Tuinal	Anesthetic, anticonvulsant, sedative, hypnotic	
Glutethimide	Doriden	Sedative, hypnotic	

Table 7-1, cont'd

Drugs	Trade or Common Names	Medical Uses	Possible Effects
Methaqualone	Optimil, Parest, Quaalude, Somnafec, Sopor	Sedative, hypnotic	
Benzodiazepines	Ativan, Azene, Clonopin, Dalmane, diazepam, Librium, Serax, Tranxene, Valium, Verstran	Antianxiety, anti-convulsant, seda-tive, hypnotic	
Other depres-sants	Equanil, Miltown, Noludar, Placidyl, Valmid	Antianxiety, seda-tive, hypnotic	
Hallucinogens			
LSD	Acid, microdot	None	Delusions and hallucinations, poor perception of time and distance
Mescaline and peyote	Mesc, buttons, cactus	None	
Amphetamine variants (designer drugs)	2,5-DMA, DOM, DOP, MDA, MDMA, PMA, STP, TMA	None	
Phencyclidine	Angel dust, hog, PCP	Veterinary anesthetic	
Phencyclidine analogs	PCE, PCPy, TCP	None	
Other hallucino-gens	Bufotenin, DMT, DET, ibogaine, psilo-cybin, psilocyn	None	
Cannabis			
Marijuana	Acapulco gold, grass, pot, reefer, sin-semilla, Thai sticks	Under investigation	Euphoria, relaxed inhibitions, increased appetite, disoriented behavior
Tetrahydro-cannabinol	THC	Under investigation	
Hashish	Hash	None	
Hashish oil	Hash oil	None	
Narcotics			
Opium	Dover's powder, paregoric, Parapec-tolin	Analgesic, antidiar-rheal	Euphoria, drowsiness, respira-tory depression, constricted pupils, nausea
Morphine	Morphine, Pectoal syrup	Analgesic, antitus-sive	
Codeine	Codeine, Empirin compound with codeine, Robitussin A-C	Analgesic, antitus-sive	
Heroin	Diacetylmorphine, horse, smack	Under investigation	
Hydromorphone	Dilaudid	Analgesic	
Meperidine (pethidine)	Demerol, Pethadol	Analgesic	
Methadone	Dolophine, Methadone, Methadose	Analgesic, heroin substitute	
Other narcotics	Darvon,† Dromoran, Fentanyl, LAAM, Leitine, Levo-Dromoran, Percodan, Tussionex, Talwin,† Lomotil	Analgesic, antidiar-rheal, antitussive	
Inhalants			
Anesthetic gases	Aerosols, petroleum products, solvents	Surgical anesthesia	Intoxication, excitation, disorien-tation, aggression, hallucina-tion, variable effects
Vasodilators (amyl nitrite, butyl nitrite)	Aerosols, petroleum products, solvents	None	

*Designated a narcotic under the Controlled Substances Act.
†Not designated a narcotic under the Controlled Substances Act.

Table 7-2   Caffeine Content of Beverages, Food, and Drug Preparations

Coffee (5 oz cup)	Caffeine (mg)	Soft Drinks (12 oz)	Caffeine (mg)	Pain Relievers	Caffeine (mg)
Drip method	110-150	Mountain Dew	54	Anacin	32
Percolated	64-124	Mello Yello	52	Excedrin	65
Instant	40-108	TAB	46	Midol	32
Decaffeinated	2-5	Coca-Cola	46	Plain aspirin	0
		Diet Coke	46	Vanquish	33
Tea (5 oz cup)		Shasta Cola	44		
1-min brew	9-33	Mr. Pibb	40	**Diuretics**	
3-min brew	20-46	Dr. Pepper	40	Aqua Ban	100
5-min brew	20-50	Diet Dr. Pepper	40		
Instant tea	12-28	Pepsi Cola	38	**Cold Remedies**	
Iced tea (12 oz)	22-36	Diet Pepsi	36	Coryban-D	30
Cocoa				Dristan	0
Made from mix	6	**Stimulants**		Triaminicin	30
Milk chocolate (1 oz)	6	NoDoz tablets	100	**Weight-Control Aids**	
Baking chocolate	35	Vivarin tablets	200	Dexatrim	200
				Prolamine	140
				Prescription Pain Relievers	
				Cafergot	100
				Darvon compound	32
				Fiorinal	40
				Migralam	100

amphetamine, dextroamphetamine, and methamphetamine. These compounds do not have any natural sources and are completely manufactured in the laboratory. Medical use of amphetamines is limited primarily to the treatment of obesity, **narcolepsy,** and **attention deficit disorder (ADD).**

Amphetamines can be ingested, injected, or snorted (inhaled). At low-to-moderate doses, amphetamines elevate mood and increase alertness and feelings of energy by stimulating receptor sites for two naturally occurring neurotransmitters. They also slow the activity of the stomach and intestine and decrease hunger. In the 1960s and 1970s, in fact, amphetamines were commonly prescribed for dieters, but when it was discovered that the appetite suppression effect of amphetamines lasted only a few weeks, most physicians stopped prescribing them. At high doses, amphetamines can increase heart rate and blood pressure to dangerous levels. As amphetamines are eliminated from the body, the user becomes tired.

When chronically abused, amphetamines produce rapid tolerance and strong psychological dependence.

Other effects of chronic use include impotence and episodes of psychosis. When use is discontinued, periods of depression may develop.

Today the abuse of amphetamines is a more pressing concern than it has been in the recent past. Underlying this sharp increase in abuse is methamphetamine. Known by a variety of names and forms, including "crank," "ice," "crystal," "meth," "speed," "crystal meth," and "Zip," methamphetamine is produced in illegal home laboratories.

Ice

Crystal meth or ice is among the most recent and dangerous forms of methamphetamine. Ice is a very pure form of methamphetamine that looks like rock candy. When smoked, the effects of ice are felt in about 7 seconds as a wave of intense physical and psychological exhilaration. This effect lasts for several hours (much longer than the effects of *crack*) until the user becomes physically exhausted. Chronic use leads to nutritional difficulties, weight loss, reduced resistance to infection, and damage to the liver, lungs, and kidneys. Psychological dependence is quickly estab-

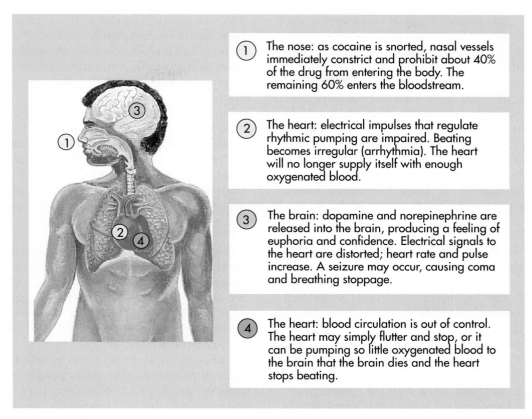

1. The nose: as cocaine is snorted, nasal vessels immediately constrict and prohibit about 40% of the drug from entering the body. The remaining 60% enters the bloodstream.

2. The heart: electrical impulses that regulate rhythmic pumping are impaired. Beating becomes irregular (arrhythmia). The heart will no longer supply itself with enough oxygenated blood.

3. The brain: dopamine and norepinephrine are released into the brain, producing a feeling of euphoria and confidence. Electrical signals to the heart are distorted; heart rate and pulse increase. A seizure may occur, causing coma and breathing stoppage.

4. The heart: blood circulation is out of control. The heart may simply flutter and stop, or it can be pumping so little oxygenated blood to the brain that the brain dies and the heart stops beating.

Figure 7-2   Cocaine's effects on the body.

Inhalation of "lines" of cocaine was the primary route of administration in the 1980s.

lished. Withdrawal causes acute depression and fatigue but not significant physical discomfort.

Cocaine

Cocaine, perhaps the strongest of the stimulant drugs, has received much media attention. Cocaine is the primary psychoactive substance found in the leaves of the South American coca plant. The effects of cocaine are brief—from 5 to 30 minutes (Figure 7-2). Regardless of the form in which it is consumed, cocaine produces an immediate, near-orgasmic "rush," or feeling of exhilaration. This euphoria is quickly followed by a period of marked depression. Used only occasionally as a topical anesthetic, cocaine is usually inhaled (snorted), injected, or smoked (as *freebase* or crack). There is overwhelming scientific evidence that users quickly develop a strong psychologi-

narcolepsy (**nar** co lep see)
A sleep-related disorder in which a person has a recurrent, overwhelming, and uncontrollable desire to sleep.

attention deficit disorder (ADD)
Above-normal rate of physical movement; often accompanied by an inability to concentrate well on a specified task; also called *hyperactivity*.

cal dependence to cocaine. There is considerable evidence that physical dependence also rapidly develops. However, physical dependence on cocaine does not lead to death on withdrawal.

The status of cocaine as a substitute for amphetamines (during the 1960s), as a recreational drug for the wealthy (during the 1970s), and as a widely abused drug by many segments of society (during the 1980s) is well documented. During the 1990s, overall cocaine use has decreased, although heavy use has increased. Today, freebasing and the use of crack have replaced the inhalation of "lines" of cocaine, which was the primary route of administration in the 1980s.

Freebasing

Freebasing and the use of crack cocaine are the most recent techniques for maximizing the psychoactive effects of the drug. Freebasing first requires that the common form of powdered cocaine (cocaine hydrochloride) be chemically altered (alkalized). This altered form is then dissolved in a solvent, such as ether or benzene. This liquid solution is heated to evaporate the solvent. The heating process leaves the freebase cocaine in a powder form that can then be smoked, often through a water pipe. Because of the large surface area of the lungs, smoking cocaine facilitates fast absorption into the bloodstream.

One danger of freebasing cocaine is the risk related to the solvents used. Ether is a highly volatile solvent capable of exploding and causing serious burns. Benzene is a known carcinogen associated with the development of leukemia. Clearly, neither solvent can be used without increasing the level of risk normally associated with cocaine use. This method of making smokeable cocaine led to a new epidemic of cocaine use, smoking crack.

Crack

In contrast to freebase cocaine, crack is made by combining cocaine hydrochloride with common baking soda. When this pastelike mixture is allowed to dry, a small rocklike crystalline material remains. This crack is heated in the bowl of a small pipe, and the vapors are inhaled into the lungs. A single dose of crack currently sells for $20 to $30. Some crack users spend hundreds of dollars a day to maintain their habit.

The effect of crack is almost instantaneous. Within 10 seconds after inhalation, cocaine reaches the CNS and influences the action of several neurotransmitters at specific sites in the brain. As with the use of other forms of cocaine, convulsions, seizures, respiratory distress, and cardiac failure have been reported with this sudden, extensive stimulation of the nervous system.

Within about 6 minutes, the stimulating effect of crack has been completely expended, and users frequently become depressed. Dependence develops within a few weeks, since users consume more crack in response to the short duration of stimulation and rapid onset of depression.

Intravenous administration has been the preferred route for cocaine users who are also regular users of heroin and other injectable drugs. Intravenous injection results in an almost immediate high, which lasts about 10 minutes. A "smoother ride" is said to be obtained from a "speedball," the injectable mixture of heroin and cocaine (or methamphetamine).[4]

Cocaine and society

It is beyond the scope of this book to chronicle the way in which cocaine use has profoundly damaged our nation. However, we encourage students to watch or read the daily media reports about this topic. A few of the central reasons why civic and government leaders have declared war on the use of illicit drugs, especially cocaine, follow.

Although cocaine use hurts people from all walks of life, it most critically affects people from inner-city minority groups and the urban poor.[7] Cocaine use provides an instant temporary escape from an unpromising future. For many inner-city youths, selling cocaine or crack is the easiest way to escape poverty. However, drug dealing also brings with it an escalation of involvement in street gangs, crime, and violence.[8] Crack houses are also notorious for promoting the spread of HIV infection and other serious diseases. Tragically, a high percentage of babies born in large city hospitals are addicted to cocaine and have both physical and neurological difficulties. Some are born with an HIV infection that soon leads to AIDS. Indeed, the personal and social cost of cocaine use is enormous.

Depressants

Depressants (or sedatives) sedate the user, slowing down CNS function. Drugs included in this category are alcohol (see Chapter 8), barbiturates, and tranquilizers. Depressants produce tolerance in abusers, as well as strong psychological and physical dependence.

Barbiturates

Barbiturates are the so-called sleeping compounds that function by enhancing the effect of inhibitory neurotransmitters. They depress the CNS to the point where the user drops off to sleep or, as is the case with surgical anesthetics, the patient becomes anesthetized. Medically, barbiturates are used in widely varied dosages as anesthetics and for treatment of anxiety, insomnia, and epilepsy.[3] Regular use of a barbiturate quickly produces tolerance—eventually such a high dose is required that the user still feels the effects of the drug throughout the next morning. Some abusers then begin to alternate barbiturates with stimulants, producing a vicious circle of dependence. Other misusers combine alcohol and barbiturates or tranquilizers, inadvertently producing toxic or even lethal results. Abrupt withdrawal from barbiturate use frequently produces a withdrawal syndrome that can involve seizures, delusions, hallucinations, and even death.

Methaqualone (Quaalude, "ludes," Sopor) was developed as a sedative that would not have the dependence properties of other barbiturates.[3] Although this did not happen, Quaaludes were occasionally prescribed for anxious patients. Today, compounds resembling Quaaludes are manufactured in home laboratories and sold illegally so that they can be combined with small amounts of alcohol for an inexpensive, drunklike effect.

Tranquilizers

Tranquilizers are depressants that are intended to reduce anxiety and to relax people who are having problems managing stress. They are not specifically designed to produce sleep but rather to help people cope during their waking hours. Such tranquilizers are termed *minor tranquilizers,* of which diazepam (Valium) and chlordiazepoxide (Librium) may be the most commonly prescribed examples. Unfortunately, some people become addicted to these and other prescription drugs (see the article on pp. 175-176).

Some tranquilizers are further designed to control hospitalized psychotic patients who may be suicidal or who are potential threats to others. These *major tranquilizers* subdue people physically but permit them to remain conscious. Their use is generally limited to institutional settings. All tranquilizers can produce physical and psychological dependence and tolerance.

Hallucinogens

As the name suggests, hallucinogenic drugs produce hallucinations—perceived distortions of reality. Also known as *psychedelic* drugs or *phantasticants,* **hallucinogens** reached their height of popularity during the 1960s (see the Learning from All Cultures box at right). At that time, young people were encouraged to use hallucinogenic drugs to "expand the mind," "reach an altered state," or "discover reality." Not all of the reality distortions, or "trips," were pleasant. Many users reported "bummers," or trips during which they perceived negative, frightening distortions.

LEARNING from ALL CULTURES

Hallucinogens and Religious Ceremonies

Hallucinogens became very popular in the United States in the 1960s, and they are still used today. Some of these substances have been fairly recently discovered, whereas others have been used for hundreds of years by certain societies. Some forms have been and continue to be used by Native Americans as part of their religious ceremonies.[4]

Mescaline is a hallucinogen derived from the peyote cactus. Native American tribes in Mexico used peyote in religious ceremonies many years ago to enhance the spiritual experience. The practice then spread to Native American tribes in the United States. Today, the Native American Church of North America still uses peyote in religious ceremonies.[4]

Some tribes have had to change their practices of peyote use because of state laws. The legality of using peyote for religious ceremonies is a state decision. A Supreme Court ruling in favor of the state of Oregon, prohibiting the use of peyote, stated that Native American tribes must comply with the state laws concerning the use of peyote in religious rituals. However, 23 other states allow ceremonial peyote use by the Native American Church.[14]

Other religious practices, such as the sacrifice of animals, have been questioned by some state governments. How much authority should the government have in regulating the ceremonial rituals of religious groups?

Hallucinogenic drugs include laboratory-produced lysergic acid diethylamide (LSD), mescaline (from the peyote cactus plant), and psilocybin (from a particular genus of mushroom). Consumption of hallucinogens seems to produce not physical dependence but mild levels of psychological dependence. The development of tolerance is questionable. *Synesthesia,* a sensation in which users report hearing a color, smelling music, or touching a taste, is sometimes produced with hallucinogen use.

The long-term effects of hallucinogenic drug use are not fully understood. Questions about genetic

hallucinogens
Psychoactive drugs capable of producing hallucinations (distortions of reality).

abnormalities in offspring, fertility, sex drive and performance, and the development of personality disorders have not been fully answered. One phenomenon that has been identified and documented is the development of *flashbacks*—the unpredictable return to a psychedelic trip that occurred months or even years earlier. Flashbacks are thought to result from the accumulation of a drug within body cells.

LSD

The most well-known hallucinogen is lysergic acid diethylamide. LSD is a drug that helped define the counterculture movement of the 1960s. During the 1970s and the 1980s, this drug lost considerable popularity. However, in the 1990s, LSD is making a comeback, with some studies showing that about 1 in 10 high school students and 1 in 20 college students has experimented with LSD. Fear of cocaine and other powerful drugs, boredom, low cost, and an attempt to revisit the culture of the '60s are thought to have increased LSD's attractiveness to today's young people.

LSD is manufactured in home laboratories and frequently distributed in blotter paper decorated with cartoon characters. Users place the paper on their tongue or chew the paper to ingest the drug. LSD can produce a psychedelic (mind-viewing) effect that includes altered perception of shapes, images, time, sound, and body form. Synesthesia is common to LSD users. Ingested in doses known as "hits," LSD produces a 6- to 9-hour experience. Hits range in price from $3 to $5.[9]

Although the hits today are about half as powerful as those in the 1960s, users still tend to develop high tolerance to LSD. Physical dependence does not occur. Not all LSD trips are pleasant. Hallucinations produced from LSD can be frightening and dangerous. Users can injure or kill themselves accidentally during a bad trip. Dangerous side effects include panic attacks, flashbacks, and occasional prolonged psychosis.

Designer drugs

In recent years, chemists who produce many of the illicit drugs in home laboratories have designed versions of drugs listed on **FDA Schedule 1.** These *designer drugs* are similar to the controlled drugs on the FDA Schedule 1 but are sufficiently different so that they escape governmental control. The designer drugs are either newly synthesized products that are similar to already outlawed drugs but against which no law yet exists, or they are reconstituted or renamed illegal substances. Designer drugs are said to produce effects similar to their controlled drug counterparts.

People who use designer drugs do so at great risk because the manufacturing of these drugs is unregulated. The neurophysiological effect of these homemade drugs can be quite dangerous. So far, a synthetic heroin product (MPPP) and several amphetamine derivatives with hallucinogenic properties have been designed for the unwary drug consumer.

DOM (STP), MDA (the "love drug"), and MDMA ("ecstasy" or "XTC") are examples of amphetamine-derivative, hallucinogenic designer drugs. These drugs produce mild LSD-like hallucinogenic experiences, positive feelings, and enhanced alertness. They also have a number of potentially dangerous effects. Experts are particularly concerned that MDMA can produce strong psychological dependence and can deplete serotonin, an important excitatory neurotransmitter associated with a state of alertness. Permanent brain damage is possible.[3]

Phencyclidine

Phencyclidine (PCP, "angel dust") has been classified variously as a hallucinogen, a stimulant, a depressant, and an anesthetic. PCP was studied for years during the 1950s and 1960s and was found to be an unsuitable animal and human anesthetic. PCP is an extremely unpredictable drug. Easily manufactured in home laboratories in tablet or powder form, PCP can be injected, inhaled, taken orally, or smoked. The effects vary. Some users report mild euphoria, although most report bizarre perceptions, paranoid feelings, and aggressive behavior. PCP overdose may cause convulsions, cardiovascular collapse, and damage to the brain's respiratory center.

In a number of cases the aggressive behavior caused by PCP has led users to commit brutal crimes against both friends and innocent strangers. PCP accumulates in cells and may stimulate bizarre behavior months after initial use.

Cannabis

Cannabis (marijuana) has been labeled a mild hallucinogen for a number of years. However, most experts now consider it to be a drug category in itself. Marijuana produces mild effects like those of stimulants and depressants. The recent implication of marijuana in a large number of traffic fatalities makes this drug one whose consumption should be carefully considered. Marijuana is actually a wild plant (*Cannabis sativa*) whose fibers were once used in the manufacture of hemp rope. When the leafy material and small stems are dried and crushed, users can smoke the mixture in rolled cigarettes ("joints") or pipes. The resins collected from scraping the flowering tops of the plant yield a mari-

Smoking pot.

juana product called *hashish,* or *hash,* commonly smoked in a pipe.

The potency of marijuana's hallucinogenic effect is determined by the percentage of the active ingredient tetrahydrocannabinol (THC) present in the product. Based on the analysis of samples from drug seizures and street buys in the United States, the concentration of THC averages about 3.5% for marijuana, 7% to 9% for higher-quality marijuana (sinsemilla), 8% to 14% for hashish, and as high as 50% for hash oil.

THC is a fat-soluble substance and thus is absorbed and retained in fat tissues within the body. Before being excreted, THC can remain in the body for up to a month. With the sophistication of today's drug tests, trace amounts of THC can be detected for up to 3 weeks after consumption.[3] It is possible that the THC that comes from passive inhalation (for example, during an indoor rock concert) can also be detected for a short time after exposure.

Once marijuana is consumed, its effects vary from person to person. Being "high" or "stoned" or "wrecked" means different things to different people. Many people report heightened sensitivity to music, cravings for particular foods, and a relaxed mood. There is widespread consensus that marijuana's behavioral effects includes four probabilities: (1) users must learn to recognize what a marijuana high is like, (2) marijuana impairs short-term memory, (3) users overestimate the passage of time, and (4) users lose the ability to maintain attention to a task.[3]

The long-term effects of marijuana use are still being studied. Chronic abuse may lead to an *amotivational syndrome* in some people. The irritating effects of marijuana smoke on lung tissue are more pronounced than those of cigarette smoke, and some of the over 400 chemicals in marijuana are now linked to lung cancer development. In fact, one of the most

potent carcinogens, benzopyrene, is found in higher levels in marijuana smoke than in tobacco smoke. Marijuana smokers tend to inhale deeply and hold the smoke in the lungs for long periods. It is likely that at some point the lungs of chronic marijuana smokers will be damaged.

Long-term marijuana use is also associated with damage to the immune system and to the male and female reproductive systems and with an increase in birth defects in babies born to mothers who smoke marijuana. Chronic marijuana use lowers testosterone levels in men, but the effect of this change is not known. The effect of long-term marijuana use on a variety of types of sexual behavior is also not fully understood.

Because the drug can distort perceptions and thus perceptual ability (especially when combined with alcohol), its use by automobile drivers clearly jeopardizes the lives of many innocent people.

The only medical uses for marijuana are to relieve the nausea caused by chemotherapy, to improve appetites in AIDS patients, and to ease the pressure that builds up in the eyes of glaucoma patients. However, a variety of other drugs, many of which are nearly as effective, are also used for these purposes.

One particularly alarming statistic concerning marijuana use emerged in late 1995 with the release of the 1994 National Household Survey on Drug Abuse.[10] This national report indicated that marijuana use among 12- to 17-year-olds had nearly doubled in a 2-year period. In 1992, 4% of this age group reported monthly marijuana use, yet by 1994, 7.3% indicated monthly marijuana use.

Along with this increase in marijuana use was the finding that fewer American youths perceived great risk of harm in using marijuana occasionally.[10] Why do you think that today's young people believe that marijuana use is not dangerous?

Narcotics

The **narcotics** are among the most dependence-producing drugs. Medically, narcotics are used to relieve pain and induce sleep. On the basis of origin,

---

FDA Schedule 1
A list of drugs that have a high potential for abuse but no medical use.

narcotics
Opiates; psychoactive drugs derived from the Oriental poppy plant; narcotics relieve pain and induce sleep.

narcotics can be subgrouped into the natural, quasi-synthetic, and synthetic narcotics.

Natural narcotics

Naturally occurring substances derived from the Oriental poppy plant include opium (the primary psychoactive substance extracted from the Oriental poppy), morphine (the primary active ingredient in opium), and thebaine (a compound not used as a drug). Morphine and related compounds have medical use as analgesics in the treatment of mild to severe pain.

Quasisynthetic narcotics

Quasisynthetic narcotics are compounds created by chemically altering morphine. These laboratory-produced drugs are intended to be used as analgesics, but their benefits are largely outweighed by a high dependence rate and a great risk of toxicity. The best known of the quasisynthetic narcotics is heroin. Although heroin is a fast-acting and very effective analgesic, it is extremely addictive. Once injected into a vein or "skin-popped" (injected beneath the skin surface), heroin produces dreamlike euphoria and, like all narcotics, strong physical and psychological dependence and tolerance.

As with the use of all other injectable illegal drugs, the practice of sharing needles increases the likelihood of transmission of various communicable diseases, including HIV (see Chapter 12). Abrupt withdrawal from heroin use is rarely fatal, but the discomfort during **cold turkey** withdrawal is reported to be overwhelming. The use of heroin has increased during the last decade. The purity of heroin has improved while the price has dropped. Cocaine abusers may use heroin to "come down" from the high associated with cocaine.

Synthetic narcotics

Meperidine (Demerol) and propoxyphene (Darvon), common postsurgical painkillers, and methadone, the drug prescribed during the rehabilitation of heroin addicts, are *synthetic narcotics*. These opiate-like drugs are manufactured in medical laboratories. They are not natural narcotics or quasisynthetic narcotics because they do not originate from the Oriental poppy plant. Like true narcotics, however, these drugs can rapidly induce physical dependence. One important criticism of methadone rehabilitation programs is that they merely shift the addiction from heroin to methadone.

Inhalants

Inhalants are a class of drugs that includes a variety of volatile (quickly evaporating) compounds that generally produce unpredictable, drunklike effects in users. Users of inhalants may also have some delusions and hallucinations. Some users may become quite aggressive. Drugs in this category include anesthetic gases (chloroform, nitrous oxide, and ether), vasodilators (amyl nitrite and butyl nitrite), petroleum products and commercial solvents (gasoline, kerosene, plastic cement, glue, typewriter correction fluid, paint, and paint thinner), and certain aerosols (found in some propelled spray products, fertilizers, and insecticides).

Most of the danger in using inhalants lies in the damaging, sometimes fatal effects on the respiratory system. Furthermore, users may unknowingly place themselves in dangerous situations because of the drunklike hallucinogenic effects. Aggressive behavior might also make users a threat to themselves and others.

COMBINATION DRUG EFFECTS

Drugs taken in various combinations and dosages can alter and perhaps intensify effects.

A **synergistic drug effect** is a dangerous consequence of taking different drugs in the same general category at the same time. The combination exaggerates each individual drug's effects. For example, the combined use of alcohol and tranquilizers produces a synergistic effect greater than the total effect of each of the two drugs taken separately. In this instance a much-amplified, perhaps fatal sedation will occur. In a simplistic sense, "one plus one equals four or five."

When taken at or near the same time, drug combinations produce a variety of effects. Drug combinations have additive, potentiating, or antagonistic effects. When two or more drugs are taken and the result is merely a combined total effect of each drug, the result is an **additive effect.** The sum of the effects is not exaggerated. In a sense, "one plus one plus one equals three."

When one drug intensifies the action of a second drug, the first drug is said to have a **potentiated effect** on the second drug. One popular drug-taking practice during the 1970s was the consumption of Quaaludes and beer. Quaaludes potentiated the inhibition-releasing, sedative effects of alcohol. This particular drug combination produced an inexpensive but potentially fatal drunklike euphoria in the user.

An **antagonistic effect** is an opposite effect one drug has on another drug. One drug may be able to reduce another drug's influence on the body. Knowledge of this principle has been useful in the medical treatment of certain drug overdoses, as in the use of tranquilizers to relieve the effects of LSD or other hallucinogenic drugs.

SOCIETY'S RESPONSE TO DRUG USE

During the last 20 years, society has responded to illegal drug use with growing concern. Most adults see drug abuse as a clear danger to society. This position has been supported by the development of community, school, state, and national organizations interested in the reduction of illegal drug use. These organizations have included such diverse groups as Parents Against Drugs, Parents for a Drug-Free Youth, Mothers Against Drunk Driving (MADD), Narcotics Anonymous, and the federal Drug Enforcement Administration. Certain groups have concentrated their efforts on education, others on enforcement, and still others on the development of laws and public policy.

The personal and social issues related to drug abuse are very complex. Innovative solutions continue to be devised. Some believe that only through early childhood education will people learn alternatives to drug use. Starting drug education in the preschool years may have a more positive effect than waiting until the upper elementary or junior high school years. Recently, the focus on reducing young people's exposure to so-called **gateway drugs** (especially tobacco, alcohol, and marijuana) may help slow down the move to other addictive drugs. Some people advocate much harsher penalties for drug use and drug trafficking, including extreme measures such as public executions.

Others support legalizing all drugs and making governmental agencies responsible for drug regulation and control, as is the case with alcohol. Advocates of this position believe that drug-related crime and violence would virtually cease once the demand for illegal products is reduced. Sound arguments can be made on both sides of this issue. What is your opinion?

Unless significant changes in society's response to drug use take place soon, the disastrous effects of virtually uncontrolled drug abuse will continue to be felt. Families and communities will continue to be plagued by drug-related tragedies. Law enforcement officials will be pressed to the limits of their resources in their attempts to reduce drug flow. Our judicial system will be heavily burdened by thousands of court cases. Health care facilities could face overwhelming numbers of patients.

In comparison with other federally funded programs, the "war on drugs" is less expensive than farm support, food stamps, Medicare, and national defense. However, it remains to be seen whether any amount of money spent on enforcement, without adequate support for education, treatment, and poverty reduction, can reduce the illegal drug demand and supply. Currently, $12 billion is spent to fight the drug war in the United States: $8 billion is spent on law enforcement, and $4 billion is spent on education, prevention, and treatment.

Drug Testing

Society's response to concern over drug use includes the development and growing use of drug tests. At present, the five largest drug-testing laboratories in the United States process over 1 million urine specimens per month combined.[11] Most of the specimens come from corporations that screen employees for commonly abused drugs. Among these are amphetamines, barbiturates, benzodiazepines (the chemical bases for prescription tranquilizers such as Valium and Librium), cannabinoids (THC, hashish, and marijuana), methaqualone, opiates (heroin,

---

cold turkey
Immediate, total discontinuation of use of a drug; associated withdrawal discomfort.

inhalants
Psychoactive drugs that enter the body through inhalation.

synergistic drug effect (sin er **jist** ick)
Heightened, exaggerated effect produced by the concurrent use of two or more drugs.

additive effect
The combined (but not exaggerated) effect produced by the concurrent use of two or more drugs.

potentiated effect (poe **ten** she ay ted)
Phenomenon whereby the use of one drug intensifies the effect of a second drug.

antagonistic effect
Effect produced when one drug reduces or offsets the effects of a second drug.

gateway drug
An easily obtainable legal or illegal drug that represents a user's first experience with a mind-altering drug.

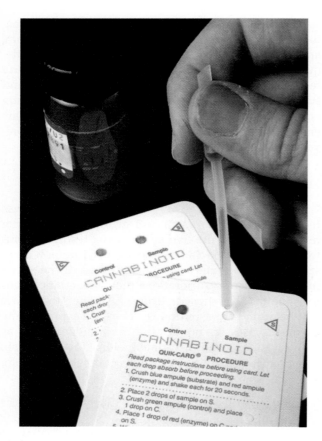

A drug test.

codeine, and morphine), and PCP. With the exception of marijuana, most traces of these drugs are eliminated by the body within a few days after use. Marijuana can remain detectable for weeks after use.

How accurate are the results of drug testing? At typical cutoff standards, drug tests will likely identify 90% of recent drug users. This means that about 10% of recent users will pass undetected. (These 10% are considered false negatives.) Nonusers whose drug tests indicate drug use (false positives) are quite rare. (Follow-up tests on these false positives would nearly always show negative results.) Human errors are probably more responsible than technical errors for inaccuracies in drug tests.[11]

Recently, scientists have been refining procedures that use hair samples to detect the presence of drugs.[12] These procedures seem to hold much promise, although certain technical obstacles remain. Watch for refinements in hair-sample drug testing in the near future.

Most Fortune 500 companies, the armed forces, various government agencies, and nearly all athletic organizations have already implemented mandatory drug testing. Corporate substance abuse policies are being developed, with careful attention to legal and ethical issues.

Do you think that the possibility of having to take a drug test would have any effect on college students' use of drugs?

COLLEGE AND COMMUNITY SUPPORT SERVICES FOR DRUG DEPENDENCE

Students who have drug problems and realize they need assistance might select assistance based on the services available on campus or in the surrounding community and the costs they are willing to pay for treatment services.

One recently developed approach to convince drug-dependent people to enter treatment programs is the use of *confrontation*. People who live or work with chemically dependent people are being encouraged to confront them directly about their addiction. Direct confrontation helps chemically dependent people realize the effect their behavior has on others. Once chemically dependent people realize that others will no longer tolerate their behavior, the likelihood of their entering treatment programs is increased significantly. Although effective, this approach is very stressful for family members and friends and requires the assistance of professionals in the field of chemical dependence. These professionals can be contacted at a drug treatment center in your area.

Treatment

Comprehensive drug treatment programs are available in very few college or university health centers. College settings for drug dependence programs are more commonly found in the university counseling center. At such a center the emphasis will probably be not on the medical management of dependence but on the behavioral dimensions of drug abuse. Trained counselors and psychologists who specialize in chemical dependence counseling will work with students to (1) analyze their particular concerns, (2) establish constructive ways to cope with stress, and (3) search for alternative ways to achieve new "highs" (see the Personal Assessment on p. 171).

Medical treatment for the management of drug problems may need to be obtained through the services of a community treatment facility administered by a local health department, community mental health center, private clinic, or local hospital. Treatment may be on an inpatient or outpatient basis. Medical management

PERSONAL ASSESSMENT

Getting a Drug-Free High

Experts agree that drug use provides only short-term, ineffective, and often destructive solutions to problems. We hope that you have found (or will find) innovative, invigorating drug-free experiences that make your life more exciting. Circle the number for each activity that reflects your intention to try that activity. Use the following guide:

1 No intention of trying this activity
2 Intend to try this within 2 years
3 Intend to try this within 6 months
4 Already tried this activity
5 Regularly engage in this activity

1.	Learn to juggle	1	2	3	4	5
2.	Go backpacking	1	2	3	4	5
3.	Complete a marathon race	1	2	3	4	5
4.	Start a vegetable garden	1	2	3	4	5
5.	Ride in a hot air balloon	1	2	3	4	5
6.	Snow ski or water ski	1	2	3	4	5
7.	Donate blood	1	2	3	4	5
8.	Go river rafting	1	2	3	4	5
9.	Learn to play a musical instrument	1	2	3	4	5
10.	Cycle 100 miles	1	2	3	4	5
11.	Go skydiving	1	2	3	4	5
12.	Go rockclimbing	1	2	3	4	5
13.	Play a role in a theater production	1	2	3	4	5
14.	Build a piece of furniture	1	2	3	4	5
15.	Solicit funds for a worthy cause	1	2	3	4	5
16.	Learn to swim	1	2	3	4	5
17.	Overhaul a car engine	1	2	3	4	5
18.	Compose a song	1	2	3	4	5
19.	Travel to a foreign country	1	2	3	4	5
20.	Write the first chapter of a book	1	2	3	4	5

Your total points _____

Interpretation

61-100   You participate in many challenging experiences

41-60   You are willing to try some challenging new experiences

20-40   You take few of the challenging risks described here

To Carry This Further . . .

Looking at your point total, were you surprised at the degree to which you are aware of alternative activities? What are the top five activities, and can you understand their importance? What activities would you add to this list?

National Anti–Drug Abuse Groups and Hot Lines

National Groups

- PRIDE (Parent's Resource Institute for Drug Education): Atlanta (404) 577-4500; in Georgia (900) 998-7743
- National Federation of State High School Associations Target Programs: Kansas City, Mo (816) 464-5400
- National Health Information Clearinghouse: (800) 336-4797
- National Clearinghouse for Alcohol and Drug Information: Silver Spring, Md (800) 729-6686; (301) 468-2600
- Narcotics Anonymous: Van Nuys, Calif (818) 780-3951
- Toughlove: Doylestown, Penn (215) 348-7090
- Alcoholics Anonymous, P.O. Box 459, Grand Central Station, New York, NY, 10163 (212) 686-1100

Hot Lines

- National Institute on Alcohol and Drug Abuse Hot Line: (800) 662-HELP
- National Cocaine Hot Line: (800) COCAINE
- Alcohol Hot Line: (800) ALCOHOL
- Cocaine Abuse Hot Line: (800) 888-9383; (800) 234-0420

Cocaine Anonymous (Central Offices)

- National Office: Culver City, Calif (213) 839-1141
- California: Los Angeles (800) 347-8998
  Los Angeles area (818) 447-2887
  San Francisco (415) 821-6155
  Solana Beach (619) 268-9109
- Connecticut: New Haven (203) 387-1664
- Georgia: Atlanta (404) 255-7787
- Illinois: Chicago (312) 202-8898
- New Jersey: Summit (908) 273-4530
- New York: Manhattan (212) 496-4266
- Tennessee: Nashville (615) 747-5483

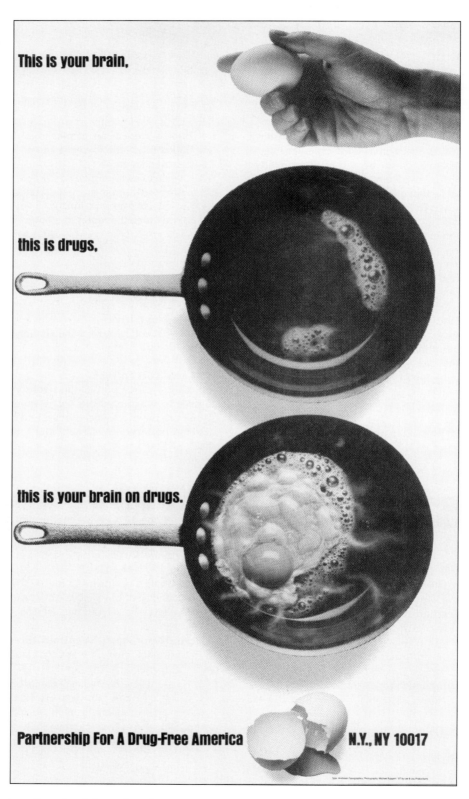

Will this approach reduce the rate of drug abuse?

might include detoxification, treatment of secondary health complications and nutritional deficiencies, and therapeutic counseling related to chemical dependence.

Some communities have voluntary health agencies that deliver services and treatment programs for drug-dependent people. Check your telephone book for listings of drug-treatment facilities. Some communities have drug hot lines that offer advice for people with questions about drugs (see the Star Box on p. 171 for a list of anti–drug abuse organizations and hot line numbers).

Costs of treatment for dependence

Drug-treatment programs that are administered by colleges and universities for faculty and students usually require no fees. Local agencies may provide either free services or services based on a **sliding scale.** Private hospitals, physicians, and clinics are the most expensive forms of treatment. Inpatient treatment at a private facility may cost as much as $1000 per day. Since the length of inpatient treatment averages 3 to 4 weeks, a patient can quickly accumulate a very large bill. However, with many types of health insurance policies now providing coverage for alcohol and other drug dependences, even these services may not require additional out-of-pocket expenses.

> **sliding scale**
> A method of payment by which patient fees are scaled according to income.

Summary

- Drug abuse has a devastating effect on society.
- Drug use, drug abuse, tolerance, and dependence are important terms to understand.
- A drug affects the CNS by altering neurotransmitter activity on the neuron.
- Drugs can be placed into six categories: stimulants, depressants, hallucinogens, cannabis, narcotics, and inhalants.

- Combination drug effects include synergistic, additive, potentiated, and antagonistic effects.
- Society's response to drug abuse has been widely varied and has included education, enforcement, treatment, testing, and the search for drug-free ways to achieve highs.
- Drug testing is becoming increasingly common in our society.

Review Questions

1. How is the term *drug* defined in this chapter? What are psychoactive drugs? How do medicines differ from drugs?
2. Explain what *dependence* means. Identify and explain the two types of dependence.
3. Define the word *tolerance.* What does *cross-tolerance* mean? Give an example of cross-tolerance.
4. Differentiate between drug misuse and drug abuse.
5. Identify some reasons commonly given for why people use psychoactive drugs.

6. Describe how neurotransmitters work.
7. List the six general categories of drugs. For each category, give several examples of drugs and explain the effects they would have on the user. What are designer drugs?
8. What is the active ingredient in marijuana? What are its common effects on the user? What are the long-term effects of marijuana use?
9. Explain the terms *synergistic effect, additive effect, potentiated effect*, and *antagonistic effect.*
10. How accurate is drug testing?

💡 Think About This . . .

- Are there any drugs on which you may have developed either a physical or psychological dependence?
- Do you find that you now require a larger dose of a particular drug to reach a high or low that you once felt with a smaller dose?

- Evaluate your own use of drugs, including caffeine, tobacco, and OTC pain medication. Do you consider your drug use to be a problem?
- Think about your own life experiences. What things have you done that have produced drug-free highs?

References

1. Office of the National Drug Control Policy: *1992 national drug control strategy: a nation responds to drug use,* Washington, DC, January 1992, US Government Printing Office.
2. US Department of Health and Human Services: *Smoking, drinking, and illicit drug use among American secondary school students, college students, and young adults 1975-1992, vol 2,* NIH Pub No BKD-124, Washington, DC, 1992, US Government Printing Office.
3. Ray O, Ksir C: *Drugs, society, & human behavior,* ed 7, St Louis, 1996, Mosby.
4. Pinger RR, Payne WA, Hahn DB, Hahn EJ: *Drugs: issues for today,* ed 2, St Louis, 1995, Mosby.
5. Thibodeau GA: *Structure & function of the body,* ed 9, St Louis, 1992, Mosby.
6. Armstrong BG, McDonald AD, Sloan M: Cigarette, alcohol, and caffeine consumption and spontaneous abortion, *Am J Public Health* 82(1):85-87, 1991.
7. Cocaine: the first decade, *Rand Drug Policy Research Center Issue Paper* 1(1):1-4, 1992.
8. US Department of Justice, Bureau of Justice Statistics: *Drugs and crime facts, 1994,* Washington, DC, 1994, US Government Printing Office.
9. Urban J: Thirty years later, LSD again becoming the drug of choice, *The Muncie Star,* p. 6B, March 21, 1993.
10. U.S. Department of Health and Human Services, Substance Abuse and Mental Health Services Administration: *National drug survey results released with new youth public education materials,* (press release), pp 1-3, Sept 12, 1995.
11. Ackerman S: Drug testing: the state of the art, *Am Sci* 77:19-23, 1989.
12. Mieczkowski T: New approaches in drug testing: a review of hair analysis, *Ann Am Acad Pol Soc Sci* 521:132-150, 1992.
13. *Comprehensive procedures for drug testing in the workplace,* DHHS Pub No (ADM) 91-1731, Washington, DC, 1991, National Institute on Drug Abuse.
14. Religious liberties, *Time,* p 85, April 30, 1990.

Suggested Readings

Almy G, Almy CT: *Addicted to recovery,* Eugene, Ore, 1994, Harvest House Publishers.
Two physicians write about their belief that the recovery movement does not deliver all that it promises. The Almys contend that the long-term answer to stress, insecurity, and harmful habits comes through a more focused relationship with God, primarily through Biblical counseling.

St. James E: *Inner simplicity: 100 ways to regain peace and nourish your soul,* New York, 1995, Hyperion.
This best-selling author shows readers a drug-free way to reduce the frantic nature of their lives, to work less, and to enjoy life more. Includes a series of brief essays to help people rethink their lives and tap into their creativity.

Wiley J: *Power recovery: the twelve steps for a new generation,* New York, 1995, Paulist Press.
This is a companion book for people going through a 12-step drug, alcohol, or compulsive behavior program. Aimed at young people born in the late '60s and in the '70s and '80s. Includes the personal impressions of people going through recovery programs.

 AS WE GO TO PRESS...

Actor Woody Harrelson was arrested in Lee County, Kentucky, on misdemeanor charges of cultivating marijuana. Harrelson, an advocate for the commercialization of industrial hemp, planted four seeds of industrial hemp in a public protest of a Kentucky law that considers industrial hemp the same as marijuana. Industrial hemp, grown in many parts of the world, is used for the production of paper and cloth products and contains little of the THC responsible for marijuana's high.

Prescription Drug Abuse

Lucy, a 35-year-old mother of two, seems like a typical suburban homemaker. She attends church regularly, belongs to the PTA, and volunteers at the local battered women's shelter. Her husband is a well-respected businessman and her children are honor students at the local high school. In short, life seems perfect for Lucy and her family, at least on the outside. However, Lucy has a secret that few outside her family know about.

Lucy's children and husband regularly come home to a disheveled household, finding Lucy passed out somewhere in the house or sometimes even on the back porch. Lucy's mood swings are unpredictable. One day, she will be a loving, devoted wife and mother; the next, she will talk rapidly and endlessly to whomever she can get to listen; still later, her speech will slur and she will seem incoherent. All this usually occurs whenever a stressful or unpleasant situation comes up in her life with which she cannot cope. Lucy's family never knows what to expect from one day to the next. The children have moved in and out of the home to live with their grandparents dozens of times over the past several years, and Lucy's husband has threatened her with divorce. Lucy has been to inpatient detoxification programs three times, only to "fall off the wagon" whenever a stressful event occurs.

You would probably guess that Lucy is an alcoholic or an illegal drug addict; however, Lucy's drugs of choice are all legal and all readily available to her from any one of a number of reputable physicians she visits. She uses a combination of drugs that range from sedatives to tranquilizers to antidepressants. Lucy is a prescription drug addict. Her suppliers are unwitting physicians who have no idea that she is seeing other doctors.

The reported numbers on the abuse of prescription drugs are alarming. In 1993 there were an estimated 7.9 million prescription drug abusers in the United States, with 125,000 deaths per year attributed to prescription drug abuse.[1] Over 100,000 prescription drug overdoses were reported in 1993, compared with fewer than 62,000 reported heroin overdoses.[2] Approximately 245,000 senior citizens are hospitalized each year for abuse of prescription drugs.[2] It is estimated that up to 50% of all prescriptions are used incorrectly.[1,2]

Most people would be surprised to learn that according to the Drug Enforcement Administration, 12 of the top 20 most abused controlled substances are prescription drugs.[1] These drugs fall into the following categories:

- *Opioids.* These drugs are narcotics typically prescribed to relieve acute or chronic pain. Common prescription drugs include Demerol, Darvocet, Vicodin, and drugs with codeine.
- *Stimulants.* These drugs affect the central nervous system and increase mental alertness, decrease fatigue, and produce a sense of well-being. They are usually prescribed for appetite suppression, attention deficit disorder, and narcolepsy. Common prescription drugs include Dexedrine, Ritalin, Fastin, and Cyclert.
- *Sedatives.* These drugs depress the central nervous system and are frequently used to treat anxiety, panic disorder, and insomnia. They may be dispensed for either daytime or nighttime use. Common prescription drugs include Xanax, Valium, Ativan, Dalmane, and Halcion.

Under certain conditions, nearly anybody could wind up abusing a prescription drug, but there are particular groups of people who are at high risk for prescription drug abuse. People with a family history of depression, smokers, and excessive drinkers are more likely to become addicted to prescription drugs, as are those with a history of abusing illegal drugs. Stress from traumatic experiences can also make a person more likely to abuse prescription drugs, and people who are hyperactive, obese, or who suffer from chronic pain are also at risk. Health care professionals are considered to be a high-risk group,[2,3] and older people have a greater tendency to abuse prescription drugs.[4]

A patient can become physiologically dependent on a drug, which is considered to be a more manageable condition than addiction. Physiological dependence, which involves the body's adaptation to a drug over time, is considered a temporary, benign condition. Physiological dependence is usually treated by gradual reductions in use of the drug, and although there may be withdrawal symptoms during this period, there is not normally a relapse afterward. The gradual reduction in dosage can be handled with medical supervision, and the patient does not normally need to enter a substance abuse program. Addiction involves a continued need to use a drug for psychological effects or mood alteration, and the patient goes to great lengths to obtain the drug even if its effects become harmful to him or her. Addiction is considered a chronic, complex problem and is usually handled with specific chemical dependence treatment.[1]

Abuse is often caused or continued because of deliberate deception on the part of the patient, but misuse of a prescription drug can start innocently enough. A patient may be receiving several prescriptions that have the same effect, or a patient may have several doctors prescribing the same medication. Prescription drugs may react with each other and cause different effects than intended. Sometimes communication problems between patient and physician cause errors in prescription dispensation. The patient may unintentionally use the prescription incorrectly. One of these situations or a combination of factors can start prescription drug abuse.[4] Often a single prescription drug, such as a painkiller or sedative, is enough to start the process of dependence.

Older people are considered at high risk for prescription drug abuse for several reasons. The process of aging or the transition to retirement can leave a person with symptoms of depression or anxiety, and illnesses can also increase as a person gets older. Many people see multiple doctors as they get older and thus may wind up getting several prescriptions for the same drug under different brand names without realizing it. Sometimes physicians give older patients the same dosages as younger patients. Body functions slow and change with age, and when this occurs, the duration and intensity of drug effects can change as well.[4] Such conditions can increase the risk of drug abuse among the elderly.

If addiction starts, older people may then resort to the same tactics as any prescription drug addict. They may begin to "doctor-hop" (moving from one doctor to the next without informing the doctors) to get multiple prescriptions, or they may go to an emergency room to get a quick fix of a particular drug. Patients may also hoard pills or swap pills with friends to cut costs and ensure availability of their drug of choice. In the United States, it is estimated that 2 million older adults are at risk of addiction or are addicted to tranquilizers or sleeping pills.[4]

Health care professionals are also at high risk for prescription drug abuse. Physicians are five times more likely than the general population to take sedatives or tranquilizers without another doctor's supervision. The high stress of the job and the availability of drugs are both believed to be contributing factors to abuse among health care professionals. However, studies suggest that those physicians who are psychologically sound had little problem handling the stress of their jobs and generally resisted the temptation of readily available drugs. Those physicians considered to have psychological problems were more likely to be abusers.[3]

Effects of Abuse

As abuse of a drug continues, the tolerance of the body to that drug increases, which can lead to stronger self-dosing. As use increases, the detoxification process can become more difficult. In some cases, people refuse to believe they are addicted, and older people who are isolated from others do not even realize they are hooked.[4] Physicians may inadvertently promote the abuse by failing or refusing to acknowledge the signs of addiction in a patient.

If a person admits he or she has a problem with a drug, the recovery process can begin, but trying to kick the habit without professional help may only make things worse. If the person tries to cut back or stop use of the drug, withdrawal symptoms may occur. These symptoms include pain, nausea, sleeplessness, nervousness, irritability, hallucinations, and confusion, and can be quite severe. Sometimes other underlying psychological problems (for example, depression) must also be dealt with to prevent a relapse.[4] In short, recovery from prescription drug abuse becomes as difficult as recovery from abuse of illegal drugs. For these reasons, professional help is usually necessary for a full recovery from prescription drug abuse.

If you or someone you know is abusing prescription drugs, help is available. Many hospitals that sponsor detoxification programs for alcoholics and illegal drug addicts also have programs for individuals who are addicted to prescription drugs. Often, insurance will cover the costs of these programs. After detoxification the individual will need to continue recovery through a program such as Alcoholics Anonymous (the principles used for recovery from alcoholism are also applicable to recovery from drug addiction), Narcotics Anonymous, or Benzodiazepine Anonymous. These organizations can be found in the white pages of any local telephone directory. If the addicted person has family or close friends who are being seriously affected by addiction issues, they may want to try Al-Anon, Alateen, or Adult Children of Alcoholics support groups. Finally, individual or family counseling may be of value in helping to sort out emotional issues that lie behind the addiction. A certified addictions counselor may be the most helpful person to an addict, or the family may choose a psychiatrist, psychologist, or social worker who has knowledge of addiction issues.

Although prescription drug addicts will always be "recovering" rather than "recovered," they can still lead relatively normal lives with proper physical and psychological treatment. However, there are no quick fixes or easy answers. Recovery is an ongoing process for both the addict and his or her family.

For Discussion . . .

Do you know of anyone who has intentionally abused prescription drugs? Have you ever taken a prescription drug in a different way than it was prescribed? Have you ever taken someone else's prescription drug, and if so, why did you do it? Can you think of a case where use of another person's prescription drug can be justified?

References

1. Colvin R: *Prescription drug abuse: the hidden epidemic*, Omaha, Neb, 1995, Addicus Books.
2. Colvin R: I tried to be my brother's keeper: one family's battle with prescription drug abuse, *Family Circle*, 108(13), Sep 19, 1995.
3. Vaillant GE: Physician, cherish thyself: the hazards of self prescribing, *JAMA* 267(17), 1992.
4. Chastain S: The accidental addict: are you hooked on your prescriptions? *Modern Maturity*, 35(1), Feb-Mar 1992.

Taking Control of Alcohol Use

Healthy People 2000 Objectives

The Healthy People 2000 Midcourse Review highlights significant progress toward achieving several important alcohol-related objectives. The most notable and encouraging change is the reduction in the number of alcohol-related traffic fatalities. The 1990 goal has been easily surpassed in this area. This success is largely attributable to the passage of state laws that revoke drunk drivers' automobile licenses and lower the legal limit for blood alcohol concentration from .10% to .08%.

The number of deaths caused by cirrhosis (alcohol-related liver disease) has declined, and per capita alcohol consumption has dropped. We are now about halfway toward reaching the specific targets for these two objectives. If these goals can be fully achieved, the number of alcohol-related deaths each year is expected to decline from the current figure of 100,000.

Reducing binge drinking (measured by the number of people who reported heavy drinking during the past 2 weeks) among high school and college students has occurred, according to the Midcourse Review. However, the gains made by high school students in reducing binge drinking far exceed those made by college students.

The push for zero tolerance laws, the tightening of standards for determining legal intoxication, and the growing influence of national groups concerned with alcohol misuse indicate that our society is more sensitive than ever to the growing misuse of alcohol.

People are concerned about the consequences of drunk driving, alcohol-related crime, and lowered job productivity. National data indicate that per capita alcohol consumption has gradually dropped in the United States.[1] Alcohol use remains the preferred form of drug use for most adults (including college students), but as a society, we are increasingly uncomfortable with the ease with which alcohol can be misused.

CHOOSING TO DRINK

Clearly, people drink for many different reasons (see the Star Box at right). We believe that most people drink because alcohol is an effective, affordable, and legal substance for altering the brain's chemistry. As **inhibitions** are removed by the influence of alcohol, behavior that is generally held in check is expressed. At least temporarily, drinkers become a different version of themselves—more outgoing, relaxed, and adventuresome. If alcohol did not make

Why Do I Choose an Alcoholic Beverage?
- I think alcoholic beverages are more thirst quenching than nonalcoholic alternatives.
- Alcoholic beverages taste better—their flavor is unique and satisfying.
- My friends always choose alcoholic beverages—I've learned to do the same.
- Alcoholic drinks are an important part of the larger statement I am making about myself. They reflect that I am an adult.
- Drinking alcoholic beverages makes me feel different—I like the changes that come about when I drink.

these changes in people, it would not be consumed as much. Do you agree or disagree?

ALCOHOL USE PATTERNS

From magazines to billboards to television, alcohol is one of the most heavily advertised consumer products in the country.[2] You cannot watch television,

LEARNING from ALL CULTURES

Alcohol Use

Whether or not people use alcohol is often a reflection of attitudes developed through the culture in which they live. How much they drink, what they drink, when they drink, and why they drink are all habits derived from their particular environments. Attitudes that a particular culture develops also influence rates of alcoholism. Times change, however, and countries are less isolated than they once were. Those cultural attitudes of a generation ago probably had more influence on behavior, such as drinking alcohol, than they do today. Still, culture does play a role in developing attitudes and behavior concerning alcohol consumption.

Italy is the second largest wine-producing country in the world, and Italians have historically enjoyed drinking wine. Yet a generation ago, Italy's rates of alcoholism were low. Most Italians drank wine and approved of the practice. They typically drank wine with the noon and evening meals. Excessive drinking and drunkenness, however, were unacceptable.[5]

Jews, like Italians, have had low rates of alcoholism. Their attitudes toward drinking and drinking habits have been very similar to those of Italians.[5]

Attitudes continue to change in different cultures, but there are a few factors that seem to affect the rate of alcoholism. In societies in which alcohol is introduced to children in small amounts on special occasions and within a sound family structure, the rates of alcoholism are low. This is also true when drinking is not the main focus of entertainment but accompanies another activity. Conversely, high rates of alcoholism are common in cultures that seem to have no standards about how to drink and how much to drink.[5]

Consider the attitudes toward drinking within your culture and family. How do these attitudes and practices influence your own opinions toward alcohol use?

Do you see this kind of behavior frequently on your campus?

Moderate Drinking Redefined

Alcohol Alert, a publication of the National Institute on Alcohol Abuse and Alcoholism (NIAAA), indicates that moderate drinking can be defined as no more than two drinks each day for most men and one drink each day for women.[12] These cutoff levels are based on the amount of alcohol that can be consumed without causing problems, either for the drinker or society. (The gender difference is due primarily to the higher percentage of body fat in women and to the lower amount of an essential stomach enzyme in women.) Elderly people are limited to no more than one drink each day, again due to a higher percentage of body fat.

These consumption levels are applicable to most people. Indeed, people who plan to drive, women who are pregnant, people recovering from alcohol addiction, people under age 21, people taking medications, and those with existing medical concerns should not consume alcohol. Additionally, although some studies have shown that low levels of alcohol consumption may have minor psychological and cardiovascular benefits, the NIAAA does not advise nondrinkers to start drinking.

listen to the radio, or read a newspaper without being encouraged to buy a particular brand of beer, wine, or liquor. The advertisements create a warm aura about the nature of alcohol use. The implications are clear: alcohol use will bring you good times, handsome men or seductive women, exotic settings, and a chance to forget the hassles of hard work and study.

Perhaps as a consequence of the many pressures to drink, it is not surprising that most adults drink alcoholic beverages. Two thirds of all American adults are classified as drinkers. Yet one in three adults does not drink. In the college environment, where surveys indicate that 85% to 90% of all students drink, it is difficult for many students to imagine that every third adult is an abstainer. Complete the Personal Assessment on p. 181 to rate your own alcohol use.

Alcohol consumption figures are reported in many different ways, depending on the researchers' criteria. Figures from various sources support the contention that about one third of adults 18 years of age and older are abstainers, about one third are light drinkers, and one third are moderate-to-heavy drinkers (see the Star Box at right). As a single category, heavy drinkers make up about 10% of the adult drinking population. Students who drink in college tend to classify themselves as light-to-moderate drinkers. It comes as a shock to students, though, when they read the criteria for each drinking classification. According to the combination of quantity of alcohol consumed per occasion and the frequency of drinking, these criteria are established as shown in Table 8-1.

In a recent unpublished survey of our undergraduate health science classes, we found that 37% of the 200 students met the criteria for heavy drinking, 26%

met the criteria for moderate drinking, 13% met the criteria for light drinking, 11% were infrequent drinkers, and 13% were abstainers.[3] It is not surprising that many students, faculty, and administrators believe that alcohol abuse is a serious problem on their campuses.

Binge Drinking

Alcohol abuse by college students usually takes place through a drinking pattern called *binge drinking*. Binge drinking refers to the consumption of five drinks in a row, at least once during the previous 2-week period.[4] College students who fit the category of "heavy drinkers" rarely consume small amounts of alcohol each day but instead binge on 1 or 2 nights a week. Some students in our classes openly admit that they plan to "get really drunk" on the weekend. They plan to binge drink.

By its very nature, binge drinking can be dangerous. Drunk driving, physical violence, property destruction, date rape, police arrest, and lowered academic performance are all highly associated with binge drinking. Reducing binge drinking is one of the Healthy People 2000 objectives. The direct correlation between the amount of alcohol consumed and lowered academic performance is crystal clear (Figure 8-1). Frequently,

PERSONAL ASSESSMENT

How Do You Use Alcoholic Beverages?

Answer the following questions about your own alcohol use. Record your number of "yes" and "no" responses in the box at the end of the questionnaire.

Do you: **Yes**   **No**

1. Drink more often than you did a year ago?

2. Drink more heavily than you did a year ago?

3. Plan to drink, sometimes days in advance?

4. Gulp or "chug" your drinks, perhaps in a contest?

5. Set personal limits on the amount you plan to drink but then consistently disregard these limits?

6. Drink at a rate greater than two drinks per hour?

7. Encourage or even pressure others to drink with you?

8. Frequently want a nonalcoholic beverage but then end up drinking an alcoholic drink?

9. Drive your car while under the influence of alcohol or ride with another person who has been drinking?

10. Use alcoholic beverages while taking prescription or OTC medications?

11. Forget what happened while you were drinking?

12. Have a tendency to disregard information about the effects of drinking?

13. Find your reputation fading because of alcohol use?

                                       TOTAL _____ _____

Interpretation

If you answered "yes" to any of these questions, you may be using alcohol irresponsibly. Two or more "yes" responses indicate an unacceptable pattern of alcohol use and may reflect problem drinking behavior.

To Carry This Further . . .

Ask your friends or roommates to take this assessment. Are they willing to take this assessment and then talk about their results with you? Be prepared to discuss any follow-up questions they might have about their (or your) alcohol consumption patterns. Your willingness to talk about drinking behavior might help someone realize that this topic can and should be discussed openly. Finally, be aware of how people in your area can get professional help with drinking or other drug concerns. ☑

---

the social costs of binge drinking can be very high, especially when intoxicated people demonstrate their level of immaturity. How common is binge drinking on your campus?

For large numbers of students who drink, the college years are a time when they will drink more heavily than at any other period during their lifetime. Some will suffer serious consequences as a result

(Figure 8-2). These years will also mark the entry into a lifetime of problem drinking for some.

inhibitions
Inner controls that prevent a person from engaging in certain types of behavior.

Table 8-1　Criteria for Drinking Classifications

Classification	Alcohol-Related Behavior
Abstainers	Do not drink or drink less often than once a year
Infrequent drinkers	Drink once a month at most and drink small amounts per typical drinking occasion
Light drinkers	Drink once a month at most and drink medium amounts per typical drinking occasion, or drink no more than three to four times a month and drink small amounts per typical drinking occasion
Moderate drinkers	Drink at least once a week and small amounts per typical drinking occasion or three to four times a month and medium amounts per typical drinking occasion or no more than once a month and large amounts per typical drinking occasion
Moderate/heavy drinkers	Drink at least once a week and medium amounts per typical drinking occasion or three to four times a month and large amounts per typical drinking occasion
Heavy drinkers	Drink at least once a week and large amounts per typical drinking occasion

NOTE: Small amounts = One drink or less per drinking occasion

Medium amounts = Two to four drinks per drinking occasion

Large amounts = Five or more drinks per drinking occasion (binge drinking)

Drink = 12 fluid oz of beer, 4 fluid oz of wine, or 1 fluid oz of distilled spirits

THE NATURE OF ALCOHOLIC BEVERAGES

Alcohol (also known as *ethyl alcohol* or *ethanol*) is the principal product of **fermentation.** In this process, yeast cells act on the sugar content of fruits and grains to produce alcohol and carbon dioxide.

The alcohol concentration in distilled beverages (such as whiskey, gin, rum, and vodka) is expressed by the term *proof*, a number that is twice the percentage of alcohol by volume in a beverage. Thus 70% of the fluid in a bottle of 140 proof gin is pure alcohol.

Most proofs in distilled beverages range from 80 to 160. The familiar, pure *grain alcohol* that is often added to fruit punches and similar beverages has a proof of almost 200 (see Table 8-2).

The nutritional value of alcohol is extremely limited. Alcoholic beverages produced today through modern processing methods contain nothing but empty calories—about 100 calories per fluid ounce of 100-proof distilled spirits and about 150 calories per each 12-ounce bottle or can of beer.[5] Clearly, alcohol consumption is a significant contributor to the additional pounds of fat that many college students accumulate. Pure alcohol contains only simple carbohydrates; it has no vitamins and minerals, and no fats or protein.

"Lite" beer and low-calorie wines have been intro-duced in response to concerns about the number of calories that alcoholic beverages provide. These "lite" beverages are not low-alcohol beverages but merely low-calorie beverages. Only beverages marked "low alcohol" contain a lower concentration of alcohol than the usual beverages of that type (see the Star Box on p. 184). In fact, the popular new ice beers actually contain a higher percentage of alcohol than other types of beer (see the Star Box on p. 185).

THE PHYSIOLOGICAL EFFECTS OF ALCOHOL

First and foremost, alcohol is classified as a drug—a very strong CNS depressant. The primary depressant effect of alcohol is seen in the brain and spinal cord. Many people think of alcohol as a stimulant because of the way most users feel after consuming a serving or two of their favorite drink. Any temporary sensations of jubilation, boldness, or relief are attributable to alcohol's ability as a depressant drug to release personal inhibitions and provide temporary relief from tension.

Factors That Influence the Absorption of Alcohol

The **absorption** of alcohol is influenced by several factors, most of which can be controlled by the individual. These factors include the following:

- *Strength of the beverage.* The stronger the beverage, the greater the amount of alcohol that will accumulate within the digestive tract.
- *Number of drinks consumed.* As more drinks are consumed, more alcohol is absorbed.
- *Speed of consumption.* If consumed rapidly, even relatively few drinks will result in a large con-

Figure 8-1   Average number of drinks consumed per week by grade point average.

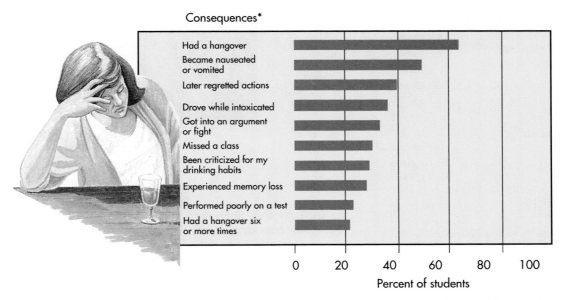

Figure 8-2   Negative consequences of alcohol and drug use as reported by college students. (*Occurred at least once in the past year.)

centration gradient that will lead to high blood alcohol concentration.

- *Presence of food.* Food can compete with alcohol for absorption into the bloodstream, thus slowing the absorption of alcohol. By slowing alcohol absorption, removal of the alcohol already in the bloodstream can occur. Slow absorption favors better control of blood alcohol concentration.
- *Body chemistry.* Each person has an individual pattern of physiological functioning that may affect the ability to process alcohol. For example, in some conditions, such as that marked by "dumping syndrome," the stomach empties more rapidly than is normal, and alcohol seems

fermentation
A chemical process whereby plant products are converted into alcohol by the action of yeast cells on carbohydrate materials.

absorption
The passage of nutrients or alcohol through the walls of the stomach or intestinal tract into the bloodstream.

Table 8-2   Categories of Alcohol Beverages*

Alcohol Beverage	Alcohol Content (%)†	Normal Measure
Beer		
Ale	5	12-oz bottle
Ice beer	5.5	12-oz bottle
Malt liquor	7	12-oz bottle
Lite beer	4	12-oz bottle
Regular beer	4	12-oz bottle
Low-alcohol beer	1.5	12-oz bottle
Wine		
Fortified: port, sherry, muscatel, etc.	18	3-oz glass
Natural: red/white	12	3-oz glass
Champagne	12	4-oz glass
Wine cooler	6	12-oz bottle
Cider (Hard)	10	6-oz glass
Liqueurs		
Strong: sweet, syrupy	40	1-oz glass
Medium: fruit brandies	25	2-oz glass
Distilled Spirits		
Brandy, cognac, rum, scotch, vodka, whiskey	45	1-oz glass
Mixed Drinks and Cocktails		
Strong martini, manhattan	30	3½-oz glass
Medium: old-fashioned, daiquiri, Alexander	15	4-oz glass
Light: highball, sweet and sour mixes, tonics	7	8-oz glass

*In all major alcohol beverages—beer, table wines, cocktail and dessert wines, liqueurs and cordials, and distilled spirits—the significant ingredient is identical: alcohol. The typical drink, half an ounce of pure alcohol, is provided by a shot of spirits, a glass of fortified wine, a larger glass of table wine, or a bottle of beer.

†In addition, these beverages contain other chemical constituents. Some come from the original grains, grapes, or other fruits; others are produced during the chemical processes of fermentation, distillation, and storage. Some are added as flavoring or coloring. These nonalcohol substances contribute to the effects of certain beverages either by directly affecting the body or by affecting the rates at which alcohol is absorbed into the blood.

to be absorbed more quickly. The emptying time may be either slowed or quickened by anger, fear, stress, nausea, and the condition of the stomach tissues.

- *Gender.* A significant study published in the *New England Journal of Medicine* reported that women produce much less alcohol dehydroge-

The Perfect Alternative?

Many low-alcohol and nonalcoholic malt beverages have entered the marketplace. Do you believe that these products will have much influence on the beer industry? Would you consider using these beverages as an alternative to alcoholic beverages at a party you were hosting? Why or why not?

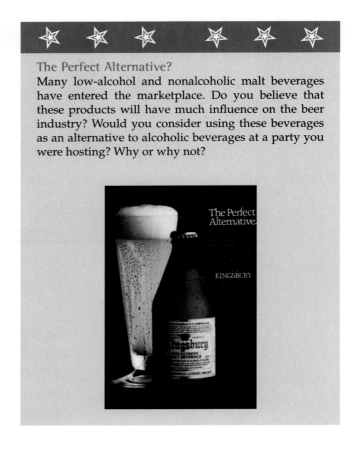

nase than men do.[6] This enzyme is responsible for breaking down alcohol in the stomach. With less alcohol dehydrogenase action, women absorb about 30% more alcohol into the bloodstream than men, despite an identical number of drinks and equal body weight.

Three other reasons help explain why women tend to absorb alcohol more quickly than men of the same body weight: (1) Women have proportionately more body fat than men. Since alcohol is not very fat soluble, it enters the bloodstream relatively quickly. (2) Women's bodies have proportionately less water than men's bodies of equal weight. Thus alcohol consumed does not become as diluted as in men. (3) Alcohol absorption is influenced by a woman's menstrual cycle. Alcohol is more quickly absorbed during the premenstrual phase of a woman's cycle. Also, there is evidence that women using birth control pills absorb alcohol faster than usual.[5]

With the exception of a person's body chemistry and gender, all factors that influence absorption can be moderated by the alcohol user.

Ice Beer

Recently a new brew has entered the marketplace and has been very popular—ice beer. The term *ice* refers to the manner in which this beer is brewed and processed. After brewing and fermentation, it is deep-chilled at 24° to 28° F, which causes ice crystals to form in the mixture. When these ice crystals are removed, the remaining liquid contains a higher percentage of alcohol.

Most regular beers and lite beers typically contain less than 5% alcohol, whereas ice beers generally contain 5% to 6% alcohol. Do you think beer drinkers are choosing this beer for its reportedly "rich, flavor" or simply because it contains more alcohol?

Blood Alcohol Concentration

A person's **blood alcohol concentration (BAC)** rises when alcohol is consumed faster than it can be removed (oxidized) by the liver. A fairly predictable sequence of events takes place when a person drinks alcohol at a rate faster than one drink every hour. When the BAC reaches 0.05%, initial measurable changes in mood and behavior take place. Inhibitions and everyday tensions appear to be released, while judgment and critical thinking are somewhat impaired. This BAC would be achieved by a 160-pound person taking about two drinks in an hour.

At a level of 0.10% (one part alcohol to 1000 parts blood), the drinker typically loses significant motor coordination. Voluntary motor function becomes quite clumsy. At this BAC, most states consider a drinker legally intoxicated and thus incapable of safely operating a vehicle. Although physiological changes associated with this BAC do occur, certain users do not feel intoxicated or do not outwardly appear to be impaired.

As a person continues to elevate the BAC from 0.20% to 0.50%, the health risk of acute alcohol intoxication increases rapidly. A BAC of 0.20% is characterized by the loud, boisterous, obnoxious drunk person who staggers. A 0.30% BAC produces further depression and stuporous behavior, during which time the drinker becomes so confused that he or she may not be capable of understanding anything. The 0.40% or 0.50% BAC produces unconsciousness. At this BAC a person can die, since brain centers that control body temperature, heartbeat, and respiration may be virtually shut down.

An important factor influencing the BAC is the individual's blood volume. The larger the person, the greater the amount of blood into which alcohol can be distributed. Conversely, the smaller person has less blood into which alcohol can be distributed, and as a result, a higher BAC will develop.

Sobering Up

Alcohol is removed from the bloodstream principally through the process of **oxidation.** Oxidation occurs at a constant rate (about ¼ to ⅓ oz of pure alcohol per hour) that cannot be appreciably altered. Since each typical drink of beer, wine, or distilled spirits contains about ½ oz of pure alcohol, it takes about 2 hours for the body to fully oxidize one typical alcoholic drink.[7]

Although people have attempted to sober up by drinking hot coffee, taking cold showers, or exercising, the oxidation rate of alcohol is unaffected. Thus far the FDA has not approved any commercial product that can help people achieve sobriety. Passage of time remains the only effective remedy for diminishing alcohol's effects.

First Aid for Acute Alcohol Intoxication

Not everyone who goes to sleep, passes out, or even becomes unconscious after drinking has a high BAC. People who are already sleepy, have not eaten well, are sick, or are bored may drink a little alcohol and quickly fall asleep. However, people who drink heavily in a rather short time may be setting themselves up for an extremely unpleasant, toxic, potentially life-threatening experience because of their high BAC.

Although responsible drinking would prevent **acute alcohol intoxication** (poisoning), such responsi-

---

blood alcohol concentration (BAC)
The percentage of alcohol in a measured quantity of blood; BACs can be determined directly through the analysis of a blood sample or indirectly, through the analysis of exhaled air.

oxidation
The process that removes alcohol from the bloodstream.

acute alcohol intoxication
A potentially fatal elevation of the BAC, often resulting from heavy, rapid consumption of alcohol.

ble drinking will never be a reality for everyone. As caring adults, what should we know about this health emergency that may help us save a life—perhaps even a friend's life?

The first real danger sign we need to recognize are the typical signs of **shock.** By the time these signs are evident, a drinker will already have become unconscious. He or she cannot be aroused from a deep stupor. The person will probably have a weak, rapid pulse (over 100 beats per minute). Skin will be cool and damp, and breathing will be increased to once every 3 or 4 seconds. These breaths may be shallow or deep but will certainly occur in an irregular pattern. Skin will be pale or bluish. (In the case of a person with dark skin, these color changes will be more evident in the fingernail beds or in the mucous membranes inside the mouth or under the eyelids.) Whenever any of these signs is present, seek emergency medical help immediately (see the Health Action Guide below for a summary of these signs).

Involuntary regurgitation (vomiting) can be another potentially life-threatening emergency for a person who has drunk too much alcohol. When a drinker has consumed more alcohol than the liver can oxidize, the pyloric valve at the base of the stomach tends to close. Additional alcohol remains in the stomach. This alcohol irritates the lining of the stomach so much that involuntary muscle contractions force the stomach contents to flow back through the esophagus. By removing alcohol from the stomach, vomiting may be a life-saving mechanism for conscious drinkers.

HEALTH Action Guide

Alcohol Intoxication

You should seek emergency help for acute alcohol intoxication when you find that a person drinking heavily:
- Cannot be aroused
- Has a weak, rapid pulse
- Has an unusual or irregular breathing pattern
- Has cool (possibly damp), pale, or bluish skin

An unconscious drinker who vomits may be lying in such a position that the airway becomes obstructed with the vomitus from the stomach. This person is in great risk of dying from **asphyxiation.** As a first-aid measure, unconscious drinkers should always be rolled onto their sides to minimize the chance of airway obstruction. If you are with a person who is vomiting, make certain that his or her head is positioned lower than the rest of the body. This position minimizes the chance that vomitus will obstruct the air passages.

It is also important to keep a close watch on anyone who passes out from heavy drinking. Unfortunately, party goers sometimes make the mistake of carrying these people to bed and then forgetting about them. We should do our best to monitor the physical condition of anyone who becomes unconscious from heavy drinking because of the risks of death. If you really care about these people, you will observe them at regular intervals until they appear to be clearly out of danger. Although this may mean an evening of interrupted sleep for you, you might save a friend's life.

ALCOHOL-RELATED HEALTH PROBLEMS

The relationship of chronic alcohol use to the structure and function of the body is reasonably well understood. Heavy alcohol use causes a variety of changes to the body that lead to an increase in morbidity and mortality. Figure 8-3 describes these changes. Some of these health problems are specifically addressed in the Healthy People 2000 objectives.

Research clearly shows that chronic alcohol use also damages the immune system and the nervous system. Thus chronic users are at high risk for a variety of infections and neurological complications.[1]

Fetal Alcohol Syndrome and Fetal Alcohol Effects

A growing body of scientific evidence indicates that alcohol use by pregnant women can result in birth defects in unborn children. When alcohol crosses the **placenta,** it enters the fetal bloodstream in a concentration equal to that in the mother's bloodstream. Because of the underdeveloped nature of the fetal liver, this alcohol is oxidized much more slowly than the alcohol in the mother. During this time of slow detoxification, the developing fetus is certain to be

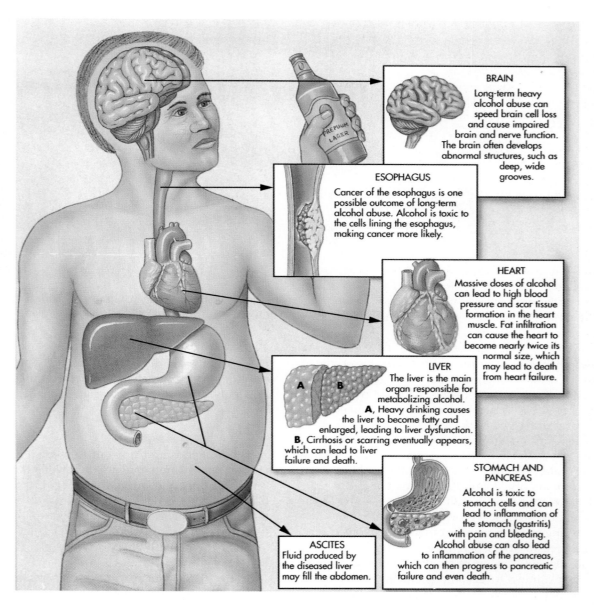

Figure 8-3   Effects of alcohol use on the body. The mind-altering effects of alcohol begin soon after it enters the bloodstream. Within minutes, alcohol numbs nerve cells in the brain. The heart muscle strains to cope with alcohol's depressive action. If drinking continues, the rising BAC causes impaired speech, vision, balance, and judgment. With an extremely high BAC, respiratory failure is possible. Over time, alcohol abuse increases the risk for certain forms of heart disease and cancer and makes liver and pancreas failure more likely.

overexposed to the toxic effects of alcohol. Mental retardation frequently develops.

This exposure has additional disastrous consequences for the developing fetus. Low birth weight, facial abnormalities (e.g., small head, widely spaced eyes), and heart problems are often seen in such infants (Figure 8-4). This combination of effects is called **fetal alcohol syndrome.** Recent estimates indi-

cirrhosis (sir **oh** sis)
Pathological changes to the liver resulting from chronic, heavy alcohol consumption; a frequent cause of death among heavy alcohol users (see Figure 8-3).

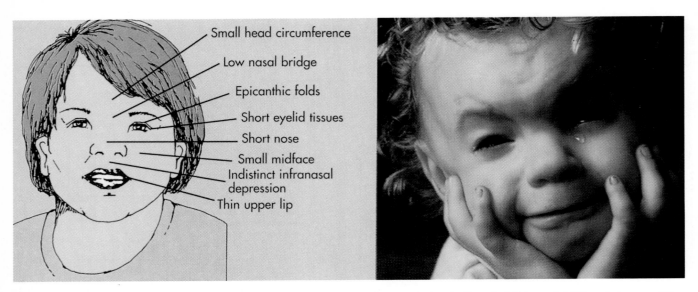

Figure 8-4   Fetal alcohol syndrome. The facial features shown are characteristic of affected children. Additional abnormalities in the brain and other internal organs accompany fetal alcohol syndrome but are not obvious from simply looking at the child.

In the illustration, the labeled facial features are:
- Small head circumference
- Low nasal bridge
- Epicanthic folds
- Short eyelid tissues
- Short nose
- Small midface
- Indistinct infranasal depression
- Thin upper lip

cate that the full expression of this syndrome occurs at a rate of between 1 and 3 per 1000 births. Partial expression (fetal alcohol effects [FAE]) can be seen in 3 to 9 per 1000 live births.[1] In addition, it is likely that many cases of FAE go undetected.

Is there a safe limit to the number of drinks a woman can consume during pregnancy? Since no one can accurately predict the effect of drinking even small amounts of alcohol during pregnancy, the wisest plan is to avoid alcohol altogether.

Because of the critical growth and development that occur during the first months of fetal life, women who have any reason to suspect they are pregnant should stop all alcohol consumption. Furthermore, women who are planning to become pregnant and women who are not practicing effective contraception must also consider keeping their alcohol use to a minimum.

ALCOHOL-RELATED SOCIAL PROBLEMS

Beyond personal health problems, alcohol abuse is related to a variety of social problems. These problems affect the quality of interpersonal relationships, employment stability, and the financial security of both the individual and family. Clearly, alcohol's negative social consequences lower our quality of life. In financial terms the cost of alcohol abuse and dependence has been estimated at $150 billion for 1995.[1]

The effect of alcohol consumption on several problems was summarized in the *7th Special Report to the U.S. Congress on Alcohol and Health.*[1] This important publication documented reported findings related to accidents, crime and violence, and suicide.

Accidents

The four leading causes of accidental death in the United States (motor vehicle collisions, falls, drownings, and fires and burns) have significant statistical connections to alcohol use. Approximately 40% of all fatal traffic crashes are alcohol related. Further, the likelihood of being involved in a fatal collision is about eight times higher for a drunk driver (0.10% BAC) than for a sober one.

Many people are surprised to learn that falls are the second leading cause of accidental death in the United States, with about 13,000 deaths per year. Alcohol use increases the risk for falls. Various studies suggest that alcohol is involved in between 17% and 53% of deadly falls and between 21% and 77% of non-fatal falls.

Drownings are the third leading cause of accidental death in the United States. Studies have shown that alcohol use is implicated in approximately 38% of these deaths. Over one third of boaters have been found to drink alcohol while boating.

Fires and burns are responsible for an estimated 6000 deaths each year in the United States, the fourth leading cause of accidental death. This cause is also connected to alcohol use: studies indicate that nearly half of burn victims have BACs above the legal limit.

Crime and Violence

You may have noticed at your college that most of the violent behavior and vandalism on campus is related to alcohol use. Indeed, the connection of alcohol to crime has a long history. Prison populations have large percentages of alcohol abusers and alcoholics: people who commit crimes are more likely to have alcohol problems than people in the general population. This is especially true for young criminals. Furthermore, alcohol use has been reported in 67% of all homicides, with either the victim, the perpetrator, or both found to have been drinking. In rape situations, rapists are intoxicated 50% of the time and victims 30% of the time.[5]

Because of research methodological problems, pinpointing alcohol's connection to family violence is difficult.[1] However, it seems clear that among a large number of families, alcohol is associated with violence and other harmful behavior, including physical abuse, child abuse, psychological abuse, and abandonment.[5] The article on pp. 199-200 explores the link between alcohol and violence.

Suicide

The 1990 *7th Special Report to the U.S. Congress on Alcohol and Health* points out alcohol's relationship to suicide. Between 20% and 36% of suicide victims have a history of alcohol abuse or were drinking shortly before their suicides. Also, alcohol use is associated with impulsive suicides rather than with premeditated ones. Drinking is also connected with more violent and lethal means of suicide, such as the use of firearms.[1]

For many of these social problems, alcohol use impairs critical judgment and allows a person's behavior to quickly become reckless, antisocial, and deadly. Because most of us wish to minimize problems associated with alcohol use, acting responsibly when we host a party is a first step in this direction.

HOSTING A RESPONSIBLE PARTY

Some people might say that no party is totally safe when alcohol is served. These people are probably right, considering the possibility of unexpected **drug synergism,** overconsumption, and the consequences of released inhibitions. Fortunately, an increasing awareness of the value of responsible party hosting seems to be spreading among college communities. The impetus for this awareness has come from various sources, including respect for an individual's right to choose not to drink alcohol, the growing

recognition that many automobile accidents are alcohol related, and the legal threats posed by **host negligence.**

For whatever reasons, responsibly hosting parties at which alcohol is served is becoming a trend, especially among college-educated young adults. The Education Commission of the States' Task Force on Responsible Decisions about Alcohol has generated a list of guidelines for hosting a social event at which alcoholic beverages are served. The list includes the recommendations shown in the Star Box on p. 190.

In addition to these suggestions, the use of a **designated driver** is an important component of responsible alcohol use. By planning to abstain from alcohol or to carefully limit their own alcohol consumption, designated drivers are able to safely transport friends who have been drinking. Have you noticed an increased use of designated drivers in your community? Would you be willing to be a designated driver?

shock
Profound collapse of many vital body functions; evident during acute alcohol intoxication and other serious health emergencies.

asphyxiation
Death resulting from lack of oxygen to the brain.

placenta
The structure through which nutrients, metabolic wastes, and drugs (including alcohol) pass from the bloodstream of the mother into the bloodstream of the developing fetus.

fetal alcohol syndrome
Characteristic birth defects noted in the children of some women who consume alcohol during their pregnancies.

drug synergism (sin er jism)
Enhancement of a drug's effect as a result of the presence of additional drugs within the system.

host negligence
A legal term that reflects the failure of a host to provide reasonable care and safety for people visiting the host's residence or business.

designated driver
A person who abstains from or carefully limits alcohol consumption to be able to safely transport other people who have been drinking.

Guidelines for Hosting a Responsible Party[8]

- Provide other social activities as a primary focus when alcohol is served.
- Respect an individual's decision about alcohol if that decision is either to abstain or to drink responsibly.
- Recognize the decision not to drink and the respect it warrants by providing equally attractive and accessible nonalcohol drinks when alcohol is served.
- Recognize that drunkenness is neither healthy nor safe. One should not excuse otherwise unacceptable behavior solely because of "too much to drink."
- Provide food when alcohol is served.
- Serve diluted drinks, and do not urge that glasses be constantly full.

- Keep the cocktail hour before dinner to a reasonable time and consumption limit.
- Recognize your responsibility for the health, safety, and pleasure of both the drinker and the nondrinker by avoiding intoxication and helping others do the same.
- Make contingency plans for intoxication. If it occurs in spite of efforts to prevent it, assume responsibility for the health and safety of guests—for example, by providing transportation home or overnight accommodations.
- Serve or use alcohol only in environments conducive to pleasant and relaxing behavior.

ORGANIZATIONS THAT SUPPORT RESPONSIBLE DRINKING

The serious consequences of the irresponsible use of alcohol have led to the formation of a number of concerned-citizen groups. Although each organization has a unique approach, all attempt to deal objectively with two indisputable facts: alcohol use is part of our society, and irresponsible alcohol use can be deadly.

Mothers Against Drunk Driving

Mothers Against Drunk Driving (MADD) is a national network of over 400 local chapters in the United States and Canada. MADD attempts to educate people about alcohol's effects on driving and to influence legislation and enforcement of laws related to drunk drivers. MADD clearly had a strong influence on the passage of a federal law requiring states to raise the drinking age to 21 or risk the loss of federal highway funds.

Students Against Driving Drunk

Students Against Driving Drunk (SADD) is an organization composed primarily of high school students whose goal is to reduce alcohol-related deaths among teenagers. Founded in 1981, SADD now has approximately 15,000 chapters and about 4 million members. In this organization, students help educate other students about the consequences of combining drinking and driving. One interesting practice of this organization's effort is to encourage students and their parents to sign a "contract" to provide transportation for each other if either is unable to drive

safely after consuming alcohol. This pact also stipulates that no consequences are to be discussed until the following day.

Boost Alcohol Consciousness Concerning the Health of University Students

BACCHUS is an acronym for Boost Alcohol Consciousness Concerning the Health of University Students. Run by student volunteers, this college-based organization promotes responsible drinking among university students who choose to drink. BACCHUS supports responsible party hosting, including providing quantities of food and nonalcoholic beverages. The individual chapters of BACCHUS (which now total well over 200) are encouraged to use a number of innovative educational approaches to promote alcohol awareness.

Other Approaches

Other responsible approaches to alcohol use are surfacing nearly every day. Even among college fraternity organizations, attitudes toward the indiscriminate use of alcohol are changing. Most fraternity rush functions are now conducted without the use of alcohol.

Another encouraging sign seen on college campuses is the increasing number of alcohol use task forces. Although each of these study committees has its own focus and title, many of these groups are meeting to discuss alcohol-related concerns on their particular campus. These task forces often attempt to formulate detailed, comprehensive policies for alcohol use across the entire campus community.

Membership on these committees often includes students (on-campus and off-campus, graduate and undergraduate), faculty and staff members, academic administrators, residence hall advisors, university police, health center personnel, alumni, and local citizens. Does your college have such a committee?

PROBLEM DRINKING AND ALCOHOLISM

Problem Drinking

At times the line separating **problem drinking** from alcoholism is difficult to distinguish (see the Star Box below). There may be no true line, with the exception that an alcoholic is unable to stop drinking. Problem drinking is a pattern of alcohol use in which a drinker's behavior creates personal difficulties or difficulties for other people. What are some of these behaviors? Examples might be drinking to avoid life stressors, going to work intoxicated, drinking and driving, becoming injured or injuring others while drinking, solitary drinking, morning drinking, an occasional **blackout,** and being told by others that you drink too much. For college students, two clear indications of problem drinking are missing classes and lowered academic performance caused by alcohol involvement. The Health Action Guide at right offers suggestions that can help you keep drinking under control.

Problem drinkers are not always heavy drinkers; they might not be daily or even weekly drinkers. Unlike alcoholics, problem drinkers do not need to drink to maintain "normal" body functions. However, when they do drink, they (and others around them) experience problems . . . sometimes with tragic conse-

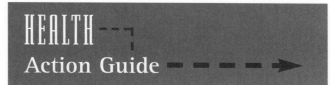

HEALTH
Action Guide

Tips to Help You Keep Drinking Under Control

- Do not drink before a party.
- Avoid drinking when you are anxious, angry, or depressed.
- Measure the liquor you put in mixed drinks (use only 1-1½ oz).
- Eat ample amounts of food and drink lots of water before and during the time you are drinking.
- Avoid salty foods that may make you drink more than you had planned.
- Drink slowly.
- Do not participate in drinking games.
- Do not drive after drinking; use a designated non-drinking driver.
- Consume only a predetermined number of drinks.
- Stop alcohol consumption at a predetermined hour.

problem drinking
An alcohol use pattern in which a drinker's behavior creates personal difficulties or difficulties for other people.

blackout
A temporary state of amnesia experienced by an alcoholic; an inability to remember events that occurred during a period of alcohol use.

Progressive Stages of Alcohol Dependence

Early	Middle	Late
• Escape drinking	• Loss of control	• Prolonged binges
• Binge drinking	• Self-hate	• Alcohol used to control withdrawal symptoms
• Guilt feelings	• Impaired social relationships	• Alcohol psychosis
• Sneaking drinks	• Changes in drinking patterns (more frequent binge drinking)	• Nutritional disease
• Difficulty stopping once drinking has begun	• Temporary sobriety	• Frequent blackouts
• Increased tolerance	• Morning drinking	
• Preoccupation with drinking	• Dietary neglect	
• Occasional blackouts	• Increased blackouts	

quences. It is not surprising that problem drinkers are more likely than other drinkers to eventually develop alcoholism. Are there people around you that you believe show signs of problem drinking?

Alcohol and Driving

Reports indicate that the percentage of traffic deaths resulting from alcohol use has dropped to well below 50%. However, the 20,000 deaths attributed annually to drunk driving remains an unacceptably high number, and the additional number of serious injuries is great. All states have raised the legal drinking age to 21 years. Most states have set 0.10% as the BAC at which drivers are considered to be legally drunk (Figure 8-5). However, more than 10 states have lowered this standard to 0.08%, and legislative efforts are being made in many other states to follow this lead. By midsummer 1995, 29 states had enacted **zero tolerance laws** to help prevent underage drinking and driving.[9] These laws may help the United States achieve some of its major health objectives for the year 2000.

Other programs and policies are being implemented that are designed to prevent intoxicated people from driving. Included are efforts to educate bartenders to recognize intoxicated customers, to encourage people to establish designated drivers, to use off-duty police officers as observers in bars, to use police roadblocks, and to develop mechanical devices that prevent intoxicated drivers from starting their cars.

Alcoholism

In 1992 a revised definition of **alcoholism** was established by a joint committee of experts on alcohol

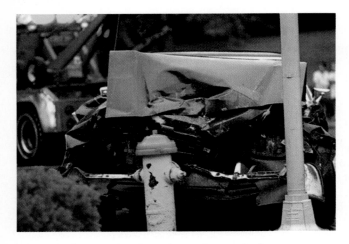

Drinking drivers often hurt themselves and others.

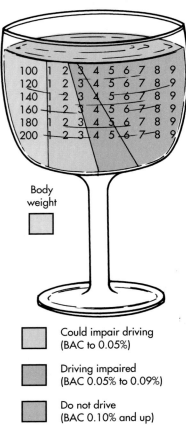

Number of drinks in 2-hour period (1½-oz 86-proof liquor or 12-oz beer)

	1	2	3	4	5	6	7	8	9
100	1	2	3	4	5	6	7	8	9
120	1	2	3	4	5	6	7	8	9
140	1	2	3	4	5	6	7	8	9
160	1	2	3	4	5	6	7	8	9
180	1	2	3	4	5	6	7	8	9
200	1	2	3	4	5	6	7	8	9

Body weight

Could impair driving (BAC to 0.05%)

Driving impaired (BAC 0.05% to 0.09%)

Do not drive (BAC 0.10% and up)

Figure 8-5 For most states, a BAC of 0.10% constitutes legal intoxication. However, a BAC as low as 0.05% can impair functioning enough to cause a serious accident.

dependence.[10] This committee defined alcoholism as follows:

> Alcoholism is a primary, chronic disease with genetic, psychosocial, and environmental factors influencing its development and manifestations. The disease is often progressive and fatal. It is characterized by impaired control over drinking, preoccupation with the drug alcohol, use of alcohol despite adverse consequences, and distortions in thinking, most notably denial. Each of these symptoms may be continuous or periodic.

This definition incorporates much of the knowledge gained from addiction research during the last two decades. It is well recognized that alcoholics do not drink for the pleasurable effects of alcohol but to escape being sober. For alcoholics, being sober is stressful.

Unlike problem drinking, alcoholism involves a physical addiction to alcohol. For the true alcoholic, when the body is deprived of alcohol, physical and mental withdrawal symptoms become evident. These withdrawal symptoms can be life threatening. Uncontrollable shaking can progress to nausea, vomiting, hallucinations, shock, and cardiac and pulmonary arrest. Uncontrollable shaking combined with irrational hallucinations is called *delirium tremens* (DT), an occasional manifestation of alcohol withdrawal.

The complex reasons for the physical and emotional dependence of alcoholism have not been fully explained. Why, when more than 100 million adults use alcohol without becoming dependent on it, do 10 million or more others become unable to control its use?

Could alcoholism be an inherited disease? Studies in humans and animals have provided strong evidence that genetics plays a role in some cases of alcoholism. Two forms of alcoholism are thought to be inherited: type I and type II. Type I is thought to take years to develop and may not surface until midlife. Type II is a more severe form and appears to be passed primarily from fathers to sons. This form of alcoholism frequently begins earlier in a person's life and may even start in adolescence.

Genetics may also help protect some Asians from developing alcoholism. About half of all Far East Asians produce low levels of an important enzyme that helps metabolize alcohol. These people cannot tolerate even small amounts of alcohol. Genetic factors pertaining to the absorption rates of alcohol in the intestinal tract have been hypothesized to predispose some Native Americans to alcoholism. It is likely that more research will be undertaken concerning the role of genetic factors in all forms of chemical dependence.

The role of personality traits as conditioning factors in the development of alcoholism has received considerable attention. Factors ranging from unusually low self-esteem to an antisocial personality have been implicated. Additional factors making people susceptible to alcoholism may include excessive reliance on denial, hypervigilance, compulsiveness, and chronic levels of anxiety. Always complicating the study of personality traits is the uncertainty of whether the personality profile is a predisposing factor (perhaps from inheritance) or is caused by alcoholism.

Denial and Enabling

Problem drinkers and alcoholics frequently use the psychological defense mechanism of *denial* to maintain their drinking behavior. By convincing themselves that their lives are not affected by their drinking, problem drinkers and alcoholics are able to maintain their drinking patterns. A person's denial is an

unconscious process that is apparent only to rational observers.

Formerly, it was up to alcoholics to admit that their denial was no longer effective before they could be admitted to a treatment program. This is not the case today. Currently, family members, friends, or coworkers of alcohol-dependent people are encouraged to intervene and force an alcohol-dependent person into treatment.

During treatment, it is important for chemically dependent people to break through the security of denial and to admit that alcohol controls their lives. This process will be demanding and often time consuming, but no alternative exists if they are to recover.

For family and friends of chemically dependent people, denial is part of a process known as *enabling*. In this process, people close to the problem drinker or alcoholic inadvertently support drinking behavior by denying that a problem really exists. Enablers unconsciously make excuses for the drinker, try to keep the drinker's work and family life intact, and in effect make the continued abuse of alcohol possible. For example, college students enable problem drinkers when they clean up a drinker's messy room, lie to professors about a student's class absences, and provide class notes or other assistance to a drinker who cannot keep up academically. In fact, even the use of designated drivers has been criticized as enabling behavior (see the Star Box on p. 194).

Alcohol counselors contend that enablers are an alcoholic's worst enemy because they can significantly delay the onset of effective therapy. Do you know of a situation in which you or others have enabled a person with alcohol problems?

Alcoholism and the Family

There is considerable disruption in the families of alcoholics, not only by the consequences of the drinking behavior (such as violence, illness, and unemployment), but also by the uncertainty of the family's role

---

zero tolerance laws
Laws that severely restrict the right to operate motor vehicles for underage drinkers who have been convicted of driving under any influence.

alcoholism
A primary, chronic disease with genetic, psychosocial, and environmental factors influencing its development and manifestations.

in causing and prolonging the situation. Family members often begin to adopt a variety of new roles that will allow them to cope with the presence of the alcoholic in the family. Among the more commonly seen roles are the family hero, the lost child, the family mascot, and the scapegoat.[5] Unless family members receive appropriate counseling, these roles may remain intact for a lifetime.

Once an alcoholic's therapy has begun, family members are encouraged to participate in many aspects of the recovery. This participation will also help them understand the ways in which they are affected by alcoholism. If therapy and aftercare include participation in Alcoholics Anonymous (AA), family members will be encouraged to become affiliated with related support groups.

Codependence

Within the last decade, a new term has been used to describe the relationship between drug-dependent people and those around them—*codependence*. This term implies a kind of dual addiction. The alcoholic and the person close to the alcoholic are both addicted, one to alcohol and the other to the alcoholic. People who are codependent often find themselves denying the addiction and enabling the alcohol-dependent person.

Unfortunately, this kind of behavior damages both the alcoholic and the codependent. The alcoholic's intervention and treatment may be delayed for a considerable time. Codependent people often pay a heavy price as well. They often become drug or alcohol dependent themselves, or they may suffer a variety of psychological consequences related to guilt, loss of self-esteem, depression, and anxiety. Codependents may be at increased risk for physical and sexual abuse.

Fortunately, researchers continue to explore this dimension of alcoholism. Many students have found some of the sources listed on p. 196 and at the end of this chapter to be especially helpful.

Helping the Alcoholic: Rehabilitation and Recovery

Once an alcoholic realizes that alcoholism is not a form of moral weakness but rather a clearly defined illness, the chances for recovery are remarkably good. It is estimated that as many as two thirds of alcoholics can recover. Recovery is especially enhanced when the addicted person has a good emotional support system, including concerned family members, friends, and employer. When this support system is not well

Are Designated Drivers "Enablers"?

In recent years the number of deaths resulting from drunk driving has declined. This decline can be partially attributed to the use of designated drivers. This is the good news.

However, there may be a down side. Some health professionals are concerned that the use of designated drivers allows the nondrivers to drink more heavily than they might otherwise. In effect, designated drivers "enable" drinkers to be less responsible for their own behavior. The concern is that this freedom from responsibility might eventually lead to further problems for the drinkers. What do you think?

established, the alcoholic's chances for recovery are considerably lower.

AA is a voluntary support group of recovering alcoholics who meet regularly to help each other get and stay sober. Over 19,000 groups exist in the United States. AA encourages alcoholics to admit their lack of power over alcohol and to turn their lives over to a higher power (although the organization is nonsectarian). Members of AA are encouraged not to be judgmental about the behavior of other members. They support anyone with a problem caused by alcohol.

Al-Anon and Alateen are parallel organizations that give support to people who live with alcoholics. Al-Anon is geared toward spouses and other relatives, whereas Alateen focuses on children of alcoholics. Both organizations help members realize that they are not alone and that successful adjustments can be made to nearly every alcoholic-related situation. AA, Al-Anon, and Alateen chapter organizations are usually listed in the telephone book or in the classified sections of local newspapers.

For people who feel uncomfortable with the concept that their lives are controlled by a higher power, *secular recovery programs* are becoming popular. These programs maintain that sobriety comes from within the alcoholic. Secular programs strongly emphasize self-reliance, self-determination, and rational thinking about one's drinking. Secular Organizations for Sobriety (SOS) and Rational Recovery are examples of secular recovery programs.

New Drug to Treat Alcoholism

Could there be a medical cure for alcoholism? For nearly 50 years, the only prescription drug physicians could use to help drinkers stop drinking was

Problem drinkers and alcoholics need professional help.

Antabuse. Antabuse would cause drinkers to become extremely nauseated whenever they used alcohol.

In 1995 the Food and Drug Administration approved a drug (naltrexone) that works by reducing the craving for alcohol and the pleasurable sensations felt when drinking. Combining naltrexone with conventional behavior modification has been shown to reduce alcohol relapse significantly. It will be interesting to see how effective this drug will be on a long-term basis.

CURRENT ALCOHOL CONCERNS

Adult Children of Alcoholic Parents

In recent years a new dimension of alcoholism has been identified—the unusually high prevalence of alcoholism among adult children of alcoholics (ACOAs). It is estimated that these children are about four times more likely to develop alcoholism than children whose parents are not alcoholics. Even the ACOAs who do not become alcoholics may have a difficult time adjust-

ing to everyday living. Janet Geringer Woititz, author of the best-selling book *Adult Children of Alcoholics*,[11] describes 13 traits that, to some degree, most ACOAs exhibit (see the Star Box on p. 196).

In response to this concern, support groups have been formed to prevent the adult sons and daughters of alcoholics from developing the condition that afflicted their parents (see the Star Box on p. 196). If a stronger link for an inherited genetic predisposition to alcoholism is found, these groups may play an even greater role in the prevention of alcoholism.

Women and Alcohol

For decades, women have consumed less alcohol and had fewer alcohol-related problems than men. As we move through the 1990s, evidence is mounting that a greater percentage of women are choosing to drink and that some subgroups of women, especially young women, are drinking more heavily. An increased number of admissions of women to treat-

Common Traits of ACOAs
Adult children of alcoholics may:
- Have difficulty identifying normal behavior
- Have difficulty following a project from beginning to end
- Lie when it would be just as easy to tell the truth
- Judge themselves without mercy
- Have difficulty having fun
- Take themselves very seriously
- Have difficulty with intimate relationships
- Overreact to changes over which they have no control
- Constantly seek approval and affirmation
- Feel that they are different from other people
- Be super-responsible or super-irresponsible
- Be extremely loyal, even in the face of evidence that the loyalty is undeserved
- Tend to lock themselves into a course of action without considering the consequences

ment centers may also reflect that alcohol consumption among women is on the rise.[1]

Studies indicate that there are now almost as many female as male alcoholics. However, there appear to be differences between men and women when it comes to alcohol abuse[5]: (1) More women than men can point to a specific triggering event (such as a divorce, death of a spouse, a career change, or children leaving home) that started them drinking heav-

ily. (2) Alcoholism among women often starts later and progresses more quickly than alcoholism among men. (3) Women tend to be prescribed more mood-altering drugs than men. Thus women face greater risk of drug interaction or cross-tolerance. (4) Nonalcoholic men tend to divorce their alcoholic spouses nine times more often than nonalcoholic women divorce their alcoholic spouses. Thus alcoholic women are not as likely to have a family support system to aid them in their recovery attempts. (5) Female alcoholics do not tend to receive as much social support as men in their treatment and recovery. (6) Unmarried, divorced, or single-parent women tend to have significant economic problems that may make entry into a treatment program especially difficult.[5] In light of the generally recognized educational, occupational, and social gains made by women during the last two decades, it will be interesting to see whether these male-female differences continue. What's your best guess?

Alcohol Advertising

Every few years, careful observers can see subtle changes in the ways the alcoholic beverage industry markets its products (see the Health Action Guide on p. 197).

Recently, the marketing push appears to be directed toward minorities (through advertisements for malt liquor and fortified wines), women (through wine and wine cooler ads), and youth (through trendy, young adult–oriented commercials).

Resources for Adult Children of Alcoholics
Experts agree that adult children of alcoholics who believe they have come to terms with their feelings sometimes face lingering problems. It can prove worthwhile to seek help if you experience the following:
- Difficulty in identifying your needs
- Persistent anger or sadness
- Inability to enjoy your successes
- Willingness to tolerate inappropriate behavior
- Continual fear of losing control

Support groups to contact for more information are listed below:

Al-Anon Adult Family Groups
P.O. Box 862 Midtown Station
New York, NY 10018-0862
(212) 302-7240

Al-Anon Adult Children Groups
One Park Avenue
New York, NY 10016
(212) 302-7240

Children of Alcoholics Foundation, Inc.
200 Park Avenue, 31st Floor
New York, NY 10010
(212) 351-2680

National Council on Alcoholism and Drug Dependence
12 West 21st Street
New York, NY 10010
(212) 206-6770
(800) NCA-CALL (800-622-2255)

On the college campus, aggressive alcohol campaigns have used rock stars, beach party scenes, athletic event sponsorships, and colorful newspaper supplements as vehicles to encourage the purchase of alcohol. Critics claim that most of the collegiate advertising is directed at the "below age 21" crowd and that the prevention messages are not strong enough to offset the potential health damage to this population. As a college student, how do you feel about alcohol advertising on your campus? If you are a nontraditional student, do you find the advertising campaigns amusing or potentially dangerous?

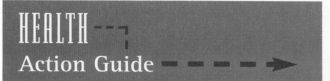

HEALTH
Action Guide

Advertising Ploys

The next time you watch television and see a beer commercial, you and your friends might analyze the commercial by considering the three following points:
- How attractive are the actors in the commercial?
- What type of environment (or atmosphere) is presented?
- To what extent is responsible drinking encouraged?

Summary

- Alcohol is the drug of choice among college students and the rest of American society.
- Many factors affect the rate of absorption of alcohol into the bloodstream.
- As BAC rises, predictable depressant effects take place.
- People with acute alcohol intoxication must receive first-aid care immediately.
- The health effects of chronic alcohol abuse are quite serious.
- Problem drinking reflects an alcohol use pattern in which a drinker's behavior creates personal difficulties or problems for others.
- Alcoholism is a primary, chronic disease with a variety of possible causes and characteristics.
- Denial, enabling, codependence, ACOAs, and alcohol advertising are current issues related to alcohol abuse in the United States.
- Recovery and rehabilitation programs can be effective in helping alcoholics become sober.
- Antabuse and naltrexone are drugs prescribed by physicians to help alcoholics stop drinking.

Review Questions

1. What percentage of American adults consume alcohol? Approximately what percentage of adults are classified as abstainers? What percentage of college students drink?
2. What is binge drinking?
3. What is meant by the term *proof*?
4. What is the nutritional value of alcohol? How do "lite" and low-alcohol beverages compare?
5. Identify and explain the various factors that influence the absorption of alcohol. Why is it important to be aware of these factors?
6. What is BAC? Describe the general sequence of physiological events that takes place when a person drinks alcohol at a rate faster than the liver can oxidize it.
7. What are the signs and symptoms of acute alcohol intoxication? What are the first-aid steps you should take to help a person with this problem?
8. Describe the characteristics of fetal alcohol syndrome and fetal alcohol effects.
9. Explain the differences between problem drinking and alcoholism.
10. What roles do denial and enabling play in alcoholism? What is codependence?
11. What are some common traits of ACOAs?
12. What unique alcohol-related problems exist for women?

Think About This . . .

- How much is your decision to drink or not drink influenced by those around you?
- Did you know that drinking alcohol in cold weather actually causes heat loss? The feeling of warmth results from the loss of body heat caused by the dilation of blood vessels under the skin. In effect, you may feel warmer but are actually getting colder.
- This chapter refers to data indicating that about one third of college drinkers can be considered heavy drinkers. Do you think this is true at your college?
- What role should men play in the prevention of fetal alcohol syndrome?
- How can you tell whether you and your friends are drinking responsibly?
- Do you believe it is your responsibility to make sure friends do not drink and drive?
- Do you think your drinking pattern will change when you are out of college?

References

1. US Department of Health and Human Services: *Alcohol and health: seventh special report to the US Congress,* DHHS Pub No (ADM) 90-1656, Washington, DC, 1990, US Government Printing Office.
2. US Bureau of the Census: *Statistical abstract of the United States, 1994,* annual, ed 114, Washington, DC, 1995, US Government Printing Office.
3. Payne WA, Hahn DB: *Alcohol consumption of students in the personal health class,* 1995, unpublished research.
4. Presley CA, Meilman PW: *Alcohol and drugs on American college campuses: a report to college presidents, June 1992,* US Department of Education, Drug Prevention in Higher Education Program (FIPSE Grant), Southern Illinois University Student Health Program Wellness Center.
5. Kinney J, Leaton G: *Loosening the grip: a handbook of alcohol information,* ed 5, St Louis, 1995, Mosby.
6. Frezza M et al: High blood alcohol levels in women: the role of decreased gastric alcohol dehydrogenase activity and first-pass metabolism, *N Engl J Med* 322:(4) 95-99, 1990.
7. Ray O, Ksir C: *Drugs, society, and human behavior,* ed 7, St Louis, 1996, Mosby.
8. Task Force on Responsible Decisions about Alcohol: *Interim report no 2,* Denver, Education Commission of the States.
9. Marshall S: Zero tolerance sobering for teen drivers, *USA Today,* p 1-A, June 19, 1995.
10. Morse RM et al: The definition of alcoholism, *JAMA* 268(8): 1012-1014, 1992.
11. Woititz JG: *Adult children of alcoholics,* Pompano Beach, Fla, 1983, Health Communications Inc.
12. US Department of Health and Human Services: *NIAAA Alcohol Alert,* No 13 (PH 297), Washington, DC, July 1991, US Government Printing Office.

Suggested Readings

Kinney J, Leaton G: *Loosening the grip: A handbook of alcohol information,* ed 5, St Louis, 1995, Mosby.
A comprehensive resource about alcohol and alcohol dependence and recovery. A highly recommended text for college students and all who work in the alcohol recovery field (physicians, nurses, counselors, social workers, and clergy).

Kishline A: *Moderate drinking: the new option for problem drinkers,* Tucson, Ariz, 1994, See Sharp Press.
This is a self-help book for problem drinkers who want to reduce their drinking. This is the official handbook of Moderation Management, the first support group in the United States that helps problem drinkers moderate their drinking.

Tate P: *Alcohol—how to give it up and be glad you did: a sensible approach,* Altamonte Springs, Fla, 1993, Rational Self-Help Press.
Using the rational emotive therapy approach, Tate presents a series of steps to assist people in overcoming their alcohol addiction. Tate encourages the transition from irrational beliefs about drinking and recovery to rational beliefs.

ON...

Alcohol and Violence

In recent years, there has been an increase in public service messages to raise awareness about driving under the influence of alcohol. In fact, the massive campaign against drinking and driving has been quite successful in reducing the number of drunk-driving accidents and fatalities. However, people may think that as long as a person doesn't get behind the wheel, it's okay to drink. But there are other potential dangers to the abuse of alcohol. One particular problem that perhaps has not been stressed enough in the media is the link between alcohol use and violent crime.

The Link Between Alcohol and Violence

The first question that arises when discussing the relationship between alcohol use and violence is whether there is a link at all. Obviously, not everyone who drinks becomes violent, but in many violent crimes at least one person involved has been drinking. The answer is perhaps that alcohol by itself is not enough to cause violence, but use of alcohol may be one of several factors that act in combination to cause violent behavior in some instances.[1]

Who is most likely to be involved in an alcohol-related violent crime? A 9-year study of over 4000 Los Angeles homicide victims suggests that men are much more likely to be involved than women. In the study, 51.3% of the male victims had detectable blood alcohol concentrations compared with 25.8% of the female victims.[1] Other studies have shown that young people under age 30 are more likely than older people to be involved in both sexual and nonsexual assault when alcohol is a factor. Data on race and ethnicity are inconclusive; some studies show that whites are more likely to be involved in alcohol-related homicides, whereas others show that African-Americans are. In the Los Angeles study, 38.2% of Hispanic homicide victims had detectable blood alcohol concentrations; this places them between the percentage figures for male victims and female victims and thus shows no tendency for or against involvement in alcohol-related violence. Alcohol-related homicides and assaults are more likely to occur on weekends than weekdays in part because more people tend to drink on weekends.[1]

Alcohol and Types of Violent Crime

The risk of a person's perpetrating a violent event is higher among heavy drinkers than light drinkers. Heavy drinkers are also at higher risk of being victims of violent crime and are also more likely to inflict and to receive violent injuries.[2] A Johns Hopkins University study shows that being a victim of sexual abuse or assault is also linked to high rates of alcohol use.[3] An environment where alcohol is prevalent is a risk factor associated with gun injuries, particularly deaths among youths.[4] Alcohol-related violence tends to be more prevalent in urban environments. It is estimated that eliminating the glut of inner city alcohol outlets could cut the U.S. homicide rate by 10% and could save 2000 lives annually.[5]

Alcohol plays a significant role in various types of violent crime. Substantial numbers of sexual-assault victims and offenders were drinking before their crime occurred. Alcohol use is present in over half of all domestic violence cases, and frequency of drunkenness for husbands appears to be associated with spouse abuse.[1] One study estimated that incidence of spouse abuse were almost 15 times higher for households where husbands were described as often drunk as opposed to never drunk. And drinking may also increase the risk of becoming a robbery victim.[1]

Campus Crime and the Effects of Alcohol

Of particular interest to college students are the data linking campus crimes to alcohol use. A USA Today study of 13,000 students suggests that as many as 4 out of 5 campus crimes committed by students are related to alcohol or drug use or both. The attitudes of college students may be a contributing factor to alcohol abuse on campus; 85% of freshmen in the survey condoned binge drinking (defined in this study as over 5 drinks in a continuous period). Victims of violent crime on campus generally reported heavier drinking habits than nonvictims,[6] and this parallels data from the general population.[1] When sexual assaults and rapes were reported, both the perpetrator and the victim had typically been drinking.[6]

So why is alcohol a contributing factor in violent crime? Alcohol acts as a depressant, which can reduce reaction time, impair coordination, and cloud judgment. Such impairment could decrease the chances of avoiding personal injury once a physical altercation begins. Alcohol also decreases inhibitions and may increase aggressive behavior. It also may increase the likelihood of inflicting or receiving a severe injury during a violent act and has been shown to increase the severity of injuries obtained in violent acts. Alcohol impairs cognitive abilities and may increase the chances for miscommunication or misinterpretation during verbal conflicts.[1,2]

What You Can Do

Although alcohol alone may not cause violence, when alcohol is introduced into a situation that has the potential to become violent, it can increase the chances that violence will occur. As the number of drunk drivers on the road has decreased, so has the number of drunk-driving accidents and fatalities. It seems logical to assume that if alcohol is kept out of the hands of people who are predisposed to violence, the number of alcohol-related crimes may also decrease. This is not always possible, but it is possible for you to use good common sense when you are drinking or if you are with people who are drinking. Try to avoid potentially violent situations, and avoid people drinking around you who are acting in a reckless or violent manner. Drink in moderation, and help your companions recognize when they have had too much. Perhaps you or one of your companions can remain sober (a "designated thinker") to help avoid potentially dangerous situations and stay safe while partying.

For Discussion . . .

Have you ever encountered an angry drinker? Is there a safe way to handle a person who is drunk and intending to do harm to someone? If you have ever been drunk, do you feel that you could have controlled your actions in a confrontation while you were drunk?

References

1. Messerschmidt PM: Epidemiology of alcohol related violence, *Alcohol Health and Research World*, 17(2), 1993.
2. Cherpitel CJ: What emergency room studies reveal about alcohol involvement in violence-related injuries, *Alcohol Health and Research World*, 17(2), 1993.
3. Violence, drugs, alcohol spur decline of youth health across U.S., study says, *Jet*, 88(7), June 26, 1995.
4. Voelker R: Taking aim at handgun violence, *JAMA* 273(22), 1995.
5. Abramson H: Quick fix for violence: cut back on liquor stores, *Nation's Cities Weekly*, 18(3), 1995.
6. Siegel D: What is behind the growth of violence on college campuses? *USA Today Magazine*, 122(2588), May 1994.

Rejecting
Tobacco Use

Healthy People 2000 Objectives

Several Healthy People 2000 objectives were established in an effort to reduce the use of all tobacco products, especially cigarettes. Prevention of heart disease, stroke, and cancer and promotion of physical activity, fitness, and oral health depend to varying degrees on reducing the extent to which tobacco products are used.

One important specific objective was to slow the rate of increase in smoking-related lung cancer deaths. The Midcourse Review does not assess progress in this area. However, information from other sources indicates that the death rate in this category has continued to rise. Another key objective was to slow the increase in cases of chronic obstructive lung disease (COLD) caused by cigarette smoking. Again, information from other sources suggests that little or no progress has been made in this area because of continuing cigarette use by men and the only recently apparent effects of tobacco use in women. In addition, the rapid increase in cigarette use by young people ages 14 to 19 does not bode well for reducing respiratory tract illnesses in the future.

Decreasing the prevalence of smoking among young adults ages 20 and over was another important initial objective. The Midcourse Review reports some headway in this area, although progress has been uneven among various educational, occupational, and age subgroups.

Today the evidence linking tobacco use to impaired health is beyond any serious challenge.[1] The regular user of tobacco products, particularly cigarettes, is more likely to become sick, remain sick for extended periods, and die prematurely than a nonuser. It is estimated that tobacco use, and cigarette smoking in particular, will result in 2 million deaths between 1986 and the year 2000,[1] with 419,000 in 1996 alone. Consequently, any contention made by the tobacco industry suggesting that tobacco use is not dangerous is little more than a groundless statement that ignores the growing weight of scientific evidence.

TOBACCO USE IN AMERICAN SOCIETY

On the basis of a variety of currently available statistics, less than 26% of all adults smoke cigarettes.[2] Further, data on smoking reveal that since 1964 the percentages of men and women who smoke cigarettes have declined steadily. For example, in 1965, 52.4% of adult men (age 20 and over) smoked compared with 28.1% in 1991. Among women, 34.1% smoked in 1965 compared with 23.5% in 1991.[3]

Use among Adolescents

As encouraging as it is that adults have moved away from smoking in recent decades, the most current data about smoking by adolescents are discouraging. On the basis of 1994 statistics, 19% of eighth-grade students and 31% of high school seniors reported smoking at least once within the past month, and 9% of eighth-grade students and 19% of high school seniors describe themselves as smoking daily.[4] Since 14- to 17-year-old young people model most closely the behavior of 18- to 24-year-olds, this upward trend in the oldest student group does not bode well for the future.

The Influence of Education

In spite of the trend seen in today's students, for adults a greater amount of formal education completed is associated with a lower rate of smoking. Among those with less than 12 years of formal education, 32% smoked during 1991, whereas only 13.6% of those with 16 or more years of education were cigarette smokers.[2] Clearly, education appears to assist people in understanding the risks of cigarette smoking. In contrast to the general population, where higher percentages of men than women smoke, col-

lege women are more likely to smoke than college men, perhaps since they wish to control their weight. Approximately 16% of college women smoke, whereas only 12% of college men smoke.[5] At this time the group least likely to smoke cigarettes is African-American men enrolled in predominately black colleges. On the basis of the current trend among public school students, the level of smoking among college students will likely increase.

How much do you know about cigarette smoking? Find out by completing the Personal Assessment on pp. 204-205.

In recent years the type of cigarettes preferred by smokers has changed. Today only a small percentage of all cigarette smokers prefer the small unfiltered cigarettes that were popular before and just after World War II. Even the king-sized filtered cigarettes popular during the 1960s are losing popularity. High-tar and high-nicotine cigarettes have been replaced by low- and ultralow-tar and nicotine brands. Today *low-tar and low-nicotine* brands (15 mg of tar or less) and *ultralow-tar and ultralow-nicotine* brands (less than 4 mg of tar) have the major share of the total cigarette market. In regard to these cigarettes, however, it should be noted that documents from inside the tobacco industry obtained by *USA Today* indicate that tar levels may be understated because of the method of testing used by the Federal Trade Commission.[6]

Advertising Approaches

The change in the American public's preference in cigarettes is a reflection of the strength of the tobacco industry in shaping demand for their products. Through continuous product development, skilled marketing, aggressive political lobbying, and diversification, the industry has managed to remain viable in the face of overwhelming evidence that their products are life threatening. Several of their survival techniques are:

- Reducing the number of cigarettes per pack to reduce the price per pack, making the product more affordable for youths and the poor
- Continued marketing of generic brands under the label of "value brands"
- Lowering the price of brand-name cigarettes to compete with value brands
- Carefully targeted advertising, particularly to women, minorities, and less-educated young adults
- Youth-oriented advertisements (while simultaneously supporting public policy statements to control minors' access to cigarettes)

★ ★ ★ ★ ★ ★   ★ ★ ★ ★ ★ ★

Surgeon General's Warnings

One of four surgeon general's warnings must appear on every package of cigarettes sold in the United States, as well as in every cigarette advertisement and on most promotional items, such as the hot air balloon pictured at right. The four warnings are listed below:

- Quitting smoking now greatly reduces serious risks to your health.

- Cigarette smoke contains carbon monoxide.

- Smoking by pregnant women may result in fetal injury, premature birth, and low birth weight.

- Smoking causes lung cancer, heart disease, emphysema, and may complicate pregnancy.

Canada's health warning, "Smoking can kill you," is more forceful and thus more likely to be remembered than the U.S. warnings.[7]

- Increased marketing of tobacco products overseas where health restrictions are less forceful (see the Learning from All Cultures box on p. 206)
- Acquiring non–tobacco-related companies (corporate diversification) to minimize the loss of revenues from decreased sales of tobacco products
- Marshalling tobacco users into a "grass roots" effort to counter the growing political power of antismoking groups

Clearly, the tobacco industry remains healthy and their products remain life threatening to smokers and nonsmokers alike.

Pipe and Cigar Smoking

Many people believe that pipe or cigar smoking is a safe alternative to cigarette smoking. Unfortunately, this is not the case. All forms of tobacco present users with a series of health threats.

When compared with cigarette smokers, pipe and cigar smokers have cancer of the mouth, throat, larynx (voice box), and esophagus at the same frequency. Cigarette smokers are more likely than pipe and cigar smokers to have lung cancer, chronic obstructive lung

disease (COLD), and heart disease. However, the incidence of respiratory disease and heart disease in pipe and cigar smokers is still greater than that among nonusers of tobacco.

THE DEVELOPMENT OF DEPENDENCE ON TOBACCO PRODUCTS

Dependence can imply both a physical and psychological relationship. Particularly with cigarettes, *physical dependence* or *addiction*, with its associated *tolerance*, *withdrawal*, and **titration**, is strongly developed by nearly one half of all smokers. Most of the remaining population of smokers will experience lesser degrees of physical dependence.[8] *Psychological dependence* or

titration (tie **tray** shun)
Particular level of a drug within the body; adjusting the level of nicotine by adjusting the rate of smoking.

PERSONAL ASSESSMENT

How Much Do You Know about Cigarette Smoking?

Assumption

1. There are now safe cigarettes on the market.

2. A small number of cigarettes can be smoked without risk.

3. Most early changes in the body resulting from cigarette smoking are temporary.

4. Filters provide a measure of safety to cigarette smokers.

5. Low-tar, low-nicotine cigarettes are safer than high-tar, high-nicotine brands.

6. Mentholated cigarettes are better for the smoker than are nonmentholated brands.

7. It has been scientifically proven that cigarette smoking causes cancer.

8. No specific agent capable of causing cancer has ever been identified in the tobacco used in smokeless tobacco.

9. The cure rate for lung cancer is so good that no one should fear developing this form of cancer.

10. Smoking is not harmful as long as the smoke is not inhaled.

11. The "smoker's cough" reflects underlying damage to the tissue of the airways.

12. Cigarette smoking does not appear to be associated with damage to the heart and blood vessels.

13. Because of the design of the placenta, smoking does not present a major risk to the developing fetus.

14. Women who smoke cigarettes and use an oral contraceptive should decide which they wish to continue because there is a risk in using both.

15. Air pollution is a greater risk to our respiratory health than is cigarette smoking.

16. Addiction, in the sense of physical addiction, is found in conjunction with cigarette smoking.

Discussion

F   Depending on the brand, some cigarettes contain less tar and nicotine; none are safe, however.

F   Even a low level of smoking exposes the body to harmful substances in tobacco smoke.

T   Some changes, however, cannot be reversed—particularly changes associated with emphysema.

T   However, the protection is far from adequate.

T   Many people, however, smoke low-tar, low-nicotine cigarettes in a manner that makes them just as dangerous as stronger cigarettes.

F   Menthol simply makes cigarette smoke feel cooler. The smoke contains all of the harmful agents found in the smoke from regular cigarettes.

T   Particularly lung cancer and cancers of the larynx, esophagus, oral cavity, and urinary bladder.

F   Unfortunately, smokeless tobacco is no safer than the tobacco that is burned. The user of smokeless tobacco swallows much of what the smoker inhales.

F   Approximately 10% of people who have lung cancer will live the 5 years required to meet the medical definition of "cured."

F   Because of the toxic material in smoke, even its contact with the tissue of the oral cavity introduces a measure of risk in this form of cigarette use.

T   The "cough" occurs in response to an inability to clear the airway of mucus as a result of changes in the cells that normally keep the air passages clear.

F   Cigarette smoking is in fact the single most important risk factor in the development of cardiovascular disease.

F   Children born to women who smoked during pregnancy show a variety of health impairments, including smaller birth size, premature birth, and more illnesses during the first year of life. Smoking women also have more stillbirths than nonsmokers.

T   Women over 35 years of age, in particular, are at risk of experiencing serious heart disease should they continue using both cigarettes and an oral contraceptive.

F   Although air pollution does expose the body to potentially serious problems, the risk is considerably less than that associated with smoking.

T   Dependence, including true physical addiction, is widely recognized in cigarette smokers.

17. Among the best "teachers" a young smoker has are his or her parents.

T There is a strong correlation between cigarette smoking of parents and the subsequent smoking of their children. Parents who do not want their children to smoke should not smoke.

18. Nonsmoking and higher levels of education are directly related.

T The higher one's level of education, the less likely one is to smoke.

19. About as many women smoke cigarettes as do men.

T Although in the past, more men smoked than did women, the gap is narrowing.

20. Fortunately, for those who now smoke, stopping is relatively easy.

F Unfortunately, relatively few smokers can quit. The best advice is never to begin smoking.

To Carry This Further . . .
Were you surprised at the number of items that you answered correctly? In what areas did you hold misconceptions regarding cigarette smoking? Do you think that most university students are as knowledgeable as you?

Where do you see the general public in terms of its understanding of cigarette smoking? How can the health care community do a better job in educating the public about tobacco use?

habituation, with its accompanying psychological *compulsion* and *indulgence,* is frequently seen.

Compulsion is a strong emotional desire to continue tobacco use despite restrictions on smoking and the awareness of health risks. Very likely, the user is "compelled" to engage in uninterrupted tobacco use in fear of the unpleasant physical, emotional, and social effects that result from discontinuing use. In compulsion, indulgence is seen as "rewarding" oneself for aligning with a particular group or behavior pattern. Indulgence is made possible by the existence of various reward systems built around the use of tobacco.

Much to the benefit of the tobacco industry, dependence on tobacco is easily established. Many experts believe that physical dependence on tobacco is far more easily established than is dependence on alcohol, cocaine (other than crack), or heroin. Of all people who experiment with cigarettes, 85% develop various aspects of a dependent relationship.

A small percentage of smokers, known as "chippers," can smoke a few cigarettes on a daily basis without becoming dependent. Experts believe that they are less likely to use cigarettes to influence their mood and thus do not "require" cigarettes to feel a sense of pleasure.[9] They may, in fact, be truly "social smokers" in that they smoke only with a few selected friends or in a very limited number of places. Unfortunately, many inexperienced smokers feel that they too are only "social smokers"; however, a few additional months of this type of occasional smoking could be a transitional period into a dependence pattern of tobacco use.

Physiological Factors

In the brain, **nicotine** stimulates the production of excitatory neurotransmitters, including norepinephrine, dopamine, acetylcholine, and serotonin, that generate a pleasurable sensation of arousal. Wanting to maintain this feeling of arousal, the smoker inhales again and again. Several hundred puffs per day quickly establish the schedule necessary to maintain the desired effect.

Beyond the action described above, nicotine may also stimulate the release of adrenocorticotropic hormone (ACTH) from the pituitary gland (see Chapter 3). In response to ACTH, beta endorphins (naturally occurring opiate-like chemicals) are produced in specific areas of the brain, leading to mild feelings of euphoria. Perhaps this stresslike response mechanism involving ACTH may also account for the increased energy expenditure seen in smokers and thus their tendency to maintain lower body weight than nonsmokers.

When these physiological responses are viewed collectively, nicotine may be seen as biochemically influencing brain activity by enhancing the extent and strength of various forms of "communication" between different brain areas.[10] If this is the case, it is apparent why once addicted, the functioning of the

nicotine
Physiologically active, dependence-producing drug found in tobacco.

LEARNING *from* ALL CULTURES

Tobacco Use

American cigarette companies are coping with the declining U.S. cigarette consumption by increasing their sales abroad, especially in developing nations. In the industrialized world, smoking is decreasing about 1% each year. However, in Asia and Latin America the incidence of smoking is growing 7% faster than the population. In Africa, it is growing 18% faster.

Even with the availability of low- and ultralow-tar and low- and ultralow-nicotine cigarettes, given enough time, the health effects of cigarette smoking will begin to be seen in these countries. Who will take responsibility for the sickness and death that will occur?

Although the tobacco industry continues to advertise in developing countries, some governments of the Latin American countries are passing legislation restricting advertising and promotion of tobacco products. Fifteen Latin American countries have enacted legislation to discourage the use of cigarettes by adolescents and children, and 13 of those countries have restricted the kind of advertising that targets young people. In six Latin American countries, it is illegal to sell tobacco products to minors.

Will legislation in these countries help reduce the use of tobacco? Is legislation that limits marketing and sales going to be enough? What else do these developing countries need to do to substantially reduce the use of tobacco products?

smoker's nervous system is much altered in comparison with that of nonsmokers.

Yet another explanation, called *self-medication*, suggests that nicotine, through the effects of mood-enhancing neurotransmitters, may allow smokers to "treat" feelings of tiredness and lack of motivation. In other words, a "smoke" lifts the spirits, if only briefly. Eventually, however, smokers become dependent on tobacco as a "medication" to make them feel better. Because tobacco is a legal drug, it becomes "preferred" over equally effective illegal drugs such as cocaine and stimulants.

Eventually for almost all smokers to some degree, smoking behavior is adjusted to maintain titration and prevent the uncomfortableness of withdrawal. Thus for most smokers, the desire to not experience withdrawal is as important as the arousal produced by nicotine.

Nicotine as an Addictive Drug

A great deal of interest and controversy now exists regarding information contained in documents released by people once inside the tobacco industry pertaining to the addictive nature of nicotine. Included among these issues are the extent to which the tobacco industry was aware of the addictive nature of nicotine and the appropriateness of studies conducted by the tobacco industry to determine whether young children would become future smokers. Further issues include allegations that the tobacco industry adjusted the pH levels of smokeless tobacco brands to alter nicotine levels and that research was conducted by the industry regarding nicotine enhancement of cigarettes.[11-13] Many people believe that if tobacco companies knew of the dangers of smoking and nevertheless encouraged nicotine addiction, they should compensate smokers or their families for losses resulting from smoking-related illnesses. This topic is discussed in the Star Box below.

Although these issues are far from resolved and a lawsuit has been won by the tobacco industry against the American Broadcasting Corporation for publicizing aspects of these documents, the FDA and various other health organizations remain convinced that tobacco products are, in fact, drug delivery systems intended to deliver a powerfully addictive drug, nicotine.[14] If this latter contention is supported by the U.S. Congress, the FDA could be given the power to regulate the availability of tobacco products.

Psychosocial Factors

In the view of behavioral scientists, dependence on tobacco can also be explained on the basis of psy-

chosocial factors. Both research and general observation support many of the powerful influences these factors have on the beginning smoker.

Modeling

Because tobacco use is a learned behavior, it is reasonable to accept that *modeling* acts as a stimulus to experimental smoking. Modeling suggests that susceptible people smoke to emulate, or model their behavior after, smokers whom they admire or with whom they share other types of social or emotional bonds. Particularly for young adolescents (ages 14 to 17), smoking behavior correlates with the smoking behavior of slightly older peers and very young adults (ages 18 to 22), older siblings, and to some degree, parents. Is it possible that the very young and attractive models used in tobacco (and beer) advertisements may be seen by young adolescents as being closer to their own age than they really are?

Modeling is particularly evident when smoking is a central factor in peer group formation and peer

Tobacco Industry Liability

For years, ill and dying smokers (and their survivors) have been suing, without success, tobacco companies for damages resulting from tobacco-induced illnesses. The success for the industry in countering these suits has been built around the contention that before 1964, they were unaware of any suspected dangers, and since 1966, they have warned smokers of the dangers they faced when using cigarettes. Accordingly, smokers were found to be responsible for their own poor judgment and the tobacco companies free of liability because of their compliance with mandates to warn smokers.

For the first time, in a recent Supreme Court ruling on June 24, 1992, the door has been opened for smokers (or their families) to attempt to prove that the smoking-induced illness resulted because smokers were enticed into smoking by the tobacco industry in spite of its compliance with governmental mandates to warn smokers of the risk of cigarette smoking. In other words, the court is allowing plaintiffs to attempt to prove that the tobacco companies said one thing (our products are potentially dangerous) and did another (make smoking appear safe and attractive). Only time will tell whether plaintiffs will be successful. Expert opinion is clearly divided on the issue of their success.

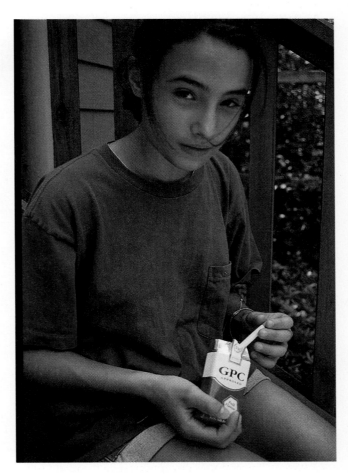

Does smoking make young people appear older?

group association and can lead to a shared behavioral pattern, which differentiates the group from others and from adults. Further, when risk-taking behavior and disregard for authority are common to the group, smoking becomes the behavioral pattern that most consistently identifies and bonds the group. Particularly for those young people who lack self-directedness or the ability to resist peer pressure, initial membership in a tobacco-using peer group may become inescapable.

Further, when adolescents have lower levels of self-esteem and are searching for an avenue to improve self-image, a role model who smokes is often seen as tough, sociable, and sexually attractive.[15] The latter two traits have been played up by the tobacco industry in their carefully crafted advertisements.

Manipulation

In addition to tobacco use's psychosocial link with modeling, tobacco use may meet the beginning smoker's need to physically manipulate something and at the same time provide the manipulative "tool" necessary to offset boredom, feelings of depression, or

social immaturity. The ability to take out a cigarette or fill a pipe adds a measure of structure and control to situations in which they might otherwise feel somewhat ill at ease. The cigarette becomes a readily available and dependable "friend" to turn to during stressful moments.

Susceptibility to advertising

The images of the smoker's world portrayed in tobacco advertisements can be attractive. For adolescents, women, minorities, and other carefully targeted groups of adults, the tobacco industry has associated the suggestion of a better life with the use of their products (see the Star Box below). Young and potential users are told that using tobacco products is associated with a sense of power, liberation, affluence, sophistication, and adult status. The message they are told (or sold) is that smoking will allow them to achieve things for which most people must work a long time.

A second aspect of the tobacco advertising strategy is giving away "free" products by the tobacco companies. Clearly in terms of college students, the readily

Cigarette Advertising Approaches
As the incidence of smoking declines within the general population, the tobacco industry has altered its advertising approaches to attract new markets and solidify their position in other markets. One tobacco company has attempted to target two groups: minorities from inner cities and undereducated "virile females," a term used to describe 18- to 20-year old women who have limited formal education and traditionally male occupations and interests. The R.J. Reynolds company unsuccessfully tried to test market a brand called Uptown. This cigarette was aimed principally at urban minorities. Test marketing of this brand was discontinued. Reynolds also introduced a cigarette called Dakota. The group targeted for this cigarette was "virile females."

Philip Morris Tobacco Company targeted a different group with its super-thin, low-smoke cigarette Superslims. Apparently, marketing of Superslims has been aimed at a more sophisticated woman who is so concerned about her weight that she is willing to disregard the health risks of smoking in an attempt to remain thin.

Misty is a value-brand (lower-cost) cigarette being marketed to young women who are just beginning their professional careers. By producing this "fashionably inexpensive" cigarette, American Tobacco is offering a more affordable alternative to Virginia Slims and Slims. Of course, the model, Misty, appearing in the brand's initial advertisements, is thin. Although these brands are

advertised to mature young women, their appeal has been primarily to female adolescents.

Macho men are not being spared the attention of tobacco companies either. Brands including Magna, Bucks, and a new version of Bull Durham appeared in 1990. As more highly educated men continue to move away from tobacco use, these brands are designed to appeal to younger, less highly educated men.

Cartoon characters make seductive models. R.J. Reynolds' Joe Camel campaign has been so successful that Joe is a familiar face to American youngsters, rivaling Mickey Mouse. Some health experts even suggest that Joe is largely responsible for adding 3000 new (adolescent age) smokers into the pipeline every day—the number needed by the tobacco industry to replace smokers who die or give up smoking. Regardless of whether they are new smokers or crossovers, preference for the Camel brand among younger smokers has increased from 2% to nearly 30%—five times the market share of the adult population. Advertising experts suggest that the more Joe is criticized, the more attractive he will be to adolescents.

Reynolds, along with Phillip Morris, the makers of Marlboro, uses another marketing ploy to appeal to youth: the sale of promotional items such as magazines, calculators, T-shirts, caps, can holders, and posters. In the case of Camel cigarettes, these items can be bought with "Camel Cash" coupons that accompany every package of Camel cigarettes purchased.

available cap, T-shirt, beverage can carrier, or light-weight jacket, all with logos, indicate social affiliation and serve as "a little reward" for doing nothing more than smoking a particular brand. Of course, long after the products have worn out or been lost, the dependence on tobacco remains.

In spite of the psychological needs that are met through continuing to use tobacco, approximately 90% of adult smokers have, on at least one occasion, expressed a desire to quit, and 80% have actually attempted to become nonsmokers.

Preventing Teen Smoking

August 1995 marked the beginning of an aggressive effort on the part of the FDA to discourage cigarette smoking among America's teens. Should efforts prove effective, it is hoped that 50% fewer adolescents will smoke in the year 2002 than do today. Specific aspects of the program include the following[16]:

- Limit tobacco advertising in publications that appeal to teens and restrict billboards with tobacco-related content to no closer than 1000 feet of schools and playgrounds. (An August 1995 study in California found that stores near schools displayed significantly more tobacco-related advertisements than those farther from schools.)
- Require merchants to obtain proof of age when selling tobacco products to adolescents. (Indiana has begun levying fines against both the owner and employee of a store that fails to require proof of age.)
- Bar certain sources of access to tobacco products, such as mail-order sales, the distribution of free samples, and vending machines.
- Halt sponsorship of high-visibility events such as auto racing and athletic contests in which brand names appear on highly televised surfaces (hoods, fenders, uniforms, and arena sign boards).

By the end of 1995, implementing many of these changes began, including the removal of tobacco-related advertisements from the rink boards in NHL arenas, the removal of Joe Camel billboards (see the Star Box at right), and the prosecuting of merchants who failed to restrict the sale of tobacco products to minors. By December 1995, Joe Camel billboards reappeared carrying a seasonal message. During the first week of 1996 the tobacco industry announced that they would fight in the courts any attempt to restrict their advertising, as well as any attempt on the part of the FDA to classify nicotine as an addictive agent or the cigarette as a drug delivery system.

Joe Camel . . . That "Smooth Character"

In spite of claims by the tobacco industry that it only attempts to challenge brand loyalty of established smokers through its advertisements, antismoking groups believe that children are its real targets. At no time has this disagreement been more in evidence than in conjunction with R.J. Reynolds' use of the cartoon character Joe Camel. A "smooth character," his escapades chronicle the "good life" enjoyed by attractive, affluent, sexually appealing young adults who just happen to smoke cigarettes.

In a report on three studies that looked at the influence of Joe Camel on people of various ages, the *Journal of the American Medical Association* reported the following:

- 33% of 3 year olds and 91% of 6 year olds could match Joe Camel with a picture of a cigarette.
- In terms of name recognition, 6 year olds were as familiar with Joe Camel as they were with Mickey Mouse.
- 98% of teenagers could identify the brand of cigarettes associated with Joe Camel advertisements (vs. 67% of an adult sample).

Further support for the position of the antismoking groups was seen when sales for Camel brand cigarettes to people under the age of 18 increased from less than 1% of the brand's total sales (before Joe Camel's appearance) to more than 30% of total sales. These data were disturbing enough for both the Surgeon General of the United States and the American Medical Association to request that R.J. Reynolds discontinue the use of their smooth character.

In October 1995, R.J. Reynolds agreed to discontinue the use of billboard advertisements featuring Joe Camel. Promotional material and print media will, however, still feature the suave cigarette-smoking character. The Centers for Disease Control and Prevention estimates that 500,000 smokers under the age of 18 have been influenced by the appeal and recognition of Joe.

TOBACCO: THE SOURCE OF PHYSIOLOGICALLY ACTIVE COMPOUNDS

When burned, the tobacco in cigarettes, cigars, and pipe mixtures is a source of an array of physiologically active chemicals, many of which are closely linked to significant changes in normal body structure and function. With each puff of smoke the body is exposed to over 4000 chemical compounds, hundreds of which are known to be physiologically active, toxic, and carcinogenic. An annual 50,000 puffs taken in by the one-pack-a-day cigarette smoker results in a regularly occurring environment that makes the most polluted urban environment seem clean in comparison.

Cigarette, cigar, and pipe smoke can be described on the basis of two phases or components: the particulate phase and the gaseous phase. The **particulate phase** includes nicotine, water, and a variety of powerful chemical compounds known collectively as *tar*. Tar includes phenol, cresol, pyrene, DDT, and a benzene-ring group of compounds that includes benzo[*a*]pyrene. A person who smokes one pack of cigarettes per day will cause the collection of 4 oz of tar in the lungs in one year.[15] As tar is drawn down the airway, the larger particles settle along its length, while the smaller particles reach the alveoli, or small saclike ends of the airway, where air comes in close association with the bloodstream. Most carcinogenic (cancer-causing) compounds are found within the tar.

The **gaseous phase** of tobacco smoke, like the particulate phase, is composed of a variety of physiologically active compounds, including carbon monoxide, carbon dioxide, ammonia, hydrogen cyanide, isoprene, acetaldehyde, and acetone. At least 43 of these compounds have been determined to be carcinogenic.[17] *Carbon monoxide* is the most damaging compound found in this component of tobacco smoke. Its effects are discussed shortly.

Nicotine

Nicotine is a powerful psychotropic (psychoactive) chemical agent found in the particulate phase of tobacco smoke. When drawn into the lungs, about one fourth of the nicotine in the inhaled smoke passes into the circulation and into the brain within 10 seconds of inhalation. *Nicotine receptors* within the brain are activated and produce a variety of responses, most of which are stimulating (see the discussion of nicotine addiction on pp. 205-207). High levels of nicotine, however, depress the CNS and result in the relaxation associated with heavy smoking.

The remaining nicotine absorbed into the blood travels throughout the body to nicotinic receptors located in a variety of tissues. Among the presently understood additional effects of nicotine are the reduction of intestinal activity, the release of epinephrine from the adrenal glands, the release of **norepinephrine** from peripheral nerves, increase in heart rate, the constriction of peripheral blood vessels, and the dilation of airways within the respiratory system.

Nicotine that enters the body by routes other than inhalation produces similar effects but at a much slower rate. Smokeless tobacco, for example, reaches its fullest physiological effect by the end of 20 minutes, nicotine-containing gum within 30 minutes, and transdermal nicotine patches within several hours.

Carbon Monoxide

Burning tobacco forms **carbon monoxide (CO)** gas. Carbon monoxide is one of the most harmful components of tobacco smoke.

Carbon monoxide is a colorless, odorless, tasteless gas that possesses a very strong physiological attraction for hemoglobin, the oxygen-carrying component of each red blood cell. When carbon monoxide is inhaled, it quickly bonds with hemoglobin and forms a new compound, *carboxyhemoglobin*. In this form, hemoglobin is unable to transport oxygen to the tissues and cells where it is needed.

The presence of excessive levels of carboxyhemoglobin in the blood of smokers leads to shortness of breath and lowered endurance. Brain function may be reduced, reactions and judgment are dulled, and, of course, cardiovascular function is impaired. Fetuses are especially at risk for this oxygen deprivation because fetal development is so critically dependent on a sufficient oxygen supply from the mother.

ILLNESS, PREMATURE DEATH, AND TOBACCO USE

For people who begin tobacco use as adolescents or young adults, smoke heavily, and continue to smoke, the likelihood of premature death is virtually ensured. Two-pack-a-day cigarette smokers can expect to die 7 to 8 years earlier than their nonsmoking counterparts. Only nonsmoking-related deaths that can afflict both smokers and nonsmokers alike, such as automobile accidents, keep the difference at this level rather than much higher. Not only will these people die sooner, but they also will probably be plagued with painful, debilitating illnesses for an extended time.

Cardiovascular Disease

Cardiovascular disease is the leading cause of death among all adults, accounting for 939,180 deaths in the United States in 1994.[18] Tobacco use, and cigarette smoking in particular, is clearly one of the major factors contributing to this cause. So important is tobacco use as a contributing factor in deaths from heart disease that cigarette smokers double the risk of experiencing a **myocardial infarction** and increase their risk of **sudden cardiac death** by two to four times. Fully one third of all cardiovascular disease can be traced to cigarette smoking. The relationship between tobacco use and cardiovascular disease is centered on two major components of tobacco smoke: nicotine and carbon monoxide.

Nicotine and cardiovascular disease

The influence of nicotine on the cardiovascular system occurs when it stimulates the nervous system to release norepinephrine. This powerful stimulant increases the rate at which the heart contracts. The extent to which this is dangerous depends in part on the ability of the heart's own blood supply system to provide blood to the working heart muscle.

In addition to its influence on heart rate, nicotine is also a powerful constrictor of blood vessels throughout the body. As vessels constrict, the pressure within them goes up. This resultant high blood pressure adds to any existing high blood pressure from other causes.

Nicotine also increases blood **platelet adhesiveness.** *Platelets* are the components of blood that causes it to clot, or coagulate, after an injury. Nicotine makes these platelets more likely to adhere to one another, or "clump," which can cause blood clots to develop in the arteries. Heart attacks occur when clots form within the coronary arteries (see Chapter 10) or are transported to the heart from other areas of the body.

In addition to other influences on the cardiovascular system, nicotine possesses the ability to decrease the proportion of high-density lipoproteins (HDLs) and to increase the proportion of low-density lipoproteins (LDLs) and very-low-density lipoproteins that make up the body's blood cholesterol. (See Chapter 10 for further information about cholesterol's role in cardiovascular disease.)

Carbon monoxide and cardiovascular disease

Carbon monoxide, a second substance contributed by tobacco, influences the type and extent of cardiovascular disease found among tobacco users. Carbon monoxide interferes with oxygen transport within the circulatory system.

As described previously, carbon monoxide is a component of the gaseous phase of tobacco smoke and readily attaches to the hemoglobin of the red blood cells. Once attached, carbon monoxide makes the red blood cell permanently weaker in its ability to transport oxygen. These red blood cells remain relatively useless during the remainder of their 120-day life. Levels of carboxyhemoglobin in heavy smokers are associated with significant increases in the incidence of heart attack.

When a person has impaired oxygen-transporting abilities, physical exertion becomes increasingly demanding on both the heart and the lungs. The cardiovascular system will attempt to respond to the body's demand for oxygen, but these responses are themselves impaired as a result of the influence of nicotine on the cardiovascular system. If tobacco does create the good life, as advertisers claim, it also unfortunately lowers ability to participate actively in that life.

Cancer

Data supplied by the American Cancer Society (ACS) indicate that during 1995 an estimated 1,252,000 Americans were diagnosed with cancer.* These cases were nearly equally divided between the genders and will eventually result in approximately 547,000 deaths.[1] In the opinion of the ACS, 30% of all cancer cases are heavily influenced by tobacco use. Lung cancer alone accounted for about 169,900 of the new cancer cases and 157,400 deaths in 1995. Fully 85% of male lung cancer victims were cigarette smokers. Cancer of the respiratory system, including lung cancer and cancers of the mouth and throat,

---

*Excluding about 800,000 cases of nonmelanoma skin cancer.

particulate phase
Portion of the tobacco smoke composed of small suspended particles.

gaseous phase
Portion of the tobacco smoke containing carbon monoxide and many other physiologically active gaseous compounds.

norepinephrine (nor epp in **eff** rin)
Adrenaline-like chemical produced within the nervous system.

carbon monoxide (CO)
Chemical compound that can "inactivate" red blood cells.

myocardial infarction
Heart attack; the death of heart muscle as a result of a blockage in one of the coronary arteries.

sudden cardiac death
Immediate death resulting from a sudden change in the rhythm of the heart.

platelet adhesiveness
Tendency of platelets to clump together, thus enhancing the speed at which the blood clots.

accounted for about 186,300 new cases of cancer and 162,900 deaths.[1] Despite these high figures, not all smokers develop cancer. Perhaps the extent to which the body's cancer suppressor genes are influenced by carcinogenic substances in tobacco smoke makes some smokers at greater risk for tobacco-related cancer than others.[19]

Recall that tobacco smoke has both a gaseous phase and a particulate phase. The particulate phase contains the tar fragment of tobacco smoke. This rich chemical environment contains over 4000 known chemical compounds, hundreds of which are known as possible carcinogens.

In the normally functioning respiratory system, particulate matter suspended in the inhaled air settles on the tissues lining the airways and is trapped in **mucus** produced by specialized *goblet cells* (Figure 9-1). This mucus, with its trapped impurities, is continuously swept upward by the beating action of hairlike **cilia** of the cells lining the air passages. On reaching the throat, this mucus is swallowed and eventually removed through the digestive system.

When tobacco smoke is drawn into the respiratory system, however, its rapidly dropping temperature allows the particulate matter to accumulate. This brown, sticky tar contains compounds known to harm the ciliated cells, goblet cells, and the *basal cells* of the respiratory lining. As the damage from smoking increases, the cilia becomes less effective in sweeping mucus upward to the throat. When cilia can no longer clean the airway, tar accumulates on the surfaces and brings carcinogenic compounds into direct contact with the tissues of the airway.

At the same time that the sweeping action of the lining cells is being slowed, substances in the tar are stimulating the goblet cells to increase the amount of mucus they normally produce. The "smoker's cough" is an attempt to remove this excess mucus.

With prolonged exposure to the carcinogenic materials in tar, predictable changes will begin to occur within the respiratory system's *basal cell layer* (see Figure 9-1). The basal cells begin to display changes characteristic of all cancer cells. In addition, an abnormal accumulation of cells occurs. Collectively these changes in the basal cell layer signal the beginning of lung cancer (Figure 9-2).

By the time lung cancer is usually diagnosed, its development is so advanced that the chance for recovery is very poor. Only 13% of all lung cancer victims survive for 5 years or more after diagnosis.[1] Most die in a very agonizing, painful way.

Cancerous activity in other areas of the respiratory system, including the *larynx,* and within the oral cavity (mouth) follows a similar course. In the case of oral cavity cancer, carcinogens found within the smoke and within the saliva are involved in the can-

Figure 9-1   Histological (tissue) changes associated with bronchogenic carcinoma.

Figure 9-2   **A,** Normal lung. **B,** Cancerous lung.

cerous changes. Tobacco users, such as pipe smokers, cigar smokers, and the users of smokeless tobacco, have a very high rate of cancer of the mouth, tongue, and voice box.

In addition to drawing smoke into the lungs, tobacco users swallow saliva that contains an array of chemical compounds from tobacco. As this saliva is swallowed, carcinogens are absorbed into the circulatory system and transported to all areas of the body. The filtering of the blood by the liver, kidneys, and bladder may account for the higher than normal levels of cancer in these organs among smokers.

Chronic Obstructive Lung Disease

Chronic obstructive lung disease (COLD) is a chronic disorder in which air flow in and out of the lungs becomes progressively limited. COLD is a disease state that is made up of two separate but related diseases: **chronic bronchitis** and **pulmonary emphysema.**

With chronic bronchitis, excess mucus is produced in response to the effects of smoking on airway tissue, and the walls of the bronchi become inflamed and infected. This produces a characteristic narrowing of the air passages. Breathing becomes difficult, and activity can be severely restricted. People who stop smoking can reverse chronic bronchitis.

For college students who have only recently begun smoking, the chronic nature of bronchitis may not yet be in place. Be forewarned, however, that the now occasional episodes of airway inflammation and congestion will occur on a more regular basis, and eventually the foundation on which COLD is built will be in place.

Pulmonary emphysema causes damage to the tiny

---

mucus
Clear, sticky material produced by specialized cells within the mucous membranes of the body; mucus traps much of the suspended particulate matter within tobacco smoke.

cilia (sill ee uh)
Small, hairlike structures that extend from cells that line the air passages.

chronic bronchitis
Persistent inflammation and infection of the smaller airways within the lung.

pulmonary emphysema
Irreversible disease process in which the alveoli are destroyed.

air sacs of the lungs, the **alveoli,** that cannot be reversed. Chest pressure builds when air becomes trapped by narrowed air passages (chronic bronchitis), and the thin-walled sacs rupture. Emphysema patients often develop a "barrel chest" as they lose the ability to exhale fully. You have most likely seen people with this condition in shopping malls and other locations as they walk slowly by, carrying or pulling behind them their portable oxygen tanks.

More than 10 million Americans have COLD. It is responsible for a greater limitation of physical activity than any other disease, including heart disease.[20] COLD patients tend to die a very unpleasant, prolonged death, often from a general collapse of normal cardiorespiratory function that results in *congestive heart failure* (see Chapter 10).

Additional Health Concerns

In addition to the serious health problems stemming from tobacco use already described, other health-related changes that are routinely seen include a generally poor state of nutrition, the gradual loss of the sense of smell, and premature wrinkling of the skin. Tobacco users are also more likely to experience strokes (a potentially fatal condition), lose bone mass leading to osteoporosis, experience more back pain and muscle injury, and find that fractures heal more slowly. Further, smokers who have surgery spend more time in the recovery room. Although not perceived as a "health problem" by people who continue smoking to control weight, smoking does appear to minimize weight gain. In studies using male identical twins, the siblings who smoked were 6 to 8 pounds lighter than their nonsmoking siblings.[21]

TOBACCO AND CAFFEINE USE

As discussed in Chapter 7, caffeine is the psychotropic drug in coffee, tea, cocoa, many soft drinks, and several nonprescription drugs, and it produces a stimulatory effect on the CNS. Because of caffeine's presence in such widely used and legal products, it may be the most used (and potentially misused) drug in this country. Refer back to Table 7-2, which depicts the amount of caffeine in various soft drinks, the major sources of caffeine for children and for many adults.

Think about how often you see someone light up a cigarette while enjoying a cup of coffee. The exact action of caffeine on the body is not fully understood, but its stimulatory effects are widespread. In low doses, consumption results in increased mental

awareness, alertness, and a quickening of thought processes. At higher doses, restlessness, agitation, tremors, and cardiac dysrhythmia occur. Dependence on caffeine, including addiction and habituation, develops rapidly (some studies suggest within a matter of a few days). Unpleasant withdrawal symptoms develop within several hours after the end of consumption. For those who smoke, this becomes a second dependence added to their nicotine addiction.

Chronic heavy consumption of caffeine is called *caffeinism* and is associated with a number of physiological indicators including nervousness, irritability, tremors, insomnia, heart palpitation, and gastrointestinal disturbances.[22] Efforts have been made to link caffeine consumption to coronary heart disease, pancreatic cancer, fibrocystic breast disease, and most recently, bone loss. To date, there has been little conclusive evidence relating serious health problems and caffeine consumption. However, caffeine does appear to be associated with a risk for miscarriage during pregnancy and should not, therefore, be consumed by women during pregnancy.[23] Regardless, for other adults, caffeine should most likely be consumed in moderation, particularly in light of its widespread presence in foods and products.

SMOKING AND REPRODUCTION

In all of its dimensions the reproductive process is impaired by the use of tobacco, particularly cigarette smoking. Problems can be found in association with infertility, problem pregnancy, breastfeeding, and the health of the newborn.

Infertility

Recent research indicates that cigarette smoking by both men and women can reduce levels of fertility. Among men, smoking adversely affects sperm motility and sperm shape and can inhibit sperm production. Among women, lower levels of estrogen (a hormone necessary for uterine wall development), a reduced ability to conceive, and a somewhat earlier onset of menopause appear to be related to cigarette smoking.

Problem Pregnancy

The harmful effects of tobacco smoke on the course of pregnancy are principally the result of the carbon monoxide and nicotine to which the mother and her fetus are exposed. Carbon monoxide is carried to the placenta, where it "locks up" fetal hemoglobin. As a

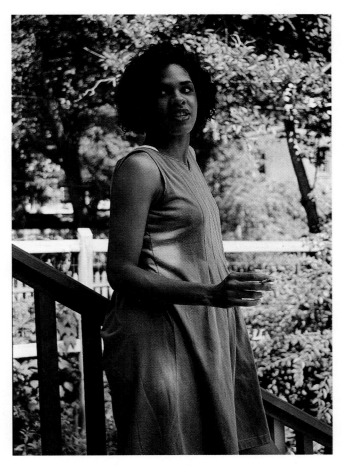

Tobacco use during pregnancy is harmful to the fetus.

result of this exposure to carbon monoxide, the fetus is deprived of normal oxygen transport and in effect suffocates.

Nicotine also exerts its influence on the developing fetus. Thermographs of the placenta and fetus show signs of marked constriction of blood vessels within a few seconds after inhalation by the mother. This constriction further reduces oxygen supplies. In addition, nicotine stimulates the mother's stress response, placing the mother and fetus under the potentially harmful influence of elevated epinephrine and corticoid levels (see Chapter 3). Any fetus exposed to all of these agents is more likely to be *miscarried* or *stillborn*. Children born to mothers who smoked during pregnancy often have low birth weights and may show other signs of having had a stressful life in the uterus.

Breastfeeding

Women who smoke while they breastfeed their infants will continue to expose their children to the

harmful effects of tobacco smoke. Mothers who stop smoking during pregnancy should be encouraged to continue to refrain from smoking while they are breastfeeding.

Health Problems among Infants

Babies born to women who smoked during pregnancy will, on average, be shorter and have a lower birth weight than children born to nonsmoking mothers. During the earliest months of life, babies born to mothers who smoke experience an elevated rate of death caused by sudden infant death syndrome.[24] Statistics also show that these infants are more likely to develop chronic respiratory problems, be hospitalized, and have poorer overall health during their early years of life. Additionally, children exposed to the influences of tobacco prenatally may hold a greater chance of developing attention deficit disorder (ADD). These problems are compounded when the children are exposed to involuntary smoking in the household environment (see pp. 216-217).

Parenting, in the sense of assuming responsibility for the well-being of a child, begins before birth, especially in the case of smoking. A pregnant woman who continues to smoke is disregarding the well-being of the child she is carrying. Other family members, friends, and co-workers who subject pregnant women to cigarette, pipe, or cigar smoke are, in a sense, contributing a measure of their own disregard for the health of the next generation.

ORAL CONTRACEPTIVES AND TOBACCO USE

Women who smoke and use oral contraceptives are placing themselves at a much greater risk of experiencing a fatal cardiovascular accident (heart attack, stroke, or **embolism**) than oral contraceptive users who do not smoke. This risk of cardiovascular complications is further increased for oral contraceptive

---

alveoli (al vee oh lie)
Thin, saclike terminal ends of the airways; the site at which gases are exchanged between the blood and inhaled air.

embolism (em boe liz um)
Potentially fatal condition in which a circulating blood clot lodges itself in a smaller vessel.

users 35 years of age or older. Women who both smoke and use oral contraceptives are four times more likely to die from myocardial infarction (heart attack) than women who only smoke.[25] Because of this adverse relationship, *it is strongly recommended that women who smoke not use oral contraceptives.*

SMOKELESS TOBACCO USE

As the term implies, smokeless tobacco is not burned; rather, it is placed into the mouth. Once in place, the physiologically active nicotine and other soluble compounds are absorbed through the mucous membranes and into the blood. Within a few minutes, chewing tobacco and snuff generate blood levels of nicotine in amounts equivalent to those seen in cigarette smokers.

Chewing tobacco is taken from its foil pouch, formed into a small ball (called a "wad," "chaw," or "chew"), and placed into the mouth. Once in place, the ball of tobacco is sucked and occasionally chewed but not swallowed. Some users develop great skill at spitting the copious dark brown liquid residue into an empty coffee can, out a car window, or on the sidewalk.

Snuff, a more finely shredded smokeless tobacco product, is marketed in small, round cans. Snuff is formed into a small mass (or "quid"). The quid is "dipped," or placed between the jaw and the cheek; the user sucks the quid and spits out the brown liquid.

Although smokeless tobacco would seem to free the tobacco user from many of the risks associated with smoking, chewing and dipping are not without their own substantial risks. The presence of leukoplakia (white spots) and erythroplakia (red spots) on the tissues of the mouth indicate precancerous changes (see the Health Action Guide at right). In addition, an increase in **periodontal disease** (with the pulling away of the gum from the teeth and later tooth loss), the abrasive damage to the enamel of the teeth, and the high concentration of sugar in processed tobacco all contribute to health problems seen among users of smokeless tobacco.

In addition to the damage done to the tissues of the mouth, the need to process the inadvertently swallowed saliva that contains dissolved carcinogens places both the digestive and urinary systems at risk of cancer.

In the opinion of health experts the use of smokeless tobacco and its potential for life-threatening disease is presently at the place cigarette smoking was 40 years ago. Consequently, television advertisement has been banned, and one of the following warnings appears on every package of smokeless tobacco:

WARNING: THIS PRODUCT MAY CAUSE MOUTH CANCER.

WARNING: THIS PRODUCT MAY CAUSE GUM DISEASE AND TOOTH LOSS.

WARNING: THIS PRODUCT IS NOT A SAFE ALTERNATIVE TO CIGARETTE SMOKING.

Clearly, smokeless tobacco is a dangerous product. There is little doubt that continued use of tobacco in this form is a serious problem to health in all of its dimensions.

INVOLUNTARY (PASSIVE) SMOKING

The smoke generated by the burning of tobacco can be classified as either **mainstream smoke** (the smoke inhaled and then exhaled by the smoker) or **sidestream smoke** (the smoke that comes from the burning end of the cigarette, pipe, or cigar). When either form of tobacco smoke is diluted and stays within a common source of air, it is referred to as **environmental tobacco smoke.** All three forms of tobacco smoke lead to involuntary smoking and can present health problems for both nonsmokers and smokers.

Surprisingly, mainstream smoke makes up only 15% of our exposure to involuntary smoking. This is because much of the nicotine, carbon monoxide, and particulate matter are retained within the active smokers.

HEALTH Action Guide

Smokeless Tobacco Use

If you use smokeless tobacco, you are at risk for serious health problems. If you have any of the following signs, see your dentist or physician immediately:

- Lumps in the jaw or neck area
- Color changes or lumps inside the lips
- White, smooth, or scaly patches in the mouth or on the neck, lips, or tongue
- A red spot or sore on the lips or gums or inside the mouth that does not heal in 2 weeks
- Repeated bleeding in the mouth
- Difficulty or abnormality in speaking or swallowing

Sidestream smoke is responsible for 85% of our involuntary smoke exposure. Because it is not filtered by the tobacco, the filter, or the smoker's lungs, sidestream smoke contains more free nicotine and produces higher yields of both carbon dioxide and carbon monoxide. Much to the detriment of nonsmokers, sidestream smoke has 20 to 100 times the quantity of highly carcinogenic substances (N-nitrosamines) that mainstream smoke has.

Current scientific opinion suggests that smokers and nonsmokers are exposed to very much the same smoke when tobacco is used within a common airspace. The important difference is the quantity of smoke inhaled by smokers and nonsmokers. It is likely that for each pack of cigarettes smoked by a smoker, nonsmokers who must share a common air supply with the smokers will involuntarily smoke the equivalent of three to five cigarettes per day. Because of the small size of the particles produced by burning tobacco, environmental tobacco smoke cannot be completely removed from an indoor site by even the most effective ventilation system.

On the basis of recently reported research, involuntary smoke exposure may be responsible for between 10,000 and 20,000 premature deaths per year among nonsmokers in the United States (other estimates range upward to 53,000 premature deaths).[26] In addition, large numbers of people exposed to involuntary smoke develop eye irritation, nasal symptoms, headaches, and a cough. Furthermore, most nonsmokers dislike the odor of tobacco smoke.

For these reasons, state, local, and private-sector initiatives to restrict smoking have been introduced. Most buildings in which people work, study, play, reside, eat, or shop now have some smoking restrictions. Some have complete smoking bans. The most highly visible of these bans occurred in 1994 when McDonald's announced that all 1400 company-owned restaurants were smoke-free. Franchised-owned stores began the movement to smoke-free environments in the belief that such an environment is in the best interest of children and is preferred by adults. Arby's and Wendy's have banned smoking in some stores as well. Nowhere is smoking more noticeably prohibited than in the U.S. airline industry. Currently, smoking is banned on all domestic plane flights. American Airlines has extended the ban on smoking to selected international flights as well.

Involuntary smoking poses serious threats to nonsmokers within residential settings.[27] Spouses and children of smokers are at greatest risk from involuntary smoking. Scientific studies suggest that nonsmokers married to smokers are three times more likely to experience heart attacks than nonsmoking

spouses of nonsmokers, and they have a 30% greater risk of lung cancer than nonsmoking spouses of nonsmokers.

The children of parents who smoke are twice as likely as children of nonsmoking parents to experience bronchitis or pneumonia during the first year of life. In addition, throughout childhood, these children will experience more wheezing, coughing, and sputum production than children whose parents do not smoke.[27] Of course, the impact on children who have two parents who smoke is greater than on children who have only one parent who smokes.

STOPPING WHAT YOU STARTED

As in the case of weight reduction, there are several ways to attempt to stop smoking. Among these are the *cold turkey* approach, a gradual reduction in cigarette use, organized smoking cessation programs, and the use of medically prescribed and OTC drug treatment. For those who fear the discomfort of going cold turkey, a more gradual approach can be attempted. The Health Action Guide on p. 218 provides several suggestions for quitting smoking or cutting down on tobacco consumption until stopping totally is possible.

Although it is far from easy to stop smoking, most of the 1.3 million people who quit smoking each year do so by throwing their cigarettes away and going cold turkey.[28] After days, weeks, or even months of discomfort, the body will eventually begin functioning normally without nicotine. Respiratory capacity will return, the ability to taste will return, and, if undertaken soon enough, tissues of the airways will begin returning to a more normal appearance. On a less pleasant note, it may take years before the mental

periodontal disease (pare ee oh **don** tal)
Destruction to soft tissue and bone that surround the teeth.

mainstream smoke
Smoke inhaled and then exhaled by a smoker.

sidestream smoke
Smoke that comes from the burning end of a cigarette, pipe, or cigar.

environmental tobacco smoke
Tobacco smoke that is diluted and stays within a common source of air.

pictures of "smoking pleasures" have faded. For most, some weight will be gained (about 6 to 8 pounds), but this represents a minimal health risk in comparison with the benefits of not smoking. The Health Action Guide on p. 219 offers tips for avoiding weight gain when you quit smoking.

As mentioned above, many group-based smoking cessation programs exist. These programs are usually operated by hospitals, universities, health departments, voluntary health agencies, private physicians, and even local churches. Perhaps the best that can be said is that the better programs will have limited success—a 20% to 50% success rate as measured over 1 year—whereas the remainder will have even poorer levels of success.

Two approaches for weaning smokers from cigarettes to a nontobacco source of nicotine dependency are nicotine-containing chewing gum (Nicorette) and the transdermal nicotine patches (Nicoderm, Habitrol, Prostep) that allow nicotine to slowly diffuse through the skin surface into the body. The chewing gum has been on the market for a number of years and, when used correctly along with smoking cessation counseling, has demonstrated a success rate of 40% or more. Correct use of nicotine-containing chewing gum requires an immediate cessation of smoking, a determination of the initial dosage (4 mg or 2 mg of nicotine per piece), the manner of chewing each piece (rate of chewing and the avoidance of certain foods or beverages), the number of pieces to be chewed each day (usually 9 to 12), and the individual manner of withdrawal from chewing the gum after 2 to 3 months of its use.[29] In 1996 a nonprescription version of Nicorette became available.

In comparison with nicotine-containing chewing gum, the more recently developed transdermal nico-

HEALTH
Action Guide

Quitting or Reducing Smoking

Instead of reaching for a cigarette, reach out for life and health. The suggestions below, many of which are recommended by the American Cancer Society, will help you make a concerted effort to stop smoking. Are you ready to try?

- Get mad at yourself for having become less fully self-directed than you could be. Few smokers can contend that they are fully self-directed when they can barely function in the absence of their cigarettes.
- Think of one sentence that expresses your personal reason for wanting to quit smoking. Repeat the sentence to yourself often.
- Observe nonsmokers. Note that nonsmokers are not missing out on anything as the result of not smoking. Recognize that the price you will pay for no longer smoking is not as high as it might have first appeared.
- Pick a quit day, sometime within the next 2 weeks. Plan either to stop cold turkey or to cut down gradually.
- Plan ahead for how you will handle tough times in your first few days off cigarettes.
- Stock up on low- or no-calorie snacks.
- On your quit day, drink a lot of water and keep busy.
- Limit your contact with other cigarette smokers. Keep in mind that once you quit, smokers won't go out of their way to assist you in your efforts.

- Stay clear, as much as possible, of the locations and activities that are now associated with your smoking. Old habits will be hard to break, but at least you do not have to be constantly reminded by their presence.
- Establish a series of rewards that you will give yourself as you progress through your smoking cessation program.
- Call the American Cancer Society for more information about quitting: self-help, how-to's, and group sessions in your community.

An alternative to total cessation is, of course, to reduce exposure to tobacco. This reduction can be accomplished through one or more of the following approaches:

- Reduce the consumption of your present high-tar and high-nicotine brand by smoking fewer cigarettes, inhaling less often and less deeply, and by smoking the cigarette only halfway down.
- Switch to a low-tar and low-nicotine brand of cigarette. However, you must not compensate for this change by smoking more cigarettes or by inhaling more deeply and frequently. Instead, try to reduce the number of cigarettes smoked and the depth and number of inhalations, and smoke only a limited portion of each cigarette.
- Switch to a smokeless form of tobacco, but be prepared for the potential problems that were discussed earlier in this chapter.

HEALTH
Action Guide ----▶

Avoiding Weight Gain When You Stop Smoking

For many smokers, particularly women, an important "plus" for smoking is weight management. In their minds the risks associated with tobacco use are more than offset by the cigarette's ability to curb appetite and thus serve as an aid in restricting caloric intake. Accordingly, the fear of weight gain frequently prevents any serious attempts at stopping smoking or permits easy relapse back into cigarette use.

The fear described above is in fact true. Most people who quit smoking do gain weight during the 10 years after cessation and in amounts greater than that seen in people who continue smoking or who have never smoked. It is also true, however, that this weight gain is relatively small (2.4 pounds for women and 3.8 pounds for men) and only slightly greater than that experienced by age mates who smoke or have never smoked. Certainly, the weight gained is a minimal health risk compared with the risks associated with continued smoking.

The keys to minimizing weight gain after smoking ces-sation are centered in two areas: (1) the ability to manage the "smoking urges" associated with the first several months of being a former smoker without resorting to eating and (2) the willingness to adopt healthy eating and exercise behaviors.

In regard to the management of smoking urges, people who are attempting to quit smoking should recognize that these powerful urges are very temporary, usually lasting only about 2 minutes. During these periods of intense desire for a cigarette, coping activities such as taking a short walk, drinking water or a diet beverage, or talking with a co-worker or family member will distract the mind from a cigarette until the urge has passed. If one "must" eat during these times, then healthy low-calorie snacks, such as apple slices, should be selected.

To minimize weight gain (or actually achieve a lower weight than when smoking) in the years after stopping smoking, a serious wellness-oriented lifestyle change involving both exercise and diet should be implemented. Specific information regarding adult fitness and sound nutrition can be found in Chapters 4 and 5, respectively.   ◀------▶

---

tine patches appear to be somewhat less effective than the chewing gum but easier to use. The use of a transdermal nicotine patch, such as Nicoderm, must be supervised by a physician. Because transdermal patches come in three dosages (21 mg, 14 mg, and 7 mg per day), a determination must be made as to the appropriate initial dosage, the length of time at that dosage and lower dosages, and the manner of withdrawal after the usual 8 to 12 weeks of patch wearing. Most patients begin the regimen with a 21-mg-per-day patch and use it for the first 6 weeks, followed by the use of 14-mg-per-day and 7-mg-per-day patches for 2 weeks each.[30] Concern about fatal heart attacks in people who use the nicotine patches and continue

A transdermal nicotine patch or nicotine-containing gum can be part of an effective smoking cessation program.

to smoke has been recently reviewed by the FDA. Currently, the transdermal nicotine patches remain on the market as prescription items intended to be used under close medical supervision and with other smoking cessation approaches.

A third approach to transferring nicotine dependence from cigarettes to a nontobacco source is through nicotine inhalation. Although still being clinically tested, this system, which uses the same extensive absorptive surface of the lungs as smoking, is seen as a promising tool in weaning smokers from their cigarettes.

TOBACCO USE: A QUESTION OF RIGHTS

Let us offer two simple questions concerning the issues of smokers' vs. nonsmokers' rights:
- To what extent should smokers be allowed to pollute the air and endanger the health of nonsmokers?
- To what extent should nonsmokers be allowed to restrict the personal freedom of smokers, particularly since tobacco products are sold legally?

At this time, answers to these questions are only partially available, but one trend is developing: the tobacco user is being forced to give ground to the nonsmoker. Today, in fact, it is becoming more a matter of when the smoker will be allowed to smoke rather than a matter of when smoking will be restricted. Increasingly, smoking is tolerated less and less. The health concerns of the majority are prevailing over the dependence needs of the minority. See article on pp. 224-226 for a fuller explanation of this topic.

IMPROVING COMMUNICATION BETWEEN SMOKERS AND NONSMOKERS

Exchanges between smokers and nonsmokers are sometimes strained, and in many cases, friendships are damaged beyond the point of repair. As you have more than likely observed, roommates are changed, dates are refused, and memberships in groups are withheld or rejected because of the opposing rights of these two groups.

Recognizing that social skill development is an important task for young adults, the following simple considerations or approaches for smokers can reduce some conflict presently associated with smoking.
- Ask whether smoking would bother others near you.

- When in a neutral setting, seek physical space in which you will be able to smoke and in a reasonable way not interfere with nonsmokers' comfort.
- Accept the validity of the nonsmoker's statement that your smoke causes everything and everyone to smell.
- Respect stated prohibitions against smoking.
- If a nonsmoker requests that you refrain from smoking, respond with courtesy, regardless of whether you intend to comply.
- Practice "civil smoking" by applying a measure of restraint when you recognize that smoking is offensive to others. Particularly, respect the aesthetics that should accompany any act of smoking—ashes on dinner plates and cigarette butts in flower pots are hardly popular with others.

The suggestions above can become skills for the social dimension of your health that can be applied to other social conflicts. Remember that as a smoker, you are part of a statistical minority living in a society that often makes decisions and resolves conflict based on majority rule.

For those of you who are nonsmokers, we would suggest several approaches we believe will make you more sensitive and skilled in dealing with smoking behavior:
- Attempt to develop a feeling for or a sensitivity to the power of the dependence that smokers have on their cigarettes.
- Accept the reality of the smoker's sensory insensitivity—an insensitivity that is so profound that the odors you complain about are not even recognized by the smoker.
- When in a neutral setting, allow smokers their fair share of physical space in which to smoke. As long as the host does not object to smoking, you as a guest do not have the right to infringe on a person's right to smoke.
- When asking a person to not smoke, use a manner that reflects social consideration and skill. State your request clearly, and accept a refusal gracefully.
- Respond with honesty to inquiries from the smoker as to whether the smoke is bothering you.

For those who are contemplating smoking, we ask you to explore closely whether the social isolation that appears to be more and more common for smokers will be offset by the benefits you might receive from cigarettes. The ability to find satisfaction through social contact may be one of the most important dimensions in a productive and satisfying adult life.

Summary

- The percentage of American adults who smoke is continuing to decline.
- The incidence of adolescent and young-adult smoking is increasing.
- The federal government has proposed a broadly based program intended to reduce the use of cigarettes by adolescents.
- In spite of denial by the tobacco industry, tobacco-related advertisements appear to be directed to adolescents and very young adults.
- Dependence, including addiction and habituation, is established quickly through tobacco use.
- Nicotine is the addictive agent in tobacco whose level in tobacco products can be modified.
- Modeling, self-reward, and self-medication play important roles in the development of tobacco dependence.
- The tobacco industry is constantly targeting new markets, such as women, minorities, and adolescents, through a variety of techniques, including the sale of logo-bearing products and an appealing cartoon character, Joe Camel.
- Tobacco smoke can be divided into gaseous and particulate phases. Each phase has its unique chemical composition.
- Nicotine, carbon monoxide, and phenol have damaging effects on various body tissues. Several hundred carcinogenic agents are found in tobacco smoke.
- Nicotine has predictable effects on the function of the cardiovascular system when used at relatively low doses.
- Most forms of cancer are worsened by tobacco use. Lung cancer progresses in a predictable fashion.
- Chronic obstructive lung disease (COLD) is a likely consequence of long-term cigarette smoking, with early symptoms appearing shortly after beginning regular smoking.
- Caffeine consumption in combination with smoking produces predictable changes in nervous system function, but its long-term effect on health is uncertain.
- Smoking alters normal structure and function of the body, as seen in premature wrinkling, diminished ability to smell, and bone loss leading to osteoporosis.
- Several areas of reproductive health are negatively influenced by tobacco use. Cigarette smoking and long-term use of oral contraceptives are not compatible.
- Smokeless tobacco carries its own health risks, including oral cancer.
- Involuntary smoke carries with it a wide variety of threats to the spouse, children, and co-workers of the smoker.
- Stopping smoking can be undertaken in any one of several ways, including going cold turkey.
- Nicotine gum and patches can be effective in a smoking cessation program.
- Both smokers and nonsmokers have certain rights regarding the use of tobacco. Effective communication can be established between smokers and nonsmokers.

Review Questions

1. What percentage of the American adult population smokes? In what direction has change been occurring? What is the current direction that adolescent smoking is taking? What factors may account for this newly observed trend?
2. In what way do modeling and advertising explain the development of emotional dependency on tobacco? How do self-esteem, self-image, and self-directedness relate to tobacco use?
3. How is the federal government attempting to limit the exposure that children and adolescents currently have to tobacco products and tobacco advertisements? What techniques have been developed by the tobacco industry to market their products to children and adolescents, in spite of their contentions to the contrary?
4. What are the principal components of the gaseous and particulate phases of tobacco smoke?
5. What are the specific influences of nicotine, carbon monoxide, and phenol on the normal function of the body?
6. In what ways does cigarette smoking contribute to cardiovascular disease? What effect does nicotine have on the cardiovascular system?
7. To what extent is tobacco use a factor in cancer? What specific airway tissues are involved in lung cancer?
8. What is the traditional progression of chronic

obstructive lung disease? In what ways does tobacco use impair reproductive health?

9. In what ways is smokeless tobacco equal to smoking in the development of serious health concerns?

10. What is our current understanding about chronic caffeine consumption and smoking as a health problem?

11. What is involuntary smoking? Why is there growing concern about the effects of involuntary smoke on spouses and children?

12. What is the most effective way to stop smoking? What is the average weight gain after stopping smoking? How effective are other approaches to stopping smoking? What are the principal nicotine replacement systems in use today?

13. What rights do smokers and nonsmokers have in public places? How can communication be enhanced between smokers and nonsmokers?

 ## Think About This . . .

• Why do proportionally more highly educated women than highly educated men smoke cigarettes?
• If you saw a minor being sold cigarettes, would you feel comfortable mentioning your concern to the merchant?

• If you are a smoker, do you understand why you are more "winded" than nonsmokers with whom you try to compete athletically?
• If you are a smoker, have you ever been asked to extinguish your cigarette? How did you react? How did you feel about this?

References

1. *Cancer facts & figures—1996,* Atlanta, Ga, 1996, American Cancer Society.
2. Current trends: cigarette smoking among adults—United States, 1991, *MMWR* 42(12):230-232, 1993.
3. US Department of Health and Human Services: *Preventing tobacco use among young people: a report of the Surgeon General,* Atlanta, Ga, 1994, US Department of Health and Human Services, Public Health Service, Centers for Disease Control and Prevention, National Center for Chronic Disease Prevention and Health Promotion, Office on Smoking and Health.
4. *The monitoring the future study,* Ann Arbor, Mich, 1995, The University of Michigan.
5. National survey results on drug use. From *The monitoring the future study,* 1975-1992, vol 11, NIH Publ No. 93-3598, Washington, DC, 1993, National Institute on Drug Abuse.
6. Levy D: Firm knew cigarette tar tested low. *USA Today,* p1D Aug 2, 1995.
7. Levy D: Youths remember tough smoking label. *USA Today,* p1D June 28, 1995.
8. Personal interview, Art Uline, MD, NBC News, New York, Nov 6, 1995.
9. Shiffman S: Chippers—individual differences in tobacco dependence, *Psychopharmacology* 97(4):539-547, 1989.
10. McGehee D: Nicotine enhancement of fast excitatory synaptic transmission in CNS by presynaptic receptors, *Science* 269: 1692-1696, Sept 22, 1995.
11. Henningfield JE, Radzius A, Cone EJ: Estimation of

available nicotine content of six smokeless tobacco products, *Tobacco Control* 4:57-61, 1995.
12. Manning A: Lawmaker: kids used in tobacco tests, *USA Today,* p1A, July 25, 1995.
13. Philip Morris raised nicotine, Rep. says, *USA Today,* p6D, Aug 1, 1995.
14. Bash A, Levy D: ABC, tobacco firms settle libel suits, *USA Today,* p1A, Aug 22, 1995.
15. Pinger R, Payne W, Hahn D, Hahn E: *Drugs: issues for today,* ed 2, St Louis, 1995, Mosby.
16. Manning A: Industry sues over teen smoking effort, *USA Today,* p1a, Aug 11, 1995.
17. Centers for Disease Control: The Surgeon General's 1989 report on reducing the health consequences of smoking: 25 years of progress (executive summary), *MMWR* 38 (suppl 5) 2:1, 1989.
18. *American Heart Association: 1995 heart and stroke facts: 1995 statistical supplement,* Dallas, 1994, The Association.
19. Brennhan J et al: Association between cigarette smoking and mutation of the p53 gene in squamous-cell carcinoma of the head and neck, *N Engl J Med* 332:712-717, 1995.
20. Crowley LV: *Introduction to human disease,* ed 3, Boston, 1992, Jones & Bartlett.
21. Eisen S, Lyon M, Goldberg J, True W: The impact of cigarette and alcohol consumption on weight and obesity: an analysis of 1911 monozygotic male twin pairs, *Arch Intern Med* 153(21):2457-2463, 1993.
22. Gilbert RJ: Caffeine: The most popular stimulant. In

Encyclopedia of psychoactive drugs, New York, 1986, Chelsea House.

23. Caffeine during pregnancy: grounds for concern? *JAMA* 270(24):2973, 1993 (editorial).

24. Klonoff-Cohen HS et al: The effect of passive smoking and tobacco exposure through breast milk on sudden infant death syndrome, *JAMA* 273(10):795-798, 1995.

25. Hatcher RA et al: *Contraceptive technology, 1994,* ed 18, New York, 1994, Irvington Publishers.

26. Glantz SA, Parmely WW: Passive smoking and heart disease: epidemiology, physiology, and biochemistry, *Circulation* 83(1):1-12, 1991.

27. Overpeck MD, Moss AJ: Children's exposure to environmental cigarette smoke before and after birth: United States, 1988, *Advanced data from vital and health statistics, no 202,* Hyattsville, Md, 1991, National Center for Health Statistics.

28. Fiore MC et al: Methods used to quit smoking in the United States, *JAMA* 263(20):2760-2765, 1990.

29. Nicorette and Nicorette DS. Product information insert, Uppsala, Sweden, 1992, Kab; Pharmacia AB.

30. Nicoderm. Product information insert, Palo Alto, Calif, January 1992, ALZA Corporation.

Suggested Readings

Delaney S: *Women smokers can quit—a different approach,* Evanston, Ill, 1990, Women's Healthcare Press.
    Written by a former heavy smoker, this book details information about the special concerns women have when they try to stop smoking. Emphasis is on quitting smoking without gaining weight and on learning new ways of coping with stress.

Douville JA: *Active and passive smoking in the workplace,* New York, 1990, Von Nostrand Reinhold.
    A chemist and information scientist clearly explains the health effects of environmental tobacco smoke. This is an excellent guide for employers who must provide a healthful workplace. The author examines programs that have worked in different companies.

King S: *Nightmares and dreamscapes,* New York, 1993, Viking Penguin.
    A futuristic account of smokers as a subtribe of people whose habit limits their involvement with society.

Today Show: *Quit Smoking with Today,* New York, 1995, NBC (videotape).
    Although not a "suggested reading" in the traditional sense, this excellent new video program for home use provides detailed instructions for implementing a 4-day smoking cessation program. An accompanying stress reduction program can be used to assist with the stress of withdrawal.

 AS WE GO TO PRESS . . .

California health officials are concerned with an apparent recent increase in smoking among the state's adult population. In the first 6 months of 1995, state surveys indicated that 15.5% of adults in California smoked. This was an all-time low for the state. However, in the last 6 months of 1995, 17.9% of adults surveyed indicated that they smoked.

Smokers vs. Nonsmokers: A Question of Rights

A quiet battle is being waged in the United States over smoking, an activity that was once universally accepted. Within the last decade, regulations restricting the act of smoking have affected stores, restaurants, offices, and public buildings. It is difficult these days to find a place of business in the United States where smoking is totally unrestricted. Some of these restrictions are put in place by law or municipal ordinances; some are placed voluntarily by business management. However, it is clear that the voices of nonsmokers, long silent and largely ignored by society, are finally being heard and are behind the recent increase in restrictions on smoking.

As antismokers have made progress in cutting back on unwanted environmental smoke, smokers have begun to fight back. As restrictions have mounted, they have united and mobilized to prevent themselves from being pushed to the fringes of society. The two sides have sparked a debate that goes to the heart of the American value system and is questioning the way we think about the rights of the individual.

Changing attitudes

For decades, there was no debate or controversy. People smoked whenever and wherever they wished. Smoking was glamorized in the movies, on television, and in print throughout most of the twentieth century. Famous athletes and movie stars could be found in cigarette advertisements. Some ads even promoted the "health benefits" of smoking. Although there were a few people who felt that smoking was dangerous, their voices had little effect on society's acceptance of tobacco use. Gradually, however, attitudes began to change. As data from medical studies began to accumulate on the dangers of tobacco, antismoking advocates started to achieve some victories in society and in public policy.

Restrictions on tobacco use

In the 1980s, restrictions on smoking greatly increased. In 1987, smoking was banned on all domestic airplane flights of less than 2 hours; in 1990, this ban was later increased to all domestic flights of less than 6 hours.[1] A growing number of state and local laws curtailing or banning smoking in places of business have been enacted. For example, Maryland has banned smoking in all workplaces except those with a sealed, separately ventilated room for smokers,[2] and in the state of Washington, smoking is prohibited in all enclosed public and private offices.[2] Many businesses that were not forced by law to restrict smoking did so anyway, citing public sentiment in favor of such regulations. Smoking is prohibited on over 80% of Amtrak trains, and 1400 company-owned McDonald's restaurants are now smoke free.[2]

As a result of these restrictions, smoking areas in places of business are shrinking in size or are being eliminated. Congregations of smokers outside of office buildings have become a common sight. Some smokers have taken the changes in stride. Others have cut back on smoking or have quit smoking altogether. Many, however, are not happy about having to step outside in all kinds of weather to smoke. They feel ostracized and are speaking out against what they perceive as an outright attack on their personal freedoms.

The prosmoker defense

In response to these perceived attacks, smokers have started to become organized on a worldwide level and within individual communities and workplaces. They are clearly worried that this trend of restricting tobacco use will not stop until smoking is eliminated everywhere and the use of tobacco becomes illegal.

Groups such as the British-based Freedom Organisation for the Right to Enjoy Smoking Tobacco (FOREST) have actively pushed smokers' rights and have espoused the "benefits" of smoking.[3] They cite controversial scientific studies demonstrating that smokers are less likely to develop Alzheimer's disease and Parkinson's disease and that teen acne is "almost exclusively" a nonsmokers' affliction.[3]

Smokers are also worried about how their smoking activities are perceived by employers and insurers. Companies are growing less tolerant of unhealthy activities by their employees, since they have to pay increased insurance costs for treatment. Many fear that insurance companies will begin to refuse treatment to smokers who continue to smoke. They cite cases such as one from the United Kingdom in which a cardiac patient was refused treatment because he continued to smoke and had a poor prognosis for recovery.[4] Talk of changing the U. S. health care system to a more European-style system has smoking activists worried that such treatment refusals could become commonplace here.

Some companies in the United States have gone as far as to conduct breath tests to determine if employees have been smoking away from the workplace.[3] Smoking activists feel that what employees do in the privacy of their own home is their own business and that these tests are akin to urine tests for illegal drugs. Some fear that restrictions will continue to reach into the home setting.

As a result, smoking activists have teamed up with the tobacco industry and the American Civil Liberties Union to convince states to adopt laws prohibiting companies from discriminating against smokers. These lobbying activities have been successful in 28 states.[5]

The worst-case scenario for smokers is that their smoking will be restricted even at home. "What if the government starts keeping us from having kids because we smoke?" worries "Earl," a two-pack a day smoker. "I've heard tell that we could have our kids taken away because we smoke at home. Do we have to step outside of our own homes to smoke?"[6]

Fighting for clean air

Many nonsmokers are just as adamant about defending their side, saying that smokers have been subjecting them to cancer-causing agents for decades and that the restrictions are long overdue. They are tired of having smoke blown in their faces in public. Antismoking activists find the "individual freedom" argument of smokers objectionable. "What about my right to breathe?" asks "Stan," an office worker who is subjected to smoke from nearby cubicles. "The management, most of whom smoke, have decided that since we don't deal directly with the public, smoking is okay," he complains.[7]

Many nonsmoking activists feel that it is in the public's best interest to restrict exposure to tobacco smoke and to cut back on tobacco use as a whole. They are angered not only that they have to be exposed to it, but that a good chunk of their insurance premiums is going toward health care costs from smoking. It is estimated that $65 billion a year goes to treat tobacco-related diseases, roughly one fourth of all money spent on health care in the United States each year.[8] The groundswell of support for tobacco regulations may be happening in response to the growing number of medical studies that show the dangers of tobacco use. The Centers for Disease Control and Prevention estimate that 418,000 deaths per year can be attributed to tobacco smoke, and approximately 3000 nonsmokers die yearly from lung cancer caused by exposure to tobacco smoke.[2] As the data accumulate on the hazards of smoking, many nonsmokers are becoming concerned about their exposure to secondhand smoke. They are also worried about the addictive properties of nicotine and are concerned that their children may get hooked.

Though they have had much success in getting restrictions adopted, antismoking activists have also faced defeat in the legislatures as well. Municipalities in North Carolina can no longer pass local laws restricting smoking, thanks to a preemptive state law passed on July 15, 1993.[9] HB 957 allows local regulations adopted before October 15, 1993, to remain in effect, but it bans any future regulations from being adopted. The 3-month period between passage of the bill and the regulation deadline left a very short window of time for local bodies to organize, debate, and vote on smoking restrictions. As a result, 59% of workers in North Carolina have no legal protection at all from exposure to tobacco smoke.[9]

Even without the health problems posed by tobacco smoke, many nonsmokers feel that it should be curtailed simply because of its unpleasant smell. Since smoking is not a self-contained activity, smoke diffuses far away from the smoker, often offending people many feet away. "What good does it do to seat a nonsmoker next to the smoking section in a restaurant?" notes "Irina," an avid antismoking activist.[10] "The smoke just drifts over anyway. It stinks, and not just during the meal. It gets into your clothes and hair and stays with you all day. Why must we tolerate smoke?"

What the future may hold

Such arguments may open the door to more restrictions on smoking, a possibility that has smokers' rights advocates angry. Many are convinced that antismoking forces want nothing less than a total ban on tobacco use. Although this scenario is highly unlikely, more regulations may be on the way. FDA head David Kessler is considering a proposal that would eliminate cigarette vending machines (an easy tobacco source for juveniles) and restrict tobacco advertisements near schools.[2] The group Action on Smoking and Health has petitioned the Occupational Safety and Health Administration to ban all workplace smoking.[11] The EPA has labeled secondhand smoke as a Class A carcinogen.[11] The restrictions reach into the home as well, since some child custody cases are being decided (at least in part) by the smoking habits of the adults involved,[11] and some physicians now consider exposure to smoke in the home a form of child endangerment.

Antismoking advocates do not see these regulations as restrictions on individual freedom. Instead, they see these regulations as a means of liberation from decades of exposure to smoke with little or no means of legal recourse. Many nonsmokers feel that they should not be forced to breathe in smoke simply because someone wants to light up. Advocates for these regulations claim that tobacco-related illnesses increase health care costs for everyone. They also complain that their tax dollars are being used to subsidize the tobacco industry, so that in effect they are paying to be exposed to the smoke of others. Restrictions on smoking are a welcome means of relief for those nonsmokers with lung diseases or allergies to tobacco as well.

Since smoking by its very nature is not a self-contained activity, conflicts are bound to happen, but perhaps some acceptable middle ground can be reached between smokers and nonsmokers both in law and in society.

For Discussion . . .
Have you ever asked someone not to smoke near you or been asked not to smoke around someone? Should taxpayers be responsible for taking on the burden of those being treated for smoking-related diseases? Are the individual freedoms of smokers being infringed on by smoking regulations? Are the individual freedoms of nonsmokers being violated by smokers? Is smoking at home around your children a form of child endangerment?

References
1. The tyranny of the majority, *The Economist* 313(7626), Oct 28, 1989.
2. Farley CJ, Toufexis A: The butt stops here, 143(16), *Time* Apr 18, 1994.
3. Platt S: Ashes to ashes, *New Statesman and Society* 7(289), Feb 11, 1994.
4. McNulty K: A smoky issue, *Science World* 50(11), Mar 11, 1994.
5. A get-tough approach can pose pitfalls, *Nation's Business* 83(9), Sept 1995.
6. Anonymous, personal communication, January 1996.
7. Anonymous, personal communication, June 1994.
8. What are they smoking? *FW* 161(5), Mar 3, 1992.
9. Conlisk E et al: The status of local smoking regulations in North Carolina following a state preemption bill, *JAMA* 273(10), 1995.
10. Anonymous, personal communication, March 1996.
11. Holt TH: Pests' attacks on smoking threaten individual freedoms, *Insight, vol. 42*, Oct 18, 1993.

PART 4

DISEASES

Reducing Your Risk of Cardiovascular Disease

Healthy People 2000 Objectives

The Midcourse Review reports that we have successfully moved toward achieving 15 of the 17 Healthy People 2000 objectives in the priority area of cardiovascular disease. This is not surprising, since widespread public education programs have been developed and implemented during the last 25 years. Measures to identify high-risk groups have been initiated and refined. The ability to control high blood pressure and blood cholesterol levels has improved markedly. A great deal of evidence now indicates that heart disease can indeed be prevented through lifestyle changes.

Nevertheless, cardiovascular disease remains the nation's number-one cause of death and disability, considerably outdistancing the number two cause. The Midcourse Review reminds us that premature morbidity (sickness) is devastating for many heart disease patients. Affected people often cannot participate fully in daily activities, and many become unable to function independently. The annual economic impact of heart disease is estimated to be $190 billion, which includes health care expenses, medications, and lost work productivity resulting from disability and death.

This section of the book contains three chapters that deal with diseases. It is not surprising that diseases and adverse health conditions can be major obstacles to a healthy life. Although uninformed people claim that "there is nothing you can do to avoid disease," there is ample evidence that positive personal health choices can help reduce the chances of developing many diseases, from cardiovascular disease to cancer to sexually transmitted diseases, including HIV and AIDS.

Look at the progress made with respect to **cardiovascular** disease (CVD), the focus of this chapter. Although heart disease continues to be the number one killer of Americans, between 1982 and 1992 the death rates from CVD declined 24.5%.[1] The American Heart Association, in its *1995 Heart and Stroke Facts*, credits this reduction to a combination of (1) changing American lifestyles and (2) medical advances in the diagnosis and treatment of CVD.[1]

This chapter provides you with material to help you understand how the heart works. Beyond this, it will help you identify your CVD risk factors and suggest ways you can alter certain lifestyle behaviors to reduce the risk of developing heart disease.

PREVALENCE OF CARDIOVASCULAR DISEASE

Cardiovascular diseases are directly related to over 40% of deaths in the United States and indirectly related to a large percentage of additional deaths.[1]

Heart disease, stroke, and related blood vessel disorders combined to kill nearly 1 million Americans in 1992 (Figure 10-1). This figure represents more deaths than were caused by cancer, accidents, pneumonia, influenza, lung diseases, diabetes, and AIDS combined. Indeed, cardiovascular disease is our nation's number one "killer" (see the Star Box on p. 230).

NORMAL CARDIOVASCULAR FUNCTION

The cardiovascular or circulatory system uses a muscular pump to send a complex fluid on a continuous trip through a closed system of tubes. The pump is the heart, the fluid is blood, and the closed system of tubes is the network of blood vessels.

The Vascular System

The term *vascular system* refers to the body's blood vessels. Although we might be familiar with the arteries (vessels that carry blood away from the heart) and the veins (vessels that carry blood toward the heart), arterioles, capillaries, and venules are also included in

> **cardiovascular**
> Pertaining to the heart (cardio) and blood vessels (vascular).

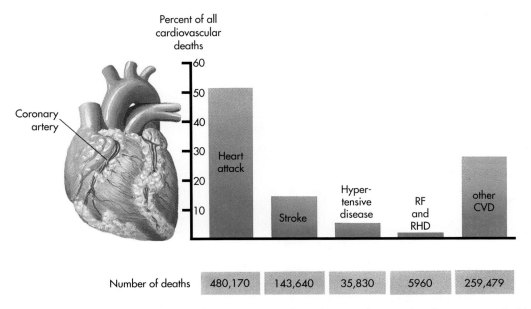

Figure 10-1   Of the 925,079 deaths in the United States in 1992 resulting from cardiovascular diseases, over half were attributable to heart attack.

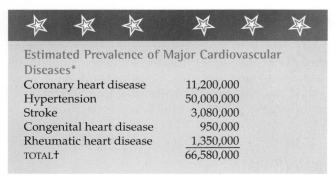

Estimated Prevalence of Major Cardiovascular Diseases*	
Coronary heart disease	11,200,000
Hypertension	50,000,000
Stroke	3,080,000
Congenital heart disease	950,000
Rheumatic heart disease	1,350,000
TOTAL†	66,580,000

*58,920,000 people total.

†The sum of the individual estimates exceeds 58,920,000 because many people have more than one cardiovascular disorder.

The Heart

The heart is a four-chambered pump designed to create the pressure required to circulate blood throughout the body. Usually considered to be about the size of a person's clenched fist, this organ lies slightly tilted between the lungs in the central portion of the **thorax.** The heart does not lie completely in the center of the chest. Rather, approximately two thirds of the heart is to the left of the body midline and one third is to the right.[2]

Two upper chambers, called *atria,* and two lower chambers, called *ventricles,* form the heart. The thin-walled atrial chambers are considered collecting chambers, whereas the thick-walled muscular ventricles are considered the pumping chambers. The right and left sides of the heart are divided by a partition called the *septum.* Study Figure 10-2 and follow the flow of blood through the heart's four chambers.

For the heart muscle to function well, it must be supplied with adequate amounts of oxygen. The two main **coronary arteries** (and their numerous branches) accomplish this. These arteries are located outside of the heart (see Figure 10-1). If the coronary arteries are diseased and not functioning well, a heart attack is possible.

Heart stimulation

The heart contracts and relaxes through the delicate interplay of **cardiac muscle** tissue and cardiac electrical centers called *nodes.* Nodal tissue generates the electrical impulses necessary to contract heart

the vascular system. Arterioles are the farther, smaller-diameter extensions of arteries. These arterioles lead eventually to capillaries, the smallest extensions of the vascular system. At the capillary level, exchanges of oxygen, food, and waste occur between cells and the blood.

Once the blood leaves the capillaries and begins its return to the heart, it drains into small veins, or venules. The blood in the venules flows into increasingly larger vessels called *veins.* Blood pressure is highest in arteries and lowest in veins, especially the largest veins, which empty into the right atrium of the heart.

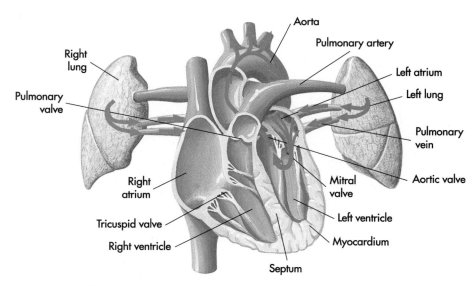

Figure 10-2   The heart functions like a complex double pump. The right side of the heart pumps deoxygenated blood to the lungs. The left side of the heart pumps oxygenated blood through the aorta to all parts of the body. Note the thickness of the walls of the ventricles. These are the primary pumping chambers.

muscle.[3] The heart's electrical activity is measured by an instrument called an *electrocardiograph* (ECG or EKG), which provides a printout called an electrocardiogram that can be evaluated to determine cardiac electrical functioning.

Blood

The average-sized adult has approximately 6 quarts of blood in his or her circulatory system. Blood's functions, which are performed continuously, are quite similar to the overall functions of the circulatory system and include the following:

- Transportation of nutrients, oxygen, wastes, hormones, and enzymes
- Regulation of water content of body cells and fluids
- Buffering to help maintain appropriate pH balance of body fluids
- Regulation of body temperature; the water component in the blood absorbs heat and transfers it
- Prevention of blood loss; by coagulating or clotting, the blood can alter its form to prevent blood loss through injured vessels
- Protection against toxins and microorganisms, accomplished by chemical substances called *antibodies* and specialized cellular elements circulating in the bloodstream

CARDIOVASCULAR DISEASE RISK FACTORS

As you have just read, the heart and blood vessels are among the most important structures in the human body. By protecting your cardiovascular system, you lay the groundwork for a more exciting, productive, and energetic life. The best time to start protecting and improving your cardiovascular system is early in life, when lifestyle patterns are developed and reinforced (see the Star Box at right). Of course, it is difficult to move backward through time, so the second best time to start protecting your heart is *today.* Improvements in certain lifestyle activities can pay significant dividends as your life unfolds. Complete the Personal Assessment on pp. 232-233 to determine your risk for heart disease.

The American Heart Association encourages people to protect and enhance their heart health by examining the 10 cardiovascular risk factors that are related to various forms of heart disease. A *cardiovascular risk factor* is an attribute that a person has or is exposed to that increases the likelihood that he or she will

Prevention of Heart Disease Begins in Childhood

For many aspects of wellness, preventive behaviors are often best learned in childhood, where they can be repeated and reinforced by family members and caregivers. This is especially true for preventive actions concerning heart disease. Although many problems related to heart disease are seen most frequently at midlife and beyond, the roots of heart disease start early in life.

The most serious childhood health behaviors associated with heart disease are poor dietary practices, lack of physical activity, and cigarette smoking. Sadly, the present state of health for America's youth shows severe deficiencies in these three areas. Children's diets lack nutrient density and remain alarmingly high in overall fat. Teenaged children are becoming increasingly overweight and obese. Studies consistently show a deterioration in the amount of physical activity by today's youth, as television and video games have become the after-school companions for large numbers of children. Sadly, cigarette smoking continues to rise among school children, especially teenagers.

These unhealthy behaviors are laying the foundation for coronary artery disease, hypertension, and stroke in the future. Rather than trying to repair sick people in their older years, increased efforts on childhood prevention should be a focus for today's adults. Those of us who are parents must make better efforts to encourage our children to eat more nutritiously and be physically active. We can discourage cigarette use. Perhaps the best thing all adults can do for our youth is to set a good example by adopting our own heart-healthy behaviors. Following the Food Guide Pyramid (p. 108) and exercising regularly are excellent strategies that can be started early in life.

thorax
The chest; portion of the torso above the diaphragm and within the rib cage.

coronary arteries
Vessels that supply oxygenated blood to heart muscle tissues.

cardiac muscle
Specialized smooth muscle tissue that forms the middle (muscular) layer of the heart wall.

PERSONAL ASSESSMENT

What Is Your Risk for Heart Disease?

Cholesterol

Your serum cholesterol level is:

0	190 or below
+ 2	191 to 230
+ 6	231 to 289
+12	290 to 319
+16	Over 320

Your HDL cholesterol is:

− 2	Over 60
0	45 to 60
+ 2	35 to 44
+ 6	29 to 34
+12	23 to 28
+16	Below 23

Smoking

You smoke now or have in the past:

0	Never smoked, or quit more than 5 years ago
+1	Quit 2 to 4 years ago
+3	Quit about 1 year ago
+6	Quit during the past year

You now smoke:

+ 9	½ to 1 pack a day
+12	1 to 2 packs a day
+15	More than 2 packs a day

The quality of the air you breathe is:

0	Unpolluted by smoke, exhaust, or industry at home **and** at work
+2	Live **or** work with smokers in unpolluted area
+4	Live **and** work with smokers in unpolluted area
+6	Live **or** work with smokers **and** live or work in air-polluted area
+8	Live **and** work with smokers **and** live and work in air-polluted area

Blood Pressure

Your blood pressure is:

0	120/75 or below
+ 2	120/75 to 140/85
+ 6	140/85 to 150/90
+ 8	150/90 to 175/100
+10	175/100 to 190/110
+12	190/110 or above

Exercise

Your exercise habits are:

0	Exercise vigorously 4 or 5 times a week
+2	Exercise moderately 4 or 5 times a week
+4	Exercise only on weekends
+6	Exercise occasionally
+8	Little or no exercise

Weight

Your weight is:

0	Always at or near ideal weight
+1	Now 10% overweight
+2	Now 20% overweight
+3	Now 30% or more overweight
+4	Now 20% or more overweight and have been since before age 30

Stress

You feel overstressed:

0	Rarely at work or at home
+ 3	Somewhat at home but not at work
+ 5	Somewhat at work but not at home
+ 7	Somewhat at work **and** at home
+ 9	Usually at work **or** at home
+12	Usually at work **and** at home

Diabetes

Your diabetic history is:

0	Blood sugar always normal
+2	Blood glucose slightly high (prediabetic) or slightly low (hypoglycemic)
+4	Diabetic beginning after age 40 requiring strict dietary or insulin control
+5	Diabetic beginning before age 30 requiring strict dietary or insulin control

Alcohol

You drink alcoholic beverages:

0	Never or only socially, about once or twice a month, or only one 5-ounce glass of wine or 12-ounce glass of beer or 1½ ounces of hard liquor about 5 times a week
+2	Two to three 5-ounce glasses of wine or 12-ounce glasses of beer or 1½-ounce cocktails about 5 times a week
+4	More than three 1½-ounce cocktails or more than three 5-ounce glasses of wine or 12-ounce glasses of beer almost every day

Continued

Interpretation
Add all sources and check below
0 to 20: Low risk. Excellent family history and lifestyle habits.
21 to 50: Moderate risk. Family history or lifestyle habits put you at some risk. You might lower your risks and minimize your genetic predisposition if you change any poor habits.
51 to 74: High risk. Habits and family history indicate high risk of heart disease. Change your habits now.

Above 75: Very high risk. Family history and a lifetime of poor habits put you at very high risk of heart disease. Eliminate as many of the risk factors as you can.

To Carry This Further . . .
Were you surprised with your score on this assessment? What were your most significant risk factors? Do you plan to make any changes in your lifestyle to reduce your cardiovascular risks? Why or why not?

develop some form of heart disease. Three risk factors are ones you will be unable to change. An additional four risk factors are ones you can clearly change. Three final risk factors are ones that are thought to be contributing factors to heart disease. These risk factors are summarized in the Star Box below. Let's look at these three groups of risk factors separately.

Risk Factors That Cannot Be Changed

The three risk factors that you cannot change are increasing age, male gender, and heredity. Despite the fact that these risk factors cannot be changed, your knowledge that they might be an influence in your life should encourage you to make a more serious commitment to the risk factors you *can* change.

Increasing age

Heart diseases tend to develop gradually over the course of one's life. Although we may know of a person or two who experienced a heart attack in their thirties or forties, most of the serious consequences of heart disease are evident in older ages. For example, approximately 80% of people who die from heart attack are age 65 and older.

Male gender

Young women have lower rates of heart disease than young men. Yet when women move through menopause (typically in their fifties), their rates of heart disease are similar to men's rates (see the Star Box on p. 234). It is thought that women are somewhat more protected from heart disease than men because of their natural production of the hormone estrogen during their fertile years.

Heredity

Obviously, you have no input in determining whom your biological parents are. Like increasing age and male gender, this risk factor cannot be changed.

By the luck of the draw, some people are born into families where heart disease has never been a serious problem, whereas others are born into families where heart disease is quite prevalent. In this latter case, children are said to have a genetic predisposition (tendency) to develop heart disease as they grow and develop throughout their lives. These people have every reason to be highly motivated to reduce the risk factors they can control.

Race is also a consideration related to heart disease. African-Americans have moderately high blood pressure at rates twice that of whites and severe hypertension at rates three times higher than whites (for a detailed discussion of this topic, see "Focus on . . . Hypertension among African-Americans," pp. 247-248). Hypertension significantly increases the risk of both heart disease and stroke. Fortunately, as you will soon read, hypertension can be controlled through a variety of methods. It is especially impor-

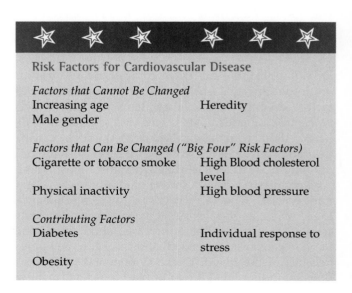

Risk Factors for Cardiovascular Disease

Factors that Cannot Be Changed
Increasing age   Heredity
Male gender

Factors that Can Be Changed ("Big Four" Risk Factors)
Cigarette or tobacco smoke   High Blood cholesterol
                                  level
Physical inactivity   High blood pressure

Contributing Factors
Diabetes   Individual response to
                                  stress
Obesity

Women and Heart Disease

Do you think heart disease is a problem just for men? You might be surprised to discover that data from the American Heart Association indicate that 52% of all cardiovascular disease deaths are in women. 20,800 women under the age of 65 die from heart attack each year and 29% of women who die from coronary artery disease are under age 55. Also, 44% of women who have a heart attack will die within 1 year, compared with 27% of men. A total of 60% of the deaths from stroke and high blood pressure are in women, compared with 40% in men. Women who smoke and also take oral contraceptives are 39 times more likely to have a heart attack and 22 times more likely to have a stroke than women who neither smoke nor use oral contraceptives.[1]

For many years, it was thought that men were at much greater risk than women for the development of cardiovascular problems. It is now known that younger men are more prone to heart disease than young women, yet once women reach menopause (usually in their early middle 50s), their rates of heart-related problems quickly equal those of men.

The protective mechanism for young women seems to be the female hormone estrogen. Estrogen appears to help women maintain a beneficial profile of blood fats. When the production of estrogen is severely reduced at menopause, this protective factor no longer exists. This is one of the reasons that increasing numbers of physicians are prescribing estrogen replacement therapy (ERT) for many postmenopausal women.

Of course, young women should not rely solely on naturally-produced estrogen to prevent heart disease. The general recommendations for maintaining heart health through a good diet, adequate physical activity, monitoring blood pressure and cholesterol levels, controlling weight, avoiding smoking, and managing stress will benefit women at every stage of life.

---

tant for African-Americans to take advantage of every opportunity to have their blood pressure measured so that preventive actions can be started immediately if necessary.

Risk Factors That Can Be Changed

There are four cardiovascular risk factors that are influenced, in large part, by our lifestyle choices. These risk factors are cigarette/tobacco smoke, physical inactivity, high blood pressure, and high blood cholesterol level. Healthful behavior changes you make concerning these "big four" risk factors can help you protect and enhance your cardiovascular system.

Cigarette or tobacco smoke

Although the other three controllable risk factors are important, this one may be the most critical risk factor. Smokers have a heart attack risk that is over twice that of nonsmokers. Smoking cigarettes is *the* major risk factor associated with sudden cardiac death. In fact, smokers have two to four times the risk of dying from sudden cardiac arrest than nonsmokers.

Cigarette or tobacco smoke also adversely affects nonsmokers who are exposed to environmental tobacco smoke. Studies suggest that the risk of death caused by heart disease is increased about 30 percent in people exposed to secondhand smoke in the home.[5] Because of the health threat to nonsmokers, restrictions on indoor smoking in public areas and business settings are increasing tremendously in every part of the country.

For years the notion was that if you had smoked for many years, it was pointless to try to quit; the damage to one's health could never be reversed. However, the American Heart Association now indicates that by quitting smoking, regardless of how long or how much you have smoked, your risk of heart disease declines rapidly. For people who have smoked a pack or less of cigarettes per day, within 3 years after quitting smoking, their heart disease risk is virtually the same as those who never smoked.

This news is exciting and should encourage people to quit smoking, regardless of how long they have smoked. Of course, if you have started to smoke, the healthy approach would be to *quit now* . . . before the nicotine controls your life and damages your heart. (For additional information about the health effects of tobacco, see Chapter 9.)

Physical inactivity

Lack of exercise is a significant risk factor for heart disease. Regular aerobic exercise (discussed in Chapter 4) helps strengthen the heart muscle, maintain healthy blood vessels, and improve the ability of the vascular system to transfer blood and oxygen to all parts of the body. Additionally, physical activity helps lower overall blood cholesterol levels for most people, encourages weight loss and retention of lean muscle

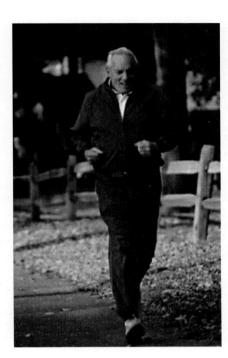

Regular aerobic exercise helps maintain cardiovascular health.

mass, and allows people to moderate the stress in their lives.

With all the benefits that come with physical activity, it amazes health professionals that so many Americans refuse to participate in regular exercise. Perhaps people feel that they do not have enough time or that they must work out strenuously. However, you will recall from Chapter 4 that only 20 to 60 minutes of moderate aerobic activity three to five times each week is recommended. This is not a large price to pay for a lifetime of cardiovascular health. Find a partner and get started!

If you are middle-aged or older and have been inactive, you should consult with a physician before starting an exercise program. Also, if you have any known health condition that could be aggravated by physical activity, check with a physician first.

High blood cholesterol level

The third controllable risk factor for heart disease is high blood cholesterol level. Generally speaking, the higher the blood cholesterol level, the greater the risk for heart disease. When high blood cholesterol levels are combined with other important risk factors, the risks become much greater.

Fortunately, blood cholesterol levels are relatively easy to measure. Many campus health and wellness centers provide cholesterol screenings for employees and students. These screenings help identify people whose cholesterol levels (or profiles) may be potentially dangerous. Medical professionals have been able to determine the link between a person's diet and his or her cholesterol levels (see the Learning from All Cultures box on p. 236). People with high blood cholesterol levels are encouraged to consume a heart-healthy diet (see Chapter 5) and to become physically active. In recent years a variety of cholesterol-lowering drugs have also been developed that are very effective at lowering cholesterol levels. In an upcoming section in this chapter, you will read more about cholesterol.

High blood pressure

The fourth of the "big four" cardiovascular risk factors is high blood pressure, or hypertension. You will soon be reading more about hypertension, but for now, suffice it to say that high blood pressure can seriously damage a person's heart and blood vessels. High blood pressure causes the heart to work much harder, eventually causing the heart to enlarge and weaken. High blood pressure increases the chances for stroke, heart attack, congestive heart failure, and kidney disease.

When high blood pressure is seen with other risk factors, the risk for stroke or heart attack is increased tremendously. As you will soon see, this "silent killer" is easy to monitor and can be effectively controlled using a variety of approaches. This is the positive message about high blood pressure.

Other Risk Factors That Contribute to Heart Disease

The American Heart Association identifies three other risk factors that are associated with an increased risk of heart disease. These risk factors are diabetes, obesity, and stress.

Diabetes

Diabetes mellitus (discussed in detail on pp. 266-269) is a debilitating chronic disease that has a significant effect on the human body. In addition to increasing the risks of developing kidney disease, blindness, and nerve damage, diabetes increases the likelihood of developing heart and blood vessel diseases. Over 80% of people with diabetes die of some type of heart or blood vessel disease. The cardiovascular damage is thought to occur when diabetes begins to alter normal cholesterol and blood fat levels. With weight management, exercise, dietary changes, and drug therapy, diabetes can be relatively well controlled in most people. Despite

LEARNING *from* ALL CULTURES

Diet and Coronary Heart Disease

Lifestyle and culture affect your risk for coronary heart disease. For example, Japanese people who live in the United States have a greater risk of developing heart disease than Japanese people who live in Japan. Diet seems to be the most important factor. People who eat a low-fat diet experience fewer incidences of heart disease, regardless of where they live. Conversely, individuals who maintain a diet high in saturated fats, wherever they live, have a higher incidence of coronary heart disease.[15]

Developed Western countries seem to have a fairly high incidence of coronary heart disease, some of which can be attributed to lifestyle and diet. Early evidence of this was reported in a 5-year study of middle-aged men in the late 1950s and early 1960s. The Seven Countries Study reported that the death rate from heart attacks was 3 to 10 times greater for men from Finland, the United States, and the Netherlands than for men from Greece, Yugoslavia, Italy, and Japan. Some of the difference was explained by determining blood cholesterol levels; they were much higher for men in the United States, Finland, and the Netherlands than for men from the other four countries. Men from the three high-risk countries consumed greater amounts of saturated fats in their diets than those from Japan and the Mediterranean countries.[15]

Consider your risk factors that can be changed. Then consider your lifestyle. Are your eating habits typical of those of a number of Americans, too high in saturated fats? What kinds of changes have you made or could you make to lower your risk factor of lifestyle and culture?

careful management of this disease, diabetic patients remain quite susceptible to eventual heart and blood vessel damage.

Obesity

Even if they have no other risk factors, obese people are more likely than nonobese people to develop heart disease and stroke. Obesity places considerable strain on the heart, and it tends to influence both blood pressure and blood cholesterol levels. Also, obesity tends to trigger diabetes in predisposed people. The importance of maintaining body weight within a desirable range minimizes the chances of obesity ever happening. To accomplish this, you can elect to make a commitment to a reasonably sound diet and an active lifestyle.

Individual response to stress

Unresolved stress over a long period may be a contributing factor to the development of heart disease. Certainly, people who are unable to cope with stressful life experiences are more likely to develop negative dependence behaviors (for example, smoking, underactivity, poor dietary practices), which can then lead to cardiovascular problems through changes in blood fat profiles, blood pressure, and heart workload. To discover ways of coping with stress, you might wish to return to the discussion in Chapter 3.

FORMS OF CARDIOVASCULAR DISEASE

The American Heart Association describes the five major forms of CVD as coronary heart disease, hypertension, stroke, congenital heart disease, and rheumatic heart disease.[1] A person may have just one of these five diseases or a combination of forms at the same time. Each form exists in varying degrees of severity. All forms are capable of causing secondary damage to other body organs and body systems.

Coronary Heart Disease

This form of CVD, also known as *coronary artery disease*, involves damage to the vessels that supply blood to the heart muscle. The bulk of this blood is supplied by the coronary arteries. Any damage to these important vessels can cause a reduction of blood (and its vital oxygen and nutrients) to specific areas of heart muscle. The ultimate result of inadequate blood supply is a heart attack.

Atherosclerosis

The principal cause for the development of coronary heart disease is atherosclerosis (Figure 10-3). **Atherosclerosis** produces a narrowing of the coronary arteries. This narrowing stems from the long-term buildup of fatty deposits, called *plaque*, on the

Connective tissue
Smooth muscle
Endothelial cell
Lumen
Plaque accumulation

Figure 10-3 Progression of atherosclerosis. This diagram shows how plaque deposits gradually accumulate to narrow the lumen (interior space) of an artery. Although enlarged here, coronary arteries are only as wide as a pencil lead.

inner walls of the arteries. This buildup reduces the blood supply to specific portions of the heart. Some arteries of the heart can become so blocked (occluded) that all blood supply is stopped. Heart muscle tissue begins to die when it is deprived of oxygen and nutrients. This damage is known as **myocardial infarction.** In lay terms, this event is called a *heart attack.* The Health Action Guide on p. 238 explains how to recognize the signs of a heart attack and what to do next.

Cholesterol and lipoproteins. For many years, scientists have known that atherosclerosis is a complicated disease that has many causes. Some of these causes are not well understood, but others are clearly understood. *Cholesterol,* a soft, fatlike material, is manufactured in the liver and small intestine and is necessary in the formation of sex hormones, cell membranes, bile salts, and nerve fibers. Elevated levels of serum cholesterol (200 mg/dl or more for adults age 20 and older, and 170 mg/dl or more for young people below age 20) are associated with an increased risk for developing atherosclerosis[1] (see the Health Action Guide on p. 239).

Some 52% of American adults age 20 and older exceed the "borderline high" 200 mg/dl cholesterol level. It is estimated that nearly 40% of American youth age 19 and below have "borderline high" cholesterol levels of 170 mg/dl and above. About one out of five American adults has a "high" blood cholesterol level, that is, 240 mg/dl or greater.[1]

Initially, most people can help lower their serum cholesterol level by adopting three dietary changes: lowering the intake of saturated fats, lowering the intake of dietary cholesterol, and lowering caloric intake to a level that does not exceed body requirements. The aim is to reduce excess fat, cholesterol, and calories in our diet while promoting sound nutrition. By carefully following such a diet plan, people with elevated serum cholesterol levels typically are able to reduce their cholesterol levels by 30 to 55 mg/dl.[4] However, dietary changes do not affect people equally; some will experience greater reductions than others. Some will not respond at all to dietary changes and may need to take cholesterol-lowering medications and increase physical activity.

Cholesterol is attached to structures called *lipoproteins.* Lipoproteins are particles that circulate in the blood and transport lipids (including cholesterol).[5] Two major classes of lipoproteins exist: **low-density lipoproteins (LDLs)** and **high-density lipoproteins (HDLs).** A person's total cholesterol level is determined by the amount of the LDLs and HDLs in a measured sample of blood. (For example, a person's total cholesterol level of 200 mg/dl could be represented by an LDL level of 160 and an HDL level of 40, or an LDL level of 140 and an HDL level of 60.)

After much scientific study, it has been determined that high levels of LDL are a significant cause of atherosclerosis. This makes sense because LDLs carry the greatest percentage of cholesterol in the bloodstream. LDLs are more likely to deposit excess cholesterol into the artery walls. This contributes to plaque formation.

atherosclerosis
Buildup of plaque on the inner walls of arteries.

myocardial infarction
Heart attack; the death of part of the heart muscle as a result of a blockage in one of the coronary arteries.

low-density lipoprotein (LDL)
The type of lipoprotein that transports the largest amount of cholesterol in the bloodstream; high levels of LDL are related to heart disease.

high-density lipoprotein (HDL)
The type of lipoprotein that transports cholesterol from the bloodstream to the liver, where it is eventually removed from the body; high levels of HDL are related to a reduction in heart disease.

HEALTH
Action Guide ------→

Recognizing Signs of a Heart Attack and Taking Action

Warning Signs of a Heart Attack
- Uncomfortable pressure, fullness, squeezing, or pain in the center of your chest lasting 2 minutes or longer
- Pain spreading to your shoulders, neck, or arms
- Severe pain, dizziness, fainting, sweating, nausea, or shortness of breath

Not all of these warning signs occur with every heart attack. If some start to occur, don't wait. Get help immediately!

What to Do in an Emergency
- Find out which hospitals in your area have 24-hour emergency cardiac care.
- Determine (in advance) the hospital or medical facility that is nearest your home and office, and tell your family and friends to call this facility in an emergency.
- Keep a list of emergency rescue service numbers next to your telephone and in your pocket, wallet, or purse.
- If you have chest discomfort that lasts for 2 minutes or more, call the emergency rescue service.
- If you can get to a hospital faster by going yourself and not waiting for an ambulance, have someone drive you there.

Be a Heart Saver
- If you are with someone experiencing the signs of a heart attack and the warning signs last for 2 minutes or longer, act immediately.
- Expect a "denial." It is normal for someone with chest discomfort to deny the possibility of something as serious as a heart attack. Don't take "no" for an answer. Insist on taking prompt action.
- Call the rescue service (911), or get to the nearest hospital emergency room that offers 24-hour emergency cardiac care.
- Give CPR (mouth-to-mouth breathing and chest compression) if it is necessary and if you are properly trained. ◄------•

For this reason, LDLs are often called the "bad cholesterol."[6] High LDL levels are determined partially by inheritance, but they are also clearly associated with smoking, poor dietary patterns, obesity, and lack of exercise.

On the other hand, high levels of HDLs are related to a decrease in the development of atherosclerosis. HDLs are thought to transport cholesterol out of the bloodstream. Thus HDLs have been called the "good cholesterol." Certain lifestyle alterations, such as quitting smoking, reducing obesity, increasing physical activity, and decreasing dietary fats, help many people increase their level of HDLs.

Reducing total serum cholesterol levels is a significant step in reducing the risk of death from coronary heart disease. For people with elevated cholesterol levels, a 1% reduction in serum cholesterol level yields about a 2% reduction in the risk of death from heart disease. Thus a 10% to 15% cholesterol reduction can reduce risk by 20% to 30%.[7] Study Table 10-1 for cholesterol classifications and current recommended follow-up.

Angina pectoris. When coronary arteries become narrowed, chest pain, or *angina pectoris,* is often felt. This pain results from a reduced supply of oxygen to heart muscle tissue. Usually, angina is felt when the patient becomes stressed or exercises too strenuously. Angina reportedly can range from a feeling of mild indigestion to a severe viselike pressure in the chest. The pain may extend from the center of the chest to the arms and even up to the jaw. Generally, the more severe the blockage, the more pain is felt.

Table 10-1   Classification and Recommended Follow-up Based on Total Cholesterol Level

Total Cholesterol Level	Classification	Recommended Follow-up
<200 mg/dl	Desirable blood cholesterol level	Repeat test within 5 years
200-239 mg/dl	Borderline-high blood cholesterol level	*Without* definite CHD or two other CHD risk factors (one of which may be male gender): dietary modification and annual retesting *With* definite CHD or two other CHD risk factors: lipoprotein analysis; further action based on LDL-cholesterol level
≤240 mg/dl	High blood cholesterol level	Lipoprotein analysis; further action based on LDL-cholesterol level

Some cardiac patients relieve angina with the drug *nitroglycerin,* a powerful blood vessel dilator. This prescription drug, available in slow-release transdermal patches or small pills that are placed under the patient's tongue, causes the coronary arteries to dilate and allow a greater flow of blood into heart muscle tissue. Other cardiac patients may be prescribed drugs such as **calcium channel blockers** or **beta blockers.**

Emergency response to heart crises

Heart attacks are not always fatal. The consequences of any heart attack depend on the location of the damage to the heart, the extent to which heart muscle is damaged, and the speed with which adequate circulation is restored. Injury to the ventricles may very well prove fatal unless medical countermeasures are immediately undertaken. The recognition of heart attack is critically important (see the Health Action Guide on p. 238).

Cardiopulmonary resuscitation (CPR) is one of the most important immediate countermeasures that trained people can use when confronted with a victim of heart attack. Public education programs sponsored by the American Red Cross and the American Heart Association teach people how to recognize, evaluate, and manage heart attack emergencies. CPR trainees are taught how to restore breathing (through mouth-to-mouth resuscitation) and circulation (through external chest compression) in people who require such emergency countermeasures. Frequently, colleges offer CPR classes through health science or physical education departments. We encourage each student to enroll in a CPR course.

Diagnosis and coronary repair

Once a person's vital signs have stabilized, further diagnostic examinations can reveal the type and extent of damage to heart muscle. Initially an ECG might be taken. This test analyzes the electrical activity of the heart. *Heart catheterization,* also called *coronary arteriography,* is a minor surgical procedure that starts by placing a thin plastic tube into an arm or leg

HEALTH Action Guide

Monitoring Your Cholesterol Level

The next time you get your blood cholesterol level checked, try to find out more than just your total cholesterol level. Ask for the following three measurements, and compare them with the desirable measurements for adults, listed below.

Readings for	Your measurement	Desirable measurement
HDL level:	_____	Above 45 mg/dl
LDL level:	_____	Below 130 mg/dl
Total level:	_____	Below 200 mg/dl

How do your measurements compare with the desirable measurements? If they are not satisfactory, refer to Table 10-1 and the discussion on pp. 237-238 to improve your levels.

calcium channel blockers
Drugs that prevent arterial spasms; used in the long-term management of angina pectoris.

beta blockers
Drugs that prevent overactivity of the heart, which results in angina pectoris.

artery. This tube, called a *catheter,* is guided through the artery until it reaches the coronary circulation, where a *radiopaque dye* is then released. X-ray pictures called *angiograms* then record the progress of the dye through the coronary arteries. Areas of blockage are relatively easily identified.

Once the extent of damage is identified, a physician or team of physicians can decide on a medical course of action.[14] Currently popular is an extensive form of surgery called **coronary artery bypass surgery.** An estimated 468,000 bypass surgeries were performed in 1992.[1] The purpose of such surgery is to detour (bypass) areas of coronary artery obstruction by using a section of a vein from the patient's leg (often the saphenous vein) or an artery from the patient's chest (the internal mammary artery) and grafting it from the aorta to a location just beyond the area of obstruction. Multiple areas of obstruction result in double, triple, or quadruple bypasses.

Angioplasty. *Angioplasty,* an alternative to bypass surgery, involves the surgical insertion of a dough-nut-shaped "balloon" directly into the narrowed coronary artery (Figure 10-4). When this balloon is inflated, plaque and fatty deposits are compressed against the artery walls, widening the space through which blood flows. These balloons usually remain within the artery for less than 1 hour. Renarrowing of the artery will occur in about one quarter of angioplasty patients. Nearly 400,000 angioplasty procedures were performed in 1992.[1] Balloon angioplasty can be used for blockages in the heart, kidneys, arms, and legs. The decision whether to have angioplasty or bypass surgery can be a difficult one to make.[8]

In 1990 the FDA approved a new device for clearing heart and leg arteries. This device is called a *motorized scraper.*[9] Inserted through a leg artery and held in place by a tiny inflated balloon, this motor-driven cutter shaves off plaque deposits from inside the artery. A nose cone in the scraper unit stores the plaque until the device is removed.

The use of laser beams to dissolve plaque that blocks arteries has been slowly evolving. The FDA has approved three laser devices for use in clogged leg arteries. In February 1992 the FDA approved the use of an excimer laser for use in coronary arteries.[10]

Aspirin. Studies released in the late 1980s highlighted the role of aspirin in reducing the risk of heart attack in men who had no history of previous attacks. Specifically, the studies concluded that for men with hypertension, elevated cholesterol levels, or both, taking one aspirin per day was a significant factor in reducing their risk of heart attack. Aspirin works by making the blood less able to clot. This reduces the likelihood of blood vessel blockages. Presently, there is differing opinion regarding the age at which this preventive action should begin. The safest advice is to check with your physician before starting aspirin therapy.[11] Hopefully, studies on the role of aspirin therapy involving women will appear in the near future.

Alcohol. For years, scientists have been uncertain about the extent to which alcohol consumption is related to a reduced risk for heart disease. The current thinking is that moderate drinking (defined as no more than two drinks per day for men and one drink per day for women) is related to a lower heart disease risk. However, the benefit is much smaller than proven risk reduction behavior such as stopping smoking, reducing cholesterol level, lowering blood pressure, and increasing physical activity. Experts caution that heavy drinking increases cardiovascular risks and that nondrinkers should not start to drink just to reduce heart disease risk.

Heart transplants and artificial hearts. For approximately 30 years, surgeons have been able to surgically replace a person's damaged heart with that of another human being. Although very risky, these transplant operations have added years to the lives of a number of patients who otherwise would have lived only a short time. In 1993, 2298 heart transplants were performed in the United States.[1]

A   B

Figure 10-4   Angioplasty. **A,** A "balloon" is surgically inserted into the narrowed coronary artery. **B,** The balloon is inflated, compressing plaque and fatty deposits against the artery walls.

Artificial hearts have also been developed and implanted in humans. These mechanical devices have extended the lives of patients and have also served as temporary hearts while patients are waiting for a suitable donor heart. One of the important difficulties with artificial heart implantation has been the control of blood clots that may form, especially around the artificial valves.

Hypertension

Just as your car's water pump recirculates water and maintains water pressure, your heart recirculates blood and maintains blood pressure. When the heart contracts, blood is forced through your arteries and veins. Your blood pressure is a measure of the force that your circulating blood exerts against the interior walls of your arteries and veins.

Blood pressure is measured with a *sphygmomanometer*. A sphygmomanometer is attached to an arm-cuff device that can be inflated to stop the flow of blood temporarily in the brachial artery. This artery is a major supplier of blood to the lower arm. It is located on the inside of the upper arm, between the biceps and triceps muscles.

A physician, nurse, or technician using a stethoscope will listen for blood flow while the pressure in the cuff is released. Two pressure measurements will be recorded: the **systolic pressure** is the blood pressure against the vessel walls when the heart contracts, and the **diastolic pressure** is the blood pressure against the vessel walls when the heart relaxes (between heartbeats). Expressed in millimeters of mercury displaced on the sphygmomanometer, blood pressure is recorded in the form of a fraction, for example, 115/82. Because blood pressure drops when the heart relaxes, the diastolic pressure is always lower than the systolic pressure.

Although many people still consider 120/80 as a "normal" or safe blood pressure for a young adult, variations from this figure do not necessarily indicate a medical problem. In fact, many young college women of average weight will indicate blood pressures that seem to be relatively low (100/60, for example), yet these lowered blood pressures are quite "normal" for them. Any wide deviation from 120/80 in your blood pressure should be discussed with a physician.

Hypertension refers to a consistently elevated blood pressure. Generally, concern about a young adult's high blood pressure begins when he or she has a systolic reading of 140 or above or a diastolic reading of 90 or above.[5] Approximately 50 million American adults and children have hypertension. The American Heart Association reports that African-Americans, Puerto Ricans, Cuban-Americans, and Mexican-Americans have significantly higher rates of high blood pressure than white Americans.[1] Asian-Americans and Pacific Islanders have significantly lower rates of hypertension, however.[1]

Although the reasons for 90% to 95% of the cases of hypertension are not known, the health risks produced by uncontrolled hypertension are clearly understood. Throughout the body, hypertension makes arteries and arterioles become less elastic and thus incapable of dilating under a heavy workload. Brittle, calcified blood vessels can burst unexpectedly and produce serious strokes (brain accidents), kidney failure (renal accidents), or eye damage (**retinal hemorrhage).** Furthermore, it appears that blood and fat clots are more easily formed and dislodged in a vascular system affected by hypertension. Thus hypertension can be a cause of heart attacks. Clearly, hypertension is a potential killer.

Ironically, despite its deadly nature, hypertension is referred to as "the silent killer" because people with hypertension often are not aware that they have the condition. People with this disorder cannot feel the sensation of high blood pressure. The condition does not produce dizziness, headaches, or memory loss unless one is experiencing a medical crisis. Because it is a silent killer, it is estimated that nearly 35% of the people who have hypertension do not realize they have it.[1] Many who are aware of their hypertension do little to control it. Only a small percentage (21%) of people who have hypertension control it adequately, generally through dietary control, supervised fitness, relaxation training, and drug therapy.

Hypertension is not thought of as a curable disease; rather, it is a controllable disease. Once therapy is stopped, the condition returns. As a responsible adult, use every opportunity you can to measure your blood pressure on a regular basis.

---

coronary artery bypass surgery
Surgical procedure designed to improve blood flow to the heart by providing alternative routes for blood to take around points of blockage.

systolic pressure (sis tol ick)
Blood pressure against blood vessel walls when the heart contracts.

diastolic pressure (dye uh stol ick)
Blood pressure against blood vessel walls when the heart relaxes.

retinal hemorrhage
Uncontrolled bleeding from arteries within the eye's retina.

Prevention and treatment. Weight reduction, physical activity, moderation in alcohol use, and sodium restriction are often used to reduce hypertension. For overweight or obese people, a reduction in body weight may produce a significant drop in blood pressure. Physical activity helps lower blood pressure by expending calories (which leads to weight loss) and improving overall circulation. Reducing alcohol consumption to less than 2 ounces daily helps reduce blood pressure in some people.

The restriction of sodium (salt) in the diet also helps some people reduce hypertension. Interestingly, this strategy is effective only for those who are **salt sensitive**—estimated to be about 25% of the population. Reducing salt intake would have little effect on the blood pressure of the rest of the population. Nevertheless, since our daily intake of salt vastly exceeds our need for salt, the general recommendation to curb salt intake still makes good sense.

Many of the stress reduction activities we discuss in Chapter 3 are receiving increased attention in the struggle to reduce hypertension. In recent years, behavioral scientists have reported the success of meditation, biofeedback, controlled breathing, and muscle relaxation exercises in reducing hypertension. Look for further research findings in these areas in the years to come.

In the late 1990s, there are literally dozens of drugs that are available for use by people with hypertension.[12] Unfortunately, many patients refuse to take their medication on a consistent basis, probably because of the mistaken notion that "you must feel sick to be sick." Nutritional supplements, such as calcium, magnesium, potassium, and fish oil, are not effective in lowering blood pressure.[13]

Stroke

Stroke is a general term for a wide variety of crises (sometimes called *cerebrovascular accidents* [CVAs]) that result from blood vessel damage in the brain. African-Americans have a 60% greater risk of stroke than white Americans do, probably because African-Americans have a greater likelihood of having hypertension than white Americans. Data for 1992 indicate that 143,640 deaths and half a million new cases of stroke occurred.[1] Just as the heart muscle needs an adequate blood supply, so does the brain. Any disturbance in the proper supply of oxygen and nutrients to the brain can pose a threat.

Perhaps the most common form of stroke results from the blockage of a cerebral (brain) artery. Similar to coronary occlusions, **cerebrovascular occlusions** can be started by a clot that forms within an artery, called a *thrombus,* or by a clot that travels from another part of the body to the brain, called an *embolus* (Figure 10-5, *A* and *B*). The resultant accidents (*cerebral thrombosis* or *cerebral embolism*) cause between 70% and 80% of all strokes. The portion of the brain deprived of oxygen and nutrients can literally die.

A third type of stroke can result from an artery that bursts to produce a crisis called *cerebral hemorrhage* (Figure 10-5, *C*). Damaged, brittle arteries can be especially susceptible to bursting when a person has hypertension.

A fourth form of stroke is a *cerebral aneurysm.* An aneurysm is a ballooning or outpouching on a weakened area of an artery (Figure 10-5, *D*). Aneurysms may occur in various locations of the body and are not always life threatening. The development of aneurysms is not fully understood, although there seems to be a relationship between aneurysms and hypertension. It is quite possible that many aneurysms are congenital defects. In any case, when a cerebral aneurysm bursts, a stroke results. See the Health Action Guide on p. 244 to learn the warning signs of stroke.

A person who reports any warning signs of stroke or any small stroke, called a **transient ischemic attack (TIA),** will undergo a battery of diagnostic tests, which could include a physical examination, a search for possible brain tumors, tests to identify areas of the brain affected, use of the electroencephalogram, cerebral arteriography, and the use of the **CAT** (computerized axial tomography) **scan** or **MRI** (magnetic resonance imaging) **scan.** Many additional tests are also available.

Treatment of stroke patients depends on the nature and extent of the damage. Some patients require surgery (to repair vessels and relieve pressure) and acute care in the hospital. Others undergo drug treatment, especially the use of anticoagulant drugs, including aspirin.

The advancements made in the rehabilitation of stroke patients are amazing. Although some severely affected patients have little hope of improvement, our increasing advancements in the application of computer technology to such disciplines as speech and physical therapy offer encouraging signs for stroke patients and their families.

Congenital Heart Disease

A congenital defect is one that is present at birth. The American Heart Association estimates that each year about 32,000 babies are born with a congenital heart defect. In 1992, 5600 children (mostly infants) died of congenital heart disease.[1]

A variety of abnormalities may be produced by congenital heart disease, including valve damage, holes in the walls of the septum, blood vessel transpo-

Thrombus
A clot that forms within
a narrowed section of a
blood vessel and remains
at its place of origin.

Embolus
A clot that moves through
the circulatory system and
becomes lodged at a nar-
rowed point within a vessel.

Hemorrhage
The sudden bursting
of a blood vessel.

Aneurysm
A sac formed when a
section of a blood vessel
thins and balloons; the
weakened wall of the sac
can burst, or rupture, as
shown here.

Figure 10-5   Causes of stroke.

sition, and an underdevelopment of the left side of the heart. All of these problems ultimately prevent a new-born baby from adequately oxygenating tissues throughout the body. A bluish skin color (cyanosis) is seen in some infants with such congenital heart defects. These infants are sometimes referred to as *blue babies*.

The cause of congenital heart defects is not clearly understood, although one cause, *rubella*, has been identified. The fetuses of mothers who contract the rubella virus during the first 3 months of pregnancy are at great risk of developing *congenital rubella syndrome (CRS)*, a catchall term for a wide variety of congenital defects, including heart defects, deafness, cataracts, and mental retardation. Other hypotheses about the development of congenital heart disease implicate environmental pollutants; maternal use of drugs, including alcohol, during pregnancy; and unknown genetic factors. (see the Star Box on p. 244)

Treatment of congenital defects usually requires surgery, although some conditions may respond well to drug therapy. Defective blood vessels and certain mal-formations of the heart can be surgically repaired. This surgery is so successful that many children respond quite quickly to the increased circulation and oxygena-tion. Many are able to lead normal, active lives.

Rheumatic Heart Disease

Rheumatic heart disease is the final stage in a series of complications started by a streptococcal infection of the throat (strep throat). The Star Box at

salt sensitive
Term used to describe people whose bodies overreact to the presence of sodium by retaining fluid and thus experience an increase in blood pressure.

cerebrovascular occlusion
(ser **ee** bro **vas** kyou lar)
Blockages to arteries supplying blood to the cerebral cortex of the brain; strokes.

transient ischemic attack (TIA) (**tran** see ent iss **key** mick)
Strokelike symptoms caused by temporary spasm of cerebral blood vessels.

CAT scan
Computerized axial tomography scan; an x-ray procedure that is designed to visualize struc-tures within the body that would not normally be seen through conventional x-ray procedures.

MRI scan
Magnetic resonance imaging scan; an imaging procedure that uses a giant magnet to generate an image of body tissue.

rheumatic heart disease
Chronic damage to the heart (especially heart valves) resulting from a streptococcal infection within the heart; a complication associated with rheumatic fever.

HEALTH
Action Guide - - - - ➤

Recognizing Warning Signs of Stroke

Although many stroke victims have little advance warning of an impending crisis, there are some warning signals of stroke that should be recognized. The American Heart Association encourages everyone to be aware of the following signs:

- Sudden, temporary weakness or numbness of the face, arm, and leg on one side of the body
- Temporary loss of speech or trouble in speaking or understanding speech
- Temporary dimness or loss of vision, particularly in one eye
- Unexplained dizziness, unsteadiness, or sudden falls

Many severe strokes are preceded by "little strokes," warning signals like the above, experienced days, weeks, or months before the more severe event. Prompt medical or surgical attention to these symptoms may prevent a fatal or disabling stroke from occurring.   ◀ - - - - -

right lists common symtoms of strep throat. This bacterial infection, if untreated, can result in an inflammatory disease called *rheumatic fever* (and a related condition, scarlet fever). Rheumatic fever is a whole-body (systemic) reaction that can produce fever, joint pain, skin rashes, and possible brain and heart damage. A person who has had rheumatic fever is more susceptible to subsequent attacks. Rheumatic fever tends to run in families. Approximately 6000 Americans died from rheumatic fever and rheumatic heart disease in 1992.[1]

Damage from rheumatic fever centers on the heart's valves. For some reason the bacteria tend to proliferate in the heart valves. Defective heart valves may fail either to open fully (*stenosis*) or to close fully (*insufficiency*). Diagnosis of valve damage might initially come when a physician hears a backwashing or backflow of blood (a **murmur**). Further tests—including chest x-rays, cardiac catheterization, and echocardiography—can reveal the extent of valve damage.[5] Once identified, a faulty valve can be replaced surgically with a metal or plastic artificial valve or a valve taken from an animal's heart.

Related cardiovascular conditions

Besides the cardiovascular diseases already discussed, the heart and blood vessels are also subject to other pathological conditions. Tumors of the heart, although rare, occur. Infectious conditions involving the pericardial sac that surrounds the heart (*pericarditis*) and the innermost layer of the heart (*endocarditis*) are more commonly seen. In addition, inflammation of the veins (*phlebitis*) is troublesome to some people.

Peripheral artery disease. Peripheral artery disease (PAD), also called *peripheral vascular disease (PVD),* is a blood vessel disease characterized by pathological changes to the arteries and arterioles in the extremities (primarily the legs and feet but sometimes the hands). These changes result from years of damage to the peripheral blood vessels. Important causes of PAD are cigarette smoking, a high-fat diet, obesity, and sedentary occupations. In some cases, PAD is aggravated by blood vessel changes resulting from diabetes.

PAD severely restricts blood flow to the extremities. The reduction in blood flow is responsible for leg pain or cramping during exercise, numbness, tingling, coldness, and loss of hair in the affected limb. The most serious consequence of PAD is the increased likelihood of developing ulcerations and tissue death. These conditions can lead to gangrene and may eventually necessitate amputation.

The treatment of PAD consists of multiple approaches and may include efforts to improve blood lipid levels (through diet, exercise, or drug therapy), reduce hypertension, reduce body weight, and

Risk Factors for Congenital and Rheumatic Heart Disease

Risk Factors for Congenital Heart Disease
Fetal exposure to rubella, other viral infections, pollutants, alcohol, or tobacco smoke during pregnancy

Risk Factors for Rheumatic Heart Disease
Streptococcal infection

Common Symptoms of Strep Throat
Sudden onset of sore throat, particularly with pain when swallowing

Fever
Swollen, tender glands under the angle of the jaw
Headache
Nausea and vomiting
Tonsils covered with a yellow or white pus or discharge

eliminate smoking. Blood vessel surgery may be a possibility.

Congestive heart failure. Congestive heart failure is a condition in which the heart lacks the strength to continue to circulate blood normally throughout the body. During congestive heart failure, the heart continues to work, but it cannot function well enough to maintain appropriate circulation. Venous blood flow starts to "back up." Swelling occurs, especially in the legs and ankles. Fluid can collect in the lungs and cause breathing difficulties and shortness of breath, and kidney function may be damaged.[5]

Congestive heart failure can result from heart damage caused by congenital heart defects, lung disease, rheumatic fever, heart attack, atherosclerosis, or high blood pressure. Generally, congestive heart failure is treatable through a combined program of rest, proper diet, modified daily activities, and the use of appropriate drugs. Without medical care, congestive heart failure can be fatal.

murmur
An atypical heart sound that suggests a backwashing of blood into a chamber of the heart from which it has just left.

peripheral artery disease (PAD)
Damage resulting from restricted blood flow to the extremities, especially the legs and feet.

congestive heart failure
Inability of the heart to pump out all the blood that returns to it; can lead to dangerous fluid accumulations in veins, lungs, and kidneys.

Summary

- Cardiovascular disorders are responsible for more disabilities and deaths than any other disease.
- The cardiovascular system consists of the heart, blood, and blood vessels. This system performs many functions.
- Our overall health depends on the health of the cardiovascular system.
- A cardiovascular risk factor is an attribute that a person has or is exposed to that increases the likelihood of heart disease.
- The "big four" risk factors are cigarette smoking, high blood pressure, high blood cholesterol level,

and physical inactivity. These are controllable risk factors.
- Heredity, male gender, and increasing age are risk factors that cannot be controlled.
- Contributing risk factors are diabetes, obesity, and individual response to stress.
- The major forms of cardiovascular disease include coronary artery disease, high blood pressure, stroke, congenital heart disease, and rheumatic heart disease. Each disease develops in a specific way and may require a highly specialized form of treatment.

Review Questions

1. Identify the principal components of the cardiovascular system. Trace the path of blood through the heart and cardiovascular system.
2. How much blood does the average adult have? What are some of the important functions of blood?
3. Define cardiovascular risk factor. What relationship do risk factors have to cardiovascular disease?
4. Identify those risk factors for cardiovascular disease that cannot be changed. Identify those risk factors that can be changed. Identify those risk factors that are contributing factors.

5. What are the major forms of cardiovascular disease? For each of these diseases, describe what the disease is, its cause (if known), and its treatment.
6. Describe how high-density lipoproteins differ from low-density lipoproteins.
7. What problems does atherosclerosis produce?
8. Why is hypertension referred to as "the silent killer"?
9. What are the warning signals of stroke?

Think About This . . .

- Have you ever considered your potential for developing heart disease?
- In the last week, what have you done to improve your cardiovascular system?
- Do you know your total cholesterol reading? Do you know your levels of LDLs and HDLs?

- When was the last time you had your blood pressure checked? What were the readings?
- What role should men play in reducing the threats of congenital heart disease?
- Are you comfortable talking with your relatives about their possible risk factors?

References

1. The American Heart Association: *Heart and stroke facts: 1995 statistical supplement,* Dallas, 1995, The Association.
2. Thibodeau GA: *Structure and function of the body,* ed 9, St Louis, 1992, Mosby.
3. Thibodeau GA, Patton KT: *The human body in health and disease,* St Louis, 1992, Mosby.
4. US Department of Health and Human Services: *Report of the expert panel on detection, evaluation, and treatment of high blood cholesterol in adults,* US Department of Health and Human Services, Public Health Service, NIH Pub No 89-2925, Washington, DC, 1989, US Government Printing Office.
5. American Heart Association: *Heart and stroke facts,* Dallas, 1995, The Association.
6. American Heart Association: *Cholesterol and your heart,* ed 4, Dallas, 1995, The Association.
7. Cholesterol: up with the good, *Harvard Heart Letter,* 5(11):3-4, 1995.
8. Best choice: bypass or angioplasty? *Johns Hopkins Medical Letter: Health After 50,* 7(5):1-2, 1995.
9. Farley D: Help for hearts and blood vessels: balloons, lasers and scrapers, *FDA Consumer* 25(3):22-27, 1991.
10. Friend T: Laser OK'd to unclog heart arteries, *USA Today,* p1D, Feb 7, 1992.
11. Husten L: Clot prevention: anticoagulants to the rescue, *Harvard Health Letter,* 20(12):6-8, 1995.
12. The best drugs for hypertension, *The Johns Hopkins Medical Letter: Health After 50,* 7(4):1-2, 1995.
13. Trials of Hypertension Prevention Collaborative Research Group: The effects of nonpharmacologic interventions on blood pressure of persons with high normal levels: results of the trials of hypertension prevention, Phase 1, *JAMA* 267(9):1213-1220, 1992.
14. Gillis J: *The heart attack prevention and recovery handbook,* Point Roberts, Wash, 1995, Hartley and Marks Publishers.
15. Klieman C, Osborne K: *If it runs in your family: heart disease: reducing your risk,* New York, 1991, Bantam Books.

Suggested Readings

Gillis J: *The heart attack prevention and recovery handbook,* Point Roberts, Wash, 1995, Hartley and Marks Publishers. Written by a cardiologist, this 150-page handbook contains information concerning cardiovascular disease risk factors, a plan for heart attack prevention, and treatment options. Also covered are CVD in women and the elderly. Easy-to-read format.

Page HC, Schroeder JS: *The Stanford life plan for a healthy heart,* San Francisco, 1996, Chronicle Books. This book explains the program developed by a team of heart specialists at Stanford University. The major focus is on diet and its connection to heart disease. Also presented is the Stanford 25 Gram Plan, a way to control saturated fat in the diet. A detailed section on fat and cholesterol is provided with a strategy for reversing heart disease. Over 200 low-fat recipes are included.

Hypertension in African-Americans

Development of disease is an area in which each societal group is disadvantaged in one way or another. Practically every group has a tendency to develop one or more afflictions at a higher rate than the general population. For the African-American community, one particular problem is hypertension.

The existing data show that hypertension is more common in African-Americans[1,2] and is more aggressive and less well-managed in African-Americans than in whites. African-Americans also have higher rates of morbidity and mortality from diseases related to high blood pressure, such as stroke and renal failure. The natural nocturnal fall in blood pressure is less pronounced in African-Americans, and their systolic blood pressure while awake is higher than in people of other races.[1]

The exact causes of these differences have not been pinpointed, but research seems to be focused in two general areas. Some research suggests that certain physical and genetic factors contribute to increased incidence of hypertension in African-Americans, whereas other studies have shown that hypertension in African-Americans is related to environmental stress. This debate involves not just medical data but socioeconomic factors as well. In short, it is a nature vs. nurture debate, and there are supporting data for both arguments.

Nature vs. nurture

Studies have shown that environmental stress may contribute to increased hypertension in African-Americans. A study conducted by Dr. Norman Anderson of Duke University[3] shows that chronic stress may lead to an increase in the release of the hormone norepinephrine to the bloodstream. Norepinephrine reduces the amount of salt eliminated from the kidneys, and the resulting increase in blood salt content can lead to increased blood pressure. This chain reaction has been shown to occur in animal studies. The high rate of chronic exposure to stress in many African-American communities has been well documented.[3] If these studies hold true for humans, it would lend credence to the idea that certain stressful factors found in some African-American communities could cause hypertension. Stressors such as poverty, unemployment, the threat of violence, and racial discrimination could be shown to cause kidneys to reduce elimination of salt and thus may also increase the risk of hypertension.[3]

Anger in response to racism may be a significant contributing factor in increased hypertension in African-Americans. A study conducted jointly at the University of Tennessee and Saint Louis University showed that blood pressure in African-Americans increased significantly when they were shown film clips of racially motivated violence.[4] The responses of African-Americans to these scenes of racial discrimination were more pronounced than their responses to viewing scenes that were anger-provoking but had no racial component. The increases in blood pressure were not into the hypertension range, but researchers believe that over time, such continued elevation of blood pressure could become dangerous.

Such conclusions seem to suggest that socioeconomic factors are the main cause of hypertension among African-Americans. A study performed on 26 African-American women on strict low-fat diets seems to support this. The data showed that women of higher socioeconomic status had more excretion of salt than those of lower status.[3] Since proportionately more African-Americans are in lower socioeconomic classes than whites, increased stress from lower status could be the main factor behind the inflated rate of hypertension among the African-American population.

But is it all due to environment? Perhaps not. Other groups of traditionally lower socioeconomic status, such Hispanics, Asians, and Native Americans, have been found to have the same incidence of hypertension as whites.[1] African-American children have been found to have higher blood pressure in general than white children[1]; it is not known whether stress plays a significant role in affecting the blood pressure of these children so early in life.

There is also evidence that African-Americans may be predisposed to hypertension at the cellular level. Microscopic studies of blood vessels in African-Americans with severe hypertension revealed that renal arterioles were thickened and had reduced flow. This thickening, not found in the renal arterioles of hypertensive whites, was caused by hypertrophy (excess growth) of smooth muscle cells in the muscle walls of the arterioles. This thickening reduced the size of the lumen (inside opening) of the vessels, and the resulting reduced blood flow may have caused increased blood pressure. The smooth muscle cells were thought to be responding abnormally to growth factors, which caused the hypertrophy to occur.[2] The reason behind this abnormal reaction was not determined, however.

The best explanation of why African-Americans are more prone to develop hypertension may not involve environment or genetics alone, but a combination of the two. Stress factors unique to the African-American community may serve to aggravate or intensify an existing physical predisposition toward hypertension. It has already been shown that the tendency toward developing hypertension can be passed from parents to their children. Add several unique stress factors to a population already predisposed to high blood pressure, and the potential exists for high numbers of people to develop hypertension. Commenting on the UT-SLU study, Dr. Elijah Saunders agreed that "racism and Black rage are emotional stressors that could worsen a physiological tendency toward hypertension."[4]

Treatment for hypertension in African-Americans

The good news is that African-Americans respond to medical treatment in a similar manner to whites. The treatment regimen for African-Americans may have to be altered somewhat, however, since they do not respond as well to some hypertension medications as people of other races. For unknown reasons, drugs such as beta-blockers and ACE (angiotensin converting enzyme) inhibitors do not work as well in African-Americans and may need to be supplemented by other medications, such as diuretics.[1]

Lifestyle changes may also be needed and may be a more effective tool in lowering blood pressure in African-Americans than in people of other races.[1] Effort should be made to exercise and lose weight if needed, since excess weight can be a contributing factor in hypertension. African-American women in particular should make a strong effort to control their weight, since data suggest that African-American women have a greater tendency to become overweight. Hypertensive African-Americans tend to have lower intakes of potassium and calcium, so diet changes should be made that ensure that these minerals are in adequate supply. A reduction in sodium may also be desirable, since research suggests that African-Americans may be more sensitive to the effects of sodium on the cardiovascular system.[1]

Although African-Americans are more likely to develop high blood pressure, prevention and treatment can help keep hypertension from becoming a deadly affliction. Proper diagnosis is essential, so people at risk should see their doctors to determine whether they have hypertension or are at risk for developing it. Through recommending lifestyle modifications, prescribing medications, or both, a physician can help manage this condition or help prevent its onset.

For Discussion . . .

Do you feel that people in lower (or higher) socioeconomic groups suffer more from everyday stress? Do you believe physiological or genetic differences may exist between different ethnic or racial groups?

References

1. Kaplan NM: Ethnic aspects of hypertension, *Lancet* 344(8920), 1994.
2. Dustan HP: Growth factors and racial differences in severity of hypertension and renal diseases, *Lancet* 339(8805), 1992.
3. Haywood RL: Why Black Americans suffer with more high blood pressure than Whites, *Jet* Dec 5, 1994, 87(5).
4. Study reveals anger over racism causes high blood pressure in Blacks, *Jet* May 14, 1990, 78(5)

Chapter

Living with Cancer and Chronic Conditions

Healthy People 2000 Objectives

Reversing the rise in the incidence of cancer-related deaths was a key objective stated in the Healthy People 2000 document. The Midcourse Review reports that some advancement was made toward this goal, but less than was desired. Information from other sources suggests that uneven progress has been made regarding particular kinds of cancer within various population subgroups.

The Midcourse Review points to encouraging success in reducing death rates from some types of cancer. For example, the death rate from breast cancer in women has been reduced. Another achievement is the reduced death rate from colorectal cancer. However, death rates from certain other kinds of cancer, such as lung cancer, have increased (see Chapter 9).

Specific national objectives were also set in regard to noncancerous chronic health conditions. One main objective was to reduce the death rate from diabetes mellitus, but the Midcourse Review reports that no progress has been made in this area.

Most people can attest to the disruptive influence an illness can have on their ability to participate in day-to-day activities. When we are ill, school, employment, and leisure activities are replaced by periods of lessened activity and even periods of bed rest or hospitalization. When an illness is **chronic,** the effect of being ill may extend over long periods, perhaps even an entire life. People with chronic illness must eventually find a balance between day-to-day function and the continuous presence of their condition. Cancer is usually an illness that is chronic in nature.

THE STATUS OF CANCER TODAY AND TOMORROW

In spite of our understanding of its relationship to human health and our ceaseless attempts to prevent and cure it, progress in cancer prevention is at best limited. Even in light of the $27 billion spent on "the war on cancer" since 1971, deaths have risen 7% and the incidence of the disease has jumped 18% during that 25-year period.[1] A single simple answer to the question, "Why has this happened?" is not possible. It could, however, be a combination of factors, including the aging of the population, our failure to curb tobacco use, the high fat content of the typical American diet, the continuing urbanization and pollution of our environment, the presence of millions of people without health insurance to pay for early diagnosis and proper treatment, or, simply, our ability to recognize its true role in deaths ascribed to other causes. Regardless, we are still challenged to bring under control the abnormal cellular activity that we call cancer.

CANCER: A PROBLEM OF CELL REGULATION

In much the same manner that a corporation depends on competent individuals to staff its various departments, the body depends on its basic units of function—the cells. Cells band together as tissues, such as muscle tissue, to perform a prescribed function. Tissues in turn join to form organs, such as the heart, and organs are assembled into the body's several organ systems, such as the cardiovascular system. Such is the "corporate structure" of the body.

If individuals and cells are the basic units of function for their respective organizations, the failure of either to perform in a prescribed, dependable manner can erode the overall organization to the extent that it might not be able to continue. Cancer, the second leading cause of death among adults, is a condition reflecting cell dysfunction in its most extreme form.[2] In cancer the normal behavior of cells ceases.

Cell Regulation

Most of the tissues of the body lose cells over time. This continual loss requires that replacement cells be brought forward from areas of young and less specialized cells. The process of *specialization* required to turn the less specialized cells into mature cells is carefully controlled by genes within the cells. On becoming specialized, these newest cells copy, or *replicate*, themselves. These two processes are carefully monitored by the cells' **regulatory genes.** Failure to regulate specialization and replication results in abnormal, or cancerous, cells.[3]

In addition to genes that regulate specialization and replication, cells also have genes designed to repair mistakes in the copying of genetic material (the basis of replication) and genes to suppress the growth of abnormal cells should they occur. Thus *repair genes* and *suppressor genes,* such as the p53 gene, join regulatory genes to prevent the development of abnormal cells.[3] Should these genes fail to function properly, resulting in the development of malignant (cancerous) cells, the immune system (see Chapter 12) will ideally recognize their presence and remove them before a clinical (diagnosable) case of cancer can develop.

Because specialization, replication, repair, and suppressor genes can become cancer-causing genes, or **oncogenes,** when not working properly, these four types of genes could also be referred to as **protooncogenes,** or potential oncogenes.[3] How protooncogenes become oncogenes is a question that cannot be completely answered at this time. Although a detailed explanation lies outside the scope of a personal health textbook, a simplified account is provided.

Oncogene Formation

Recognizing that all cells have protooncogenes, what events alter otherwise normal cancer-preventing genes so that they become cancer-causing genes? Three mechanisms, genetic mutations, viral infections, and carcinogens, have received much attention.

Genetic mutations develop when dividing cells miscopy genetic information. If the gene that is miscopied is a protooncogene, the oncogene that results will stimulate the formation of cancerous cells. A variety of factors, including aging, free radical formation, radiation, and an array of carcinogens, are associated with the miscopying of the complex genetic information that comprises the genes found within the cell, including those intended to prevent cancer.

In both animals and humans, *cancer-producing viruses,* such as the feline leukemia virus in cats and the HIV virus in humans (see Chapter 12), have been identified. These viruses seek out cells of a particular type, such as cells of the immune system, and alter their genetic material to convert these cells into virus-producing cells. In so doing, however, they change the makeup of the specialization, replication, repair, or suppressor genes, converting the protooncogenes into oncogenes. Once converted into oncogenes, the altered genes are passed on through cell division.

A third possible explanation for the conversion of protooncogenes into oncogenes involves the presence of environmental agents known as *carcinogens.* Over an extended period, carcinogens, such as chemicals found in tobacco smoke, polluted air and water, toxic wastes, and even the high fat content of foods, may convert protooncogenes into oncogenes. These carcinogens may work alone or in combination *(co-carcinogens).* Thus people might develop lung cancer only if they are exposed to the right combination of carcinogens over an extended period.

Our understanding of the role of genes in the development of cancer is expanding rapidly. In conjunction with the **Human Genome Project,** the scientific community has now identified dozens of genes that function as oncogenes in a variety of human cancers. Among these are genes involved in the development of lung cancer (p16), breast cancer (BRCA1 and BRCA2), colon cancer (MSH2 and MSH1), and a form of leukemia (ALL-1 and AF-9).[4-6] As geneticists continue to map the human genome and, in doing so, discover additional genetic links to cancer, the possibility of some form of "gene-repair" technology becomes a more realistic possibility in the war against cancer.

The Cancerous Cell

In comparison with their noncancerous cousins, cancer cells are both similar and dissimilar in terms of how they function. It is the dissimilar aspects that in most cases make them unpredictable and more difficult to manage.

Perhaps the most different aspect of cancerous cells is their infinite life expectancy. Specifically, it appears that cancerous cells can produce an enzyme, *telomerase,* that blocks the biological clock that informs normal cells that it is time to die. In spite of this ability to live forever, cancer cells do not necessarily divide more quickly than normal cells. In fact, they can divide at the same rate or even at a slower rate.[3]

Because cancerous cells do not possess the *contact inhibition* (a control mechanism that influences the

number of cells that can occupy a particular space) of normal cells, they can accumulate and eventually alter the structure of a body organ or break through its wall into neighboring areas (invasion). Additionally, the absence of *cellular cohesiveness* (a property seen in normal cells that "keeps them at home") allows cancer cells to spread through the circulatory or lymphatic system to distant points via **metastasis** (Figure 11-1). A final unique characteristic of cancerous cells is their ability to command the circulatory system to send them additional blood supply to meet their metabolic needs and to provide additional routes for metastasis. This *angiogenesis potential* of cancer cells makes them extremely hardy in comparison with noncancerous cells.

Benign Tumors

Noncancerous, or **benign,** tumors can also form in the body. These **tumors** are usually enclosed by a

---

chronic
Develops slowly and persists for a long period of time.

regulatory genes
Genes within the cell that control cellular replication or doubling.

oncogenes
Genes that are believed to activate the development of cancer.

protooncogenes (**pro** toe **on** co genes)
Normal regulatory genes that may become oncogenes.

Human Genome Project
International quest by geneticists to identify the location and composition of every gene within the human cell.

metastasis (muh **tas** ta sis)
The spread of cancerous cells from their site of origin to other areas of the body.

benign
Noncancerous; tumors that do not spread.

tumor
Mass of cells; may be cancerous (malignant) or noncancerous (benign).

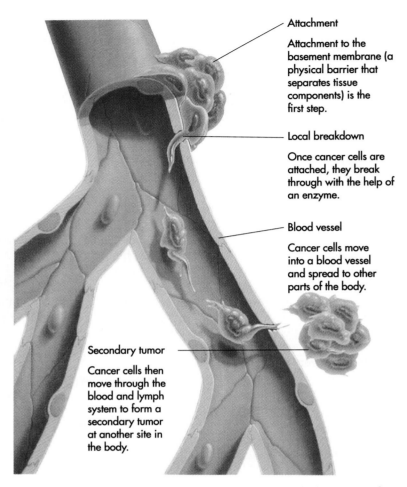

Attachment

Attachment to the basement membrane (a physical barrier that separates tissue components) is the first step.

Local breakdown

Once cancer cells are attached, they break through with the help of an enzyme.

Blood vessel

Cancer cells move into a blood vessel and spread to other parts of the body.

Secondary tumor

Cancer cells then move through the blood and lymph system to form a secondary tumor at another site in the body.

Figure 11-1   How cancer spreads. Locomotion is integral to the process of metastasis. Scientists have identified a protein that causes cancer cells to grow arms, or pseudopodia, enabling them to move to other parts of the body.

fibrous membrane and do not spread from their point of origin as cancerous tumors can. Benign tumors are dangerous, however, when they crowd out normal tissue within a confined space.

Types of Cancer and Their Locations

Cancers are named on the basis of the type of tissues in which they occur. The classifications below are used by physicians to describe malignancies to the layperson[3]:

carcinoma   Found most frequently in the skin, nose, mouth, throat, stomach, intestinal tract, glands, nerves, breasts, urinary and genital structures, lungs, kidneys, and liver; approximately 85% of all malignant tumors are classified as carcinomas

sarcoma   Formed in the connective tissues of the body; bone, cartilage, and tendons are the sites of sarcoma development; only 2% of all malignancies are of this type

melanoma   Arises from the melanin-containing cells of skin; found most often in individuals who have had extensive sun exposure, particularly a deep, penetrating sunburn; although once rare, the amount of this cancer has increased markedly in recent years; remains among the most deadly forms of cancer

neuroblastoma   Originates in the immature cells found within the central nervous system; neuroblastomas are rare; usually found in children

adenocarcinoma   Derived from cells of the endocrine glands

hepatoma   Originates in cells of the liver; although not thought to be directly caused by alcohol use, hepatomas are more frequently seen in individuals who have experienced **sclerotic changes** in the liver

leukemia   Found in cells of the blood and blood-forming tissues; characterized by abnormal, immature white blood cell formation; multiple forms found in children and adults

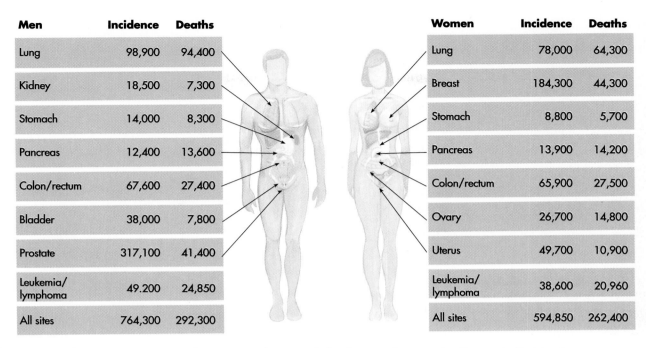

Men	Incidence	Deaths
Lung	98,900	94,400
Kidney	18,500	7,300
Stomach	14,000	8,300
Pancreas	12,400	13,600
Colon/rectum	67,600	27,400
Bladder	38,000	7,800
Prostate	317,100	41,400
Leukemia/ lymphoma	49.200	24,850
All sites	764,300	292,300

Women	Incidence	Deaths
Lung	78,000	64,300
Breast	184,300	44,300
Stomach	8,800	5,700
Pancreas	13,900	14,200
Colon/rectum	65,900	27,500
Ovary	26,700	14,800
Uterus	49,700	10,900
Leukemia/ lymphoma	38,600	20,960
All sites	594,850	262,400

Figure 11-2   These 1996 estimates of cancer incidence and deaths reveal some significant similarities between men and women. Note that lung cancer is the leading cause of cancer deaths for both genders.

lymphoma   Arises in cells of the lymphatic tissues or other immune system tissues; includes lymphosarcomas and Hodgkin's disease, characterized by abnormal white cell production and decreased resistance

Figure 11-2 presents information about the incidence of cancer and the deaths from cancer at various sites in both men and women.[7]

CANCER AT SELECTED SITES IN THE BODY

A second and more familiar way to describe cancer is on the basis of the organ (or tissue) site at which it occurs.[7] The following discussion relates to some of these more familiar sites. Regular screening procedures can lead to early identification of cancer at these sites (see the Health Action Guide on p. 254).

Lung

Lung cancer is one of the most lethal forms of cancer that is frequently diagnosed. Primarily because of the advanced stage at the time symptoms first appear, only 13% of all lung cancer victims survive 5 years beyond diagnosis.[7] By the time victims are sufficiently concerned about their persistent cough, blood-

streaked sputum, and chest pain, it is often too late for treatment to be effective.

Today it is known that a genetic predisposition is important in the development of lung cancer. Perhaps as many as 70% of the people who develop this form of cancer have an inherited "headstart."[8] When people who are genetically at risk also smoke, their level of risk for developing lung cancer is hundreds of times greater than it is for nonsmokers. About 30% of lung cancer cases appear in people who smoke but are not genetically predisposed. Environmental agents, such as radon, asbestos, and air pollutants, contribute to a lesser degree in the development of lung cancer.

According to the World Health Organization, the incidence of lung cancer has risen 200% for women, paralleling their increased smoking. Currently, lung cancer exceeds breast cancer as the leading cause of cancer deaths in women. The incidence of lung cancer has shown an encouraging decline in men while their use of tobacco drops.

sclerotic changes (skluh **rot** ick)
Thickening or hardening of tissues.

HEALTH Action Guide

Cancer-Related Checkups

Following are guidelines for the early detection of cancer in people without symptoms. Talk with your doctor—ask how these guidelines relate to you. Remember, these guidelines are not rules and apply only to people without symptoms. If you have any of the seven warning signs of cancer, see your doctor or go to your clinic without delay.

Age 20 to 40
Cancer-Related Checkup Every 3 Years
Should include the procedures listed below plus health counseling (such as tips on quitting smoking) and examinations for cancers of the thyroid, testes, prostate, mouth, ovaries, skin, and lymph nodes. *Some people are at higher risk for certain cancers and may need to have tests more frequently.*

Breast
- Examination by doctor every 3 years
- Self-examination every month
- One baseline mammogram between ages 35 and 40
Higher risk for breast cancer: personal or family history of breast cancer, never had children, first child after 30

Uterus
- Pelvic examination every 3 years

Cervix
- Pap test—after three initial negative tests 1 year apart—*at least* every 3 years; includes women under 20 if sexually active
Higher risk for cervical cancer: early age at first intercourse, multiple sex partners

Testes
- Self-examination every month
- Consult doctor when an abnormality is present
Higher risk for testicular cancer: personal or family history of testicular cancer, undescended testicles not corrected during early childhood, more prevalent in whites and in men under 35 years of age

Age 40 and Over
Cancer-Related Checkup Every Year
Should include the procedures listed plus health counseling (such as tips on quitting smoking) and examinations for cancers of the thyroid, testicles, prostate, mouth, ovaries, skin, and lymph nodes. *Some people are at higher risk for certain cancers and may need to have tests more frequently.*

Breasts
- Examination by doctor every year
- Self-examination every month
- Mammogram every year after age 50 (between ages 40 and 50, ask your doctor)
Higher risk for breast cancer: personal or family history of breast cancer, never had children, first child after 30

Uterus
- Pelvic examination every year

Cervix
- Pap test—after three initial negative tests 1 year apart—*at least* every 3 years
Higher risk for cervical cancer: early age at first intercourse, multiple sex partners

Endometrium
- Endometrial tissue sample at menopause if at risk
Higher risk for endometrial cancer: infertility, obesity, failure of ovulation, abnormal uterine bleeding, estrogen therapy

Testes
- Self-examination every month
- Consult doctor when an abnormality is present
Higher risk for testicular cancer: personal or family history of testicular cancer, undescended testicles not corrected during early childhood, more prevalent in whites, risk declines with increasing age

Colon and Rectum
- Digital (manual) rectal examination every year
- Guaiac slide test every year after age 50
- Proctoscopic exam—after two initial negative tests 1 year apart—every 3 to 5 years after age 50
Higher risk for colorectal cancer: personal or family history of colon or rectal cancer, personal or family history of polyps in the colon or rectum, ulcerative colitis

Prostate
- Digital rectal examination and PSA test every year
Higher risk for prostate cancer: a history of previous urinary tract infections and in men over 50 years of age

Breast

Surpassed only by lung cancer, breast cancer is the second leading cause of death from cancer in women. Now, nearly 1 in 8 women will develop breast cancer.[7] As they age, women are increasingly at risk for developing breast cancer. Regardless of age, however, waiting to learn whether a suspicious lump is benign or is a fluid-filled cyst will be stressful. Early detection is the key to complete recovery. In fact, 94% of women who discover their breast cancer before it has spread will survive more than 5 years.

Although all women and men are at some risk for developing breast cancer, women whose menstrual periods began when they were young and for whom menopause was late (longer exposure to higher estrogen levels), women who had no children (high risk seen later in life) or had their first child later in life (nursing helps lower risk, however), and women with a family history of breast cancer are at greater risk.[9] Also, women whose diets are high in saturated fats and who have excessive fat in the waist-hip area are more likely to develop breast cancer,[10] although the exact role of dietary fats remains contested. Alcohol consumption, use of an oral contraceptive, and use of ERT still foster controversy regarding their roles in women's risk for developing breast cancer. Most recently, the role of environmental pollutants and regional influences were introduced as causative factors in the development of breast cancer.[11,12] In the latter case, lifestyle differences may account for different breast cancer rates from region to region of the country. The incidence of breast cancer among various people and groups is discussed in the Learning from All Cultures box at right. In addition, the Personal Assessment on pp. 256-257 will help you evaluate your own risk for developing breast cancer.

Breast self-examination is recommended for women 20 years of age and older (see the Health Action Guide on p. 258). *Mammograms* are recommended every year for women 50 years of age and older, if they have had no earlier symptoms. Many physicians, however, recommend beginning mammograms as early as 35 years of age, particularly for women with earlier symptoms or a family history of breast cancer. However, there is some dispute about the effectiveness of mammography in detecting breast cancer in young women when compared with the same effectiveness that it has for women older than 50 years of age.

Regardless of age, each woman is unique in terms of her risk profile, and therefore the recommendation of her physician should be given careful consideration. Additionally, it is strongly advised that the procedure be performed in a facility that does a large number of

LEARNING from ALL CULTURES

Breast Cancer

Research on breast cancer has identified a number of risk factors, which are discussed in this text. Some of these factors can be changed or controlled, but others cannot. The following is additional information about the incidence of breast cancer. In demographic terms, breast cancer is likely to occur in the following people or groups:

1. Women much more often than men; it is 100 times more common in women.
2. Whites more often than blacks; however, one factor may be greater awareness and better access to medical resources by the white population.
3. Women over 50 more frequently than in younger women.
4. Women who are obese rather than thin.
5. Smokers rather than nonsmokers.
6. Women of Western cultures; Japanese women living in Japan seem to have a low rate of incidence. However, for those Japanese women who move to Western cultures, the rate of incidence increases. Women in the Netherlands are reported as having the highest rates of all countries.[18]

Consider this last risk factor. What can you hypothesize about the Western culture and the increased incidence of breast cancer?

mammography studies on a regular basis (with the most recent equipment, more skilled technicians, and more experienced radiologists reading the films).

In addition to breast self-examination and mammography, new techniques for detection are being considered. For example, MRI can see through dense tissue areas and collected breast fluid more effectively than x-rays.

Regardless of the method of detection, if a lump is found, a breast biopsy can determine what the lump is. If the lump is cancerous, treatment is highly effective if the cancer is found in an early stage. Since many choices exist about the type of surgery required to remove the cancer, women should seek a second opinion. The least extensive surgery, the lumpectomy, in combination with drug therapy, has proved highly effective.[13,14] However, for some women, even when their cancer is in an early stage, radical mastectomy may be the preferred route of treatment. Today, breast

PERSONAL ASSESSMENT

Are You at Risk for Skin, Breast, or Cervical Cancer?

Some people may have more than an average risk of developing particular types of cancer. These people can be identified by certain risk factors.

This simple self-testing method is designed by the American Cancer Society to help you assess your risk factors for three common types of cancer. These are the major risk factors but by no means represent the only ones that might be involved.

Check your response to each risk factor. Add the numbers in the parentheses to arrive at a total score for each cancer type. Find out what your score means by reading the information in the "Interpretation" section. You are advised to discuss the information with your physician if you are at a higher risk.

Skin Cancer

1. Frequent work or play in the sun
   a. Yes (10)   **b.** No (1)

2. Work in mines, around coal tars, or around radio activity
   a. Yes (10)   **b.** No (1)

3. Complexion—fair skin or light skin
   a. Yes (10)   **b.** No (1)

Your total points _____

Explanation

Excessive ultraviolet light causes skin cancer. Protect yourself with a sunscreen.

These materials can cause skin cancer.

Light complexions need more protection than others.

Interpretation

Numerical risks for skin cancer are difficult to state. For instance, a person with a dark complexion can work longer in the sun and be less likely to develop cancer than a light-complected person. Furthermore, a person wearing a long-sleeved shirt and a wide-brimmed hat may work in the sun and be less at risk than a person who wears a bathing suit and stays in the sun for only a short period. The risk increases greatly with age.

The key here is if you answered "yes" to any question, you need to realize that you have above-average risk.

Breast Cancer

1. Age group
   a. 20-34 (10)   **b.** 35-49 (40)   **c.** 50 and over (90)
2. Race/nationality
   a. Asian (5)   **c.** White (25)
   b. Black (20)   **d.** Mexican American (10)
3. Family history of breast cancer
   a. Mother, sister, or grandmother (30)
   b. None (10)

4. Your history
   a. No breast disease (10)
   b. Previous noncancerous lumps or cysts (25)
   c. Previous breast cancer (100)
5. Maternity
   a. First pregnancy before age 25 (10)
   b. First pregnancy after age 25 (15)
   c. No pregnancies (20)

Your total points _____

Interpretation

Under 100   Low-risk women should practice monthly breast self-examination (BSE) and have their breasts examined by a doctor as part of a cancer-related checkup.

100-199   Moderate-risk women should practice monthly BSE and have their breasts examined by a doctor as part of a cancer-related checkup. Periodic mammograms should be included as your doctor may advise.

200 or more   High-risk women should practice monthly BSE and have the examinations and mammograms described earlier.

Cervical Cancer*

1. Age group
   a. Less than 25 (10)   c. 40-54 (30)
   b. 25-39 (20)   d. 55 and over (30)

2. Race/nationality
   a. Asian (10)   d. White (10)
   b. Puerto Rican (20)   e. Mexican American (20)
   c. Black (20)

3. Number of pregnancies
   a. 0 (10)   c. 4 and over (30)
   b. 1 to 3 (20)

4. Viral infections
   a. Herpes and other viral infections or ulcer formations on the vagina (10)
   b. Never (1)

5. Age at first intercourse
   a. Before 15 (40)   c. 20-24 (20)
   b. 15-19 (30)   d. 25 and over (10)

6. Bleeding between periods or after intercourse
   a. Yes (40)   b. No (1)

Your total points _____

Explanation

The highest occurrence is in the 40-and-over age group. The numbers represent the relative rates of cancer for different age groups. A 45-year-old woman has a risk three times higher than a 20 year old.

Puerto Ricans, blacks, and Mexican Americans have higher rates of cervical cancer.

Women who have delivered more children have a higher occurrence.

Viral infections of the cervix and vagina are associated with cervical cancer.

Women with earlier intercourse and with more sexual partners are at a higher risk.

Irregular bleeding may be a sign of uterine cancer.

Interpretation/To Carry This Further . . .

40-69   This is a low-risk group. Ask your doctor for a Pap test. You will be advised how often you should be tested after your first test.

70-99   In this moderate-risk group, more frequent Pap tests may be required.

100 or higher   You are in a high-risk group and should have a Pap test (and pelvic examination) as advised by your doctor. ☑

*Lower portion of uterus. These questions would not apply to a woman who has had a complete hysterectomy.

reconstruction is often possible after more radical surgery (see the Star Box on p. 259).

Uterus

In 1996, approximately 49,700 new cases of cancer of the uterus were anticipated in the United States.[7] Included in this figure were 34,000 cases of cancer of the uterine lining (endometrial cancer) and 15,700 cases of cancer of the uterine neck (cervical cancer). Fortunately, the death rate from uterine cancer has dropped greatly since 1950, largely because of the use of the **Pap test.** This test looks for precancerous changes in the cells taken from the cervix.

The importance of women having a Pap test for cervical cancer done on a routine basis cannot be overemphasized. Without screening, a 20 year old of average risk has a 250 in 10,000 chance of getting cervical cancer and a 118 in 10,000 chance of dying from it. With screening, a 20 year old of average risk has a 35 in 10,000 chance of getting this form of cancer and only an 11 in 10,000 chance of dying from it.[15] The Pap

test is not perfect, however; about 7% of the tests will miss finding abnormal changes.[16] Further, not all women whose test results are abnormal receive adequate follow-up care, nor do they have subsequent Pap tests on a regular enough basis.[16] On a more positive note, potentially more effective computerized tests are currently awaiting FDA approval.

In addition to changes discovered by a Pap test, symptoms suggesting cancer of the uterus include abnormal bleeding between periods. Risk factors associated with developing this form of cancer include early age of first intercourse, number of sexual partners, history of infertility, human papillomavirus (HPV) infections (see p. 299 in Chapter 12), and excessive fat tissue around the waist. Women who have received ERT (see p. 72) may also have a

Pap test

A cancer screening procedure in which cells are removed from the cervix and examined for precancerous changes.

HEALTH
Action Guide ----->

Breast Self-Examination

The following explains how to do a breast self-examination:

1. *In the shower:* Examine your breasts during a bath or shower; hands glide more easily over wet skin. With your fingers flat, move gently over every part of each breast. Use right hand to examine left breast, left hand for right breast. Check for any lump, hard knot, or thickening. This self-examination should be done monthly, preferably a day or two after the end of the menstrual period.

2. *Before a mirror:* Inspect your breasts with arms at your sides. Next, raise your arms high overhead. Look for any changes in contour of each breast, a swelling, dimpling of skin, changes in the nipple. Then rest palms on hips, and press down firmly to flex your chest muscles. Left and right breast will not exactly match—few women's breasts do.

3. *Lying down:* To examine your right breast, put a pillow or folded towel under your right shoulder. Place right hand behind your head—this distributes breast tissue more evenly on the chest. With left hand, fingers flat, press gently in small circular motions around an imaginary clock face. Begin at outermost top of your right breast for 12 o'clock, then move to 1 o'clock, and so on around the circle back to 12 o'clock. A ridge of firm tissue in the lower curve of each breast is normal. Then move in an inch toward the nipple; keep circling to examine *every part of your breast,* including the nipple. This requires at least three more circles. Now slowly repeat the procedure on your left breast with a pillow under your left shoulder and left hand behind head. Notice how your breast structure feels. Finally, squeeze the nipple of each breast gently between thumb and index finger. Any discharge, clear or bloody, should be reported to your doctor immediately.

Breast cancer can occur in men too. Therefore this examination should be performed monthly by men. Regular inspection shows what is normal for you and will give you confidence in your examination.. ◄------

higher risk. A lower level of risk for uterine cancer is seen in women who have used barrier contraceptives (condoms, diaphragms, and spermicides). The Personal Assessment on pp. 256-257 will help you evaluate your risk of developing cervical cancer.

Vagina

Although rare, cancer of the vagina (the passage leading to the uterus) is of concern to a particular group of women: the daughters of over 3 million mothers who were given the drug DES (diethylstilbestrol) to prevent miscarriages. Because of the effects of DES on the fetal development of the reproductive system, these daughters now face the risk of developing a form of vaginal (and cervical) cancer called *clear cell cancer.* Since the risk was identified 30 years ago, the medical community has been following large groups of daughters to better assess their level of risk. To date, 1 in every 1000 exposed daughters has developed this form of cancer, some as early as 15 years of age.

Ovary

Since the death of actress Gilda Radner in 1996, public awareness of ovarian cancer has increased in

Breast Implants for Reconstruction and Augmentation

For a woman who must undergo **mastectomy,** the option of having breast reconstruction surgery exists. Various techniques can be used in rebuilding the breast. One is to insert packets containing silicone or saline (implants; see photo at right) within the chest wall to fashion a breast while also using tissue taken from the abdominal wall. The decision to have reconstructive surgery can be made before removal of the breast. When this is done, it is often possible for the surgeon to retain tissue that will allow reconstruction to be done immediately after removal of the breast. Surgical reconstruction can also be done later should the patient decide to wait.

A woman who undergoes mastectomy but chooses not to have reconstructive surgery has nonsurgical options available. A breast prosthesis can be worn to recreate her former appearance. A self-adhering or bra-inserted prosthesis can be purchased in stores specializing in medical supplies. Depending on the type of prosthesis being used, virtually all types of activities and styles of clothing can be accommodated. Of course, if a woman chooses, there is no need to return to the presurgical image of the chest. Once healing has occurred, normal activity can resume.

Implants have also become popular for women who wish to enlarge their breasts for cosmetic purposes (called *breast augmentation*). Today, however, women must be aware of the concerns about the safety of breast implants. An important concern is the safety of the sili-

A saline breast implant.

cone-filled implants and the possibility that they might leak at any time, rupture, become infected, stimulate an autoimmune response, or harden and obscure the tissues underlying the implants, making mammographic detection more difficult. The FDA has greatly reduced their use, allowing only a limited number to be implanted.

An alternative to the silicone implant, the saline-filled implant, has also come under closer watch. Physicians who favor saline to silicone implants believe that saline implants are less likely to harden, wrinkle, or interfere with detection of underlying breast cancer.

---

this country. In 1996, it was estimated that 26,700 new cases would be identified and 14,800 women would die. Most cases develop in women who are older than 40 years of age and who have not had children or began menstruation at an early age. The highest rate is in women over the age of 60. Today ovarian cancer causes more deaths than any form of female reproductive system cancer.

Because of its vague symptoms, ovarian cancer has been referred to as a *silent* cancer. Digestive disturbances, gas, and stomach distention are often its only symptoms. Today, diagnosis of this highly lethal cancer is made using transvaginal ultrasound and surgery. A newly discovered and approved drug, Taxol, obtained from the bark and needles of the Pacific yew tree, holds promise of being more effective than other forms of treatment.

Prostate

The prostate gland is a walnut-size gland located near the base of the penis. It surrounds the neck of the bladder

and the urethra. Cancer of the prostate is the third most common form of cancer in men and a leading cause of death from cancer in older men. On the basis of current statistics, approximately 1 out of 6 men will develop this form of cancer.[7] Men with a family history of prostate cancer are at greater risk of developing this form of cancer than men without this family history. Additionally, a link between prostate cancer and dietary patterns, such as excessive red meat and dairy product consumption, has been suggested.[17] A genetic link also appears to be a factor in the development of this form of cancer.[18]

The symptoms of prostate disease, including prostate cancer, are listed in the Star Box on p. 260. Should these symptoms appear, particularly in men 50 years of age and older, a physician should be consulted. Screening for prostate cancer should begin by age 40 and involves an annual rectal examination and

mastectomy
Removal of breast tissue.

Symptoms of Prostate Disease
- Difficulty in urinating
- Frequent urination, particularly at night
- Continued wetness for a short time after urination
- Blood in the urine
- Low back pain
- Ache in upper thighs

the prostate-specific antigen (PSA) blood test. This test may soon be replaced by a more sensitive version that can identify the "free" antigen most closely associated with prostate cancer, thus cutting down on the false positives and extensive use of biopsies of the present test. In addition, an ultrasound rectal examination will be used in men whose PSA scores are abnormally high.

Traditionally, prostate cancer has been treated through surgery or the use of radiation and chemotherapy, with a survival rate of 94% when diagnosed early and 80% overall.[7] Because this type of cancer grows slowly, it is increasingly likely that men whose cancer is very localized (Gleason's grade 1 or 2) and whose life expectancy is less than 10 years at the time of diagnosis will not receive treatment but rather will be closely monitored for any progression in the cancer.[19]

Testicle

Cancer of the testicle is among the least common forms of cancer; however, it represents the most common solid tumor in men between the ages of 20 and 34 years. Testicular cancer has a tendency to run in families and is more common in men whose testicles were undescended during childhood. The incidence of this cancer has been increasing in recent years. However, no single explanation can be given for this increase. Factors such as a difficult pregnancy, elevated temperature in the groin, mumps, or some yet identified environmental factors may be involved. White-collar workers appear to be at greater risk than people in other work sites. No association has been seen between vasectomies or electromagnetic fields (EMFs) generated by electric blankets.[20] In 1996, 7400 new cases were diagnosed and 370 deaths occurred.[7]

Symptoms of cancer of the testicles include a small, painless lump on the side of the testicle, a swollen or enlarged testicle, or heaviness or a dragging sensation in the groin or scrotum. Risk factors include confirmed injury, mumps, and hormonal treatments given to the mother before the child's birth. The importance of testicular self-examination, as well as early diagnosis and prompt treatment, cannot be overemphasized for men

in the at-risk age-group of 20 to 34 years. The Health Action Guide below explains how to perform a testicular self-examination.

Colon and Rectum

Cancer of the colon and rectum (colorectal cancer) has a combined incidence and death rate second only to that of lung cancer. Two types of tumors, carcinoma and lymphoma, can be found in both the colon and rectum. Fortunately, when diagnosed in a localized state, cancer of both the colon and rectum have relatively high survival rates (93% for colon and 87% for

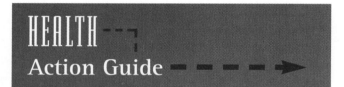

HEALTH
Action Guide

Testicular Self-Examination

Your best hope for early detection of testicular cancer is a simple 3-minute monthly self-examination. The following explains how to do a testicular self-examination. The best time is after a warm bath or shower, when the scrotal skin is most relaxed.

1. Roll each testicle gently between the thumb and fingers of both hands.

2. If you find any hard lumps or nodules, you should see your doctor promptly. They may not be malignant, but only your doctor can make the diagnosis.

After a thorough physical examination, your doctor may perform certain x-ray studies to make the most accurate diagnosis possible.

Testicular self-examinations are as important for men as breast self-examinations are for women.

rectal).[7] Genes have recently been discovered that lead to familial colon cancer and familial polyposis (abnormal tissue growth that occurs before formation of cancer) that are believed to be responsible for the tendency for colon and rectal cancer to run in families.[21] These forms of cancer are also seen in people whose diets are both high in saturated fat from red meat and low in fruits and vegetables, which contain antioxidant vitamins and fiber. Additionally, an association between colorectal cancer and smoking has been identified, suggesting that carcinogens may be ingested or pass into the digestive system from the bloodstream.

Symptoms associated with colon and rectal cancers include bleeding from the rectum, blood in the stool, or a change in bowel habits. Also, a family history of inflammatory bowel disease, polyp formation, or colorectal cancer should make one more alert to symptoms. In people over 50 years of age, any sudden change in bowel habits that lasts 10 days or longer should be evaluated by a physician. The American Cancer Society recommends preventive health care that includes digital (manual) rectal examination after age 40, a stool blood test after age 50, and proctoscopic examination every 3 to 5 years after age 50. Prompt removal of polyps has been shown to be effective in lowering the risk of developing colorectal cancer. Further, there is evidence that the development of colorectal cancer may be prevented or slowed through regular exercise and through the regular use of aspirin.[22]

The treatment of colorectal cancer involves surgery combined with the use of chemotherapy drugs. A *colostomy* is required in 15% of the cases of colon and rectal cancer.

Pancreas

Pancreatic cancer is one of the most lethal forms of cancer, with a survival rate of only 3% at 5 years after diagnosis.[7] In light of the organ's important roles in both digestion and metabolic processes (see the discussion of diabetes mellitus on pp. 266-269), its destruction leaves the body in a state incompatible with living.

In 1996, 26,300 new cases of pancreatic cancer were diagnosed.[7] The disease is more common in men than women and occurs most frequently in African-American men. Early detection of this cancer is difficult because of the absence of symptoms until late in its course. Risk of developing this form of cancer increases with age; with diabetes mellitus, pancreatitis (inflammation of the pancreas), or cirrhosis (see Chapter 8); and with diets high in fat. To date, little in the way of effective treatment has been found.

Skin

Thanks in large part to our desire for a fashionable tan, too many teens and adults are spending more time in the sun (and in tanning booths) than their skin can tolerate. As a result, skin cancer, once common only among those people who had to work in the sun, is occurring with alarming frequency. In 1996, more than 800,000 Americans developed basal or squamous cell skin cancer and 38,300 cases of highly dangerous malignant melanoma were diagnosed.[7] Severe sunburning during childhood and chronic sun exposure during adolescence and younger adulthood are responsible for these increases in skin cancer.

Although many doctors do not emphasize this point enough, the key to the successful treatment of skin cancer lies in early detection. In the case of basal cell or squamous cell cancer, the development of a pale, waxlike, pearly nodule or red, scaly patch may be the first symptom. For others, skin cancer may be noticed as a gradual change in the appearance of an already existing skin mole. If such a change is noted, a physician should be contacted. Melanoma usually

A

B

Figure 11-3 **A**, Basal cell carcinoma. Note the typical **raised, rolled edge. B**, Squamous cell carcinoma.

Figure 11-4   **A,** Normal mole. This type of lesion is often seen in large numbers on the skin of young adults and may affect any body site. Note its symmetrical shape, regular borders, uniform color, and relatively small size (about 6 millimeters). **B,** Malignant melanoma. Note its asymmetrical shape, irregular borders, uneven color, and relatively large size (about 2 centimeters).

begins as a small, molelike growth that increases progressively in size, changes color, ulcerates, and bleeds easily. For use in detecting melanoma, the American Cancer Society recommends using the guidelines below:

A   is for asymmetry
B   is for border irregularity
C   is for color (change)
D   is for a diameter greater than 6 mm

Figure 11-4 shows a mole that would be considered harmless and one that clearly demonstrates the ABCD characteristics described above. Again, it is important to be observant and not fail to recognize the changing status of a mole or other skin lesion. The Health Action Guide below depicts the steps to be taken in making a regular inspection of the skin.

When nonmelanoma skin cancer is found, an almost 100% cure rate can be expected. Treatment of these skin

HEALTH Action Guide ----->

How to look for melanoma

1. Examine your body front and back in the mirror, then right and left sides with arms raised.

2. Bend your elbows and carefully look at your palms, forearms and under your upper arms.

3. Look at the backs of your legs and feet, the spaces between your toes and the soles of your feet.

4. Examine the back of your neck and scalp with a hand mirror. Part your hair for a closer look.

5. Finally, check your back and buttocks with a hand mirror.

What to look for
Potential signs of malignancy in moles or pigmented spots:

Asymmetry
One half unlike the other half

Irregularity
Border irregular— or poorly circumscribed

Color
Color varies from one area to another; shades of tan brown or black

Size
Diameter larger than 6 mm as a rule (diameter of a pencil eraser)

cancers can involve surgical removal, destruction through burning or freezing, or the use of x-ray therapy. When the more serious melanomas are found in an early stage, a high cure rate is accomplished using the same techniques. However, when malignant melanomas are more advanced, extensive surgery and chemotherapy will be necessary, and, unfortunately, recovery is rare.

Prevention of skin cancer should be a high priority for people who enjoy the sun or must work outdoors. The use of sunscreen is of great importance. Table 11-1 provides guidance in selecting the sunscreen that is appropriate for your skin. In addition, parents can help their children prevent skin cancer later in life by restricting their outdoor play from 11:00 AM to 2:00 PM, requiring them to wear hats that shade their faces, and applying a sunscreen with SPF 15 on their children regardless of skin tone.

In spite of our long-standing attraction to a tan, it is encouraging to note that both teens and adults are beginning to take the skin cancer message seriously. As reported in 1994, 48% of adults tan less than they once did, and one third of all adults and teens do not sun at all.[23] Still, 1 of 5 adults will develop skin cancer. The Personal Assessment on pp. 256-257 will help you determine your own risk of developing this kind of cancer.

THE DIAGNOSIS OF CANCER

Is cancer survivable? The answer is, of course, yes. The chances for survival (defined as living at least 5 years after diagnosis) depend greatly on the promptness of identification, diagnosis, and treatment.

Thus the chances for recovery from cancer are best when cancer is detected early. The familiar "cancer's seven warning signals" can serve as a basis for early detection (see the Star Box at right). Also, unexplained

Cancer's Seven Warning Signs

Listed below are the seven warning signs of cancer, which the acronym **CAUTION** will help you remember:
1. **C**hange in bowel or bladder habits
2. **A** sore that does not heal
3. **U**nusual bleeding or discharge
4. **T**hickening or lump in breast or elsewhere
5. **I**ndigestion or difficulty in swallowing
6. **O**bvious change in a wart or mole
7. **N**agging cough or hoarseness
If you have a warning sign that persists for more than 5 days, see your doctor!

weight loss can be a signal for the presence of a malignancy. Weight loss, however, is not usually an early indicator of cancer. Persistent headaches and vision changes should be evaluated by a physician.

In addition to the recognition of danger signals, undergoing regularly scheduled screening for malignancy-related changes is important. Note that breast self-examination for all women over the age of 20 is recommended. Further, we strongly recommend testicular self-examination for men. Step-by-step procedures for both of these self-examinations are provided in the Star Boxes on pp. 258 and 260. The remaining screening procedures require the services of a medical practitioner.

Treatment

In today's approach to cancer treatment, proven therapies and promising new experimental approaches are often combined. The traditional thera-

Table 11-1   Sunscreen Guide

Skin Type	Pigmentation	Sunburn/Tanning History	Sun Protection Factor (SPF)
I	Very fair skin; freckling; blond, red, or brown hair	Always burns easily; never tans	15-30
II	Fair skin; blond, red, or brown hair	Always burns easily, tans minimally	15-20
III	Brown hair and eyes, darker skin (light brown)	Burns moderately, tans gradually and uniformly	8-15
IV	Light brown skin; dark hair and eyes (moderate brown)	Burns minimally; always tans well	8-15
V	Brown skin; dark hair and eyes	Rarely burns, tans profusely (dark brown)	Recommended same as skin type IV
VI	Brown-black skin; dark hair and eyes	Never burns, deeply pigmented (black)	Recommended same as skin type IV

NOTE: Although formulas as high as 60 are available, an SPF of 30 is usually appropriate for use, perhaps requiring more frequent applications. *As deterioration of the ozone layer continues, it may be necessary to use an even more protective sunscreen.*

pies are surgery, radiation, and chemotherapy. Used independently or in combination, they form the backbone of our increasingly successful efforts in treating cancer. Newer, more experimental therapies are also being used on a limited basis. One or more of these experimental approaches may combine surgery, radiation, and chemotherapy as a basis for treatment.

In the sections that follow, a brief description of each treatment is given.

Surgery

Surgical removal of tissue suspected to contain cancerous cells is the oldest approach to cancer therapy. When undertaken early in the course of the disease, surgery is particularly suited for cancers of the skin, gastrointestinal tract, breast, uterus, cervix, prostate gland, and testicle. Minimal procedures are undertaken whenever possible, and radiation or chemotherapy is often used with surgery to ensure maximum effectiveness.

Radiation

Radiation is capable of killing cancer cells by altering their genetic material while it is in an exposed state during cell division. Of course, since neighboring cells also divide, they are exposed to the damaging effects of radiation as well. However, by carefully planning the length of exposure and time of treatment, and by focusing of the radiation with precision, damage to noncancerous cells can be held to a minimum.

Chemotherapy

The important advances in successful treatment of cancer can be attributed to advances in chemotherapy, both in terms of new drugs and the more effective combination of new drugs and familiar chemotherapeutic agents. Most often, these drugs work by destroying cancer cells' ability to use important materials or carry out cell division in a normal manner. Because chemotherapy influences cell division, it will influence noncancerous cells that divide frequently. Among the cells most susceptible to this influence are those that make up bone marrow, the lining of the intestinal tract, and the hair follicles. People who are undergoing chemotherapy often have side effects directly related to these changes—immune system suppression, diarrhea, and hair loss.

Immunotherapy

Immunotherapy refers to the use of a variety of substances to trigger a person's own immune system to attack cancer cells or prevent cancer cells from becoming activated. Among these new forms of immunotherapy are the use of interferon, monoclonal antibodies, interleukin-2, tumor necrosis factor (TNF), and certain bone

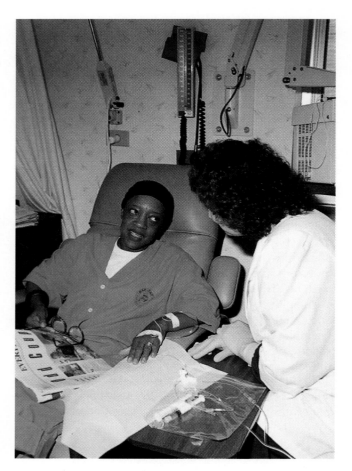

The effects of chemotherapy are carefully monitored.

marrow growth regulators. These products are being manufactured using genetic engineering technology.

Alternative (complementary) cancer therapies

In spite of advances made in the diagnosis and treatment of cancer during this century, cancer rates are climbing as we move toward the next century. In response to climbing rates and to requests made by cancer victims and many clinicians to expand the range of treatments, the National Institutes of Health[2] has begun an in-depth, $1-million study of alternative or nonconventional cancer treatments. Through the use of new and carefully controlled studies and the reassessment of research and records already available, an attempt will be made by the NIH to better understand the benefits to be derived from alternative or complementary therapies.

Among the treatments to be given closer and more careful consideration are chiropractic (the manipulation of the spine), acupressure (finger and thumb pressure to relieve pain), and acupuncture (needles inserted to relieve pain and promote the flow of energy within the body). Additional areas of investigation will include ayurveda (a traditional Indian lifestyle that involves the use of herbs and a particular diet), biofeedback (monitoring of body functions to control body processes), homeopathy (use of minuscule doses of toxic substances), and naturopathy (use of natural remedies, including sunshine and vitamins). Further focus will be directed toward oxidizing agents (substances believed to kill viruses), reflexology (the massaging of points on the feet), therapeutic touch (redirecting of "life forces" through touching areas of the body), and visualization (learning to "see" a cure occurring).

Time and study will answer many questions about the effectiveness of these methods of treating cancer. Should these areas prove to be more effective than traditional medical science now believes, their incorporation will probably be very gradual.

RISK REDUCTION

Because cancer will probably continue to be the second most common disease among adults, it is important that you explore ways to reduce your risk of developing cancer. The following factors, which could make you vulnerable to cancer, can be controlled or at least recognized.

- *Know your family history.* You are the recipient of the genetic strengths and weaknesses of your biological parents and your more distant relatives. If cancer is prevalent in your family medical history, you cannot afford to disregard this fact. It may be appropriate for you to be screened for certain types of cancer more often or at a young age.
- *Select your occupation carefully.* Because of recently discovered relationships between cancer and occupations that bring employees into contact with carcinogenic agents, you must be aware of risks with certain job selections and assignments. Worksites associated with frequent contact with pesticides, strong solvents, volatile hydocarbons, and airborne fibers could pay well but also shorten life.
- *Do not use tobacco products.* You may want to review Chapter 9 on the overwhelming evidence linking all forms of tobacco use (including smokeless tobacco) to the development of cancer. Smoking is so detrimental to health that it is considered the number one preventable cause of death.
- *Follow a sound diet.* The Health Action Guide above provides general guidelines on eating to reduce your cancer risk. In addition, review

HEALTH Action Guide

Eat to Lower Your Cancer Risk

The American Cancer Society recommends the following dietary precautions to help reduce the risk of getting cancer:
- Avoid obesity.
- Reduce total fat intake.
- Eat more high-fiber foods.
- Include foods rich in vitamins A and C in your daily diet.
- Include cruciferous vegetables in your diet.
- Avoid smoked, salt-cured, and nitrate-cured foods.
- Limit alcohol consumption.

Chapter 5 for information regarding dietary practices and the incidence of various diseases, including cancer. In that chapter the role of fruits and vegetables known to be sources of cancer-preventing phytochemicals is introduced. Table 11-2 provides a detailed listing of the phytochemicals found in a variety of foods that may play a constructive role in cancer prevention.[24] Notice that a wide variety of fruits and vegetables, particularly the cruciferous vegetables, including cauliflower, broccoli, and brussels sprouts, and the fruits that are high in beta-carotene, vitamin C, and fiber, are listed. Should research demonstrate an even clearer role for nutrients, "chemoprevention" may become an even more widely practiced component of cancer prevention.
- *Control your body weight.* Particularly for women, obesity is related to a higher incidence of cancer of the uterus, ovary, and breast. Maintaining a desirable body weight could improve overall health and lead to more successful management of cancer should it develop.
- *Exercise regularly.* Chapter 4 discusses in detail the importance of regular moderate exercise to all aspects of health, including reducing the risk of chronic illnesses. Moderate exercise increases the body's ability to deliver oxygen to its tissues and thus to reduce the formation of cancer-enhancing free radicals formed during incomplete oxidation of nutrients. Moderate exercise

Table 11-2   Phytochemicals Involved in Cancer Prevention

Phytochemical Class	Food Source
Allium compounds	Garlic, onions, chives, leeks
Carotenoids	Yellow and orange vegetables and fruits, dark green leafy vegetables
Coumarins	Vegetables and citrus fruits
Dithiolthiones	Cruciferous vegetables
Flavonoids	Most fruits and vegetables
Glucosinolates, indoles	Cruciferous vegetables, especially brussels sprouts, rutabaga, mustard greens, dried horseradish
Inositol hexaphosphate	Plant foods, especially soybeans and cereals
Isoflavones	Soybeans
Isothiocyanates	Cruciferous vegetables
Limonene	Citrus fruits
Phenols	Nearly all fruits and vegetables
Protease inhibitors	Plant foods, especially seeds and legumes, including soybeans

also stimulates the production of enzymes that remove free radicals. Some concern exists, however, that extensive exercise might actually reduce the body's ability to produce the enzymes mentioned above and thus contribute to the development of free-radical–based cellular changes, including cancer.[25]

- *Limit your exposure to sun.* It is important to heed this message, even if you enjoy many outdoor activities. Particularly for people with light complexions, the radiation received through chronic exposure to the sun may foster the development of skin cancer.
- *Consume alcohol in moderation if at all.* Heavier users of alcohol experience an increased prevalence of several types of cancer, including cancer of the oral cavity, larynx, and esophagus. Whether this results directly from the presence of carcinogens in alcohol or is more closely related to the alcohol user's tendency to smoke has not yet been established.

When the suggestions made above are given careful consideration, it should be obvious that much can be done by individuals to prevent or at least minimize the development of cancer. A wellness-oriented life style is the best weapon in your "personal war against cancer." Having said this, however, all risk factor reduction is, in the final analysis, relative in nature. Observation and experience indicate that life cannot be totally structured around the desire to achieve maximum longevity or reduce morbidity at all costs. Most people need a balance between life that is emotionally, socially, and spiritually satisfying and life that is structured solely for the purpose of living a long time and minimizing exposure to

illness. Regardless of our personal lifestyle, we can, however, educate others, give comfort and support to those who are living with cancer, and support the funding of continuing and innovative new cancer research. Resources available for people with cancer and their families are listed in the Star Box on p. 267.

CHRONIC HEALTH CONDITIONS

In addition to the two most widely recognized chronic health problems of adulthood—cardiovascular disease and cancer—aging increases the probability that the incidence of other conditions will increase as we grow older. In this section of the chapter, we examine four noncancerous, noncardiovascular chronic health conditions: diabetes mellitus, multiple sclerosis, asthma, and systemic lupus erythematosus. Of course, many additional chronic conditions are discussed in other chapters of this textbook. See the Star Box on p. 268 for information about Alzheimer's disease, a chronic illness that affects many elderly adults. See the Star Box on p. 269 for an explanation of sickle cell trait and sickle cell disease, disorders that can affect African-Americans.

Diabetes Mellitus

Diabetes mellitus is not a single condition but rather two conditions with important similarities and differences.

Non–insulin–dependent diabetes mellitus (Type II)

In people who do not have diabetes mellitus the body's need for energy is met through the "burning" of glucose (blood sugar) within the cells. Glucose is

Resources for People Living with Cancer
For people with cancer and their families, many telephone hot lines have been set up offering information and referrals:

- **American Cancer Society National Hotline:** (800) ACS-2345. Also, ACS recommends calling local ACS chapters for support group information.
- **National Cancer Institute Cancer Information Service:** (800) 4-CANCER.
- **National Coalition for Cancer Survivorship** (umbrella group for cancer survivor units nationwide): (301) 650-8868.
- **Candlelighters Childhood Cancer Foundation:** Information on support groups for children with cancer and their families: (301) 657-8401 and (800) 366-2223.

- **Surviving:** Support group. Publishes newsletter for Hodgkin's disease survivors. Stanford University Medical Center, Radiology Dept, Room C050, 300 Pasteur Dr, Stanford, CA 94305.
- **Vital Options:** Support group for people 17 to 40 who are cancer survivors: (818) 508-5657.
- **The Resource Center:** American College of Obstetricians and Gynecologists, 409 12th St. S.W., Washington, DC 20224-2188. Send a self-addressed, business-size envelope for *Detecting and Treating Breast Problems.*
- American College of Radiology, for accredited mammography centers, (800) ACR-LINE (members only) or (703) 648-8900, ask for mammography.

absorbed from the digestive tract and carried to the cells by the blood system. Passage of glucose into the cell is achieved through a transport system that moves the glucose molecule across the cell's membrane. Activation of this glucose transport mechanism requires the presence of the hormone insulin (Figure 11-5). Specific receptor sites for **insulin** can be found on the cell membrane. In addition to its role in the transport of glucose into sensitive cells, insulin is also required for the conversion of glucose into glycogen in the liver and the formation of fatty acids in adipose cells. Insulin is produced in the cells of the islets of Langerhans within the pancreas. The release of insulin from the pancreas corresponds to the changing levels of glucose within the blood.

In adults with a **genetic predisposition** for developing non–insulin-dependent diabetes mellitus a trigger mechanism (most likely obesity) begins a process through which the body cells become increasingly less sensitive to the presence of insulin, although a normal (or slightly greater than normal) amount of insulin is produced by the pancreas. The growing ineffectiveness of insulin in getting glucose into cells results in the buildup of glucose in the blood. Elevated levels of glucose give rise to *hyperglycemia,* a hallmark symptom of non–insulin-dependent diabetes mellitus.

In response to this buildup the kidneys begin the process of filtering glucose from the blood. Excess glucose then spills over into the urine. This removal of glucose in the urine demands large amounts of water, a process called *diuresis,* a second important symptom of adult-onset diabetes. Increased *thirst,* a third symptom of developing diabetes, results in response to the

movement of fluid from extracellular spaces into the circulatory system to maintain homeostasis.[26]

For many adults with diabetes, dietary modification (with an emphasis on monitoring total carbohydrate intake, not just sugar) and regular exercise is the only treatment required to maintain an acceptable level of glucose use.[27] Weight loss will improve the condition by "releasing" more insulin receptors, and exercise increases the actual number of receptor sites. With better insulin recognition, the person can return to a more normal state of functioning.

For people whose condition is more advanced, dietary modification and weight loss alone will not accomplish the level of management required, and oral drugs, including sulfonylureas and metformin, or even insulin may be necessary. For those who require insulin, management of the condition becomes much more demanding.

In addition to genetic predisposition and obesity as important factors in non–insulin-dependent diabetes mellitus, unresolved stress appears to play a role in the development of hyperglycemic states. Although stress alone probably cannot produce a diabetic condition, it

insulin
A pancreatic hormone required by the body for the effective metabolism of glucose (blood sugar).

genetic predisposition
An inherited tendency to develop a disease process if necessary environmental factors exist.

Alzheimer's Disease

Although it affects fewer than 1% to 2% of elderly people, organic brain syndrome, in either its acute or chronic form, is an incapacitating, heart-rending, and costly affliction. **Alzheimer's disease** represents the best known of the presenile dementia disorders affecting between 2 and 4 million adults. Today, more than ever before, it is *the* disease associated with those individuals who have lived a long time.

The initial indication of Alzheimer's disease is often subtle and may be confused with mild depression. At this stage of the disease process, however, the person might experience some difficulty answering questions like these:

- Where are we now?
- What month is it?
- What is today's date?
- When is your birthday?
- Who is the President?

During the ensuing months, victims experience greater memory loss, confusion, and *dementia* (or loss of reasoning). In the most advanced stage, Alzheimer's victims experience incontinence, infantile behavior, and finally total incapacitation resulting from the destruction of brain tissue. Institutionalization of people with advanced Alzheimer's disease is certain.

The precise diagnosis of Alzheimer's disease and other, similar disorders remains difficult to make before the death of the victim. At that time the characteristic *neurofibrillary tangles*, *neuritic plaques*, and loss of neurons can be identified. Before death, all other conditions capable of leading to dementia are individually ruled out. The initial diagnosis of Alzheimer's disease is made based on a process of elimination.

Several theories exist concerning the cause of Alzheimer's disease. Growing research indicates that genetic mutations in chromosomes 14, 19, or 21 may encourage the development of the disease. Additional theories suggest possible links between Alzheimer's disease and abnormal protein development, deficiencies in acetylcholine (a neurotransmitter) production, abnormal blood flow, or exposure to infectious agents or toxins.

Drugs to treat Alzheimer's disease effectively have not yet been developed. Although over 10 experimental drugs are currently being tested, none has been shown to have a significant effect on reversing the disease. One drug, tacrine (Cognex), shows minor improvements with Alzheimer's patients when used early in the disease process.

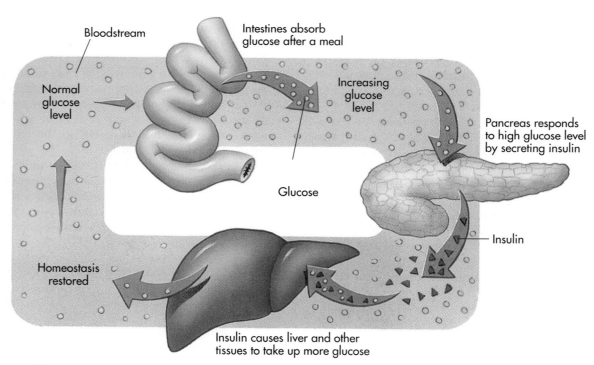

Figure 11-5   The secretion of insulin is regulated by a mechanism that tends to reverse any deviation from normal. Thus an increase in blood glucose level triggers secretion of insulin. Since insulin promotes glucose uptake by cells, blood glucose level is restored to its lower, normal level.

Sickle Cell Trait and Sickle Cell Disease

Of all the chemical compounds found within the body, few occur in as many forms as hemoglobin, which helps bind oxygen to the red blood cell. Two forms of hemoglobin are associated with sickle cell trait and sickle cell disease. African-Americans can be the recipients of either form of this abnormal hemoglobin. Those who inherit the trait-form do not develop the disease but are capable of transmitting the gene for abnormal hemoglobin to their offspring. Those people who inherit the disease-form face a shortened life characterized by periods of pain and impairment.

Approximately 8% of all African-Americans have the gene for sickle cell trait; they experience little impairment, and they can transmit the gene to their children.

For approximately 1.5% of African-Americans, sickle cell disease is a painful, incapacitating, and life-shortening disease. Red blood cells are elongated, crescent-shaped (or sickled), and unable to pass through the body's minute capillaries. The body responds to the presence of these abnormal red blood cells by removing them very quickly. This sets the stage for anemia—thus the condition is often called *sickle cell anemia*. In addition to anemia, this form of the condition is associated with many serious medical problems, including impaired lung function, congestive heart failure, gallbladder infections, bone changes, and possible abnormalities of the eye and skin. Living beyond early adulthood may not be possible.

If a key exists for preventing the occurrence of sickle cell trait and disease, it lies in the area of genetic counseling to help in making decisions regarding reproduction, including pregnancy termination. The decision to have children and perhaps risk passing on the gene for defective hemoglobin to the next generation is one that must be carefully made.

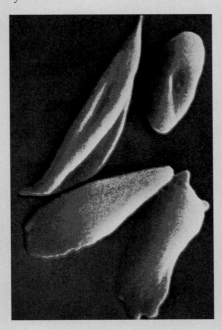

---

is likely that stress can create a series of endocrine changes that can lead to a state of hyperglycemia.

Diabetes can cause serious damage to several important structures within the body. The rate and extent to which people with diabetes develop these pathological changes can be markedly influenced by the nature of their particular condition and the type of management with which they comply. For those who already have diabetes, an understanding of the condition and a commitment to management are important elements in living with diabetes mellitus.

Insulin-dependent diabetes mellitus (Type I)

A second type of diabetes mellitus is insulin-dependent diabetes mellitus, or Type I diabetes. The onset of this type of diabetes generally occurs before the age of 35, most often during childhood. In contrast to Type II diabetes, in which insulin is produced but is ineffective because of insensitivity, in Type I diabetes the body does not produce insulin at all. Destruction of the insulin-producing cells of the pancreas by the person's immune system (possibly in search of a viral infection

within the islet cells of the pancreas) accounts for this sudden and irreversible loss of insulin production.[28]

In most ways the two forms of diabetes are similar, with the important exception that insulin-dependent diabetes mellitus requires the use of insulin from an outside source (see the Star Box on p. 270, top). Today this insulin is obtained either from animals or through genetically engineered bacteria and is taken by injection (one to four times per day) or through the use of an insulin pump that provides a constant supply of insulin to the body. Development of the glucometer, a highly accurate device for measuring the amount of glucose in the blood, allows for sound management of this condition and a life expectancy that is essentially

Alzheimer's disease
Gradual development of memory loss, confusion, and loss of reasoning; can eventually lead to total intellectual incapacitation, brain degeneration, and death.

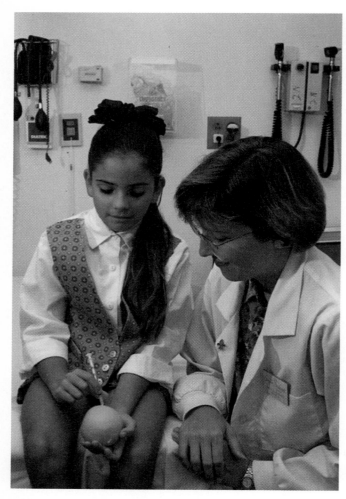

Learning to self-inject insulin.

normal. Of course, with both forms of diabetes mellitus, sound dietary practice, planned activity, and control of stress are important for keeping blood glucose levels within normal ranges. In the absence of good management of diabetes mellitus, several serious problems can result, including blindness, gangrene of the extremities, kidney disease, and heart attack. These and other common complications of diabetes are listed in the Star Box at the right. People who cannot establish good control are likely to live a shorter life than those who can.

Multiple Sclerosis

For proper nerve conduction to occur within portions of the brain and spinal cord, an insulating sheath of *myelin* must surround *neurons*. In the progressive disease multiple sclerosis (MS), the cells that produce myelin are destroyed and myelin production ceases. This disruption of normal neurological functioning eventually reaches an extent to which vital functions of the body can no longer be carried out.

Differences between Types of Diabetes Mellitus

Insulin-Dependent (Type I)
(These symptoms usually develop rapidly.)
- Extreme hunger
- Extreme thirst
- Frequent urination
- Extreme weight loss
- Irritability
- Weakness and fatigue
- Nausea and vomiting

Non–Insulin-Dependent (Type II)
(These symptoms usually develop gradually.)
- Any of the symptoms for insulin-dependent diabetes
- Blurred vision or a change in sight
- Itchy skin
- Tingling or numbness in the limbs

If you notice these symptoms occurring, bring them to the attention of your physician.

The cause of MS is not fully understood. Research continues to focus on virus-induced **autoimmune** mechanisms in which T cells attack viral-infected myelin-producing cells.[28]

Multiple sclerosis is a disease that most often appears for the first time during the young adult years—the traditional college years. After its onset, the disease progresses off and on over the next 20 to 25 years. The initial symptoms of the condition are often visual impairment, prickling and burning in the extremities, or an altered **gait.** Deterioration of nervous system function occurs in various forms during the course of MS. In the disease's most advanced stages, movement is greatly impaired, and mental deterioration may be present.

Common Complications of Diabetes
- Cataract formation
- Glaucoma
- Blindness
- Dental caries
- Stillbirths/miscarriages
- Neonatal deaths
- Congenital defects
- Cardiovascular disease
- Kidney disease
- Gangrene
- Impotence

Treatment for MS involves attempts to reduce the severity of the symptoms and extend the periods of remission. Today a variety of therapies are used, including immune system–targeted drugs, steroid drugs, drugs to relieve muscle spasms, injections of nerve blockers, and physical therapy.

The development of immune system–related agents is very much at the center of the fight against MS. Betaseron, a genetically engineered form of interferon, is a drug that effectively reduces the symptoms of MS but may not slow the progression of the disease. Betaseron is currently used by 40,000 people. Most recently, Avonex and Copolymer 1, drugs that slow the development of lesions and delay periods of relapse, have been given approval by FDA advisory panels. These drugs too are modified forms of interferon.

In addition to drug therapy, psychotherapy is an important adjunct to the treatment of MS. Profound periods of depression often accompany the initial diagnosis of this condition. Emotional support is helpful in dealing with the progressive impairment associated with the condition.

Asthma

Bronchial asthma is a chronic respiratory disease characterized by acute attacks of breathlessness and wheezing caused by narrowing of the bronchioles.

Two main types of the asthma have been identified: *extrinsic* and *intrinsic*. In extrinsic asthma, allergens such as pollen, house dust, house-dust mites, animal fur, and feathers produce sudden and extensive bronchoconstriction that narrows the airways. Increased sputum production further narrows the bronchioles and restricts the passage of air. This narrowing fosters the development of chronic inflammation of the airways, which is the most damaging aspect of asthma. Wheezing is most pronounced when the victim attempts to exhale air through the narrowed air passages. For many asthmatic people, exercise, cigarette smoke, and particular foods or drugs can cause an asthma attack.

Intrinsic asthma, the least common form, displays similar symptoms but is caused by stress or is a consequence of frequent respiratory tract infections. Allergens as such are not involved in this form of asthma.

Prevention and effective management of asthma is often possible through the use of a combination of approaches. Most basic, of course, is the maintenance of high-level wellness through a healthful lifestyle that includes sound diet, exercise, and stress management. In this approach, exercises that are well tolerated, such as swimming, have proved beneficial in maintaining a more normal level of respiratory function.[29] Secondly, *immunotherapy,* in which the patient is desensitized through injections of weakened aller-

gens, is a frequently attempted form of prevention. In addition, the careful use of corticosteroid drugs several times per day reduces inflammation and thus minimizes the likelihood of attacks occurring.

Once an attack has started, people with asthma routinely use bronchodilator drugs delivered through an inhaler. After inhalation, normal breathing is restored within several minutes. Each year in this country, however, several thousand people die as the result of asthma attacks. Some experts believe that this number could be reduced if physicians were more aggressive in their treatment of the bronchial inflammation component of the condition.

For people with exercise-induced asthma (EIA), one of the more frequently seen forms, several important steps should be taken when attempting to exercise (see the Health Action Guide below).[29]

Regardless of the potential seriousness of asthma, however, many people who experience asthma during childhood can manage well with the proper use of exercise and medication and may experience less asthma, or none at all, as they reach adulthood.

HEALTH Action Guide

Tips for Controlling Exercise-Induced Asthma

- Obtain a treatment and prevention plan from your physician.
- Alert instructors and coaches about the existence of any treatment plan.
- Medicate before exercising according to your physician's instruction.
- Warm up slowly to increase heart rate gradually and cool down slowly after exercise.
- Carry your bronchodilator with you at all times if one was prescribed.
- Wear a scarf or mask over your mouth and nose during cold weather to warm and moisten the air you breathe.
- Wear an allergy mask over the mouth and nose when exercising during pollen season.

autoimmune
An immune response against the cells of a person's own body.

gait
Pattern of walking.

Systemic Lupus Erythematosus

Systemic lupus erythematosus (SLE), or simply *lupus,* is perhaps the most familiar of a class of chronic conditions known as autoimmune disorders, or *connective tissue disorders.* Collectively, these conditions reflect an extensive and inappropriate attack by the body's immune system on its own tissues, which then serve as *self-antigens* (see Chapter 12 for a discussion of the immune response).

The name *systemic lupus erythematosus* reflects the widespread (systemic) destruction of fibrous connective tissue and other tissues and the appearance of a reddish rash (erythematosus) that imparts a characteristic "mask" to the face. SLE is most often seen in women who developed the condition during young adulthood. The course of the condition is gradual, with intermittent periods of inflammation, stiffness, fatigue, pleurisy (chest pain), and discomfort over wide areas of the body, including muscles, joints, and skin. Similar changes may also occur with tissue of the nervous system, kidneys, and heart. Diagnosis is made on the bases of a number of laboratory tests, including the identification of SLE factor in the blood.

The reason the immune system turns on the body in such a widely based and aggressive manner is not fully understood. It is likely, however, that a combination of genetic predisposition and an earlier viral infection may be involved in its development. Episodes (called *flares*) of lupus often follow exposure to the sun, periods of fatigue, or an infectious disease; all these should be avoided to the fullest extent possible. Management of the condition generally involves the long-term (and low-dose) use of prednisone (a corticosteroid) to suppress the adrenal gland's cortisone. In some cases the immune system itself may be medically suppressed as well. These treatments must be managed carefully because they carry serious side effects.[30]

Summary

- The "war on cancer" has made gains in many areas, but it is far from being won, with overall death rates having climbed since 1971.
- Cancer is a condition reflecting the body's inability to control the growth and specialization of cells.
- Genes that control replication, specialization, repair, and suppression of abnormal activity hold the potential of becoming oncogenes and thus can be considered protooncogenes.
- A variety of agents, including genetic mutations, viruses, and carcinogens (and co-carcinogens) stimulate the conversion of regulatory genes (protooncogenes) into oncogenes. The identification of oncogenes continues at a rapid pace in conjunction with the Human Genome Project.
- Cancer cells demonstrate a variety of interesting characteristics in comparison with normal cells of the same type. Benign tumors, made up of noncancerous cells, can present serious health problems.
- Cancer can be described on the basis of the type of tissue in which it has its origin—carcinoma, sarcoma, melanoma, etc.
- Cancer can be described on the basis of its location within the body—lung, breast, prostate, etc.
- Cigarette smoking and having a genetic predisposition are both related to the development of lung cancer.
- Breast cancer demonstrates clear familial patterns that suggest a genetic predisposition. Mammograms are recommended as an important component of breast cancer identification. Important options should be considered before the treatment of breast cancer.
- Regular use of Pap tests is related to the early detection of uterine (cervical) cancer. A group of middle-aged women who are the daughters of mothers given the drug DES during pregnancy have high levels of vaginal cancer. Ovarian cancer is often "silent" in its presentation of symptoms.
- The PSA test improves the ability to diagnose prostate cancer. A more sensitive PSA test will soon be available.
- Regular self-examination of the testicles leads to early detection of testicular cancer.
- Colon and rectal cancers have strong familial links and are seen in populations that consume diets high in fat and low in fruits and vegetables.
- Pancreatic cancer is very difficult to survive, in part because of the absence of symptoms early in the disease's course.
- Skin cancer prevention requires protection from excessive sun exposure.
- Early detection based on self-examination and screening is the basis for the identification and successful treatment of many cancers. Conventional and alternative treatment methods can be used to treat cancer.
- Cancer risk reduction techniques should be practiced on a regular basis.
- Diabetes mellitus, in both of its forms, is a chronic condition reflecting the body's inability to use glucose in a normal manner.
- Multiple sclerosis involves the autoimmune destruction of the insulating cover of neurons.
- Asthma may be a response to extrinsic factors such

as pollen, dust, or exercise. Factors such as stress or chronic respiratory infections are the basis of a less commonly seen form of asthma called *intrinsic asthma.*

- Autoimmune disorders, such as SLE, reflect the

immune system's failure to recognize the body's own tissue as being "self." Flares involving episodes of inflammation, swelling, pain, and discomfort occur periodically in conjunction with the disease.

Review Questions

1. What is the relationship between regulatory genes and tumor suppressor genes in the development of cancer? Why are regulatory genes called both *protooncogenes* and *oncogenes*?
2. What are some of the major types of cancer, based on the tissue in which they have their origin?
3. What are the principal factors that contribute to the development of lung cancer? Of breast cancer?
4. When should regular use of mammography begin, and which women should begin using it earliest?
5. How does the PSA test contribute to the early detection of prostate cancer?
6. What signs indicate the possibility that a skin lesion has become cancerous?
7. What important information can be obtained with the use of Pap tests?
8. What are the steps for effective self-examination of the breasts and testicles?
9. Why is ovarian cancer described as a "silent" cancer?
10. What are the conventional and alternative cancer treatments most often used in the treatment of cancer?
11. What are the risk reduction activities identified in this chapter?
12. How do non–insulin-dependent and insulin-dependent diabetes mellitus differ? How are they similar?
13. What is the role of the immune system in multiple sclerosis?
14. How do chronic respiratory tract inflammation and airway constriction relate to asthma? What is the role of exercise in both the cause and the prevention of asthma?
15. What is the role of the immune system is connective tissue disorders such as SLE? What factors are associated with the development of the disorder? Why does treatment involving immune system depression carry risks for people with SLE?

Think About This . . .

- Do you believe you could cope with a significant health problem at this time in your life?
- Do you know anyone who has or has had cancer? How did cancer affect that person's life?
- How regularly do you perform either breast or testicular self-examination?

- If you were diagnosed as having a terminal illness, how willing would you be to serve as a subject in a research project that tested a potentially toxic experimental drug?
- Which conditions in this chapter are you likely to develop, and which are you not likely to develop?

References

1. Levy D: USA 'losing ground' in cancer war, *USA Today,* Sept 30, 1994.
2. US Bureau of the Census: *Statistical abstract of the United States: 1995,* annual ed 115, Washington, DC, 1995, US Department of Commerce.
3. Songer J, oncologist, personal interview, December 1995.
4. Marx J: New tumor suppressor may rival p53 (Research News), *Science* 264(5157):344-345, 1994.
5. Wooster R et al: Identification of the breast cancer susceptibility gene BRCA2, *Nature* 378(6559):789-792, 1995.
6. Eastman P: The cancer genetics revolution: science and ethics at the crossroads, *Oncology Times* 16(8), August 1994.
7. American Cancer Society: *Cancer facts and figures: 1995,* Atlanta, 1995, The Society.
8. Sellers TA et al: Evidence of Mendelian inheritance in the pathogenesis of lung cancer, *J Natl Cancer Inst* 82(15):1272-1279, 1990.
9. Sellers TA et al: Effect of family history, body-fat distribution, and reproductive factors on the risk of postmenopausal breast cancer, *New Engl J Med* 326(20):1323-1329, 1992.
10. Ballard-Barbash R et al: Body fat distribution and breast cancer in the Framingham study, *J Natl Cancer Inst* 82(24):1943-1944, 1990.
11. Kliewer EV, Smith KR: Breast cancer mortality among immigrants in Australia and Canada (reports), *J Natl Cancer Inst* 87(15):1161, 1995.
12. Blot WJ, McLaughlin JK: Geographic patterns of breast cancer among American women, *J Natl Cancer Inst* 87(24):1819-1820, 1995.

13. Jacobson JA et al: Ten-year results of a comparison of conservation with mastectomy in the treatment of stage I and II breast cancer, *N Engl J Med* 332(14)907-911, 1995.
14. Fisher BF et al: Reanalysis and results after 12 years follow-up in a randomized clinical trial comparing total mastectomy with lumpectomy with or without irradiation in the treatment of breast cancer, *N Engl J Med* 333(22):1456-1461, 1995.
15. Eddy DM: Screening for cervical cancer, *Ann Intern Med* 113(7):560-561, 1990.
16. Janerich DT et al: The screening histories of women with invasive cervical cancer, Connecticut, *Am J Public Health* 85(6):791-794, 1995.
17. Gann PH et al: Prospective study of plasma fatty acids and risk of prostate cancer (Reports), *J Natl Cancer Inst* 86(4):281-286, 1994.
18. Lee W et al: Cytidine methylation of regulatory sequences near the class glutathione S-transferase gene accompanies human prostatic cancer, *Proc Natl Acad Sci USA* 91(24):11733-11737, 1994.
19. Lu-Yao GL, Greenberg ER: Changes in prostate cancer incidence and treatment in USA, *Lancet* 343:251-254, 1994.
20. Miller BA et al: SEER cancer statistics review: 1973-1990, NIH Pub No 93-2789, 1993, National Cancer Institute.
21. McKusick V: Our genes: what the map shows, *Time*, pp 46-53, Jan 17, 1994.
22. Giovannucci E et al: Aspirin and the risk of colorectal cancer in women, *N Engl J Med* 333(10):609-614, 1995.
23. Hardy L: Years of sun take toll on baby boomers, *USA Today*, p 3D, June 28, 1995.
24. Phytochemicals in disease prevention, *Nutri-News*, January 1995.
25. Fink W, exercise physiologist, personal interview, December 1995.
26. Thibodeau G, Patton K: *Human body in health & disease*, St Louis, 1992, Mosby.
27. Crowley LV: *Introduction to human disease*, Boston, 1992, Jones & Bartlett.
28. Conrad B et al: Evidence of superantigen involvement insulin-dependent diabetes mellitus aetiology, *Nature* 371(6495):351-354, 1994.
29. *National asthma education report: expert panel report*, National Heart, Lung, and Blood Institute, 1991.
30. Price SA, Wilson L: Pathophysiology: clinical concepts of disease processes, ed 4, St Louis, 1992, Mosby.

Suggested Readings

Dravecky D: *Comeback*, San Francisco, 1990, Zondervan Books/Harper & Row.
The heroic chronicles of a major league baseball pitcher who developed bone cancer in his pitching arm. Dravecky shows that with faith and determination, the fear of cancer can be overcome.
Schapiro R: *Multiple sclerosis: a rehabilitation approach to management*, New York, 1991, Demos Publications.
A highly authoritative book dealing with all aspects of rehabilitation for people with MS. Written with 12 other contributors who are experienced in this field, the author not only describes rehabilitation strategies but also the underlying neurological basis of each.
Carroll DL, Dudley D: *Living well with multiple sclerosis: a guide for patient, caregiver and family*, New York, 1995, Harper Collins.
This book can serve as a comprehensive guide to MS on the part of all involved people. Topics covered include mail order equipment and supplies, sexual concerns, job-related issues, and the emotional aspects of the disease. Additional resources are listed.
Lawlis GF: *The cure: the hero's journey with cancer*, San Jose, Calif, 1995, Resource Publications.
Although similar to a children's book, this is an adult fable about Alex, a gray wolf, who learns about his disease and himself as he deals with his cancer. Cancer becomes not only a part of Alex's life but a stimulus for him to grow as he explores alternatives to his life before cancer.
Love S: *Susan Love's breast book*, New York, 1995, Addison-Wesley.
Now in a revised edition, this book is considered the "bible" of breast cancer–related information. From her perspective as a woman, physician, and activist, Love shares information regarding the diagnosis, treatment, management, and prevention of breast cancer, as well as our current understanding of the disease's cause.

 AS WE GO TO PRESS . . .

At the American Diabetes Association annual meeting, evidence was presented that indicated that high intake of the essential nutrient chromium could be helpful in normalizing glucose and insulin levels in people with Type II diabetes. Chromium supplements are inexpensive and readily available in health food stores. The millions of Americans who have Type II diabetes are being cautioned that chromium is not a cure for diabetes and that all treatment options should be discussed first with a physician.

ON...

Managing Chronic Pain

Carlotta loved to spend her spare time puttering around in her flower garden. Every weekend, she would work outside for hours tilling soil, putting in new plants, pruning, and landscaping. One Saturday afternoon as she was lifting some railroad ties to provide a new border for her plant paradise, she heard a loud popping noise and felt a sharp pain in her lower back. She tried aspirin, bed rest, massage, and heat, but the pain was still excruciating even after 2 weeks. She went to see her doctor, who prescribed pain medication and a brief course of physical therapy, but the pain persisted. Finally, after nearly a year passed with no relief, her doctor recommended back surgery. Carlotta spent almost 3 months recovering from the surgery, after which she hoped to be able to lead a normal, pain-free life.

Unfortunately, Carlotta's pain persists even today, almost 2 years since her initial injury. Carlotta suffers from chronic pain, a type of pain that persists beyond the expected healing time of an injury or illness. Chronic pain differs from most ordinary encounters with pain, such as pain resulting from a headache, a fall, or surgery. According to the American Pain Society, chronic pain, is difficult to treat because it does not respond to normal pain treatments. Also, some of the usual signs that accompany acute pain, such as sweating, increased heart rate, and dilated pupils, are not present in individuals with chronic pain.[1] Because physicians have difficulty in diagnosing the source of chronic pain, they have a tendency to think a patient's suffering is "all in her head." As a result, many of the 95 million chronic pain sufferers do not get the types of treatment they so desperately need.[2,3]

Causes of Chronic Pain

Chronic pain occurs as the result of one of three primary causes. In some patients, chronic pain may be linked to injuries to the central or peripheral nervous systems, according to John D. Loeser, M.D., director of the Multidisciplinary Pain Center at the University of Washington School of Medicine.[1] In these patients, no tissue damage ever occurred in the part of their body that hurts. Whenever the nervous system heals itself, the functions of the nerve cells lost in the injury are not restored during the healing process.[2] As a result, the patient's neurological functions are impaired. This type of pain can occur as a result of limb amputation, shingles, diabetes, or surgery.[1]

A second cause of chronic pain is linked to degenerative changes in joints. In these cases, tissue damage that

has occurred may not heal properly. Patients have both inflammation of the joints and chronic degenerative problems.[1] This cause of pain usually accompanies diseases such as arthritis and lupus.

The third "cause" of pain is the catchall category: "no known pathological mechanism."[1] Doctors are unsure why these patients are having pain. The one criterion used to place a patient in this category is whether the patient's pain complaints exceed the physician's expectations based on the illness or injury the patient has suffered.

Conditions Associated with Chronic Pain

Several types of conditions are commonly associated with sufferers of chronic pain, the most common being the headache. Up to 57% of men and 76% of women in the adolescent and young adult age-groups experience recurrent headaches. The National Headache Foundation estimates that 45 million Americans suffer from chronic headaches. Of these sufferers, 86% are women. Although doctors have identified 55 types of headaches, the four most commonly associated with chronic pain are tension headaches, migraines, cluster headaches, and sinus headaches.[3]

Like Carlotta in our previous example, four out of five Americans experience back pain at some point in their lives. The problem usually resolves itself for most people; however, it is estimated that more than 11 million Americans have enough back pain to cause impairment. This cause of chronic pain is particularly troublesome because of its economic impact on society. Attorney's costs for pursuing back injuries as a result of worker's compensation and other accidents approached $5 billion in 1990. The indirect costs for lost wages and homemakers' potential lost earnings are near $3.6 billion. Based on all analyses of possible cost factors, back pain costs society anywhere from $75 billion to $100 billion annually.[1]

Another debilitating condition commonly associated with chronic pain is arthritis. More than 35 million Americans have a form of this disease. Two types of arthritis exist. *Osteoarthritis* is the breaking down of the cartilage found at the ends of the long bones. Weight-bearing and frequently used joints are the areas most commonly affected. *Rheumatoid arthritis* is an autoimmune disorder in which the patient's own immune system produces antibodies that attack the tissues in the joints of the body.[1] Symptoms of both types include stiffness and swelling of the joints.

Cancer and Chronic Pain

Although cancer is one of the conditions often associated with chronic pain, pain experts put it into a class by itself because of its special circumstances. Chronic cancer pain is complex because the pain can occur as a result of bone invasion, tumors compressing nerves, tumors affecting internal organs, obstruction of blood vessels, surgery, chemotherapy, or radiation treatment.[1]

Effects of Chronic Pain

Because chronic pain is such a disruptive, ongoing phenomenon, it can affect almost every aspect of an individual's life. Richard Linchitz, M.D., a pain specialist and chronic pain sufferer, describes what his life was like after a disk in his lower back became herniated: "As bad as the pain was, the worst aspect for me was the growing and quite depressing sense that my days of vigorous exercise were over. My doctor began ruling out, one by one, the very activities—running, bicycling, weightlifting—that had become a part of my identity . . ."[4] Veronica, one of Dr. Norman J. Marcus's patients, found it difficult not only to pursue hobbies but even to complete simple everyday tasks such as washing the dishes.[3]

The devastation of losing a job is another potential effect of suffering with chronic pain. Because the pain is so invasive and persistent, it affects a person's ability to concentrate, perform essential job duties, or even go to work. Toni, another of Dr. Marcus's patients, had been the manager of a high-pressure department of a busy store. She had always been conscientious and hard working until she began having pain in her hip. Because of the pain, she had difficulty performing her job, and she also had to take time off from work frequently either because of doctor's appointments or because her pain was too severe. As a result, Toni was fired.[3]

Sleep disorders are a third potential effect of chronic pain. Sleep disorders can come about in two ways. Either a patient is unable to sleep because of the pain, or the individual becomes dependent on a pain or sleep medication that disrupts the sleep cycle. Toni, who was described in the previous paragraph, was on many medications, including both painkillers and sleeping pills, yet she "never slept." On being admitted to a pain management center, Toni was taken off all her medications and given a mild antidepressant instead. She slept for 10 hours that night, "the first good night's sleep I'd had in four years."[3]

Serious psychological problems can also result from chronic pain. Depression is one of the most common ailments. Henry, another patient at Dr. Marcus's pain clinic and a former construction worker, had always been a calm, easygoing person who got along well with others and served as the chief provider for his family. One day at work, Henry was struck in the back of the neck by a steel beam. He suffered pain not just in his neck but also throughout his body. As time went on and the pain did not improve, Henry's entire personality began to change. He went from being easygoing to being a chronic worrier because he was concerned about the family's financial security. He isolated himself from his family and friends, and he began to snap at anyone who asked him questions about his condition. The more Henry hurt, the more he worried about hurting; the more he worried about hurting, the more he hurt. Henry was caught in a downward spiral of depression that set him apart from his family and friends.[3]

The final significant side effect of chronic pain is the potential damage it can do to the immune system. This effect can be particularly troublesome in patients whose chronic pain is the result of cancer. Studies have shown that pain can suppress the immune system, thus causing cancer patients to have difficulty recovering.[5] Because of this potentially fatal problem, it is especially important for cancer patients to have their pain treated promptly and effectively.

Methods of Managing Chronic Pain

Although chronic pain has several negative side effects, many of these effects can be controlled through proper pain management methods. Most pain specialists recommend that sufferers be treated through a multidisciplinary approach that uses a combination of methods to achieve maximal relief.

One of the most common and effective methods of achieving relief of chronic pain is the use of opioid drugs, also known as *Schedule II drugs*. These drugs have been proven to provide quick relief of pain, particularly among cancer patients and headache sufferers.[5,6] However, physicians are often reluctant to prescribe these drugs for several reasons. First, doctors are afraid that if they are perceived as prescribing too many opioids, they could be reported to the medical board and ultimately lose their licenses. Second, American society in general disapproves of prescribing narcotics because of the fear of addiction and the idea that all narcotics are bad, despite their potential for providing pain relief. Finally, medical personnel tend to underestimate the amount of pain that patients suffer. Most people who suffer severe pain and request narcotics will not become addicts, but some medical personnel who work with pain sufferers have the mindset that people with chronic pain do not hurt as badly as they claim to.[5]

For chronic headache sufferers, several other types of drugs offer hope as well. Small doses of tricyclic antidepressants taken at bedtime seem to help headache sufferers sleep better and have some preventive effect during the day. Other drugs that provide relief include beta-blockers, calcium channel blockers, and anticonvulsants. Doctors may try several combinations of these drugs to see which will most effectively relieve headache symptoms, with the eventual goal of removing as many medications as possible from the patient's daily regimen.[6]

For patients with arthritis, two classes of drugs appear to offer the most relief. The first type is known as *nonsteroidal antiinflammatory drugs*, or *NSAIDs*. The most well-known types of these drugs are Advil, Nuprin, Naprosyn, and Anaprox. They provide relief within 2 hours. A second type of antiarthritic medicine is known as *slow-acting antirheumatic drugs*, or *SAARDs*. These drugs provide time-released, long-lasting relief. Other treatments that may be used in conjunction with these two types of drugs include injectable gold and corticosteroids.[7]

Surgery is another option in the array of choices for managing chronic pain. This option is most effective in helping patients with cancer. Removing diseased cells or tumors often removes the source that is causing pain for the patient.[5] Surgery may also become necessary for the arthritis pain sufferer. Replacement of cartilage or an affected joint will often help a sufferer lead a more normal, less painful life.[6] Surprisingly, however, surgery is rarely a good option for back pain sufferers. Studies of hospital records show that back surgery often does more harm than good.[2,4]

Because the mind is such a powerful instrument of healing, pain specialists often recommend that patients undertake psychological methods of pain relief in conjunction with traditional methods. For example, many headache specialists recommend biofeedback techniques so that patients can learn to control their responses to pain.[6] Pain specialists at a pain clinic in Dallas teach their patients to do deep-breathing exercises and then advance them to meditation techniques to promote relaxation.[2] Also, positive thinking about one's situation and prospects for recovery can help patients need fewer medications, according to a recent British study.[7]

Physical methods of managing pain can add another dimension to chronic pain management. One time-tested method of relief is massage.[3] Other helpful treatments include nerve blocks to the affected area, physical therapy, and exercises as prescribed by a physical therapist or physician.[2-4] Finally, a patient can make some lifestyle changes to lessen the pain. Eating regularly, getting plenty of rest, and reducing caffeine intake have all been found to be particularly helpful to headache sufferers but may also help others afflicted with chronic pain.[6]

The Future of Chronic Pain Management

Although they were virtually unheard of just a few years ago, pain clinics, or pain centers, are becoming more prevalent in the medical community.[8] These centers feature physicians and other health care professionals who use the multidisciplinary approach to pain management. Personnel on site might include physicians, physical therapists, exercise physiologists, psychologists, and psychiatrists.[3] Pain centers are also at the forefront of pain research. A pain center in Dallas is currently studying the possibility of using gene therapy to conquer chronic pain. The new genes would enable patients to grow new, undamaged nerves, which would also enhance endorphin production.[2] Whether through medication, therapy, or research, the goal of all pain centers is the same: to improve the patient's condition so that on leaving the center, the person will be able to resume normal activities, need a minimal amount of medication, and maintain a positive attitude.[3]

An additional hope for better chronic pain management comes in the form of training of tomorrow's doctors. The American Medical Association (AMA) has called for better education about pain and pain management in both undergraduate and postgraduate medical training.[8,9] In particular, the AMA hopes to make the use of opioid drugs more acceptable to health care personnel as an option for relieving pain.[8] Hospitals are also instituting quality assurance programs so that patients can be more empowered to demand and receive the pain relief they need.[9]

An option for terminal cancer patients who are in need of relief from chronic pain is the hospice movement. Hospices put into practice a philosophy that allows medical personnel to focus on the patients rather than their diseases. The main goals of hospices are to provide pain relief and to give psychological support to both the patient and his or her family. Hospices also use a multidisciplinary approach that includes physicians, nurses, social workers, physical therapists, and members of the clergy.[1] The hospice can provide the care and support that cancer sufferers and their families need as the patient nears the end of life.

Although there is not yet a cure for chronic pain, it can be managed successfully with the help of trained personnel from a variety of fields. Unfortunately, chronic pain sufferers must be vocal and persistent to get the help they desperately need. Doctors and patients alike must realize that chronic pain is not "all in the patient's head" but a real, treatable condition.

For Discussion . . .

Have you ever known someone who suffered (or still suffers) from chronic pain? What were your feelings about this person and his or her pain? If you suffered from chronic pain, what treatments do you think would be the best for you? Would you be willing to try nonconventional therapies like the ones described in this article, or would you be more comfortable with traditional methods of therapy? Why?

References

1. Cowles J: *Pain relief*, New York, 1993, Mastermedia.
2. Atkinson J: Nerve center, *Texas Monthly* p 6, June 1994.
3. Marcus NJ: *Freedom from chronic pain*, New York, 1994, Simon & Schuster.
4. Linchitz RM: *Life without pain*, New York, 1987, Addison-Wesley.
5. Buterbaugh L: Breaking through cancer pain barriers, *Medical World* p 10, Oct 15, 1993.
6. Brooks PM: Clinical management of rheumatoid arthritis, *Lancet* (341)8840, 1993.
7. Meinson M: Brain against pain, *Prevention* p 48, Jan 1, 1996.
8. Goldsmith MF: Pain speaking—and anesthesiologists answer, *JAMA* (267)12, 1992.
9. Hill CS Jr: When will adequate pain treatment be the norm? *JAMA* (274)23, 1995.

Preventing Infectious Diseases

Healthy People 2000 Objectives

Progress has been uneven in our efforts to meet the Healthy People 2000 objectives in the area of infectious disease prevention. A principal objective was to reduce to zero the incidence of vaccine-preventable infectious diseases in people under age 25. Overall, the nation has moved steadily toward achieving this goal. However, there are clear differences in the rate and amount of progress for specific conditions. For example, substantial gains have been made in the prevention of measles, rubella, and congenital rubella syndrome. In fact, the occurrence of measles in those under 25 has almost been eliminated. In contrast, progress in preventing tetanus and pertussis (whooping cough) is lagging behind.

In the minds of many, few objectives advanced in the Healthy People 2000 document are more important than that of reducing the prevalence of HIV infections. At mid-decade, however, data were too incomplete to be reported. The Midcourse Review does indicate some modest gains in increasing condom use among sexually active teens in grades 9 through 12.

INFECTIOUS DISEASES IN THE 1990s

Before the turn of the twentieth century, infectious diseases were the leading cause of death. These deaths came after exposure to the organisms that produced such diseases as smallpox, tuberculosis (TB), influenza, whooping cough (pertussis), typhoid, diphtheria, and tetanus. However, since the early 1990s, improvements in public sanitation, the widespread use of antibiotic drugs as a treatment method, and vaccinations as preventive therapy have considerably reduced the numbers of people dying from infectious diseases. People now die more often from chronic, long-term disease processes.

Today, however, we have a new respect for infectious diseases. We have learned that AIDS threatens millions of people in many areas of the world. We are witnessing the resurgence of TB. We recognize the role of pelvic infections in infertility. We also know that failure to fully immunize children has laid the groundwork for a return of whooping cough, polio, and other serious childhood diseases.

New dimensions of infectious disease have recently arisen. These include the appearance of extremely virulent viruses, such as the Ebola virus in Zaire, which is fatal to 75% of those who contract it and for which there is neither an immunization nor an understanding of its transmission, and the Sabia virus, released in a Yale laboratory accident; the increasing resistance of bacteria such as *Staphylococcus aureus, Enterococcus,* and *Mycobacterium* (which causes tuberculosis) to antibiotics as the result of overuse, improper use, and biological "redesign" of the organisms themselves; the role of a bacterium (*Helicobacter pylori)* in the development of gastric ulcers; and, finally, the growing concern over transmission of infectious organisms through contaminated food, improper preparation of food, and contamination of water. In fact, this emergence of antibiotic-resistant and "redesigned" organisms is very serious: the death rate from infectious diseases has risen 58% during the period 1980 to 1992.

INFECTIOUS DISEASE TRANSMISSION

Infectious diseases can generally be transferred from person to person, although there is not always a direct transfer from one person to another. Infectious diseases can be especially dangerous because of their ability to spread to large numbers of people, producing *epidemics* or *pandemics.*

The sections that follow explain the process of disease transmission and the stages of infection. For a discussion of preventing infectious disease transmission, turn to the article on pp. 306-307.

Pathogens

For a disease to be transferred, a person must come into contact with the disease-producing agent, or **pathogen,** such as a virus, bacterium, or fungus. When pathogens enter our bodies, they are sometimes able to resist body defense systems, flourish, and produce an illness. We commonly call this an *infection.* Because of their small size, pathogens are sometimes referred to as *microorganisms, microbes,* or *germs.* Table 12-1 describes the more familiar infectious disease agents and some of the illnesses they produce.

Chain of Infection

The transmission of a pathogenic agent through the various links in the chain of infection (Figure 12-1) forms the basis for an understanding of how diseases spread.[1] Not every pathogenic agent will move all the way through the chain of infection because various links in the chain can be broken. Therefore the presence of a pathogen creates only the potential for a disease.

Agent

The first link in the chain of infection is the disease-causing **agent.** Whereas some agents are very **virulent** and cause serious infectious illnesses such as HIV, which causes AIDS, others produce far less serious infections, as in the common cold. Through mutation, some pathogenic agents, particularly viruses, become more virulent than they once were.

Reservoir

Infectious agents must have the support and protection of a favorable environment to survive. This environment forms the second link in the chain of infection and is referred to as the *reservoir* in which the agent resides. In many of the most common infectious diseases, the reservoirs in which the pathogenic organisms live are the bodies of already infected people. Here the agents thrive before being spread to others. These infected people are, accordingly, the hosts for particular disease agents.

For other infectious diseases, however, the reservoirs in which the agents are maintained are the bodies of animals. Rabies is among the most familiar of the animal-reservoir diseases. Not in all cases will the animals be sick or show symptoms similar to those seen in infected persons.

The third type of reservoir in which disease-causing agents can reside is on or in nonliving environ-

Table 12-1 Pathogens and Common Infectious Diseases		
Pathogen	**Description**	**Representative Disease Processes**
Viruses	Smallest common pathogens; nonliving particles of genetic material (DNA) surrounded by a protein coat	Rubeola, mumps, chickenpox, rubella, influenza, warts, colds, oral and genital herpes, shingles, AIDS, genital warts
Bacteria	One-celled microorganisms with sturdy, well-defined cell walls; three distinctive forms: spherical (cocci), rod shaped (bacilli), and spiral shaped (spirilla)	Tetanus, strep throat, scarlet fever, gonorrhea, syphilis, chlamydia, toxic shock syndrome, Legionnaires' disease, bacterial pneumonia, meningitis, diphtheria, food poisoning, Lyme disease
Fungi	Plantlike microorganisms; molds and yeasts	Athlete's foot, ringworm, histoplasmosis, San Joaquin Valley fever, candidiasis
Protozoa	Simplest animal form, generally one-celled organisms	Malaria, amebic dysentery, trichomoniasis, vaginitis
Rickettsia	Viruslike organisms that require a host's living cells for growth and replication	Typhus, Rocky Mountain spotted fever, rickettsialpox
Parasitic worms	Many-celled organisms; represented by tapeworms, leeches, and roundworms	Dirofilariasis (dog heartworm), elephantiasis, onchocerciasis

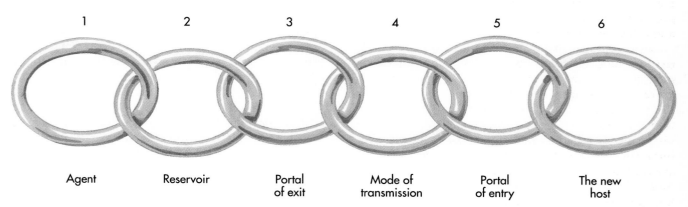

1	2	3	4	5	6
Agent	Reservoir	Portal of exit	Mode of transmission	Portal of entry	The new host

Figure 12-1   The six links in the chain of infection.

ments, such as the soil. (The spores of the tetanus bacterium can survive in soil for up to 50 years, entering the human body in a puncture wound.) Warm and moist locker-room floors are another example of this environment because the fungi that cause ringworm and jock itch can survive there.

Portal of exit

For pathogenic agents to cause diseases and illnesses in others, it is necessary that they leave their reservoirs. The third link in the chain of infection is the portal of exit, or the point at which agents leave their reservoirs.

Particularly in terms of infectious diseases that involve human reservoirs, the principal portals of exit are familiar—the digestive system, urinary system, respiratory system, reproductive system, and the blood.

Mode of transmission

The fourth link in the chain of infection is the mode of transmission, or the way that pathogens are passed from reservoirs to susceptible hosts. Two principal methods are *direct transmission* and *indirect transmission*.

pathogen
Disease-causing agent.

agent
Causal pathogen of a particular disease.

virulent (**veer** yuh lent)
Capable of causing disease.

Three types of direct transmission are observed in human-to-human transmission. These include *contact* between body surfaces (such as kissing, touching, and sexual intercourse), *droplet spread* (inhalation of contaminated air droplets), and *fecal-oral spread* (feces on the hands are brought into contact with the mouth).

Indirect transmission occurs between infected and uninfected people when infectious agents travel by means of nonhuman materials. Vehicles of transmission include *inanimate objects,* such as water, food items, soil, towels, items of clothing, and eating utensils.

A second method of indirect transmission of infectious agents occurs in conjunction with vectors. The term *vector* is related to living things, such as insects, birds, and other animals that carry diseases from human to human. An example of a vector is the deer tick that transmits Lyme disease.

Airborne indirect transmission involves the *inhalation* of infected particles that have been suspended in an air source for an extended period. Unlike droplet transmission, in which both infected and uninfected people must be in close physical proximity, noninfected people can become infected through airborne transmission by sharing air with infected people who were in the same room hours earlier. Viral infections such as German measles may be spread in this manner.

Portal of entry

The fifth link in the chain of infection is the portal of entry. As with the portals of exit, there are three primary portals of entry for pathogenic agents to enter the bodies of uninfected people. These are through the digestive system, respiratory system, and reproductive system. In addition, a break in the skin provides another portal of entry. In most infectious conditions the portals of entry prove to be within the same systems as the portals of exit were for the infected people. In the case of HIV, however, cross-system transmission is observed. Oral and anal sex allow for infectious agents to pass between the warm, moist tissues of the reproductive and digestive systems.

The new host

All people are in theory at risk for contracting infectious diseases and thus could be identified as susceptible hosts. In practice, however, factors such as overall health, acquired immunity, health care services, and health-related behavior can influence susceptibility to infectious diseases.

Stages of Infection

When a new host is assaulted by a pathogenic agent, a reasonably predictable sequence of events takes place. That is, the disease moves through five rather distinctive stages.[2] You may be able to recognize these stages of infection each time you catch a cold.

1. *The incubation stage.* This stage lasts from the time a pathogen enters the body until it multiplies enough to produce signs and symptoms of the disease. The length of this stage can vary from a few hours to many months, depending on the virulence of the organisms, the concentration of organisms, the host's level of immune responsiveness, and other health problems. This stage has been called a *silent stage.* Transmission of the pathogen to a new host is possible but not probable during this stage: a host may be infected during this stage but not infectious. HIV infection is an exception to this rule.

2. *The prodromal stage.* The incubation stage is followed by a short period during which the host may experience a variety of general signs and symptoms, including watery eyes, runny nose, slight fever, and overall tiredness. These symptoms are nonspecific in nature and may not be overwhelming enough to force the host to rest. During this stage the pathogenic agent continues to multiply. Now the host is capable of transferring pathogens to a new host. Self-imposed isolation should be practiced during this stage to protect others. Again, HIV infection is different in regard to this stage.

3. *The clinical stage.* This stage, also called the *acme* or *acute stage*, is often the most unpleasant stage for the host. At this time the disease reaches its highest point of development. All of the clinical (observable) signs and symptoms for the particular disease can be seen or analyzed by appropriate laboratory tests. The likelihood of transmitting the disease to others is highest during this peak stage; all of our available defense mechanisms are in the process of resisting further damage from the pathogen.

4. *The decline stage.* During this stage the first signs of recovery occur. The infection is ending or, in some cases, being reduced to a subclinical level. Relapse may occur if people overextend themselves. In HIV and AIDS, this is almost always the last stage before death.

5. *The recovery stage.* Also called the *convalescence stage*, this stage is characterized by apparent recovery from the invading agent. Disease transmission during this stage is possible but not probable. Until the host's overall health has been strengthened, he or she may be especially susceptible to another (perhaps different) disease pathogen. Fortunately, after the recovery stage, further susceptibility to the pathogenic agent should be reduced because of the body's buildup of immunity. This buildup of immunity is not always permanent; for example, many sexually transmitted diseases can be contracted repeatedly.

BODY DEFENSES: MECHANICAL AND CELLULAR IMMUNE SYSTEMS

Much as a military installation is protected by a series of defensive alignments, so too is the body. These defenses can be classified as being either mechanical or cellular (Figure 12-2). *Mechanical* defenses are first-line defenses, since they physically separate the internal body from the external environment. Included among these are the skin, the mucous membranes that line the respiratory and gastrointestinal tracts, earwax, the tiny hairs and cilia that filter incoming air, and even tears. These defenses serve primarily as a shield against foreign materials that may contain pathogenic agents. These defenses can, however, be disarmed, as is done when tobacco smoke kills the cilia that protect the airway, resulting in chronic bronchitis, or when contact lenses decrease tearing, leading to irritation and eye infection.

The second component of the body's protective defenses is the *cellular* system or, more commonly, the **immune system.** The cellular component is, in comparison with the mechanical defenses, far more specific, with the elimination of microorganisms, foreign proteins, and cells foreign to the body as its primary mission. A wellness-oriented lifestyle, including sound nutrition, effective stress management, and regular exercise, undergirds this important division of the immune system. The microorganism, foreign proteins, or abnormal cells whose presence activates this cellular component are identified collectively as *antigens.*[3]

Divisions of the Immune System

Closer examination of the immune system, or cellular defenses, reveals two separate but highly cooperative groups of cells. One group of cells has its origins in the fetal thymus gland and thus has become known as *T cell–mediated immunity,* or simply cell-mediated immunity. The second group of cells that make up cellular immunity are the B cells (**b**ursa of Fabricius) that are the working units of *humoral immunity.*[3] Cellular elements of both cell-mediated and humoral immunity can be found within the bloodstream, the lymphatic tissues of the body, and the fluid that surrounds body cells.

Although we are born with the structural elements of both cell-mediated and humoral immunity, the development of an immune response requires that components of these cellular systems encounter and successfully defend against specific antigens. Once this has occurred, the immune system is primed to respond quickly and effectively should the same antigens be encountered again. This confrontation results in the development of a state of **acquired immunity (AI).** As seen in Figure 12-2, the development of AI can occur in different ways.

- **Naturally acquired immunity (NAI)** occurs when the body is exposed to infectious agents.

immune system
System of cellular elements that protects the body from invading pathogens and foreign materials.

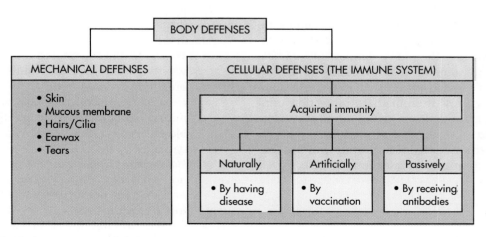

Figure 12-2 The body has a variety of defenses against invading organisms. Mechanical defenses are the first means of protection, since they separate the internal body from the external environment. Cellular defenses include chemicals and specialized cells that provide immunity to subsequent infections.

Table 12-2   Recommended Immunization Schedule*,†

	Months							Years
	Birth	1-2	2	4	6	6-18	12-15	6
Diphtheria/pertussis/ tetanus (DPT)			X	X	X		X‡	X
Polio (OPV)			X	X	X			X
Measles/mumps/ rubella (MMR)						X		X
Haemophilus influenzae (Hib)			X	X	X§		X	
Hepatitis B ǀǀ (Hep B)	X	X				X		
or:		X		X		X		

*Foreign travelers: renew immunizations for diseases prevalent in the countries of travel.

†Influenza: yearly for elderly adults, workers in occupations (such as health care workers and teachers) exposed to infected persons, and for all adults with chronic respiratory and heart disease.

‡As early as 12 months, as long as at least 6 months since last DTP dose.

§May not be required, depending on which Hib vaccine is used.

ǀǀ Anyone exposed to infected individuals or contaminated food and water, and foreign travelers and health care workers.

For referral to an immunization clinic or for other information, contact the Centers for Disease Control and Prevention National Immunization Program: (800) 232-2522 in English or TDD; (800) 232-0233 in Spanish.

Thus when we catch an infectious disease, we fight the infection and in the process become immune (protected) from developing that illness again should reinfection occur.

- **Artificially acquired immunity (AAI)** occurs when the body is exposed to weakened or killed infectious agents introduced through vaccination or immunization. As in NAI, the body engages the infectious agents and produces a record of how to fight the same battle again. Young children, older adults, and adults in high-risk occupations should consult their physicians about immunizations. Table 12-2 shows a schedule for immunization.

- **Passively acquired immunity (PAI),** a third form of immunity, results when antibodies are introduced into the body. These antibodies are for a variety of specific infections and are produced outside the body (either in animals or by the genetic manipulation of microorganisms). When introduced into the human body, they provide immediate protection until a more natural form of immunity can be developed.

Collectively, these forms of immunity can provide important protection against infectious disease.

IMMUNIZATIONS

Although the incidence of several childhood communicable diseases is at or near the lowest level ever, the risk of a resurgence of diseases such as measles, polio, diphtheria, and rubella is very real. This possible upturn in childhood infectious illnesses is based on the disturbing finding that fewer than half of American preschoolers are adequately immunized, which is principally due to a failure on the part of many parents to complete their children's immunization programs. Today a concerted effort is under way to raise the level of immunization to 90% of all children under the age of 2 years.

On the basis of current technology, vaccinations against several potentially serious infectious conditions are available and, of course, should be given. These include the following:

- *Diphtheria:* a potentially fatal illness that leads to inflammation of the membranes that line the throat, to swollen lymph nodes, and to heart and kidney failure

- *Whooping cough:* a bacterial infection of the airways and lungs that results in deep, noisy breathing and coughing

- *Hepatitis B:* a viral infection that can be transmitted sexually or through the exchange of blood or body fluids and causes serious liver damage

- *Haemophilus influenzae type B:* a bacterial infection that can damage the heart and brain, resulting in meningitis, and can produce profound hearing loss

- *Tetanus:* a fatal infection caused by bacteria found in the soil that damages the central nervous system

- *Rubella (German measles):* a viral infection of the upper respiratory tract that can cause damage to a developing fetus when the mother contracts the infection during the first trimester of pregnancy
- *Measles (red measles):* a highly contagious viral infection leading to a rash, high fever, and other upper respiratory tract symptoms
- *Polio:* a viral infection capable of causing paralysis of the large muscles of the extremities
- *Mumps:* a viral infection of the salivary glands
- *Chickenpox:* a varicella zoster virus spread by airborne droplets leading to a sore throat, rash, and fluid-filled blisters

Parents of newborns should take their infants to their family care physicians, pediatricians, or well-baby clinics operated by county health departments to begin the immunization schedule. The schedule shown in Table 12-2 is recommended by the Centers for Disease Control and Prevention (CDC). It is hoped that a single immunization to protect children against all of the infectious childhood illnesses will soon be available, perhaps only 10 years away. The newest vaccine, VariVax, a vaccine against chickenpox, is now available but has not yet been well accepted by physicians or parents. Additionally, an experimental vaccine against infant diarrhea caused by rotaviruses has also been developed, and when available, it should be an important factor in reducing infant mortality.[4]

THE IMMUNE RESPONSE

To fully understand the function of the immune system requires a substantial understanding of human biology and is beyond the scope of this text. Figure 12-3 provides a simplified view of the immune response. For a discussion of abnormal immune responses, see the Star Boxes on allergies and rheumatoid arthritis on p. 287.

When antigens (whether microorganisms, foreign substances, or abnormal cells) are discovered within the body, some antigens are confronted by various types of white blood cells and their number is initially reduced by the destructive action of these blood cells. At the same time, macrophages (a very large white blood cell) encounter other antigens and signal components of cell-mediated immunity called *helper T cells* to assist in the immune response.

Once activated by the presence of the macrophage/antigens complex, helper T cells notify a second component of cellular immunity, the killer T cells, and a component of humoral immunity, B cells. Killer T cells produce powerful chemical messengers that activate specific white blood cells that are capable of destroying antigens. At the same time, B cells are transformed into specialized cells (plasma cells) capable of producing **antibodies** and into memory cells that record information pertaining to the antigen and the appropriate immune system response.

At the same time that helper T cells and killer T cells are engaged in destroying invading antigens, two additional components of cellular immunity are formed: memory T cells and suppressor T cells. As the name suggests, the memory T cells remember additional aspects of the immune system's responses so that reinfections can be encountered even more quickly and decisively. Suppressor T cells are specialized T cells that moderate B cell activity by offsetting the action of helper T cells. Their action allows the production of antibodies to be reduced once it is apparent that the immune system has won its battle.

Clearly, without a normal immune system involving both cellular and humoral elements, we would quickly become the victims of serious and life-shortening infections and malignancies. As you will see later, this is exactly what occurs in virtually all people infected with HIV.

acquired immunity (AI)
Major component of the immune system associated with the formation of antibodies and specialized blood cells that are capable of destroying pathogens.

naturally acquired immunity (NAI)
Type of acquired immunity resulting from the body's response to naturally occurring pathogens.

artificially acquired immunity (AAI)
Type of acquired immunity resulting from the body's response to pathogens introduced into the body through immunizations.

passively acquired immunity (PAI)
Temporary immunity achieved by providing antibodies to a person exposed to a particular pathogen.

antibodies
Chemical compounds produced by the body's immune system to destroy antigens and their toxins.

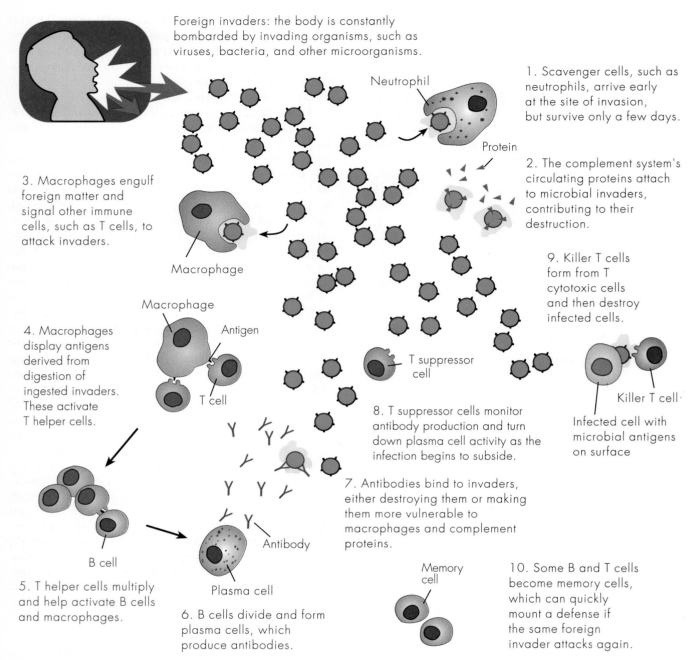

Foreign invaders: the body is constantly bombarded by invading organisms, such as viruses, bacteria, and other microorganisms.

Neutrophil

1. Scavenger cells, such as neutrophils, arrive early at the site of invasion, but survive only a few days.

Protein

2. The complement system's circulating proteins attach to microbial invaders, contributing to their destruction.

3. Macrophages engulf foreign matter and signal other immune cells, such as T cells, to attack invaders.

Macrophage

9. Killer T cells form from T cytotoxic cells and then destroy infected cells.

Macrophage

Antigen

T cell

4. Macrophages display antigens derived from digestion of ingested invaders. These activate T helper cells.

T suppressor cell

Killer T cell

Infected cell with microbial antigens on surface

8. T suppressor cells monitor antibody production and turn down plasma cell activity as the infection begins to subside.

7. Antibodies bind to invaders, either destroying them or making them more vulnerable to macrophages and complement proteins.

B cell

Antibody

Plasma cell

5. T helper cells multiply and help activate B cells and macrophages.

6. B cells divide and form plasma cells, which produce antibodies.

Memory cell

10. Some B and T cells become memory cells, which can quickly mount a defense if the same foreign invader attacks again.

Figure 12-3 Biological warfare. The body commands an army of defenders to reduce the danger of infection and guard against repeat infections. Antigens are the ultimate targets of all immune responses.

CAUSES AND MANAGEMENT OF SELECTED INFECTIOUS DISEASES

This section focuses on some of the common infectious diseases and some that, although less common, are serious when contracted. We hope this informa-

tion provides some reference points you can use to judge your own disease susceptibility.

The Common Cold

The common cold, an acute upper respiratory tract infection, must reign as humankind's supreme infec-

Allergic Disorders

People who have allergies have abnormal body reactions to certain substances called *antigens* or *allergens*. These might include certain molds, foods, plant pollens, drugs, animal hair, and insect stings. When exposed to antigens, people display allergic reactions, including nasal congestion; red, swollen, watery eyes; and sneezing. Itching of the ears, nose, throat, and mouth is often reported.

The cause of allergies lies in a disturbance in the immune system. For unknown reasons, after initial exposure to a particular antigen, some individuals' bodies prepare an overly elaborate defense system to counter later exposures to that antigen. These people have developed a hypersensitivity to the antigen. In certain extreme cases a person's body may react overwhelmingly to an antigen and produce such congestion that anaphylactic shock, asphyxiation, and death may result.

Once the antigens are identified, people can attempt to avoid exposure to them, control the symptoms if an allergic response occurs, and undergo preventive treatment called *desensitization* or *immunotherapy*.

Rheumatoid Arthritis

A commonly recognized form of arthritis is rheumatoid arthritis. Unlike osteoarthritis (see Chapter 4), rheumatoid arthritis is not the result of wear and tear but rather is caused by an autoimmune response. For unknown reasons the body's immune system attacks perfectly good cells in virtually all of the joints in the body. Approximately 2% of the population above the age of 15 has some degree of rheumatoid arthritis. Early in the condition, stiffness and joint pain are relatively common characteristics. When the condition is more advanced, swelling, redness, throbbing pain, muscle atrophy, joint deformity, and limited mobility are often reported. Significantly greater numbers of women than men develop this form of arthritis.

Interestingly, a traumatic or stressful event often triggers the onset of rheumatoid arthritis. In many cases the first symptoms are noticed in the days after a fall or a car accident. The possibility of a genetic predisposition for developing this form of arthritis is being explored.

tious disease. Also known as **acute rhinitis,** this highly contagious viral infection can be caused by any of the nearly 200 known rhinoviruses.[5] Colds are particularly common during periods in which people spend time in crowded indoor environments, such as classrooms.

The signs and symptoms of a cold are fairly predictable. Runny nose, watery eyes, general aches and pains, a listless feeling, and a slight fever may all accompany a cold in its early stages. Eventually the nasal passages swell and the inflammation may spread to the throat. Stuffy nose, sore throat, and coughing may follow. The senses of taste and smell are blocked, and appetite declines.

With the onset of symptoms, management of a cold should begin promptly. After a few days, most of the cold's symptoms subside. In the meantime, people should isolate themselves from others, drink plenty of fluids, eat moderately, and rest. Keep in mind that antibiotics are effective only against bacterial infections—not viral infections like colds.

Management of a cold can be aided by using some of the many OTC cold remedies. These remedies will not cure your cold but may lessen the discomfort associated with it. Nasal decongestants, expectorants, cough syrups, and aspirin or acetaminophen can all provide some temporary relief. Use of some of these products for more than a few days is not recommended, however, since a rebound effect may occur.

If a cold appears to become more persistent, as evidenced by prolonged chills, noticeable fever above 103° F, chest heaviness or aches, shortness of breath, coughing up rust-colored mucus, or persistent sore throat or hoarseness, a physician should be contacted.

Unfortunately, it appears to be nearly impossible to prevent colds. Since colds are now thought to be transmitted most readily by hand contact, frequent handwashing and the use of tissues are recommended.

Influenza

Influenza is also an acute, contagious disease caused by viruses. Some influenza outbreaks have produced widespread death, as seen in the influenza pandemics of 1889 to 1890, 1918 to 1919, and 1957. The viral strains that produce this infectious disease have the potential for more severe complications than the viral strains that produce the common cold. The

acute rhinitis
The common cold; the sudden onset of nasal inflammation.

viral strain for a particular form of influenza enters the body through the respiratory tract. After brief incubation and prodromal stages, the host develops signs and symptoms not just in the upper respiratory tract but throughout the entire body. These symptoms include fever, chills, cough, sore throat, headache, gastrointestinal disturbances, and muscular pain.

Except for possible secondary bacterial infections, antibiotics are not generally prescribed for people with influenza. Physicians may recommend only aspirin, fluids, and rest. Of course, parents are reminded not to give aspirin to children. Some antiviral drugs, such as amantadine, have been developed, but their use is limited. (See Table 12-3 for a comparison of influenza with the common cold.)

Most young adults can cope with the milder strains of influenza that are prevalent each winter or spring. However, pregnant women and older people—especially older people with additional health complications, such as heart disease, kidney disease, emphysema, and chronic bronchitis—are not so capable of handling this viral attack. They may quickly develop secondary bacterial complications, especially pneumonia, which can prove fatal. Flu vaccinations are routinely recommended for older people, but they have also proved effective for younger adults.[6]

Tuberculosis

Until the mid-1980s, TB, a bacterial infection of the lungs resulting in chronic coughing, weight loss, and even death, was considered to be under control in this country. Then, however, an upsurge in cases occurred, with a peak of 26,283 cases in 1992. Since that time, a decline has been noted, with 4% fewer cases (24,361) reported in 1994. However, immigration of people from areas of the world in which TB is considerably higher[7] and the emergence of drug-resistant strains of the bacterium require that continuing attention be paid to this infectious disease.

Because TB is spread through coughing, the disease thrives in crowded places where infected people are in constant contact with others. Prisons, hospitals, public housing units, and even college residence halls are places where close day-to-day contact occurs. In such settings a single infected person can spread the TB agents to many others.

When healthy people are exposed to TB agents, their immune systems generally are able to contain the bacteria in a way that both prevents the development of symptoms and reduces the likelihood of infecting others. However, when the immune system may be damaged, such as in the elderly, the malnourished, and those who are infected with HIV, the dis-

Table 12-3   Is It a Cold or the Flu?

	Cold	Flu
Symptoms		
Fever	Rare	Characteristic, high (102°-104°+ F); lasts 3-4 days
Headache	Rare	Prominent
General aches, pains	Slight	Usual; often severe
Fatigue, weakness	Quite mild	Can last up to 2-3 weeks
Extreme exhaustion	Never	Early and prominent
Stuffy nose	Common	Sometimes
Sneezing	Usual	Sometimes
Sore throat	Common	Sometimes
Chest discomfort, cough	Mild to moderate; hacking cough	Common; can become severe
Complications	Sinus congestion, earache	Pneumonia, bronchitis; can be life threatening
Prevention	Avoidance of infected people	Annual vaccination; amantadine or rimantadine (antiviral drugs)
Treatment	Temporary relief	Amantadine or rimantadine within 24-48 hours after onset of symptoms

ease can become established and eventually be transmitted to other people at risk.

As previously mentioned, multiple drug–resistant (MDR) TB has been reported. Increasingly prevalent in this country, MDR TB is the result of patients' inability to follow their physicians' instructions when initially treated (for whatever reason), inadequate treatment by physicians, and increased exposure of HIV-infected people to TB. Only 50% of people with this form of TB can be cured. Some believe that MDR TB is the next epidemic to be expected in this country.

Health officials are again requesting that TB testing programs be implemented and that those infected, once found, be isolated and brought into treatment. Newly developed diagnostic tests that are both accurate and fast have been developed and should result in more prompt treatment and effective control of the transmission of the disease.[8]

Pneumonia

Pneumonia is a general term under which a variety of infectious respiratory conditions can be placed. Bacterial, viral, fungal, rickettsial, mycoplasmal, and parasitic forms of pneumonia exist.[9] However, bacterial pneumonia is the most common form and is often seen in conjunction with other illnesses that weaken the body's immune system. This is why even healthy young people should consider colds and flu as potentially serious and treat them properly. In fact, pneumonia is so common in the frail elderly that it is often the specific condition causing death. *Pneumocystis carinii* pneumonia, a parasitic form, is of great importance today, since it is a principal opportunistic infection associated with the diagnosis of AIDS in HIV-infected people.

Among older adults with a history of chronic obstructive lung disease, cardiovascular disease, diabetes, or alcoholism, a midwinter form of pneumonia known as *acute community-acquired pneumonia* is often a serious health problem.[9] The sudden onset of chills, chest pain, and a cough producing sputum are characteristics of this condition. Additionally, a symptom-free form of pneumonia known as *walking pneumonia* is also commonly seen in adults and can become serious without warning. Individuals with the illnesses listed above should be watched carefully during the high-risk season of the year and provided with effective treatment should symptoms develop.

Mononucleosis

Of all the common infectious diseases that a college student can contract, **mononucleosis ("mono")** can

force a lengthy period of bed rest during a semester or quarter when it can least be afforded. Other common diseases that can attack you can be managed with minimal amounts of disruption. However, the overall weakness and fatigue seen in many people with mono sometimes require a month or two of rest and recuperation.

Mono is a viral infection in which the body produces an excess number of mononuclear leukocytes (a type of white blood cell). After uncertain, perhaps lengthy, incubation and prodromal stages, the acute symptoms of mono can appear, including weakness, headache, low-grade fever, swollen lymph glands (especially in the neck), and sore throat (Figure 12-4). Mental fatigue and depression are sometimes reported as side effects of mononucleosis. Usually after the acute symptoms disappear, the weakness and fatigue remain—perhaps for a few months. Mono is diagnosed on the basis of characteristic symptoms. Also, the Monospot blood smear can be used to determine the prevalence of abnormal white blood cells. In addition, an antibody test can detect activity of the immune system that is characteristic of the illness.

Since this disease is caused by a virus (Epstein-Barr virus), antibiotic therapy is not recommended. Treatment most often includes bed rest and the use of OTC remedies for fever (aspirin or acetaminophen) and sore throat (lozenges). In extreme cases, corticosteroid drugs can be used. Appropriate fluid intake and a well-balanced diet are also important in the recovery stages of mono. Fortunately, the body tends to develop NAI to the mono virus, so subsequent infections of mono are unusual.

For years, mono has been labeled the "kissing disease"; however, mono is not highly contagious and is known to be spread by direct transmission in ways other than kissing. No vaccine has been developed to confer AAI for mononucleosis. The best preventive measures include the steps that you can take to increase your resistance to most infectious diseases: (1) eat a well-balanced diet, (2) exercise regularly, (3) sleep sufficiently, (4) use health care services appropriately, (5) live in a reasonably healthful environment, and (6) avoid direct contact with infected people.

---

mononucleosis ("mono")
Viral infection characterized by weakness, fatigue, swollen glands, sore throat, and low-grade fever.

Figure 12-4   The throat of a person with mononucleosis. The tonsils are enlarged, and each is covered with a white membrane.

Chronic Fatigue Syndrome

Perhaps the most perplexing "infectious" condition seen by physicians is **chronic fatigue syndrome (CFS).** First identified in 1985, this mononucleosis-like condition is most commonly seen in women in their thirties and forties. People with CFS, many of whom are busy professional people, report flu-like symptoms, including severe exhaustion, fatigue, headaches, muscle aches, fever, inability to concentrate, allergies, intolerance to exercise, and depression. Examinations done on the first people with CFS revealed antibodies to the Epstein-Barr virus. Thus it was assumed to be an infectious viral disease (and initially called *chronic Epstein-Barr syndrome*).

In the decade since its first appearance the condition has received a great deal of attention that has resulted in considerable confusion over its exact nature. Today, opinions vary widely as to whether the condition is a specific viral infection, a condition involving both viral infections and nonviral components, or some other disorder.[10] One recent study found a strong association between CFS and neurally mediated hypotension, a condition in which blood pressure drops suddenly and substantially after long periods of standing, physical activity, or exposure to high temperatures. This disorder is easily missed using standard blood pressure screening methods because the symptoms occur only after the patient has stood for several minutes.[11] Some physicians even view CFS as a psychological disorder.

Regardless of its cause or causes, CFS is extremely unpleasant for its victims. Certainly, those experiencing the symptoms over an extended time need to be seen by a physician experienced in dealing with CFS.

Measles

Previously thought to be only a childhood disease, *red measles* (also called **rubeola** or *common measles*) has recently been seen in large numbers on some American college campuses. Red measles is the highly contagious type of measles characterized by a short-lived, relatively high fever (103° to 104° F) and a whole-body red spotty rash that lasts about a week. The other type of measles, *German measles* (**rubella,** or 3-day measles), is a much milder form of measles that has serious implications for newborn babies of mothers who contracted this disease during pregnancy.[12] Highly successful vaccines are now available for both varieties of measles and are usually given in the same injection. Women should receive these vaccinations before they become pregnant.

The outbreak of red measles among college students during each of the last several school years points to the fact that our society mistakenly believes that most infectious diseases have now been eliminated. Public health experts now realize that those who contracted the disease either had never been vaccinated or had been vaccinated with a killed variety vaccine used before 1969. Only students who had already had red measles as children or who had been vaccinated with a live virus were guaranteed full immunity against the red measles virus. Nontraditional college students in particular should attempt to determine whether their immunization status is based on use of the older, less effective vaccine.

Today, most public school systems are requiring documented proof of immunization from a physician or clinic before children can attend classes. As educated parents, you should be conscientious about adhering to immunization schedules for your children. In fact, measles immunization efforts have increased so effectively because of school and public health department involvement that the number of measles cases fell from 55,000 cases between 1989 and 1991 to 963 cases in 1994.[13]

Mumps

Mumps is one of the more familiar childhood infectious diseases. A viral illness, mumps is characterized by inflammation and swelling in one or both salivary glands at the angle of the jaw. Fever, pain, and difficulty swallowing are common symptoms associated with mumps. Treatment involves fluids, bed rest, painkillers, and, in children, a few days' absence from school.[5]

When mumps occurs in older male children, adolescents, and adults, the likelihood of infection to the testicles increases. A less common condition is inflammation of the pancreas, with abdominal pain and vomiting.

Today, protection against mumps is available with the standard childhood immunization series, measles-mumps-rubella (MMR). Those who contract mumps will develop NAI to the disease.

Lyme Disease

An infectious disease that is becoming increasingly common in Eastern, Southeastern, upper Midwestern, and West Coast states is **Lyme disease,** with 13,083 cases in 1994. This bacterial disease results when infected deer ticks, usually in the nymph (immature) state, attach to the skin and inject the infectious agent as they feed on a host's blood. Deer ticks become infected by feeding on infected white-tailed deer or white-footed mice.[14]

The symptoms of Lyme disease are variable but generally first appear within 30 days as small red bumps surrounded by a circular red rash at the site of bites. In conjunction with this phase I stage, flulike symptoms may appear, including chills, headaches, muscle and joint aches, and low-grade fever. For approximately 20% of infected people, a phase II stage develops in which nervous system or heart disorders may occur. For those who remain untreated even to this stage, a phase III stage can develop in which chronic arthritis, lasting up to 2 years, can occur. Fortunately, Lyme disease can be treated with antibiotics. Unfortunately, however, no immunity develops, so subsequent infections can occur.[14] The ability to diagnose the presence of Lyme disease in children may be more difficult than for adults.[15] Although not yet available, a Lyme disease vaccine has been successfully tested on animals.

For people living in susceptible areas, outdoor activities can expose them to the nearly invisible tick nymphs that have fallen from deer into the grass. Thus people who are active outdoors should check themselves frequently to be sure that they are tick free. Shirts should be tucked into pants, pants tucked into socks, and gloves and hats worn when possible. It is also helpful to shower after coming in from outdoors and to check clothing for evidence of ticks. Pets can carry infected ticks into the house. If ticks are found, they should be carefully removed from the skin with tweezers and the affected area washed. A physician should be consulted if symptoms appear or you are concerned that you might have been exposed.

During 1995, it was discovered that the tick that carries Lyme disease has also been responsible for a potentially fatal bacterial infection, *human granulocytic ehrlichiosis* (HGE). This disease is associated with high fever,

headache, muscle aches, and chills. Fortunately, HGE is successfully treated with doxycycline, an antibiotic that can also be used in the treatment of Lyme disease. Certainly, people with these symptoms, particularly when they are "outdoor people" and living in areas of the country in which Lyme disease is reported, should make certain that HGE is also considered in the diagnosis and treatment of their symptoms.[16]

Hantavirus Pulmonary Syndrome

Since 1993 a small but rapidly expanding number of people have died of extreme pulmonary distress caused by the leakage of plasma into the lungs. In all of the initial cases, the people lived in the Southwest, had been well until they began developing flulike symptoms over 1 or 2 days, then quickly experienced difficulty breathing, and died only hours later. Epidemiologists quickly suspected a viral agent such as the hantavirus known to exist in Asia and, to a lesser degree, in Europe. Exhaustive laboratory work led to the culturing of the virus and confirmed that all of the victims had been infected with an American version of the hantavirus. The latest infectious condition, hantavirus pulmonary syndrome, was identified.

Today the hantavirus disease described above has been reported in areas beyond the Southwest, including most of the Western states and in some of the Eastern states. The common denominator in all areas in which the hantavirus infection has occurred is the presence of deer mice. It is now known that this common rodent serves as the reservoir for the virus.

The mode of transmission of the virus from deer mice to humans involves the inhalation of dust contaminated with dried virus-rich rodent urine or saliva-contaminated materials, such as nests. In areas with deer mouse populations (most of the United States), health experts are now warning people to be extremely careful when cleaning houses and barns in

chronic fatigue syndrome
Illness that causes severe exhaustion, fatigue, aches, and depression; mostly affects women in their thirties and forties.

rubeola (roo **be** oh luh)
Red or common measles.

rubella
German or 3-day measles.

Lyme disease
Bacterial infection transmitted by deer ticks.

which deer mouse droppings are likely to be found. Should it be necessary to remove rodent nests, wear rubber gloves, pour Lysol or bleach on the nests and soak them thoroughly, and finally, pick up nests with shovels and burn or bury them in holes that are several feet deep. If done properly, these procedures should greatly minimize the airborne spread of the viral particles.[17]

There is no vaccine for hantavirus pulmonary syndrome, although the illness is now more quickly recognized. As a result of awareness of the importance of early evaluation of flulike symptoms, the death rate has begun to fall.

Toxic Shock Syndrome

Toxic shock syndrome (TSS), first reported in 1978, made front-page headlines in 1980, when it was reported by the CDC that there was a connection between TSS and the presence of a specific bacterial agent (*Staphylococcus aureus*) in the vagina associated with the use of tampons.

TSS presents the signs and symptoms listed in the Star Box below. Superabsorbent varieties of tampons apparently can irritate the vaginal lining three times more quickly than regular tampons. This vaginal irritation is enhanced when the tampons remain in the vagina for a long time (over 5 hours). Once this irritation has begun, the staphylococcal bacteria (which are commonly present in the vagina) have relatively easy access to the bloodstream. Proliferation of these bacteria in the circulatory system and their resultant toxins produce toxic shock syndrome. Left untreated, the victim can die—usually as a result of cardiovascular failure. Fortunately, less than 10% of women diagnosed as having TSS actually die.

Although the extent of this disease is still quite limited (only about 3 to 6 cases per 100,000 women per year) and the mortality figures are low (comparable with those in women who use oral contraceptives), each woman should still exercise reasonable caution in the use of tampons. Recommendations are that (1) tampons should not be the sole form of sanitary protection used, and (2) tampons should not be in place for too long. Accordingly, women should change tampons every few hours and intermittently use sanitary napkins. Tampons should not be used during sleep. Because the use of highly absorbent tampons increases the risk of TSS by 10 times over the use of regular tampons, medical experts now recommend that women use the least absorbent tampon that fits their needs.[18] Some physicians recommend that all tampon use be curtailed if a woman wants to be extraordinarily safe from TSS.

The incidence of TSS has dropped significantly since the early 1980s. Possible reasons for this decrease are the removal of some superabsorbent tampons from the market and the standardization of the labels for junior, super, and super-plus tampons that began in 1990.[19]

Hepatitis

Hepatitis is an inflammatory process in the liver and can be caused by several viruses. Types A, B, C (once called non-A and non-B), and D have been recognized. Additionally, hepatitis can result indirectly from abuse of alcohol and other drugs. General symptoms of hepatitis include fever, nausea, loss of appetite, abdominal pain, and jaundice (yellowing of the skin and eyes).[14]

Type A hepatitis is often associated with eating fecal contaminated food, such as raw shellfish, or water. Poor sanitation, particularly with the handling of food, has led to outbreaks associated with restaurants, while diaper-changing activities have resulted in outbreaks in child care centers. It is estimated that up to 200,000 people per year experience this infection, although many fewer cases (23,000 in 1992) are reported. In 1995 a vaccine, Harvix, was given FDA approval.

Type B hepatitis (HBV) is spread in various ways, including sexual contact, intravenous drug use, tattooing, and through medical and dental practice. Once spread principally through blood transfusions, this route no longer exists because of the use of effective screening tests. Chronic HBV infection has been associated with liver cirrhosis and liver cancer. The problem of HBV infection is discussed in the Learning from All Cultures box on p. 293. Type C hepatitis is contracted in similar ways as HBV (sexual contact, tainted blood, and shared needles).

Signs and Symptoms of Toxic Shock Syndrome
- Fever (102° or above)
- Headache
- Vomiting
- Sore throat
- Diarrhea
- Muscle aches
- Sunburnlike rash
- Low blood pressure
- Bloodshot eyes
- Disorientation
- Reduced urination
- Peeling of skin on the palms and soles of the feet

LEARNING *from* ALL CULTURES

Hepatitis B

Because of the AIDS epidemic, some serious diseases get little attention from the media. Hepatitis B is one of these potentially dangerous diseases. It is estimated that 200 million people in the world are chronic carriers and can therefore infect others. The virus is transmitted through blood, sexual contact, and from mother to infant.

Some people who contract hepatitis B develop chronic health problems, such as cirrhosis of the liver or liver cancer. In Asia and Africa the hepatitis B virus is believed to be a significant cause of liver cancer. The chronic effects of this virus are considered a serious world health problem. A vaccine to prevent the virus is available, but for people in developing countries, it is not widely administered.

Treatment for limiting liver damage caused by hepatitis B is currently being researched. Some folk medicines, such as the extracts of tropical weeds, are being tested. In some parts of the world these extracts are used to treat jaundice caused by some type of illness involving the liver. At the present time, treatments like this are being used on patients in India.

Considering that hepatitis B is potentially preventable, why does it remain such a worldwide health concern? What do you think the focus of research should be on hepatitis B: prevention, treatment, or cure?

The newly identified *type D (delta) hepatitis* has proven very difficult to treat but is found almost exclusively in people already suffering from type B hepatitis. Transmission of this virus, along with type B hepatitis and HIV, makes unprotected sexual contact, including anal and oral sex, very risky.[14]

AIDS

AIDS is rapidly becoming the most devastating infectious disease to have occurred in modern times. On the basis of current data, since the initial reporting of the disease in 1981, through December 1995, 513,486 Americans have been diagnosed with AIDS and 319,849 (62% of all cases) have died from the disease.[20] The Star Box on p. 294 shows the extent to which various groups of people have been affected by the disease. Furthermore, it is estimated that by the year 2000, $13.1 billion in health insurance claims will be paid for AIDS-related illnesses.[21] Today the cost of treating one AIDS patient is $119,000: $50,000 before the onset of AIDS and $69,000 thereafter.[22] The toll in human lives and the financial burden AIDS will place on our health care system make AIDS a frightening disease.

Cause of AIDS

AIDS is caused by HIV, a virus that attacks the helper T cells of the immune system (see pp. 285-286). When HIV attacks helper T cells, people lose the ability to fight off a variety of infections that normally would be easily controlled. Thus because these infections develop during a period in which people are vulnerable, they are collectively called *opportunistic infections*. HIV-infected patients become vulnerable to infection by bacteria, protozoa, fungi, and a number of viruses. Although not infections, a variety of malignancies (see Chapter 11) also develop during this period of immune system vulnerability.

During the initial years of the AIDS epidemic the presence of specific diagnosable conditions formed the basis of receiving the clinical label of HIV with AIDS. Among these were *Pneumocystis carinii* pneumonia and Kaposi's sarcoma, a rare but deadly form of skin cancer. Gradually, additional conditions were recognized as being associated with advancing deterioration of the immune system and thus were added to the list of AIDS conditions. Eventually this list contained over 25 definitive conditions, with more conditions being added as they become apparent. Among the conditions found on the current version of the list are toxoplasmosis within the brain, cytomegalovirus retinitis with loss of

toxic shock syndrome (TSS)
Potentially fatal condition resulting from the proliferation of certain bacteria in the vagina that enter the general blood circulation.

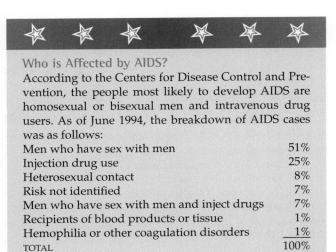

Who is Affected by AIDS?

According to the Centers for Disease Control and Prevention, the people most likely to develop AIDS are homosexual or bisexual men and intravenous drug users. As of June 1994, the breakdown of AIDS cases was as follows:

Men who have sex with men	51%
Injection drug use	25%
Heterosexual contact	8%
Risk not identified	7%
Men who have sex with men and inject drugs	7%
Recipients of blood products or tissue	1%
Hemophilia or other coagulation disorders	1%
TOTAL	100%

vision, lymphoma involving the brain, recurrent salmonella septicemia, and a wasting syndrome that includes invasive cervical cancer in women, recurrent pneumonia, and recurrent tuberculosis. Today, however, there is a growing tendency to assign the label of HIV with AIDS to HIV-infected people when their level of helper T cells drops below 200 cells per cubic millimeter, regardless of whether specific conditions are present.

Spread of HIV

HIV cannot be contracted easily. The chances of contracting HIV through casual contact with HIV-infected people at work, school, or at home are extremely rare or nonexistent. HIV is known to be spread only by direct sexual contact involving the exchange of body fluids (including blood, semen, and vaginal secretions), the sharing of hypodermic needles, transfusion of infected blood or blood products, and perinatal transmission (from an infected mother to a fetus or newborn baby). For HIV to be transmitted, it must enter the bloodstream of the noninfected person, which is done through contaminated blood or needles and tears in body tissues lining the rectum, mouth, and reproductive system. Current research also indicates that HIV is not transmitted by sweat, saliva, or tears, although the virus may be found in very low concentrations in these fluids.

Women are at much greater risk (12 times the risk) than men for the heterosexual transmission of HIV because of the higher concentration of HIV in semen than in vaginal secretions.[23] This increase is noted when comparing 1981 to 1987 levels (8%) of women infected with HIV with levels from 1988 to 1993 (12.5%), and with the most current statistic, 1993 to 1995 (19%).[20]

Signs and symptoms of HIV infection

Most people infected with HIV initially feel well and have no symptoms (that is, they are asymptomatic). The incubation period for HIV infection is generally considered to be from 6 months to 10 or more years, with the average being approximately 6 years. Despite the lengthy period between infection

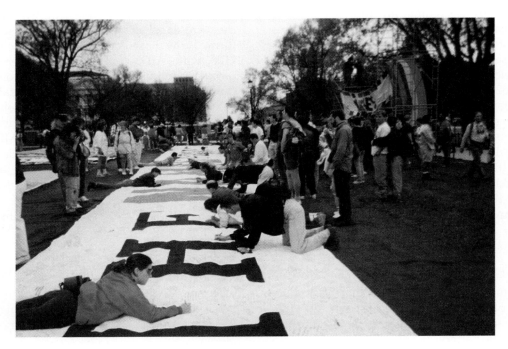

Signing of the AIDS quilt in Washington, D.C., develops community support for AIDS education.

and the first clinical observation of damage to the immune system, antibodies to HIV may appear within several weeks to 3 months of contracting the virus. This short period before the appearance of antibodies is the small "window of opportunity" that exists even to this day in terms of the blood supply. Of course, relatively few people are tested for HIV infection *at any time* during the incubation period. Thus infected people could remain in the asymptomatic state (more currently referred to as HIV+ without symptoms) and be carriers of HIV for years before they would experience signs of illness sufficient enough to warrant a physical examination.

In the absence of symptoms of immune system deterioration and of AIDS testing results, sexually active people need to redefine the meaning of *monogamous*. Today it is very possible that two people need to account for the sexual partners that they both have had over a 10-year period before it is completely safe to assume that there have been no other partners involved in their special relationship. Unfortunately, this is done, or even considered, so infrequently that some are labeling today's late adolescents and young adults as "a generation in jeopardy."

Virtually all people infected with HIV eventually develop signs and symptoms of a more advanced stage of the disease. These signs and symptoms include tiredness, fever, loss of appetite and weight, diarrhea, night sweats, and swollen glands (usually in the neck, armpits, and groin). At this point, they are said to have HIV+ with symptoms. Table 12-4 indicates that these people are infectious and have damage to the immune system.

It is estimated that given sufficient time, perhaps as long as 15 years, the vast majority (95%) of infected people will move beyond HIV with symptoms to develop one or more of the over 25 conditions whose presence leads to the label HIV with AIDS or AIDS being applied, with death following within 2 to 5 years. Although not fully understood (perhaps a suppressor compound formed by specific immune system cells), a small percentage of infected people (5%) possess an ability to hold the infection in check and have survived for two decades without developing AIDS.

As mentioned earlier, in addition to being labeled AIDS on the basis of being HIV positive and having one or more of the conditions, the label is also applied to those people whose helper T cell count falls below 200 per cubic millimeter. A normal helper T cell range is 800 to 1000. Therefore, even in the absence of specific conditions, some people will qualify for the label AIDS because of the degree of damage already done to their immune systems.

Diagnosis of HIV infection

The CDC has established specific criteria that physicians and researchers use to define HIV infection. In addition to a clinical examination and laboratory tests for accompanying infections, HIV infection is diagnosed by the use of an initial screening test, the enzyme-linked immunosorbent assay (ELISA). If antibodies to HIV are identified, a confirming test, the western blot, can be performed. At the time of this writing, a home test, Confide (Johnson & Johnson), awaits final permission for marketing. It is estimated that 1.5 to 3 million people in this country have been infected with HIV.

Table 12-4   The Spectrum of HIV Infection

	HIV+ Without Symptoms (Asymptomatic)	HIV+ With Symptoms	HIV+ With AIDS
External signs	No symptoms Looks well	Fever Night sweats Swollen lymph glands Weight loss Diarrhea Minor infections Fatigue	Kaposi's sarcoma *Pneumocystis carinii* pneumonia and/or other predetermined illnesses Neurological disorders One or more of an additional 25 + diagnosable conditions or a T4 helper cell count falls below 200 per cubic milliliter
Incubation	Invasion of virus to 10 years	Several months to 10 or more years	Several months to 10-12 or more years
Internal level of infection	Antibodies are produced Immune system remains intact Positive antibody test	Antibodies are produced Immune system weakened Positive antibody test	Immune system deficient Positive antibody test
Infectious?	Yes	Yes	Yes

There is no cure for HIV infection and AIDS. However, several drugs may be effective in reducing the rate at which helper T cells are destroyed by HIV. Among these immune system–supporting medications are AZT (azidothymidine), DDI (didanosine), ddC (didoxycytidine), and most recently 3TC (lamividudine). Today, from the very first identification of HIV infection, people are treated aggressively with a combination of AZT and one or more of the other agents. Although not a cure, this treatment delays the onset of "full-blown" AIDS, thus improving the quality, but not the length, of life.

In addition to the AZT-like family of drugs, the first approved form of proteinase inhibitors (saquinavir) is now available. Drugs of this type will alter the virus's ability to introduce its genetic material into the DNA of the host helper T cell. A final pharmacological approach to slow the progression of HIV is the use of interleukin-2, a naturally occurring immune system protein, to help protect helper T cells.

An unusual treatment approach has been the transplantation of baboon bone marrow into a human. Because baboons are naturally resistant to HIV, it was hoped that their immune system cells would transfer a protective capability to humans. Unfortunately, however, the baboon bone marrow cells failed to engraft into the human recipient.

In addition to drugs, physicians have a variety of medications that can be used in treating the symptoms associated with various infections and malignancies that comprise AIDS. As with the drugs already described, these drugs cannot reverse HIV status or cure AIDS.

In addition to the development of drugs to treat HIV and AIDS, research continues into the development of vaccines to prevent HIV infection. To date, no effective vaccine has been developed for humans. This inability to develop a safe, effective, and affordable vaccine (such as those that have been developed for other infectious diseases) is the result of the unique ability of HIV to alter its outer coat and quickly incorporate its genetic material into the host's helper T cell's genetic material, thus depriving the immune system of the ability to develop immune recognition.[24] This ability of the virus to change its appearance is so prolific that dozens of strains of HIV exist at all times in the United States. There may even be more than one version of HIV within a single individual. To date, over 20 killed-virus vaccines have been developed, but none has proven effective against this rapidly changing virus. A live-virus vaccine, although effective in animal studies, is still considered too dangerous for trials involving uninfected humans.

Can HIV infection be prevented? The answer is a definite "yes." Although HIV infection rates on college campuses are thought to be low (approximately 0.2%), students can be at risk. There are a number of steps an individual can take to reduce the risk of contracting and transmitting HIV. All of these steps involve understanding one's behavior and the methods by which HIV can be transmitted. Particularly applicable for college-aged people are *abstinence, safer sex, sobriety,* and *communication* with potential sexual partners. Excluding the recommendation to abstain from sexual activity if you desire the highest level of protection from HIV, the Health Action Guide on p. 297 lists specific points that relate to safer sex, sobriety, and the exchange of honest, accurate information regarding sexual histories.

To carry protection further, the U.S. Public Health Service has provided recommendations for the following groups: (1) the general public, (2) people at increased risk of infection (including health care workers), and (3) people with a positive HIV antibody test. The Public Health Service has a toll-free AIDS telephone hotline (1-800-342-AIDS), and local or state hotlines may exist. Keep informed about HIV infection and AIDS!

SEXUALLY TRANSMITTED DISEASES

Sexually transmitted diseases (STDs) were once referred to as venereal diseases (for Venus, the Roman goddess of love). Today the term *venereal disease* has been superseded by the broader term *sexually transmitted disease.* The current emphasis is on the successful prevention and treatment of STDs rather than on the ethics of sexuality. In conjunction with this, the following points should be remembered: (1) more than one STD can exist in a person at a given point in time; (2) the symptoms of STDs can vary over time and from person to person; (3) little immunity is developed for STDs; and (4) STDs can predispose people to additional health problems, including infertility, birth defects in their children, cancer, and long-term disability. Additionally, the risk of HIV infection is higher when sexual partners are also infected with STDs.

This section focuses on the STDs most frequently diagnosed among college students (chlamydia, gonorrhea, human papillomavirus infection, herpes simplex, syphilis, and pubic lice). A short section follows, covering common vaginal infections, some of which may occur without sexual contact. Completing the

HEALTH Action Guide

Reducing Your Risk of Contracting HIV

It is important to keep in mind that sexual partners may not reveal their true sexual history or drug habits. If you are sexually active, you can lower your risk of infection with HIV, as well as other STDs, by adopting the following safer sex practices.

- Learn the sexual history and HIV status of your sex partner.
- Limit your sex partners.
- Always use condoms correctly and consistently.
- Avoid contact with body fluids, feces, and semen.
- Curtail use of drugs that impair good judgment.
- Never share hypodermic needles.
- Refrain from sex with known injectable drug abusers.*
- Avoid sex with HIV-infected patients, those with signs and symptoms of AIDS, and the partners of high-risk individuals.*
- Get regular tests for STD infections.
- Do not insert any foreign objects into the rectum.
- Practice proper hygiene (shower before and after sex).

How easy will it be to adopt these behaviors? How real is your risk of becoming HIV positive?

*Current studies indicate that the elimination of high-risk people as sexual partners is the single most effective safer sex practice that can be implemented.

Personal Assessment on p. 298 will help you determine your own risk of contracting an STD. Also, refer to the Health Action Guide above for safer sex practices.

Chlamydia (Nonspecific Urethritis)

Chlamydia is considered the most prevalent STD in the United States today. Chlamydia infections occur an estimated 5 times more frequently than gonorrhea and up to 10 times more frequently than syphilis. However, since physicians are not required to report cases of chlamydia to the CDC, the true extent of the disease is not known.

Chlamydia trachomatis is the bacterial agent that causes the chlamydia infection. Chlamydia is the most common cause of nonspecific urethritis (NSU).[25] NSU refers to infections of the **urethra** and surrounding tissues that are not caused by the bacterium responsible for gonorrhea. Only when a culture smear test for suspected gonorrhea proves negative do clinicians diagnose NSU, usually by calling it *chlamydia*. Although not as accurate, new diagnostic tests, such as Test Pack, should allow a diagnosis to be made more quickly. About 80% of men with chlamydia indicate gonorrhea-like signs and symptoms, including painful urination and a whitish pus discharge from the penis. As in gonorrheal infections and many other STDs, most women report no overt signs or symptoms. A few women might exhibit a mild urethral discharge, painful urination, and swelling of vulval tissues. Whereas oral forms of penicillin are used in the treatment of gonococcal infections, oral tetracycline or doxycycline is prescribed for chlamydia and other NSUs.

As with all STDs, both sexual partners should receive treatment to avoid the ping-pong effect: the back-and-forth reinfection that occurs among couples when only one partner receives treatment. Furthermore, as with other STDs, having chlamydia does not effectively confer immunity.

Unresolved chlamydia can lead to the same negative health consequences that result from untreated gonorrheal infections. In men the pathogens can invade and damage the deeper reproductive structures (the prostate gland, the seminal vesicles, and Cowper's glands). Sterility can result. The pathogens can spread further and produce joint problems (arthritis) and heart complications (damaged heart valves, blood vessels, and heart muscle tissue).

In women the pathogens enter the body through the urethra or the cervical area. If not properly treated, the invasion can reach the deeper pelvic

---

sexually transmitted diseases (STDs)
Infectious diseases that are spread primarily through intimate sexual contact.

chlamydia
The most prevalent sexually transmitted disease. Caused by a nongonococcal bacterium.

urethra (yoo **ree** thra)
Passageway through which urine leaves the urinary bladder.

PERSONAL ASSESSMENT

What Is Your Risk of Contracting a Sexually Transmitted Disease?

A variety of factors interact to determine your risk of contracting a sexually transmitted disease (STD). This inventory is intended to provide you with an estimate of your level of risk.

Circle the number of each row that best characterizes you. Enter that number on the line at the end of the row (points). After assigning yourself a number in each row, total the number appearing in the points column. Your total points will allow you to interpret your risk for contracting an STD.

Age						Points
1	3	4	5	3	2	_____
0-9	10-14	15-19	20-29	30-34	35+	

Sexual Practices						
0	1	2	4	6	8	_____
Never engage in sex	One sex partner	More than one sex partner but never more than one at a time	Two to five sex partners	Five to ten sex partners	Ten or more sex partners	

Sexual Attitudes						
0	1	8	1	7	8	_____
Will not engage in nonmarital sex	Premarital sex is okay if it is with future spouse	Any kind of premarital sex is okay	Extramarital sex is not for me	Extramarital sex is okay	Believe in complete sexual freedom	

Attitudes toward Contraception						
1	1	6	5	4	8	_____
Would use condom to prevent pregnancy	Would use condom to prevent STDs	Would never use a condom	Would use the birth control pill	Would use other contraceptive measure	Would not use any-thing	

Attitudes toward STD						
3	3	4	6	6	6	_____
Am not sexually active so I do not worry	Would be able to talk about STD with my partner	Would check an infection to be sure	Would be afraid to check out an infection	Can't even talk about an infection	STDs are no problem—easily cured	

YOUR TOTAL POINTS _____

Interpretation
5-8   Your risk is well below average
9-13   Your risk is below average
14-17   Your risk is at or near average
18-21   Your risk is moderately high
22+   Your risk is high

To Carry This Further . . .
Having taken this Personal Assessment, were you surprised at your level of risk? What is the primary reason for this level? How concerned are you and your classmates and friends about contracting an STD? ☑

structures, producing a syndrome called **pelvic inflammatory disease (PID)**. The inner uterine wall (endometrium), the fallopian tubes, and any surrounding structures may be attacked to produce this painful syndrome. A variety of further complications can result, including sterility and **peritonitis.** Infected women can transmit a chlamydia infection to the eyes and lungs of newborns during a vaginal birth. For both men and women the early detection of chlamydia and other NSUs is of paramount concern.

Human Papillomavirus

With all of the concern about HIV and other STDs, the presence of an additional STD is unwanted news. Nevertheless, such is the case with **human papillomavirus (HPV).** Because HPV infections are generally asymptomatic, the exact extent of the disease is unknown. In a study with a group of sexually active college women, HPV infection was found in approximately 20% of the women. HPV-related changes to the cells of the cervix have been found in nearly 5% of the Pap smears taken from women under the age of 30. It is currently believed that for women, risk factors for HPV infection include: (1) sexual activity before age 20, (2) intercourse with three or more partners before age 35, and (3) intercourse with a partner who has three or more partners.[26] The extent of HPV infection in men is even less clearly known, but it is likely widespread.

The concern about HPV infections is centered on the ability of some of the more than 50 forms of the virus to foster precancerous changes in the cervix. In addition, HPV is associated with the development of genital warts (condyloma acuminata). These pinkish-white lesions may be found in raised clusters that resemble tiny heads of cauliflower. Found most commonly on the penis, scrotum, labia, cervix, and around the anus, genital warts are the most common symptomatic viral STD in this country. Although most genital wart colonies are small, they may become very large and block the anus or birth canal during pregnancy.

Treatment for HPV, including genital warts, may include burning, freezing, removal with a CO_2 laser, or the use of various medications. Regardless of treatment, however, return of the viral colonies will most likely occur. Condom use should be encouraged in an attempt to prevent transmission of HPV.

Gonorrhea

Another extremely common STD, gonorrhea is caused by a bacterium (*Neisseria gonorrhoea*). In men this bacterial agent can produce a milky-white discharge from the penis, accompanied by painful urination. About 80% of men who contract gonorrhea report varying degrees of these symptoms. This figure is approximately reversed for women: only about 20% of women are symptomatic and thus report varying degrees of frequent, painful urination, with a slimy yellow-green discharge from the vagina or urethra. Oral sex with an infected partner can produce a gonorrheal infection of the throat (pharyngeal gonorrhea). Gonorrhea can also be transmitted to the rectal areas of both men and women.

Diagnosis of gonorrhea is made by culturing the bacteria. Antibiotic treatment regimens include use of penicillin, tetracycline, ampicillin, or other drugs. Some strains of gonorrhea (penicillin-resistant strains) are much more difficult to treat than others.

Testing for gonorrhea is included as a part of prenatal care so that infections in mothers can be treated before birth. If the birth canal is infected, newborns could easily contract the infection in the mucous membranes of the eye. Most states still require that drops be placed in the eyes of all newborns to prevent this infection.

Herpes Simplex

Public health officials think that the sexually transmitted genital herpes virus infection rivals chlamydia as the most prevalent STD. Recent studies show that about 16% of the adult population is infected with genital herpes virus, although most people are asymptomatic for genital herpes. Herpes is really a family of over 50 viruses, some of which produce recognized diseases in humans (chickenpox, **shingles,**

pelvic inflammatory disease (PID)
Acute or chronic infection of the peritoneum or lining of the abdominopelvic cavity; associated with a variety of symptoms and a potential cause of sterility.

peritonitis (pare it ton **eye** tis)
Inflammation of the peritoneum or lining of the abdominopelvic cavity.

human papillomavirus (HPV)
Sexually transmitted virus capable of causing precancerous changes in the cervix; causative agent for genital warts.

shingles
Viral infection affecting the nerve endings of the skin.

mononucleosis, and others). One subgroup called *herpes simplex 1 virus* (HSV-1) produces an infection called *labial herpes* (oral or lip herpes). Labial herpes produces common fever blisters or cold sores seen around the lips and oral cavity. Herpes simplex 2 virus (HSV-2) is a different strain that produces similar clumps of blisterlike lesions in the genital region (Figure 12-5). Lay people have referred to this second type of herpes as the STD type, although both types produce identical clinical pictures. Both forms can exist at either site. Oral-genital sexual practices have resulted in genital herpes cases now being caused by HSV-1.

Herpes appears as a single sore or as a small cluster of blisterlike sores. These sores burn, itch, and (for some) become quite painful. The infected person might also report swollen lymph glands, muscular aches and pains, and fever. Some patients feel weak and sleepy when blisters are present. The lesions may last from a few days to a few weeks. A week is the average time for active viral shedding; then the blisters begin scabbing, and new skin is formed.

Herpes is an interesting virus for several reasons. It can lie dormant for extended periods. However, for reasons not well understood but perhaps related to stress, diet, or overall health, the viral particles can be stimulated to travel along the nerve pathways to the skin and then create an active infection. Thus herpes can be considered a recurrent infection. Fortunately for most people, recurrent infections are less severe than the initial episode and do not last as long. Herpes is also interesting because, unlike most STDs, no

treatment method has been successful at killing the virus. Acyclovir (Zovirax), in oral, ointment, and intravenous forms, has been used successfully in reducing the number and length of genital herpes infections in certain groups of patients.[27] An FDA advisory panel recently recommended that this medication be made available as an OTC product. There are also some medications that may provide symptomatic relief. Diagnosis of genital herpes is almost always made by a clinical examination.

The best prevention against ever getting a herpes infection is to avoid all direct contact with a person who has an active infection. Do not kiss someone with a fever blister—or let them kiss you (or your children) if they have an active lesion. Do not share drinking glasses or eating utensils. Check your partner's genitals. Do not have intimate sexual contact with someone who displays the blisterlike clusters or rash. (Condoms are only marginally helpful and cannot protect against lesions on the female vulva or the lower abdominal area of men). Be careful not to infect yourself by touching a blister and then touching any other part of your body. The Health Action Guide on p. 301 provides helpful advice for talking to your partner if you have genital herpes.

Newborn babies are especially susceptible to the virus should they come into contact with an active lesion during the birth process. Newborns have not developed the defense capabilities to resist the invasion. They can quickly develop a systemic, general infection (neonatal herpes) that is often fatal or local infections that produce permanent brain damage or

Figure 12-5   Herpes infections of the male (**A**) and female (**B**) genitals.

blindness. Fortunately, most of these possible problems can be prevented through proper prenatal care. If there is any chance that the viral particles may be present at birth, a cesarean delivery can be performed, although this is less commonly done today than in the past.

Syphilis

Like gonorrhea, syphilis is caused by a bacterium (*Treponema pallidum*) and is transmitted almost exclusively by sexual intercourse. The incidence of syphilis, a CDC-reportable disease, is far lower than that of gonorrhea. In 1950 a record 217,558 cases of syphilis were reported in this country. The number of cases then fell steadily to less than 80,000 cases in 1980. From 1980 through 1990 the incidence climbed, reaching nearly 140,000 cases in 1990. A subsequent decline then began, and in 1993 the number of cases dropped to 101,259. In spite of a downward trend, an alarming number of today's cases have also been associated with HIV infections. More information on this once nearly defeated disease is presented in the Star Box on p. 302. An alarming increase in infant syphilis has been noted in children born to mothers who use drugs and support their habit through sexual activity.

Pubic Lice

Three types of lice infect humans: the head louse, the body louse, and the pubic louse all feed on the blood of the host. Except for the relatively uncommon body louse, these tiny insects do not carry diseases. They are, however, quite annoying.

Pubic lice, also called *crabs*, attach themselves to the base of the pubic hairs, where they live and attach their eggs (nits). These eggs move into a larval stage after 1 week; after 2 more weeks, they develop into mature adult crab lice (Figure 12-6).

People usually notice they have a pubic lice infestation when they are confronted with intense itching in the genital region. Fortunately, both prescription and OTC creams, lotions, and shampoos are extremely effective in killing both the lice and their eggs.

Lice are not transmitted exclusively through sexual contact, but also by contact with bedsheets and clothes that may be contaminated. If you develop a pubic lice infestation, you will have to treat yourself, your clothes, your sheets, and your furniture.

Vaginal Infections

Two common pathogens produce uncomfortable vaginal infections in women. The first is the yeast or

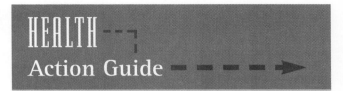

HEALTH Action Guide

Talking with Your Partner about Herpes

Although herpes rarely has serious consequences, the lesions are infectious and tend to reappear. It is important to talk openly with your partner about this sexually transmitted disease. Here are some tips to make things easier:

- *Educate yourself.*

Be aware that herpes is rarely dangerous.
Learn when the disease is most contagious (during the eruption and blister stage) and when sex is safest.

- *Choose the right time to talk.*

Discuss herpes with your partner only after you have gotten to know each other.

- *Listen to your partner.*

Be prepared to answer any questions that he or she may have.

- *Together, put things in perspective.*

Keep a positive outlook.
Remember that you are not alone.
Be aware that using a condom and abstaining from coitus during the most infectious period can prevent transmission of the disease.
Although there is no known cure, research continues on an antiviral drug.
Join a local support group together.

Figure 12-6   Human pubic louse, greatly enlarged by magnification.

Syphilis

Although we may think less often of syphilis than other sexually transmitted diseases, it remains a serious disease that if left untreated is capable of causing death. The chance of contracting syphilis during a single sexual encounter with an infected partner is now about 30%. The course taken by syphilis is well established once it is contracted.

Infection

The bacterium of syphilis, *Treponema pallidum,* a spirochete, is transmitted from an infected person to a new host through intimate contact. Moist, warm tissue, such as that lining the reproductive, urinary, and digestive systems, offers an ideal environment for the agent.

Incubation

After infection, an asymptomatic incubation period of 10 to 90 days gives way to the characteristic primary stage of the disease.

Primary Stage

Lasting 1 to 5 weeks, the primary stage of syphilis is associated with the formation of a small, raised, painless sore called a *chancre.* In 90% of women and 50% of men this highly infectious lesion is not easily identified; thus treatment is generally not sought. The chancre heals in 4 to 8 weeks.

Secondary Stage

The extremely contagious secondary stage of the disease is seen 6 to 12 weeks after initial infection. Because the infectious agents are now systemic, symptoms may include a generalized body rash, a sore throat, or a patchy loss of hair. A blood test (VDRL) will be positive, and treatment can be effectively administered. If untreated, the second stage will subside within 2 to 6 weeks. This is a stage during which syphilis can easily be transmitted by a pregnant woman to her fetus. Congenital syphilis often results in stillbirth or an infant born with a variety of life-threatening complications. Early treatment of infected pregnant women can prevent congenital syphilis.

Latent Stage

After the secondary stage subsides, an extended period of noninfectiousness is seen. The infectious agents remain dormant within the body cells, and few clinical signs exist during this stage.

Late Stage

Syphilis can recur for a third time 15 to 25 years after initial contact. In late-stage syphilis, tissue damage will be profound and irreversible. Damage to the cardiovascular system, central nervous system, eyes, and skin occurs, and death from the effects of the disease is likely.

Treatment

Syphilis is treated with penicillin, tetracycline, or erythromycin. Such treatment can kill the pathogen at any stage of the infection, but it cannot reverse the physical damage caused during the late stage of syphilis.

---

fungus pathogen *Candida (Monilia) albicans,* which produces the yeast infection often called *thrush.* These organisms, commonly found in the vagina, seem to multiply rapidly when some unusual stressor (pregnancy, use of birth control pills, diabetes, use of antibiotics) affects a woman's body. This infection, called *candidiasis,* is easily noticed by a white or cream-colored vaginal discharge that resembles cottage cheese. Vaginal itching and swelling are also commonly reported. Treatment often consists of an oral antibiotic or antibiotic douche to reduce the organisms to a normal level. Recently introduced nonprescription drugs for vaginal yeast infections allow for effective home treatment. Initial consultation with a physician is recommended before using these new products for the first time. (Men rarely report this monilial infection, although some may report mildly painful urination or a mild discharge at the urethral opening or beneath the foreskin of the penis.)

A second common agent that produces a vaginal infection is the protozoan *Trichomonas vaginalis.* This parasite can be transmitted through sexual intercourse or by contact with contaminated (often damp) objects, such as towels, clothing, or toilet seats that may contain some vaginal discharge. In women, this infection, called *trichomoniasis,* or "trich," produces a foamy, yellow-green, foul-smelling discharge that may be accompanied by itching, swelling, and painful urination. Treatment consists of a 2-week course of oral medication that helps kill the parasite. Men infrequently contract trichomoniasis but may harbor the organisms without realizing it.

Since the vagina is warm, dark, and moist, it is an ideal breeding environment for a variety of organisms. Normal hygienic measures help keep vaginal infections at a minimum. Unfortunately, use of some highly promoted commercial products seem to lead to increased incidences of vaginal infections. Among these are tight panty hose (without cotton panels), which tend to increase the vaginal temperature, and commercial vaginal douches, which can alter the acidic level of the vagina. Use of both of these products might promote infections. Women are advised to wipe from front to back after every bowel movement to reduce the opportunity for direct transmission of pathogenic agents from the rectum to the vagina. Avoiding public bath facilities is also a good suggestion. Of course, if you notice any unusual discharge from the vagina, you should report this to your physician.

Cystitis and Urethritis

Cystitis, an infection of the urinary bladder, and urethritis, an infection of the urethra, are conditions that can be caused by a sexually transmitted organism. Other modes of transmission are also associated with cystitis and urethritis, including infection with the organisms that cause vaginitis and organisms found in the intestinal tract. A culture is required to determine the specific pathogen associated with a particular case of cystitis or urethritis. The symptoms include pain when urinating, the need to urinate frequently, a dull aching pain above the pubic bone, and the passing of blood-streaked urine.

Cystitis and urethritis can be easily treated with antibiotics when the specific organism has been identified. Few complications result from infections that are treated promptly. If cystitis and urethritis are left untreated, the infectious agents could move upward in the urinary system and produce an infection of the ureters and kidneys. These upper urinary tract infections are more serious and require more extensive evaluation and aggressive treatment. It is therefore very important to obtain medical care on noticing symptoms.

Prevention of cystitis and urethritis depends to some degree on the source of the infectious agent. In a general sense, however, the incidence of infection can be lowered by urinating completely (to fully empty the urinary bladder) and by drinking ample quantities of fluids to flush the urinary tract. Whether the drinking of cranberry juice helps reduce urinary tract infections is a debatable issue.

Summary

- Progress has been made in reducing the incidence of some forms of infectious disease, but other infectious conditions are becoming more prevalent.
- A variety of pathogenic agents are responsible for infectious conditions.
- A chain of infection with six links characterizes every infectious condition.
- Infectious conditions progress through five distinct stages.
- Immunity can be acquired through both natural and artificial means. Immunization should be received on a regularly scheduled basis.
- The immune system's response to infection relies on cellular and humoral elements.
- The common cold and influenza display many similar symptoms but differ in terms of infectious agents, incubation period, prevention, and treatment.
- Tuberculosis and pneumonia are potentially fatal infections of the respiratory system.
- Mononucleosis and chronic fatigue syndrome are infections that result in chronic tiredness.
- Measles and mumps are childhood infections that can be harmful when contracted during adulthood.
- Lyme disease is a bacterial infection contracted in conjunction with outdoor activities.
- Hantavirus pulmonary syndrome is caused by a virus carried by deer mice.
- Hepatitis B (serum hepatitis) is a bloodborne infectious condition that can lead to serious liver damage. Hepatitis A, C, and D also exist.
- HIV/AIDS is a widespread, incurable viral disease transmitted through sexual activity, intravenous drug use, the use of infected blood products, or across the placenta during pregnancy.
- The definitive definition of AIDS can be based on the presence of specific conditions or the diminished number of helper T cells.
- Effective treatment of HIV and AIDS is limited, and prevention through the use of an effective vaccine is nonexistent.
- A variety of sexually transmitted conditions exists, many of which do not produce symptoms in most infected women and many infected men.
- Safer sex practices can reduce the risk of contracting STDs.

Review Questions

1. What are the agents responsible for the most familiar infectious conditions?
2. What are the six links that form the chain of infection?
3. What are the five stages that characterize the progression of infectious conditions?
4. What are the two principal components of the immune system, and how do they cooperate to protect the body from infectious agents and abnormal cells?
5. How are the common cold and influenza similar? How do they differ in terms of causative agents, incubation period, prevention, and treatment?
6. What symptoms make mononucleosis and chronic fatigue syndrome similar? What aspects of each are different?
7. Why are mumps and measles more serious conditions when they develop in adults?
8. Why is outdoor activity a risk factor in contracting Lyme disease?
9. How is hepatitis B transmitted, and which occupational group is at greatest risk of contracting this infection? How do forms A, C, and D compare with hepatitis B?
10. How is HIV transmitted? To what extent is the treatment of HIV/AIDS effective? What is meant by the term *safer sex*?
11. What specific infectious diseases could be classified as being STDs?
12. Why are women more often asymptomatic for STDs than men?
13. To what extent and in what manner can STD transmission be prevented?

Think About This . . .

- How do you feel when a classmate or co-worker comes to class or work ill? Is it fair to expose you to his or her illness?
- Which infectious disease have you had in the recent past? What impact did this infection have on your day-to-day activities?
- What diseases have you been immunized against?
- How do you feel about parents who do not have their children immunized?
- What would your initial reaction be if you found out that someone close to you had a sexually transmitted disease?

References

1. Creager J, Black J, Davinson V: *Microbiology—principles and applications,* Englewood Cliffs, NJ, 1990, Prentice Hall.
2. Hamann B: *Disease: identification, prevention and control,* St Louis, 1994, Mosby.
3. Moffett D, Moffett S, Schauf C: *Human physiology: foundations and frontiers,* ed 2, St Louis, 1993, Mosby.
4. Berstein DI et al: Evaluation of Rhesus rotavirus monovalent and tetravalent reassortant vaccines in US children, *JAMA* 273(15):1191-1196, 1996.
5. Clayman C, editor: *The American Medical Association home medical encyclopedia,* New York, 1989, Random House.
6. Nichol KI et al: The effectiveness of vaccination against influenza in healthy, working adults, *N Engl J Med* 333(14):889-893, 1995.
7. McKenna MT, McCary E, Onorato I: The epidemiology of tuberculosis among foreign-born persons in the United States, 1986 to 1993, *N Engl J Med* 332(16):1071-1076, 1995.
8. Chin DP et al: Clinical utility of a commercial test based on the polymerase chain reaction for detecting Mycobacterium tuberculosis in repiratory specimens, *Am J Respir Crit Care Med* 151:1872-1877, 1995.
9. Mandell G, Douglas GR, Bennett J: *Principles and practice of infectious diseases,* ed 3, New York, 1990, Churchill Livingstone.
10. Gold D et al: Chronic fatigue: a prospective clinical and virologic study, *JAMA* 264(1):48, 1990.
11. New treatment for chronic fatigue syndrome, *Tufts University Diet and Nutrition Newsletter* 13:12, 1996.
12. Lee S et al: Resurgence of congenital rubella syndrome

in the 1990s: report on missing opportunities and failed prevention policies among women of childbearing age, *JAMA* 267(19):2616, 1992.

13. Manning A: Measles rate going back down, *USA Today,* p1D, Oct 19, 1995.

14. Crowly L: *Introduction to human disease,* ed 3, Boston, 1992, Jones & Bartlett.

15. Feber HM, Hunt MS: Pitfalls in the diagnosis and treatment of Lyme disease in children (Brief Report), *JAMA* 274(1):66-68, 1995.

16. Gorman C: Deer ticks turn deadly, *Time* p 56, July 14, 1995.

17. Update: Hantavirus infection—United States, 1993, *MMWR* 42:517-519, 1993, as reported in *JAMA* 270(4):429-432, 1993.

18. US Department of Health and Human Services, Public Health Service: *Toxic shock syndrome is so rare you might forget it can happen,* DHHS Pub No (FDA) 90-4192, Rockville, Md, 1990.

19. Nightingala S: New requirement for tampon labeling, *Am Fam Physician* 41(3):990, 1990.

20. Centers for Disease Control and Prevention: *HIV/AIDS Surveillance Repor*t, 7(2), 1995.

21. Baumann M: AIDS cost to insurers (as reported by American Counsel of Life Insurers/Health Insurance Association of America), *USA Today,* p 1B, April 15, 1991.

22. Hellinger FJ: The lifetime cost of treating a person with HIV, *JAMA* 270(4):474-478, 1993.

23. US Department of Health and Human Services, Public Health Service, National Center for Infectious Diseases, Division of HIV/AIDS: *HIV/AIDS surveillance (third quarter edition),* Atlanta, 1993.

24. Bolognesi DP: A live-virus AIDS vaccine? Not yet, it is too early to consider use of a live-attenuated virus vaccine against HIV-1, *J NIH Res* 6:55-62, 1994.

25. Atlas RM: *Principles of microbiology,* St Louis, 1995, Mosby.

26. Ratcher R et al: *Contraceptive technology: 1994,* ed 16, New York, 1994, Irvington.

27. Jackson J: *Wellness: AIDS, STD, and other communicable diseases,* Guilford, Conn, 1992, Duskin.

Suggested Readings

Brandt A: *No magic bullet: a social history of venereal disease in the United States since 1880,* New York, 1987, Oxford University Press.

A detailed history of the social and political factors related to sexually transmitted diseases, with a chapter specifically on AIDS.

Stine GJ: *Acquired immune deficiency syndrome: biological, medical, social, and legal issues,* Englewood Cliffs, NJ, 1992, Prentice Hall.

Written for the serious student of the AIDS epidemic. Content focuses on the entire AIDS picture, including immunology, treatment, prevention, social and legal aspects, and the pandemic scope of the disease.

Fisher M: *I'll not go quietly: Mary Fisher speaks out,* New York, 1995, Scribner.

A very "normal" woman—married, mother, straight, community activist—tells of her contracting of AIDS and the path that it is taking her toward death. Her message is powerful but important: any person can contract this terrible disease, but even having done so, it is life that must be celebrated.

Close WT: *Ebola,* 1995, New York, Ivy Books.

Close, a physician, has written a novel regarding a 1976 outbreak of Ebola virus infestation closely mirroring the 1995 outbreak in Zaire. Through the writer's regard for the people of that area, the reader learns of the strength that the real victims must have brought to their situation.

 AS WE GO TO PRESS . . .

June 5, 1981, is the date identified as the start of the AIDS epidemic. June 5, 1996, marked the 15-year anniversary of the first official Centers for Disease Control and Prevention (CDC) report describing five cases of a rare pneumonia among homosexual men. Originally labeled the "gay plague," HIV and AIDS is now recognized as a disease unrelated to sexual orientation.

ON...

Controlling Infectious Disease Transmission

Ever since it was determined that microorganisms were the primary cause of communicable diseases, scientists have looked for ways to eradicate them. In the early part of the twentieth century, scientists searched for a "magic bullet" drug that would kill any organism that produced disease. Research, however, showed that disease-causing bacteria, viruses, protozoa, and other organisms were much too diverse to be wiped out with a single chemical. Still, research efforts continued to find cures for individual diseases. Slowly the significant scourges of humankind were conquered: polio, smallpox, measles, tetanus, and diphtheria. These and other killers were brought under control by the creation of various antibiotics and vaccines.[1] Starting in the 1950s, a massive campaign to immunize the world's population began, and the incidence of these diseases decreased sharply. A disease-free world seemed a real possibility.

However, that has not occurred. We underestimated the ability of these microbes to survive and adapt. Now we are continually facing the comeback of diseases we once thought were firmly under control. Outbreaks of measles, tuberculosis, and other "conquered" diseases are occurring with more frequency. To make matters worse, new disease-causing organisms that have the potential to kill on a grand scale are constantly being discovered. Why is this happening? Also, just as importantly, what can we do to bring it under control?

The Immunization Problem

Part of the problem has been our inability to continue the great strides in disease prevention made in earlier decades. Vaccination programs that were so effective in the 1960s and 1970s have not been as effective in recent years. As many as 4 million of the nation's 7.8 million 2 year olds may not be fully immunized.[2] Failure to immunize children against childhood disease is an important cause of the increase in cases of these diseases. Measles once caused up to 400,000 infections per year in the United States, but by 1983 a successful immunization campaign had reduced the number to under 1500.[3] In 1989, however, the number of infections was over 18,000.[3] The incidence of diseases such as polio and influenza is also on the rise even though there are vaccines available for them.

So why the decline in the number of immunizations? The answer is complex. Part of the reason may be the lack of accessible health care, especially for the economically disadvantaged.[4] Many families are not able to afford routine health care, and health care clinics have had to resort to extreme measures to get vaccines to children. Some clinics have vehicles that bring the vaccines to the public. Others use various means to encourage families to bring their children in for vaccinations. A clinic in Chicago went so far as to hold a car raffle for the parents of immunized children.[4] Cuts in funding have made such enticements impractical for most clinics, however.

Some parents have become fearful of the vaccines themselves. Many worry about the risk of side effects from vaccinations, even though the chances of problems occurring are remote. The pertussis (whooping cough) vaccine, for example, carries a slight risk of causing brain damage (about 1 in 300,000). Since the DPT (diphtheria-pertussis-tetanus) vaccine is given in several doses, the pertussis portion can be eliminated if the child shows signs of side effects.[4] Yet some parents think the risk is too great and therefore reject the entire series of vaccines. Thus their children miss out on the diphtheria and tetanus vaccines as well.

Children are not the only ones who suffer without proper immunizations. Adults, especially the elderly and those in high-risk groups, also need to be immunized against certain diseases. Older adults are at risk for influenza and pneumococcal disease, as are those with underlying diseases, such as heart disease or asthma.[5] Yet only about one fourth of people in these high-risk groups get immunized against influenza each year, and even fewer get immunized against pneumococcal infections.[5] Only 30% of those at risk for hepatitis B (including health care workers, homosexual men, heterosexuals with multiple partners, and IV drug users) obtain vaccinations, even though 300,000 new cases of the disease occur each year.[5]

New diseases have also caused some people to neglect vaccinations. Human immunodeficiency virus (HIV) is the most highly publicized, but others are also problematic. Before they were identified and treatments were devised, such afflictions as Lyme disease and Legionnaires' disease caused panics. Lyme disease is difficult to diagnose, and it is spread by tiny parasites known as deer ticks, which are sometimes difficult to detect on the body. Medical personnel and the general public are now more knowledgeable about ticks and the signs of the disease. The bacterium that causes Legionnaires' disease was found to thrive in places such as water from air cooling systems, so the air-handling system of a large building (such as a hotel or hospital) contaminated with this organism could potentially spread the disease to dozens of people. Managers of such facilities need to be aware of the danger from these and other organisms and need to learn how to prevent contamination.

More resistant viruses and bacteria are also causing problems. A dangerous resistant strain of pertussis broke out in Cincinnati in 1993. Many of the children who contracted the disease had already been vaccinated against the most common strain.[1] A deadly strain of the common bacterium *E. coli* wound up in the meat supply of a large fast-food restaurant chain, killing at least one child and making several other people violently ill.

Some of these new diseases are extremely frightening. For example, the Ebola virus, which kills most of those it infects, has been highly publicized in recent years. This particular virus causes devastating symptoms, including severe abdominal pain, fever, muscle aches, and hemorrhaging. Outbreaks of viruses such as Ebola have been contained successfully in fairly remote regions, but the efficiency of air travel creates the potential for an outbreak to spread quickly from one continent to another. Strains of Ebola have already been found in the United States, carried by infected primates used for research.

Staying healthy and avoiding infection is largely a matter of common sense. For an infection to occur, a disease-causing agent must be present, there must be enough of the organism to cause disease, the person must be susceptible to the disease, and the organism must have an appropriate portal of entry.[7] If one or more of these factors are eliminated, infection can be prevented. Here are a few things you can do to prevent disease:

Wash your hands. Frequent hand washing, especially with antimicrobial soap, can prevent many germs from being transmitted to you and from you to others.

Keep your vaccinations up to date. Check to make sure you and any children in your care have had all of your vaccinations, and be sure that all of your booster doses (such as tetanus vaccine) are current. Also, if you are in an at-risk group, you may want to take advantage of seasonal vaccines for diseases such as influenza. People who travel abroad in underdeveloped areas also need to be immunized against diseases they may encounter.

Cut off potential routes of transmission. Avoid making contact with any substances that may harbor bacteria. These include (but are not limited to) soiled food plates, utensils, and facial tissues and body fluids. This is especially important for those people in occupations where such contact is common (such as health care workers).

Clean and cook your food properly. Wash fresh vegetables to rid them of dirt. Be sure to cook all food thoroughly, especially foods such as meats, fish, and poultry, which are very likely to harbor harmful organisms.

Exercise and eat nutritious foods. Keeping yourself in shape and obtaining proper nutrients can help keep your immune system functioning properly and make you less susceptible to disease.

Take all of your medicine. When you do get sick, take your medicine exactly as prescribed. This is especially important when taking antibiotics. Not finishing the medication may contribute to a recurrence of the infection.

Practice safer sex. You cannot tell if a person has a blood-borne disease (such as AIDS or hepatitis B) or a sexually transmitted disease by looking at him or her. Safer sex practices can help prevent transmission of such diseases.

For Discussion . . .

Are you familiar with your immunization record? Have you ever failed to finish antibiotics that were prescribed for you? Do you feel that viruses such as Ebola are a real threat to Americans?

References

1. Lemonick MD: The killers all around: new viruses and drug-resistant bacteria are reversing human victories over infectious disease, *Time*, p11, Sept 12, 1994.
2. Standards for pediatric immunization practices (Ad Hoc Working Group for the Development of Standards for Pediatric Immunization Practices), *JAMA* 269(14), 1993.
3. Fisher LL, Douglas RG: Infectious diseases, *JAMA* 265(23), 1991 (Contempo 1991 Special Issue).
4. Levine A: Return of the old childhood scourges, *US News and World Report*, p1, June 4, 1988.
5. Eickhoff TC, Strikas, RA, Williams, WW: Update on adult immunization, *Patient Care* 26(15), 1992.
6. Preston R: *The hot zone*, New York, 1994, Random House.
7. American Red Cross: *Preventing disease transmission*, St Louis, 1993, Mosby Lifeline.

PART 5

SEXUALITY

Understanding Sexuality

Healthy People 2000 Objectives

According to the Healthy People 2000 Midcourse Review, key indicators of progress in areas related to sexuality include reducing the number of unintended pregnancies, increasing the age of initial sexual intercourse, increasing the rate of abstinence among young people who have already had sexual intercourse, and increasing the use of effective contraception (including the use of methods that also reduce the risk of various sexually transmitted diseases) among sexually active young people.

Progress toward achieving the target goals in these areas has been mixed. Despite intensive efforts to curb early sexual exploration, the age of initial sexual intercourse continues to drop. However, some small gains have been made in promoting abstinence among girls who have already been sexually active. In addition, there has been a slight increase in the percentage of teenagers who use effective contraception. We are moving away from the goal of fewer unintended pregnancies among adolescents. (Tracking data for unintended pregnancies among young adults is not available).

As we approach the year 2000, we have reached an understanding of both the biological and psychosocial factors that contribute to the complex expression of our **sexuality.** As a society, we are now inclined to view human behavior in terms of a complex script written on the basis of both biology and conditioning.

Reflecting this understanding is the way in which we use the words "male" or "female" to refer to the biological roots of our sexuality and the words "man" or "woman" to refer to the psychosocial roots of our sexuality. In this chapter, we explore human sexuality as it relates to the dynamic interplay of the biological and psychosocial bases that form your **masculinity** or **femininity.**

BIOLOGICAL BASES OF HUMAN SEXUALITY

Within a few seconds after the birth of a baby, someone (a doctor, nurse, or parent) emphatically labels the child: "It's a boy," or "It's a girl." For the parents and society as a whole, the child's **biological sexuality** is being displayed and identified. Another female or male enters the world.

Genetic Basis

At the moment of conception, a Y-bearing or an X-bearing sperm cell joins with the X-bearing ovum to establish the true basis of biological sexuality.[1] A fertilized ovum with sex chromosomes XX is biologically female, whereas fertilized ovum bearing the XY sex chromosomes is biologically male. Genetics forms the most basic level of an individual's biological sexuality.

Gonadal Basis

The gonadal basis for biological sexuality refers to the growing embryo's development of **gonads.** Male embryos develop testes about the seventh week after conception, and female embryos develop ovaries about the twelfth week after conception.

Structural Development

The development of male or female reproductive structures is initially determined by the presence or absence of hormones produced by the developing testes—androgens and müllerian inhibiting substance (MIS). With these hormones present, the male embryo starts to develop male reproductive structures (penis, scrotum, vas deferens, seminal vesicles, prostate gland, and Cowper's glands).

Because the female embryo is not exposed to these male hormones, it develops the characteristic female reproductive structures: the uterus, fallopian tubes, vagina, labia, and clitoris.

Biological Sexuality and the Childhood Years

The growth and development of the child in terms of reproductive organs and physiological processes have traditionally been thought to be "latent" during the childhood years. However, a gradual degree of growth occurs in both girls and boys. The reproductive organs, however, will undergo more greatly accelerated growth at the onset of **puberty** and will achieve their adult size and capabilities shortly.

Puberty

The entry into puberty is a gradual maturing process for young girls and boys. For young girls, the onset of menstruation, called **menarche,** occurs around age 13 but may come somewhat earlier or later.[2] Early menstrual cycles tend to be **anovulatory.** Menarche is usually preceded by a growth spurt that includes the budding of breasts and the growth of pubic and underarm hair.[3]

---

sexuality
The quality of being sexual; can be viewed from many biological and psychosocial perspectives.

masculinity
Behavioral expressions traditionally observed in males.

femininity
Behavioral expressions traditionally observed in females.

biological sexuality
Male and female aspects of sexuality.

gonads
Male or female sex glands; testes produce sperm and ovaries produce eggs.

puberty
Achievement of reproductive ability.

menarche (muh **nar** key)
Time of a female's first menstrual cycle.

anovulatory (an **oh** vyu luh tory)
Not ovulating.

Young males follow a similar pattern of maturation, including a growth spurt followed by a gradual sexual maturity. However, this process takes place about 2 years later than in young females. Genital enlargement, underarm and pubic hair growth, and a lowering of the voice commonly occur. The male's first ejaculation is generally experienced by the age of 14, most commonly through **nocturnal emission** or masturbation. For many young boys, fully mature sperm do not develop until about age 15.

Reproductive capability only gradually declines over the course of the adult years. In the woman, however, the onset of **menopause** signals a more direct turning off of the reproductive system than is the case for the male adult. By the early to mid-fifties, virtually all women have entered a postmenopausal period, but for men, relatively high-level **spermatogenesis** may continue for a decade or two.

The story of sexual maturation and reproductive maturity cannot, however, be solely focused on the changes that take place in the body. Now we discuss the psychosocial processes that accompany the biological changes.

PSYCHOSOCIAL BASES OF HUMAN SEXUALITY

If growth and development of our sexuality were to be visualized as a step ladder (Figure 13-1), one vertical rail of the ladder would represent our biological sexuality. Arising at various points along this rail would be rungs representing the sequential unfolding of the genetic, gonadal, and structural components.

Because humans, more so than any other life form, can rise above a life centered on reproduction, a second dimension or rail to our sexuality exists—our **psychosocial sexuality.** The reason we possess the ability to be more than reproductive beings is a question for the theologian or philosopher. We are considerably more complex than the functions determined by biology. The process that transforms a male into a

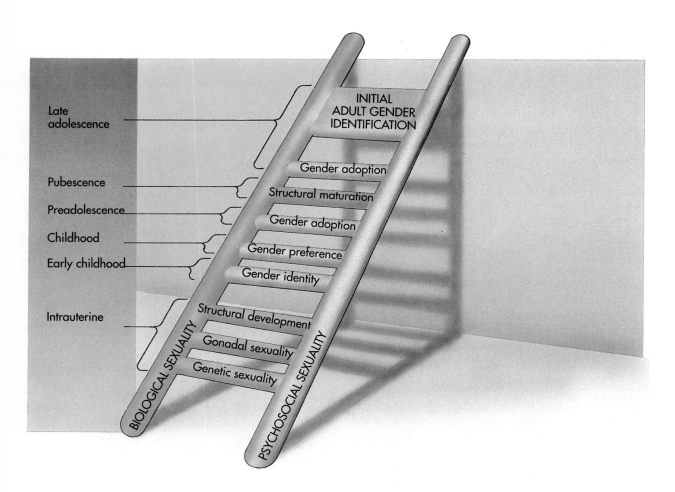

Figure 13-1   Our sexuality develops through biological and psychosocial stages.

man and a female into a woman begins at birth and continues to influence us through the course of our lives.

Gender Identity

Although expectant parents may prefer to have a child of one **gender** over the other, they frequently must wait until the birth of the baby to have their question answered. External genitals "cast the die," and femininity or masculinity begins to receive its traditional reinforcement by the parents and society in general. By the eighteenth month, typical children have both the language and the insight to correctly identify their gender. They have established a **gender identity.**[4] The first rung rising from the psychosocial rail of the ladder has been climbed.

Gender Preference

During the preschool years, children receive the second component of the *scripting* required for the full development of psychosocial sexuality—the preference for the gender to which they have been assigned. The process whereby **gender preference** is transmitted to the child is more than likely a less subtle form of the practices observed during the gender identity period (the first 18 months). Many parents begin to control the child's exposure to experiences traditionally reserved for children of the opposite gender. This is particularly true for boys; parents will stop play activities they perceive as being too feminine.

With the recent acceleration in the importance of competitive sports for women, many of the skills and experiences once reserved for boys are now being fostered in young girls. What effect, if any, this movement will have on the speed at which gender preference is reached will be a topic or further research.*

Gender Adoption

The process of reaching an initial adult gender identification requires a considerable period of time. The specific knowledge, attitudes, and behavior characteristic of adults must be observed, analyzed, and practiced. The process of acquiring and personalizing these "insights" about how men and women think, feel, and act is reflected by the term **gender adoption,**

---

*If you want to test the existence of gender preference, ask a group of first- or second-grade boys or girls if they would be happier being a member of the opposite gender. Be prepared for some frank replies.

the first and third rungs below the initial adult gender identification rail of the ladder in Figure 13-1.

In addition to the construction of a personalized version of an adult sexual identity, it is important that the child and particularly the adolescent construct a *gender schema* for a member of the opposite gender. Clearly, the world of adulthood, with its involvement with intimacy, parenting, and employment, will require that men know women and women know men. Gender adoption provides an opportunity to begin to assemble this equally valuable "picture" of what the other gender is like.

Initial Adult Gender Identification

By the time young people have climbed all of the rungs of the sexuality ladder, they have arrived at the chronological point in the life cycle when they need to construct an initial adult **gender identification.** You

---

nocturnal emission
Ejaculation that occurs during sleep; "wet dream."

menopause
Decline and eventual cessation of hormone production by the female reproductive system.

spermatogenesis (sper mat oh **jen** uh sis)
Process of sperm production.

psychosocial sexuality
Masculine and feminine aspects of sexuality.

gender
General term reflecting a biological basis of sexuality; the male gender *or* the female gender.

gender identity
Recognition of one's gender.

gender preference
Emotional and intellectual acceptance of one's own gender.

gender adoption
Lengthy process of learning the behavior that is traditional for one's gender.

gender identification
Achievement of a personally satisfying interpretation of one's masculinity or femininity.

might notice that this label seems remarkably similar to the terminology used to describe one of the developmental tasks being used in this textbook. In fact, the task of forming an initial adult identity is closely related to developing an initial adult image of oneself as a man or a woman. Although most of us currently support the concept of "person" in many gender-neutral contexts (for some very valid reasons), we still must identify ourselves as either a man or a woman.

Transsexualism

Students are often intrigued by a sexual variance that is first noticed during one or two of the psychosocial stages just discussed. Transsexualism is a sexual variance of the most profound nature because it represents a complete rejection by an individual of his or her biological sexuality. The male transsexual believes that he is female and thus desires to be the woman that he knows he is. The female transsexual believes that she is male and thus desires to become the man that she knows she should be. It should be noted that psychiatrists and sex therapists do not view transsexuals as homosexual in their sexual orientation.

For transsexuals, the periods of gender preference and gender adoption are perplexing as they attempt, with limited success, to resolve the conflict between what their mind tells them is true and what their body displays. Adolescent and young adult transsexuals often cross-dress, undertake homosexual relationships (which they view as being heterosexual relationships), experiment with hormone replacement therapy, and in some cases actively pursue a **sex reassignment operation.** Several thousand of these operations have been performed at some of the leading medical centers in the United States.

ANDROGYNY: SHARING THE PLUSES

Over the last 20 years our society has increasingly accepted an image of a person who possesses both masculine and feminine qualities. This accepted image has taken years to develop because our society traditionally has reinforced rigid masculine roles for men and rigid feminine roles for women.

In the past, from the time a child was born, we assigned and reinforced only those roles and traits that were thought to be directly related to his or her biological gender. Boys were not allowed to cry, play with dolls, or help in the kitchen. Girls were not encouraged to become involved in sports; they were told to learn to sew, cook, and baby-sit. Men were encouraged to be strong, expressive, dominant, aggressive, and career oriented, whereas women were encouraged to be weak, shy, submissive, passive, and home oriented.

These traditional biases have resulted in some interesting phenomena related to career opportunities. Women were denied jobs requiring above-average physical strength, admittance into professional schools requiring high intellectual capacities, such as law, medicine, and business, and entry into most levels of military participation. Likewise, men were not encouraged to enter traditionally feminine careers, such as nursing, clerical work, and elementary school teaching.

For a variety of reasons, the traditional picture has changed. **Androgyny,** or the blending of both feminine and masculine qualities, is more clearly evident in our society now than ever before. Today it is more acceptable to see men involved in raising children (including changing diapers) and doing routine housework. On the other hand, it is also more acceptable to see women entering the workplace in jobs traditionally managed by men and participating in sports traditionally played by men. Men are not scoffed at when they are seen crying after a touching movie. Women are not laughed at when they choose to assert themselves. The disposal of numerous sexual stereotypes has probably benefited our society immensely by relieving people of the pressure to be 100% "womanly" or 100% "macho."

Many women are now entering traditionally male professions, such as law, medicine, and business.

Research data suggest that androgynous people are more flexible, have greater self-esteem, and show more social skills and motivation to achieve.[4] This should encourage you to be unafraid to break the gender role stereotype.

REPRODUCTIVE SYSTEMS

The most familiar aspects of biological sexuality are the structures that compose the reproductive systems. Each structure contributes in unique ways to the reproductive process. Thus with these structures, males have the ability to impregnate. Females have the ability to become pregnant, give birth, and nourish infants through breast-feeding. In addition, many of these structures are associated with nonreproductive sexual behavior.

Male Reproductive System

The male reproductive system consists of external structures of genitals (the penis and scrotum) and internal structures (the testes, various passageways or ducts, seminal vesicles, the prostate gland, and the Cowper's glands) (Figure 13-2, *A*). The *testes* (also called *gonads* or *testicles*) are two egg-shaped bodies that lie within a saclike structure called the *scrotum*. During most of fetal development, the testes lie within the abdominal cavity. They descend into the scrotum during the last 2 months of fetal life. The testes are housed in the scrotum because a temperature lower than the body core temperature is required for adequate sperm development. The walls of the scrotum are composed of contractile tissue and can draw the testes closer to the body during cold temperatures (and sexual arousal) and relax during warm temperatures. Scrotal contraction and relaxation allow a constant, productive temperature to be maintained in the testes.

A cross-sectional view of a single testis reveals an intricate network of structures called *seminiferous tubules* (Figure 13-2, *B*). Within these 300 or so seminiferous tubules, the process of sperm production (spermatogenesis) takes place. Sperm cell development starts at about age 11 in boys and is influenced by the release of the hormone **ICSH (interstitial cell-stimulating hormone)** from the pituitary gland. ICSH does primarily what its name suggests: it stimulates specific cells (called *interstitial cells*) within the testes to begin producing the male sex hormone *testosterone*. Testosterone in turn is primarily responsible for the gradual development of the male secondary sex characteristics at the onset of puberty. By the time a boy is

approximately 15 years old, sufficient levels of testosterone exist so that the testes become capable of full spermatogenesis.

Before the age of about 15, most of the sperm cells produced in the testes are incapable of fertilization. The production of fully mature sperm (*spermatozoa*) is triggered by another hormone secreted by the brain's pituitary gland—**FSH (follicle-stimulating hormone)**. FSH influences the seminiferous tubules to begin producing spermatozoa that are capable of fertilization.

Spermatogenesis takes place around the clock, with hundreds of millions of sperm cells produced daily. The sperm cells do not stay in the seminiferous tubules but rather are transferred through a system of ducts that lead into the *epididymis*. The epididymis is a tubular coil that attaches to the back side of each testicle. These collecting structures house the maturing sperm cells for 2 to 3 weeks. During this period the sperm finally become capable of motion, but they remain inactive until they mix with the secretions from the accessory glands (the seminal vesicles, prostate gland, and Cowper's glands).

Each epididymis leads into an 18-inch passageway known as the *vas deferens*. Sperm, moved along by the action of hairlike projections called *cilia*, can also remain in the vas deferens for an extended time without losing their ability to fertilize an egg.

The two vasa deferens extend into the abdominal cavity, where each meets with a *seminal vesicle*—the first of the three accessory structures or glands. Each seminal vesicle contributes a clear, alkaline fluid that

---

sex reassignment operation
Surgical procedure designed to remove the external genitalia and replace them with genitalia appropriate to the opposite gender.

androgyny (an **droj** en ee)
The blending of both masculine and feminine qualities.

ICSH (interstitial cell–stimulating hormone)
(in ter **stish** ul)
A gonadotropic hormone of the male required for the production of testosterone.

FSH (follicle-stimulating hormone)
A gonadotropic hormone required for initial development of ova (in the female) and sperm (in the male).

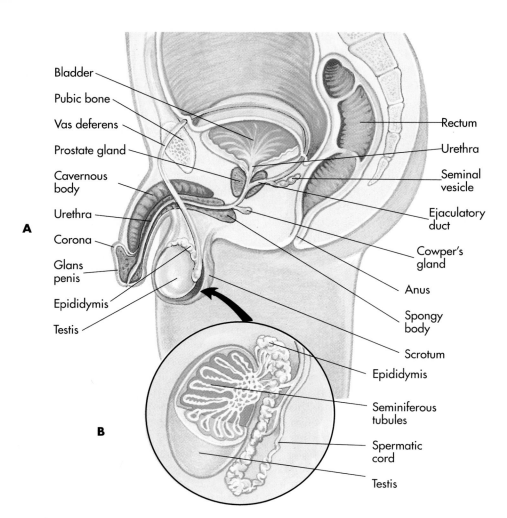

Figure 13-2 **A,** Male reproductive structures, side view. The production and delivery of sperm, as well as the production of the sex hormone testosterone, is accomplished by the male reproductive structures. **B,** Cross section of a testis.

nourishes the sperm cells with fructose and permits the sperm cells to be suspended in a movable medium. The fusion of a vas deferens with the seminal vesicle results in the formation of a passageway called the *ejaculatory duct.* Each ejaculatory duct is only about 1 inch long and empties into the final passageway for the sperm—the urethra.

This juncture takes place in an area surrounded by the second accessory gland—the *prostate gland.* The prostate gland secretes a milky fluid containing a variety of substances, including proteins, cholesterol, citric acid, calcium, buffering salts, and various enzymes. The prostate secretions further nourish the sperm cells and also raise the pH level, making the mixture quite alkaline. This alkalinity permits the sperm to have greater longevity as they are transported during ejaculation through the urethra, out of the penis, and into the highly acidic vagina.

The third accessory glands, the Cowper's glands, serve primarily to lubricate the urethra with a clear, viscous mucus. These paired glands empty their small amounts of preejaculatory fluid during the arousal stage of the sexual response cycle. Alkaline in nature, this fluid also neutralizes the acidic level of the urethra. It is hypothesized that viable sperm cells can be suspended in this fluid and can enter the female reproductive tract before full ejaculation by the male.[3] This may account for many of the failures of the "withdrawal" method of contraception.

The sperm cells, when combined with secretions from the seminal vesicles and the prostate gland, form a sticky substance called **semen.** Interestingly, the microscopic sperm actually makes up less than 5% of the seminal fluid discharged at ejaculation. Contrary to popular belief, the paired seminal vesicles contribute about 60% of the semen volume, and the prostate gland adds about 30%.[5] Thus the fear of some men that a **vasectomy** will destroy their ability to ejaculate is completely unfounded (see Chapter 14).

During *emission* (the gathering of semen in the upper part of the urethra), a sphincter muscle at the base of the bladder contracts and inhibits semen from being pushed into the bladder and urine from being deposited into the urethra.[3] Thus semen and urine rarely intermingle, even though they leave the body through the same passageway.

Ejaculation takes place when the semen is forced out of the penis through the urethral opening. The involuntary, rhythmic muscle contractions that control ejaculation result in a series of pleasurable sensations known as *orgasm*.

The urethra lies on the underside of the penis and extends through one of three cylindrical chambers of erectile tissue (two cavernous bodies and one spongy body). Each of these three chambers provides the vascular space required for sufficient erection of the penis. When a male becomes sexually aroused, these areas become congested with blood (*vasocongestion*). After ejaculation or when a male is no longer sexually stimulated, these chambers release the blood into the general circulation and the penis returns to a **flaccid** state.

The *shaft* of the penis is covered by a thin layer of skin that is an extension of the skin that covers the scrotum. This loose layer of skin is sensitive to sexual stimulation and extends over the head of the penis, except in males who have been circumcised. The *glans* (or head) of the penis is the most sexually sensitive (to tactile stimulation) part of the male body. Nerve receptor sites are especially prominent along the *corona* (the ridge of the glans) and the *frenulum* (the thin tissue at the base of the glans).

Female Reproductive System

The external structures (genitals) of the female reproductive system consist of the mons pubis, labia majora, labia minora, clitoris, and vestibule (Figure 13-3). Collectively these structures form the *vulva* or vulval area. The *mons pubis* is the fatty covering over the pubic bone. The mons pubis (or mons veneris, "mound of Venus") is covered by pubic hair and is quite sensitive to sexual stimulation. The *labia majora* are large longitudinal folds of skin that cover the entrance to the vagina, whereas the *labia minora* are the smaller longitudinal skin folds that lie within the labia majora. These hairless skin folds of the labia minora join at the top to form the *prepuce*. The prepuce covers the glans of the *clitoris,* which is the most sexually sensitive part of the female body.

A rather direct analogy can be made between the penis and the clitoris. In terms of the tactile sensitivity, both structures are the most sensitive parts of the male and female genitals. Both contain a glans and a shaft (although the clitoral shaft is beneath the skin surface). Both organs are composed of erectile tissue that can become engorged with blood. Both are covered by skin folds (the clitoral prepuce of the female and the foreskin of the male), and both structures can collect **smegma** beneath these tissue folds.[4]

The *vestibule* is the region enclosed by the labia minora. Evident here are the urethral opening and the entrance to the vagina (or vaginal orifice). Also located at the vaginal opening are the *Bartholin's glands,* which secrete a minute amount of lubricating fluid during sexual excitement.

The *hymen* is a thin layer of tissue that stretches across the opening of the vagina. Once thought to be the only indication of virginity, the intact hymen rarely covers the vaginal opening entirely. Openings in the hymen are necessary for the discharge of menstrual fluid and vaginal secretions. Many hymens are stretched or torn to full opening by adolescent physical activity or by the insertion of tampons. In women whose hymens are not fully ruptured, the first act of sexual intercourse will generally accomplish this. Pain may accompany first intercourse in females with relatively intact hymens.

The internal reproductive structures of the female include the vagina, uterus, fallopian tubes, and ovaries. The *vagina* is the structure that accepts the penis during sexual intercourse. Normally the walls of the vagina are collapsed, except during sexual stim-

---

semen
Secretion containing sperm and nutrients discharged from the urethra at ejaculation.

vasectomy
Surgical procedure in which the vasa deferens are cut to prevent the passage of sperm from the testicles; the most common form of male sterilization.

flaccid (**fla** sid)
Nonerect; the state of erectile tissue when vasocongestion is not occurring.

smegma
Cellular discharge that can accumulate beneath the clitoral hood and the foreskin of an uncircumcised penis.

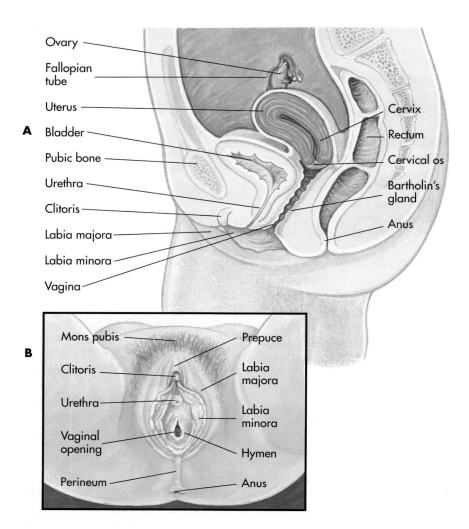

A
- Ovary
- Fallopian tube
- Uterus
- Bladder
- Pubic bone
- Urethra
- Clitoris
- Labia majora
- Labia minora
- Vagina
- Cervix
- Rectum
- Cervical os
- Bartholin's gland
- Anus

B
- Mons pubis
- Clitoris
- Urethra
- Vaginal opening
- Perineum
- Prepuce
- Labia majora
- Labia minora
- Hymen
- Anus

Figure 13-3 **A,** Female reproductive structures, side view. The formation of ova, production of the sex hormones estrogen and progesterone, and support for the developing fetus are functions of the structures of the female reproductive system. **B,** External view of the female genitals.

ulation, when the vaginal walls widen and elongate to accommodate the erect penis. Only the outer third of the vagina is especially sensitive to sexual stimulation. In this location, vaginal tissues swell considerably to form the **orgasmic platform.** This platform constricts the vaginal opening and in effect "grips" the penis—regardless of its size.[4] Thus the belief that a woman receives considerably more sexual pleasure from men with large penises is not supported from an anatomical standpoint.

The *uterus* (or *womb*) is approximately the size and shape of a small pear. This highly muscular organ is capable of undergoing a wide range of physical changes, as evidenced by its enlargement during pregnancy, its contraction during menstruation and labor, and its movement during the orgasmic phase of the female sexual response cycle. The primary func-

tion of the uterus is to provide a suitable environment for the possible implantation of a fertilized ovum, or egg. This implantation, should it occur, will take place in the innermost lining of the uterus—the *endometrium.* In the mature female, the endometrium undergoes cyclic changes as it prepares a new lining on a near-monthly basis.

The lower third of the uterus is called the *cervix.* The cervix extends slightly into the vagina. Sperm can enter the uterus through the cervical opening, or *cervical os.* Mucous glands in the cervix secrete a fluid that is thin and watery near the time of ovulation. Mucus of this consistency apparently facilitates sperm passage into the uterus and deeper structures. However, cervical mucus is much thicker during portions of the menstrual cycle when pregnancy is improbable, and during pregnancy, to protect against bacterial agents and other substances that are especially dangerous to the developing fetus.

The upper two thirds of the uterus is called the *corpus* or *body*. This is where implantation of the fertilized ovum generally takes place. The upper portion of the uterus opens into two *fallopian tubes,* or *oviducts,* each about 4 inches long. The fallopian tubes are each directed toward an *ovary.* They serve as a passageway for the ovum in its week-long voyage toward the uterus. In most cases, conception takes place in the upper third of the fallopian tubes.

The ovaries are analogous to the testes in the male. Their function is to produce the ovum, or egg. Usually, one ovary produces and releases just one egg each month. Approximately the size and shape of an unshelled almond, an ovary produces viable ova in the process known as *oogenesis.* The ovaries also produce the female sex hormones through the efforts of specific structures within the ovaries. These hormones play multiple roles in the development of female secondary sex characteristics, but their primary function is to prepare the endometrium of the uterus for possible implantation of a fertilized ovum. In the average healthy female, this preparation takes place about 13 times a year for a period of about 35 years. At menopause, the ovaries shrink considerably and stop nearly all hormonal production.

Menstrual cycle

Each month or so, the inner wall of the uterus prepares for a possible pregnancy. When a pregnancy does not occur (as is the case throughout most months of a woman's fertile years), this lining must be released and a new one prepared. The breakdown of this endometrial wall and the resultant discharge of blood and endometrial tissue is known as *menstruation* (or *menses*) (Figure 13-4). The cyclic timing of menstruation is governed by hormones released from two sources: the pituitary gland and the ovaries.

Girls generally have their first menstrual cycle, the onset of which is called *menarche,* sometime between 12 and 14 years of age. Body weight, nutrition, heredity, and overall health are factors related to menarche. Interestingly, after a girl first menstruates, she may be anovulatory for a year or longer before she releases a viable ovum during her cycle. She will then continue this cyclic activity until about age 45 to 55.

This text refers to a menstrual cycle that lasts 28 days. Be assured that few women display absolutely perfect 28-day cycles. Most women fluctuate by a few days to a week around this 28-day pattern, and some women vary extremely from this cycle.

Your knowledge about the menstrual cycle is critical for your understanding of pregnancy, contraception,

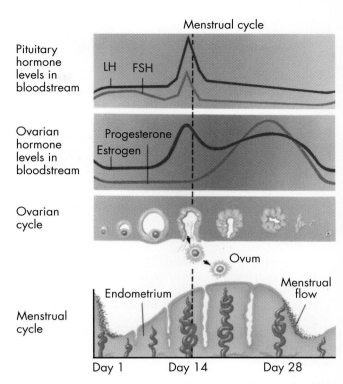

Figure 13-4 The menstrual cycle involves the development and release of an ovum, supported by hormones from the pituitary, and the buildup of the endometrium, supported by hormones from the ovary, for the purpose of establishing a pregnancy.

menopause, and issues related to the overall health and comfort of women (see the Star Box on p. 320 for a discussion of endometriosis). Although at first it may sound like a complicated process, each segment of the cycle can be studied separately for better understanding.

The menstrual cycle can be thought of as occurring in three segments or phases: the menstrual phase (lasting about 1 week), the proliferative phase (also lasting about 1 week), and the secretory phase (lasting about 2 weeks). Day 1 of this cycle starts with the first day of bleeding, or menstrual flow.

The *menstrual phase* signals the woman that a pregnancy has not taken place and that her uterine lining is being sloughed off. During a 5- to 7-day period, a woman will discharge about ¼ to ½ cup of blood and tissue. (Only about 1 ounce of the menstrual flow is actual blood.) The menstrual flow is heaviest during

orgasmic platform
Expanded outer third of the vagina that grips the penis during the plateau phase of the sexual response pattern.

Endometriosis

Endometriosis is a condition in which endometrial tissue that normally lines the uterus is found growing within the pelvic cavity. Because the tissue remains sensitive to circulating hormones, it is the source of pain and discomfort during the latter half of the menstrual cycle. Endometriosis is most commonly found in younger women and is frequently related to infertility.

In addition to discomfort before menstruation, the symptoms of endometriosis include low back pain, pain during intercourse, and a variety of lower digestive tract symptoms, such as diarrhea and constipation. As with the general pain and discomfort of endometriosis, these symptoms are also more noticeable during the latter weeks of the cycle.

Treatment of endometriosis largely depends on its extent. Drugs to suppress ovulation, including birth control pills, may be helpful in mild cases. For more severe cases, surgical removal of the tissue or a hysterectomy may be necessary. For some women, endometriosis is suppressed during pregnancy and does not return after pregnancy.

the first days of this phase. Since the muscular uterus must contract to accomplish this tissue removal, some women have uncomfortable cramping during menstruation. Most women, however, report more pain and discomfort during the few days before the first day of bleeding. (See the discussion of premenstrual syndrome [PMS] at right.)

Modern methods of absorbing menstrual flow include the use of internal tampons and external pads. Caution must be exercised by the users of tampons to prevent the possibility of toxic shock syndrome (TSS) (see Chapter 12). Since menstrual flow is a positive sign of good health, women are encouraged to be normally active during menstruation.

The *proliferative phase* of the menstrual cycle starts about the time menstruation stops. Lasting about 1 week, this phase is first influenced by the release of FSH from the pituitary gland. FSH circulates in the bloodstream and directs the ovaries to start the process of maturing approximately 20 primary ovarian *follicles*. Thousands of primary egg follicles are present in each ovary at birth. These follicles resemble shells that house immature ova. As these follicles ripen under FSH influence, they release the hormone estrogen. Estrogen's primary function is to direct the endometrium to start the development of a thick, highly vascular wall. As the estrogen levels increase, the pituitary gland's secretion of FSH is reduced. Now the pituitary gland prepares for the surge of the

luteinizing hormone (LH) required to accomplish ovulation.[6]

In the days immediately preceding ovulation, one of the primary follicles (called the *graafian follicle*) matures fully. The other primary follicles degenerate and are absorbed by the body. The graafian follicle moves toward the surface of the ovary. When LH is released in massive quantities on about day 14, the graafian follicle bursts to release the fully mature ovum. The release of the ovum is **ovulation.** Regardless of the overall length of a woman's cycle, ovulation occurs 14 days before her first day of menstrual flow.

The ovum is quickly captured by the fingerlike projections (*fimbriae*) of the fallopian tubes. In the upper third of the fallopian tubes, the ovum is capable of being fertilized in a 24- to 36-hour period. If the ovum is not fertilized by a sperm cell, it will begin to degenerate and eventually be absorbed by the body.

After ovulation, the *secretory phase* of the menstrual cycle starts when the remnants of the graafian follicle restructure themselves into a **corpus luteum.** The corpus luteum remains inside the ovary, secreting estrogen and a fourth hormone called *progesterone*. Progesterone, which literally means "for pregnancy," continues to direct the endometrial buildup. If pregnancy occurs, the corpus luteum monitors progesterone and estrogen levels throughout the pregnancy. If pregnancy does not occur, high levels of progesterone signal the pituitary to stop the release of LH and the corpus luteum starts to degenerate on about day 24. When estrogen and progesterone levels diminish significantly by day 28, the endometrium is discharged from the uterus and out the vagina. The secretory phase ends, and the menstrual phase begins. The cycle is complete.

PMS. PMS is characterized by psychological symptoms, such as depression, lethargy, irritability, and aggressiveness, or somatic symptoms, such as headache, backache, asthma, acne, and epilepsy, that recur in the same phase of each menstrual cycle, followed by a symptom-free phase in each cycle. Some of the more frequently reported symptoms of PMS include tension, tender breasts, fainting, fatigue, abdominal cramps, and weight gain.

The cause of PMS appears to be hormonal. Perhaps a woman's body is insensitive to a normal level of progesterone, or her ovaries fail to produce a normal amount of progesterone. These reasons seem plausible because PMS types of symptoms do not occur during pregnancy, during which natural progesterone levels are very high, and because women with PMS seem to feel much better after receiving high doses of natural progesterone in suppository form. When using oral contraceptives that supply synthetic progesterone at normal levels, many women report relief from some symptoms of PMS. However, the effectiveness of the most frequently used form of treatment, progesterone suppositories, is now being questioned.

Until the effectiveness of progesterone has been fully researched, it is unlikely that the medical community will deal with PMS through any approach other than a relatively conservative treatment of symptoms through the use of *analgesic drugs* (including *prostaglandin inhibitors*), diuretic drugs, dietary modifications (including restriction of caffeine and salt), vitamin B_6 therapy, exercise, and stress-reduction exercises. The exact nature of PMS has been further complicated by the classification of severe PMS as a mental disturbance by some segments of the American Psychiatric Association.

Fibrocystic breast condition. In some women, particularly those who have never been pregnant, stimulation of the breast tissues by estrogen and progesterone during the menstrual cycle results in an unusually high degree of secretory activity by the cells lining the ducts. The fluid released by the secretory lining finds its way into the fibrous connective tissue areas in the lower half of the breast, where in pocketlike cysts the fluid presses against neighboring tissues. Excessive secretory activity produces in many women a fibrocystic breast condition characterized by swollen, firm or hardened, tender breast tissue before menstruation.

Women who experience a more extensive fibrocystic condition can be treated with drugs that have a "calming" effect on progesterone production. In addition, occasional draining of the fluid-filled cysts can bring relief.

Menopause

For the vast majority of women in their late forties through their mid-fifties, a gradual decline in reproductive system function, called *menopause,* occurs. Menopause is a normal physiological process, not a disease process. It can, however, become a health concern for some middle-aged women who have unpleasant side effects resulting from this natural stoppage of ovum production and menstruation.

As ovarian function and hormone production diminish, a period of adjustment must be made by the hypothalamus, ovaries, uterus, and other estrogen-sensitive tissues. The extent of menopause as a health problem is determined by the degree to which **hot flashes,** vaginal wall dryness, depression and melancholy, breast changes, and the uncertainty of fertility are seen as problems.

In comparison with past generations, today's mid-life women are much less likely to find menopause to be a negative experience. The end of fertility, combined with children leaving the home, makes the middle years a period of personal rediscovery for many women.

For women who are troubled by the changes brought about by menopause, physicians may prescribe **estrogen replacement therapy** (ERT). This can relieve many symptoms and offer benefits to help reduce the incidence of osteoporosis (see Chapters 5 and 11) and heart disease.

HUMAN SEXUAL RESPONSE PATTERN

Although history has many written and visual accounts of the human's ability to be sexually aroused, it was not until the pioneering work of Masters and Johnson[7] that the events associated with arousal were clinically documented. Five questions posed by these researchers gave direction to a series of studies involving the scientific evaluation of human sexual response:

Is There a Predictable Pattern Associated with the Sexual Responses of Males and Females?

The answer to the first question posed by the researchers was an emphatic "yes." A predictable sexual response pattern was identified[7]; it consists of an

---

luteinizing hormone (LH) (loo ten eye zing)
A gonadotropic hormone of the female required for fullest development and release of ova; ovulating hormone.

ovulation
The release of a mature egg from the ovary.

corpus luteum (kore pus loo tee um)
Cellular remnant of the graafian follicle after the release of an ovum.

hot flashes
Temporary feelings of warmth experienced by women during and after menopause, caused by blood vessel dilation.

estrogen replacement therapy
Medically administered estrogen to replace estrogen lost as the result of menopause.

initial **excitement stage,** a **plateau stage,** an **orgasmic stage,** and a **resolution stage.** Each stage involves predictable changes in the structural characteristics and physiological function of reproductive and nonreproductive organs in both the male and female. These changes are shown in the Star Box on pp. 323-324.

Is the Sexual Response Pattern Stimuli-Specific?

The research of Masters and Johnson[7] clearly established a "no" answer to the second question concerning stimuli specificity. Their findings demonstrated that numerous senses can supply the stimuli necessary for initiating the sexual response pattern. Although touching activities might initiate arousal in most people and maximize it for the vast majority of people, in both males and females, sight, smell, sound, and *vicariously formed stimuli* can also stimulate the same sexual arousal patterns.

What Differences Occur in the Sexual Response Pattern?

Differences between males and females

In response to the third question, several differences are observable when comparing the sexual response patterns of males and females:

- With the exception of some later adolescent males, the vast majority of males are not multiorgasmic. The **refractory phase** of the resolution stage prevents most males from experiencing more than one orgasm in a short time period, even though sufficient stimulation is available.
- Females possess a **multiorgasmic capacity.** Masters and Johnson[7] found that as many as 10% to 30% of all female adults routinely experience multiple orgasms.
- Although they possess multiorgasmic potential, some 10% of all female adults are *anorgasmic*—that is, they never experience an orgasm.[7] For many anorgasmic females, orgasms can be experienced when masturbation, rather than **coitus,** provides the stimulation.
- When measured during coitus, males reach orgasm far more quickly than do females. However, when masturbation is the source of stimulation, females reach orgasm as quickly as do males.[7]

More important than any of the differences pointed out is the finding that the sexual response patterns of males and females are far more alike than they are different. Not only do males and females experience the four basic stages of the response pattern, but they also have similar responses in specific areas, including the **erection** and *tumescence* of sexual structures; the appearance of a **sex flush;** the increase in cardiac output, blood pressure, and respiratory rate; and the occurrence of *rhythmic pelvic thrusting.*[7]

Differences among subjects within a same-gender group

When a group of subjects of the same gender was studied in an attempt to answer questions about similarities and differences in the sexual response pattern, Masters and Johnson noted considerable variation. Even when variables such as age, race, education, and general health were held constant, the extent and duration of virtually every stage of the response pattern varied.

Differences within the same individual

For a given person the nature of the sexual response pattern does not remain constant, even when observed over a relatively short period. A variety of internal and external factors can alter this pattern. The aging process, changes in general health status, levels of stress, altered environmental settings, use of alcohol and other drugs, and behavioral changes in a sexual partner can cause one's own sexual response pattern to change from one sexual experience to another.[3] Sexual performance difficulties and therapies are discussed in the Star Box on p. 326.

What Are the Basic Physiological Mechanisms Underlying the Sexual Response Pattern?

The basic mechanisms in the fourth question posed by Masters and Johnson are now well recognized. One factor, *vasocongestion,* or the retention of blood or fluid within a particular tissue, is critically important in the development of physiological changes that promote the sexual response pattern.[7] The presence of erectile tissue underlies the changes that can be noted in the penis, breasts, and scrotum of the male and the clitoris, breasts, and labia minora of the female.

A second mechanism now recognized as necessary for the development of the sexual response pattern is that of *myotonia,* or the buildup of *neuromuscular tonus* within a variety of body structures.[7] At the end of the plateau stage of the response pattern, a sudden release of the accumulated neuromuscular tension gives rise to the rhythmic muscular contractions and pleasurable muscular spasms that constitute orgasm, as well as ejaculation in the male.

Sexual Response Pattern

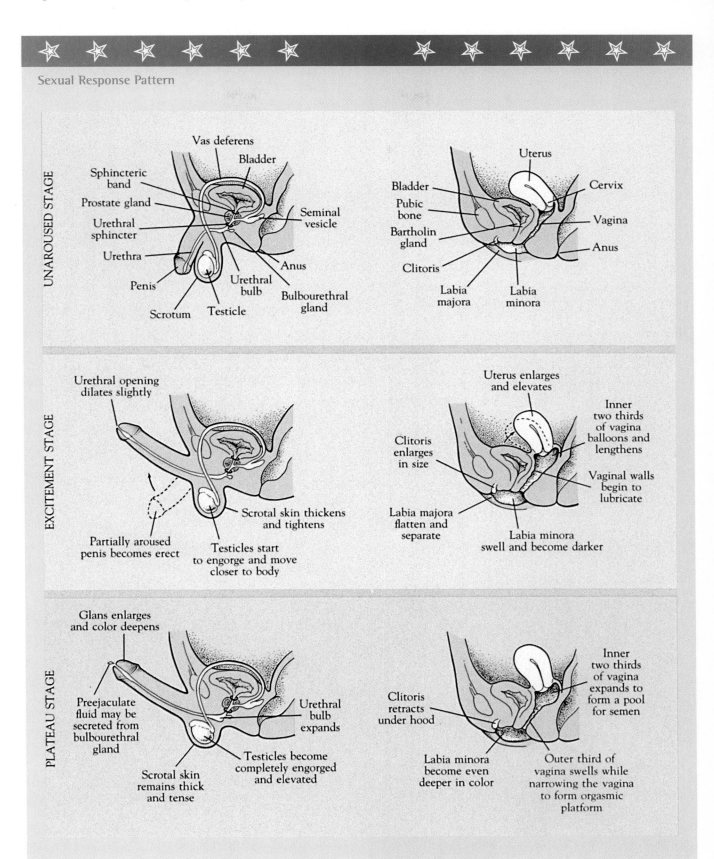

UNAROUSED STAGE

Vas deferens
Bladder
Sphincteric band
Prostate gland
Urethral sphincter
Urethra
Penis
Scrotum
Testicle
Urethral bulb
Seminal vesicle
Anus
Bulbourethral gland

Uterus
Bladder
Pubic bone
Bartholin gland
Clitoris
Labia majora
Labia minora
Cervix
Vagina
Anus

EXCITEMENT STAGE

Urethral opening dilates slightly
Partially aroused penis becomes erect
Testicles start to engorge and move closer to body
Scrotal skin thickens and tightens

Uterus enlarges and elevates
Clitoris enlarges in size
Labia majora flatten and separate
Labia minora swell and become darker
Inner two thirds of vagina balloons and lengthens
Vaginal walls begin to lubricate

PLATEAU STAGE

Glans enlarges and color deepens
Preejaculate fluid may be secreted from bulbourethral gland
Scrotal skin remains thick and tense
Testicles become completely engorged and elevated
Urethral bulb expands

Clitoris retracts under hood
Labia minora become even deeper in color
Inner two thirds of vagina expands to form a pool for semen
Outer third of vagina swells while narrowing the vagina to form orgasmic platform

Sexual Response Pattern—cont'd

ORGASMIC STAGE

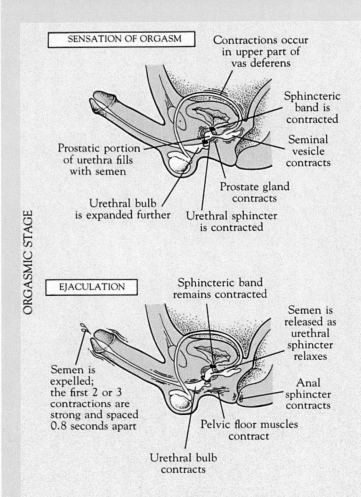

SENSATION OF ORGASM

Contractions occur in upper part of vas deferens

Sphincteric band is contracted

Seminal vesicle contracts

Prostatic portion of urethra fills with semen

Prostate gland contracts

Urethral bulb is expanded further

Urethral sphincter is contracted

EJACULATION

Sphincteric band remains contracted

Semen is released as urethral sphincter relaxes

Semen is expelled; the first 2 or 3 contractions are strong and spaced 0.8 seconds apart

Anal sphincter contracts

Pelvic floor muscles contract

Urethral bulb contracts

Uterine contractions occur

Clitoris remains under hood

Contractions occur in anal sphincter

Contractions in outer third of the vagina occur rhythmically 3 to 15 times; the first of these contractions are spread at 0.8-second intervals; latter contractions are weaker and occur more slowly

BREAST CHANGES

1 *Unaroused stage*

2 *Excitement stage*
Breast size increases; nipples become erect; veins become more visible

3 *Plateau and orgasmic stages*
Breast size increases more; areola increases in size (making nipples appear less erect); skin color may become flushed from vasocongestion

1   2   3

RESOLUTION STAGE

Rapid partial decrease in size of penis; then slow return to unaroused state and size

Scrotal skin relaxes

Testicles return to normal size and position

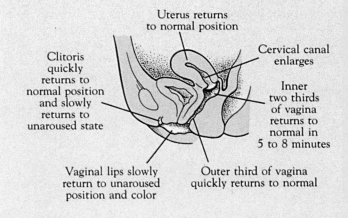

Uterus returns to normal position

Cervical canal enlarges

Clitoris quickly returns to normal position and slowly returns to unaroused state

Inner two thirds of vagina returns to normal in 5 to 8 minutes

Vaginal lips slowly return to unaroused position and color

Outer third of vagina quickly returns to normal

What Role is Played by Specific Organs and Organ Systems within the Sexual Response Pattern?

The fifth question posed by Masters and Johnson, which concerns the role played by specific organs and organ systems during each stage of the response pattern, can be readily answered by referring to the material presented in the preceding Star Box. As you study this box, remember that direct stimulation of the penis and either direct or indirect stimulation of the clitoris are the principal avenues toward orgasm. Also, intercourse represents only one activity that can lead to orgasmic pleasure.[4]

PATTERNS OF SEXUAL BEHAVIOR

Although sex researchers may see sexual behavior in terms of the human sexual response pattern just described, most people are more interested in the observable dimensions of sexual behavior. Complete the Personal Assessment on p. 327 to determine whether your own attitudes toward sexuality are traditional or nontraditional.

Celibacy

Celibacy can be defined as the self-imposed avoidance of sexual intimacy. Celibacy is synonymous with sexual abstinence. There are many reasons people could choose not to have a sexually intimate relationship. For some, celibacy is part of a religious doctrine. Others might be afraid of sexually transmitted diseases. For most, however, celibacy is preferred simply because it seems appropriate for them. Celibate people can certainly have deep, intimate relationships with other people—just not sexual relationships. Celibacy may be short-term or last a lifetime, and no identified physical or psychological complications appear to result from a celibate lifestyle.

Masturbation

Throughout recorded history, **masturbation** has been a primary method of achieving sexual pleasure. Through masturbation, people can explore their sexual response patterns. Traditionally, some societies and religious groups have condemned this behavior based on the belief that intercourse is the only "right" sexual behavior. With sufficient lubrication, masturbation cannot do physical harm. Today masturbation is considered by most sex therapists and researchers to be a normal source of self-pleasure.

Fantasy and Erotic Dreams

The brain is the most sensual organ in the body. In fact, many sexuality experts classify **sexual fantasies** and **erotic dreams** as forms of sexual behavior. Particularly for people whose verbal ability is highly developed, the ability to create imaginary scenes enriches other forms of sexual behavior.

excitement stage
Initial arousal stage of the sexual response pattern.

plateau stage
Second stage of the sexual response pattern; a leveling off of arousal immediately before orgasm.

orgasmic stage
Third stage of the sexual response pattern; the stage during which neuromuscular tension is released.

resolution stage
Fourth stage of the sexual response pattern; the return of the body to a preexcitement state.

refractory phase
That portion of the male's resolution stage during which sexual arousal cannot occur.

multiorgasmic capacity
Potential to have several orgasms within a single period of sexual arousal.

coitus (co ih tus)
Penile-vaginal intercourse.

erection
The engorgement of erectile tissue with blood; characteristic of the penis, clitoris, nipples, labia minora, and scrotum.

sex flush
The reddish skin response that results from increasing sexual arousal.

masturbation
Self-stimulation of the genitals.

sexual fantasies
Fantasies with sexual themes; sexual daydreams or imaginary events.

erotic dreams
Dreams whose content elicits a sexual response.

Sexual Performance Difficulties and Therapies

For all of the predictability of the human sexual response pattern, many people find that at some point in their lives, they are no longer capable of responding sexually. The inability of a person to perform adequately is identified as a sexual difficulty or dysfunction. Sexual difficul-ties can have a negative influence on a person's sense of sexual satisfaction and on a partner's satisfaction. Fortunately, most sexual difficulties can be resolved through strategies that use individual, couple, or group counseling. Most sexual performance difficulties stem from psychogenic factors.

Difficulty	Possible Causes	Therapeutic Approaches
Women		
Orgasmic Difficulties Inability to have orgasm	Anxiety, fear, guilt, anger, poor self-concept; lack of knowledge about female responsive-ness; inadequate sexual arousal; interper-sonal problems with partner	Counseling to improve a couple's communica-tion; educating a woman and her partner about female responsiveness; teaching a woman how to experience orgasm through masturbation
Vaginismus Painful, involun-tary contractions of the vaginal muscles	Previous traumatic experiences with inter-course (rape, incest, uncaring partners); fear of pregnancy; religious prohibitions; anxiety about vaginal penetration of any kind (including tampons)	Counseling to alleviate psychogenic causes; gradual dilation of the vagina with woman's fingers or dilators; systematic desensitiza-tion exercises; relaxation training
Dyspareunia Painful intercourse	Insufficient sexual arousal; communication problems with partner; infections, inflam-mations; structural abnormalities; insuffi-cient lubrication	Individual and couple counseling with a focus on relaxation and communication; medical strategies to reduce infections and structural abnormalities
Men		
Erectile Dysfunction Inability to achieve an erection (impotence)	Chronic diseases (including diabetes, vascular problems, and chemical dependencies); trauma; numerous psychogenic factors (including anxiety, guilt, fear, poor self-concept)	Medical intervention (including possible vas-cular surgery or the use of penile implants); couple counseling using sensate focusing, pleasuring, and relaxation strategies
Rapid Ejaculation Ejaculating too quickly after penile penetra-tion; premature ejaculation	Predominately psychogenic in origin; a man's need to prove his sexual prowess; anxiety associated with previous sexual experiences	Counseling to free the man from the anxiety associated with rapid ejaculation; altering coital position, masturbation before inti-macy; use of the squeeze technique as orgasm approaches
Dyspareunia Painful intercourse	Primarily physical in origin; inability of the penile foreskin to retract fully; urogenital tract infections; scar tissue in seminal pas-sageways; insufficient lubrication	Medical care to reduce infection or repair dam-aged or abnormal tissue; additional lubrica-tion

PERSONAL ASSESSMENT

Sexual Attitudes: A Matter of Feelings

Respond to each of the following statements by selecting a numbered response (1-5) that most accurately reflects your feelings. Circle the number of your selection. At the end of the questionnaire, total these numbers for use in interpreting your responses.

1   Agree strongly
2   Agree moderately
3   Uncertain
4   Disagree moderately
5   Disagree strongly

Men and women have greater differences than they have similarities.	1	2	3	4	5
Homosexuality and bisexuality are immoral and unnatural.	1	2	3	4	5
Our society is too sexually oriented.	1	2	3	4	5
Pornography encourages sexual promiscuity.	1	2	3	4	5
Children know far too much about sex.	1	2	3	4	5
Education about sexuality is solely the responsibility of the family.	1	2	3	4	5
Dating begins far too early in our society.	1	2	3	4	5
Sexual intimacy before marriage leads to emotional stress and damage to one's reputation.	1	2	3	4	5
Sexual availability is far too frequently the reason that people marry.	1	2	3	4	5
Reproduction is the most important reason for sexual intimacy during marriage.	1	2	3	4	5
Modern families are too small.	1	2	3	4	5
Family planning clinics should not receive public funds.	1	2	3	4	5
Contraception is the woman's responsibility.	1	2	3	4	5
Abortion is the murder of an innocent child.	1	2	3	4	5
Marriage has been weakened by the changing role of women in society.	1	2	3	4	5
Divorce is an unacceptable means of resolving marital difficulties.	1	2	3	4	5
Extramarital sexual intimacy will destroy a marriage.	1	2	3	4	5
Sexual abuse of a child does not generally occur unless the child encourages the adult.	1	2	3	4	5
Provocative behavior by the woman is a factor in almost every case of rape.	1	2	3	4	5
Reproduction is not a right but a privilege.	1	2	3	4	5

YOUR TOTAL POINTS _____

Interpretation
20-34 points	A very traditional attitude toward sexuality
35-54 points	A moderately traditional attitude toward sexuality
55-65 points	A rather ambivalent attitude toward sexuality
66-85 points	A moderately nontraditional attitude toward sexuality
86-100 points	A very nontraditional attitude toward sexuality

To Carry This Further . . .
Were you surprised at your results? Compare your results with those of a roommate or close friend. How do you think your parents would score on this assessment?

Sexual fantasies are generally found in association with some second type of sexual behavior. When occurring before intercourse or masturbation, fantasies prepare a person for the behavior that will follow. As an example, fantasies experienced while reading a book may focus your attention on sexual activity that will occur later in the day.

When fantasies occur in conjunction with another form of sexual behavior, the second behavior may be greatly enhanced by the supportive fantasy. Both women and men fantasize during foreplay and intercourse. Masturbation and fantasizing are inseparable activities.

Erotic dreams occur during sleep in both men and women. The association between these dreams and ejaculation resulting in a nocturnal emission (wet dream) is readily recognized in males. In females, erotic dreams can lead not only to vaginal lubrication but to orgasm as well.

Shared Touching

Virtually the entire body can be an erogenous zone when sensual contact between partners is involved. A soft, light touch, a slight application of pressure, the brushing back of a partner's hair, and gentle massage are all forms of communication that heighten sexual arousal.

Genital Contact

Two important uses can be identified for the practice of stimulating a partner's genitals. The first is that of being the tactile component of **foreplay.** Genital contact, in the form of holding, rubbing, stroking, or caressing, heightens arousal to a level that allows for progression into intercourse.

The second role of genital contact is that of *mutual masturbation to orgasm*. Stimulation of the genitals so that both partners have orgasm is a form of sexual behavior practiced by many people, as well as couples during the late stage of a pregnancy. For couples not desiring pregnancy, the risk of conception is virtually eliminated when this becomes the form of sexual intimacy practiced.

As is the case of other aspects of intimacy, genital stimulation is best enhanced when partners can talk about their needs, expectations, and reservations. Practice and communication can shape this form of contact into a pleasure-giving approach to sexual intimacy.

Oral-Genital Stimulation

Oral-genital stimulation brings together two of the body's most erogenous areas: the genitalia and the mouth. Couples who engage in oral sex consistently report that this form of intimacy is highly satisfactory. Some people have experimented with oral sex and found it unacceptable, and some have never experienced this form of sexual intimacy. Some couples prefer not to participate in oral sex because they consider it immoral (according to religious doctrine), illegal (which it is in some states), or unhygienic (because of a partner's unclean genitals). Some couples may refrain because of the mistaken belief that oral sex is a homosexual practice. Regardless of the reason, a person who does not consider oral sex to be pleasurable should not be coerced into this behavior.

Because oral-genital stimulation can involve an exchange of body fluids, the risk of disease transmission is real. Small tears of mouth or genital tissue may allow transmission of disease-causing pathogens. Only couples who are absolutely certain that they are free from all sexually transmitted diseases (including HIV infection) can practice unprotected oral sex. Couples in doubt should refrain from oral-genital sex or carefully use a condom (on the male) or a latex square to cover the female's vulval area. Increasingly, latex squares (dental dams) can be obtained from drug stores or pharmacies. (Dentists may also provide you with dental dams, or you can make your own latex square by cutting a condom into an appropriate shape.)

Three basic forms of oral-genital stimulation are practiced by both heterosexual and homosexual couples.[8] **Fellatio,** in which the penis is sucked, licked, or kissed by the partner, is the most common of the three. **Cunnilingus,** in which the vulva of the female is kissed, licked, or penetrated by the partner's tongue, is only slightly less frequently practiced.

Mutual oral-genital stimulation, the third form of oral-genital stimulation, combines both fellatio and cunnilingus. When practiced by a heterosexual couple, the female partner performs fellatio on her partner while her male partner performs cunnilingus on her. Homosexual couples can practice mutual fellatio or cunnilingus.

Intercourse

Sexual intercourse (coitus) refers to the act of inserting the penis into the vagina. Intercourse is the sexual behavior that is most directly associated with **procreation.** For some, intercourse is the only natural and appropriate form of sexual intimacy.

The incidence and frequency of sexual intercourse is a much-studied topic. Information concerning the percentages of people who have engaged in intercourse is readily available in textbooks used in sexuality courses. Data concerning sexual intercourse among college students may be changing somewhat because of concerns about HIV infection and other STDs, but a reasonable estimate of the percentage of college students reporting sexual intercourse is between 65% and 80%.

These percentages reflect two important concepts about the sexual activity of college students. The first is that a large majority of college students is having intercourse. The second concept is that a sizeable percentage (20% to 35%) of students is choosing to refrain from intercourse. Indeed, the belief that "everyone is doing it" may be a bit shortsighted. From a public health standpoint, we believe it is important to provide accurate health information to protect those who choose to have intercourse and to actively support a person's right to choose not to have intercourse.

Couples need to share their expectations concerning techniques and the desired frequency of intercourse. Even the "performance" factors, such as depth of penetration, nature of body movements, tempo of activity, and timing of orgasm are of increasing importance to many couples. Issues concerning sexually transmitted diseases (including HIV infection) are also critically important for couples who are contemplating intercourse. These factors also need to be explored through open communication.

There are a variety of books (including textbooks) that provide written and visually explicit information on intercourse positions. Four basic positions for intercourse—*male above, female above, side by side,* and *rear entry*—each offer relative advantages and disadvantages.

SEXUALITY AND AGING

Students are often curious about how aging affects sexuality. This is understandable because we live in a society that idolizes youth and demands performance. Many younger people become anxious about growing older because of what they think will happen to their ability to express their sexuality. Interestingly, young adults are willing to accept other physical changes of aging (such as the slowing down of basal metabolism, reduced lung capacity, and even wrinkles) but not those changes related to sexuality.

Most of the research in this area suggests that older people are quite capable of performing sexually. As with other aspects of aging, certain anatomical and physiological changes will be evident, but these changes do not necessarily reduce the ability to enjoy sexual activity.[3] Most experts in sexuality report that many older people remain interested in sexual activity. Furthermore, those who are exposed to regular sexual activity throughout a lifetime report being most satisfied with their sex lives as older adults.

As people age, the likelihood of alterations in the male and female sexual response cycles increases. In the postmenopausal woman, vaginal lubrication commonly begins more slowly, and the amount of lubrication usually diminishes. However, clitoral sensitivity and nipple erection remain the same as in earlier years. The female capacity for multiple orgasms remains the same, although the number of contractions that occur at orgasm typically is reduced.

In the older man, physical changes are also evident. This is thought to be caused by the decrease in the production of testosterone between the ages of 20 and 60 years. After age 60 or so, testosterone levels remain relatively steady. Thus many men, despite a decrease in sperm production, remain fertile into their eighties. Older men typically take longer to achieve an erection (however, they are able to maintain their erection longer before ejaculation), have fewer muscular contractions at orgasm, and ejaculate less forcefully than they once did. The volume of seminal fluid ejaculated is typically less than in earlier years, and its consistency is somewhat thinner. The resolution phase is usually longer in older men. In spite of these gradual changes, some elderly men engage in sexual intercourse with the same frequency as do much younger men.

THE DATING PROCESS

A half-century ago, the events involved in a dating relationship were somewhat predictable. People met each other through their daily activities or groups of friends, and a formal "date request" was made. Ninety-nine times out of a hundred, the requestor was male and the invitee was female. After a period of formal and informal dates, a commitment to steady dating was made or the couple decided to "date around." If the relationship progressed, further commitments were made (for example, class rings, letter

foreplay
Activities, often involving touching and caressing, that prepare individuals for sexual intercourse.

fellatio (feh **lay** she oh)
Oral stimulation of the penis.

cunnilingus (cun uh **ling** gus)
Oral stimulation of the vulva or clitoris.

procreation
Reproduction.

jackets, or other jewelry items were exchanged). After months or years of a committed relationship, the couple decided to get married. The man invariably "asked for the woman's hand" (after first receiving permission from her parents), and plans for a wedding ceremony were made.

Does this form of dating and mate selection exist as we approach the year 2000? For some couples, yes. The traditional way of dating and selecting a marriage partner works well for them. However, many young and midlife adults prefer a more flexible, less predictable format for dating and finding a person they might choose to marry. For example, more than ever, women are playing a more assertive role when it comes to initiating and establishing the ground rules for a relationship. Interestingly, a large number of our students do not even like to use the word "dating" because of its connotation to a formalized pattern of behavior used by their parents and grandparents.

What do you think? Have you recognized this more flexible dating format? Has this less traditional pattern been beneficial to couples as they make critical decisions that will influence the rest of their lives?

LOVE

Love may be one of the most elusive yet widely recognized concepts that describe some level of emotional attachment to another. Haas and Haas[3] describe five forms of love, including erotic, friendship, devotional, parental, and altruistic love. Other behavioral scientists[4] have focused primarily on two types of love most closely associated with dating and mate selection: *passionate love* and *companionate love*.

Passionate love, also described as romantic love or **infatuation,** is a "state of extreme absorption in another. It is characterized by intense feelings of tenderness, elation, anxiety, sexual desire, and ecstasy."[4] Often appearing early in a relationship, passionate love typically does not last very long. Passionate love is driven by the excitement of being closely involved with a person whose character is not fully known.

If a relationship progresses, passionate love is gradually replaced by companionate love. This type of love is "a less intense emotion than passionate love. It is characterized by friendly affection and a deep attachment that is based on extensive familiarity with the loved one."[4] This love is enduring and capable of sustaining long-term, mutual growth. Central to companionate love are feelings of empathy for, support of, and tolerance of the partner. Complete the Personal Assessment on p. 331 to determine whether you and your partner are truly compatible.

Companionate love is capable of sustaining long-term mutual growth.

FRIENDSHIP

One of the exciting aspects of college life is that you will probably meet many new people. Some of these people will become your best friends. Because of your common experiences, it is likely that you will keep in contact with a few of these friends for a lifetime. Close attachments to other people can have an important influence on all of the dimensions of your health.

What is it that draws friends together? With the exception of physical intimacy, many of the same growth experiences seen in dating and mate selection are also seen in the development of friendships. Think about how you and your best friend developed the relationship you now have. You probably became friends when you shared similar interests and experiences. Your friendship progressed (and even faltered at times) through personal gains or losses. In all likeli-

PERSONAL ASSESSMENT

How Compatible Are You?

This quiz will help test how compatible you and your partner's personalities are. You should each rate the truth of these 20 statements based on the following scale. Circle the number that reflects your feelings. Total your scores and check the interpretation following the quiz.

1   Never true
2   Sometimes true
3   Frequently true
4   Always true

Statement	1	2	3	4
We can communicate our innermost thoughts effectively.	1	2	3	4
We trust each other.	1	2	3	4
We agree on whose needs come first.	1	2	3	4
We have realistic expectations of each other and of ourselves.	1	2	3	4
Individual growth is important within our relationship.	1	2	3	4
We will go on as a couple even if our partner doesn't change.	1	2	3	4
Our personal problems are discussed with each other first.	1	2	3	4
We both do our best to compromise.	1	2	3	4
We usually fight fairly.	1	2	3	4
We try not to be rigid or unyielding.	1	2	3	4
We keep any needs to be "perfect" in proper perspective.	1	2	3	4
We can balance desires to be sociable and the need to be alone.	1	2	3	4
We both make friends and keep them.	1	2	3	4
Neither of us stays down or up for long periods.	1	2	3	4
We can tolerate the other's mood without being affected by it.	1	2	3	4
We can deal with disappointment and disillusionment.	1	2	3	4
Both of us can tolerate failure.	1	2	3	4
We can both express anger appropriately.	1	2	3	4
We are both assertive when necessary.	1	2	3	4
We agree on how our personal surroundings are kept.	1	2	3	4

YOUR TOTAL POINTS _____

Interpretation

20-35 points   You and your partner seem quite incompatible. Professional help may open your lines of communication.

36-55 points   You probably need more awareness and compromise.

56-70 points   You are highly compatible. However, be aware of the areas where you can improve.

71-80 points   Your relationship is very fulfilling.

To Carry This Further . . .

Ask your partner to take this test too. You may have a one-sided view of a "perfect" relationship. Even if you scored high on this assessment, be aware of areas where you can still improve. ☑

hood, you cared about each other and learned to share your deepest beliefs and feelings. Lastly, you cemented your friendship by transferring your beliefs into behavior.

Throughout development of a deep friendship, the qualities of trust, tolerance, empathy, and support must be demonstrated. Otherwise the friendship can fall apart. You may have noticed that the qualities seen in a friendship are very similar to the qualities noted in the description of companionate love. In both cases, people develop deep attachments through extensive familiarity and understanding.

infatuation
An often shallow, intense attraction to another person.

INTIMACY

When most people hear the word **intimacy,** they immediately think about physical intimacy. They think about shared touching, kissing, and even intercourse. However, sexuality experts and family therapists prefer to view intimacy more broadly, as any close, mutual, verbal or nonverbal behavior within a relationship. In this sense, intimate behavior can range from sharing deep feelings and experiences with a partner to sharing profound physical pleasures with a partner.

Intimacy is present in both love and friendship. You have likely shared intimate feelings with your closest friends, as well as with those you love. Intimacy helps us feel connected to others and allows us to feel the full measure of our own self-worth.

MARRIAGE

Just as there is no single best way for two people to move through dating and mate selection, marriage is an equally variable undertaking. In marriage, two people join their lives in a way that affirms each as an individual and both as a legal pair. They are able to resolve conflict constructively (see the Health Action Guide at right). However, for a large percentage of couples, the demands of marriage are too rigorous, confining, and demanding. They will find resolution for their dissatisfaction through divorce or extramarital affairs. For most, though, marriage will be an experience that alternates periods of happiness, productivity, and admiration with periods of frustration, unhappiness, and disillusionment with the partner.

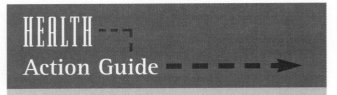

HEALTH Action Guide

Resolving Conflict

Here are some successful ways to manage conflict:

- Show mutual respect.
- Identify and resolve the real issue.
- Seek areas of agreement.
- Mutually participate in decision-making.
- Be cooperative and specific.
- Focus on the present and future—not the past.
- Don't try to assign blame.
- Say what you are thinking and feeling.
- When talking, use sentences that begin with "I."
- Avoid using sentences that start with "You" or "Why."
- Set a time limit for discussing problems.
- Accept responsibility.
- Schedule time together.

Each of you who marries will find the experience unique in every regard. The Star Box below presents some advice for improving marriage.

As we move through the mid-1990s, certain trends regarding marriage are evident. The most obvious of these is the age at first marriage. Today men are waiting longer than ever to marry. Now the average age at first marriage for men is 26 years.[9] In addition, these new

Improving Marriage

Few marital relationships are "perfect." All marriages are faced with occasional periods of strain or turmoil. Even marriages that do not exhibit major signs of distress can be improved, mostly through better communication. Marriage experts suggest that implementing some of these patterns can strengthen marriages:

- Problems that exist within the marriage should be brought into the open so that both partners are aware of the difficulties.
- Balance should exist between the needs and expectations of each partner. Decisions should be made jointly. Partners should support each other as best as they can. When a partner's goals cannot be actively supported, he or she should at least receive moral support and encouragement.

- Realistic expectations should be established. Partners should negotiate areas in which disagreement exists. They should work together to determine the manner in which resources should be shared.
- Participating in marriage counseling and marriage encounter groups can be helpful.

Beyond the patterns listed above, a sense of permanence helps sustain a marriage over the course of time. If the partners are convinced that their relationship can withstand difficult times, then they are more likely to take the time to make needed changes. Couples can develop a sense of permanence by implementing some of the patterns described above.

LEARNING *from* ALL CULTURES

Marriage Customs

The institution of marriage is found in many societies, although the rules, practices, and laws can be very different. In the United States and other Western nations, marriage is a reflection of the Judeo-Christian heritage. Monogamy is practiced, fidelity is emphasized, and the permanence of marriage is stressed.[13]

In primitive societies, marriage practices greatly vary. Some accepted forms are arranged marriages, bride abductions, and bride payments. Polygyny (having two or more wives) is common, although monogamy is also practiced, especially when economic conditions make it difficult for a man to have more than one wife.[13]

In nations in which the Islamic faith is practiced, polygyny is accepted. In countries such as India and China, parents choose marriage partners for their children or the unions are arranged. The practice of choosing one's own mate, however, is becoming more acceptable in those countries.[13]

In view of the high divorce rate in the United States, are arranged marriages any less successful than our own practices? How can men and women make wise choices in deciding on a marriage partner?

husbands are better educated than in the past and are more likely to be established in their careers. Women are also waiting longer to get married and tend to be more educated and career oriented. Recent statistics indicate that the average age at first marriage is 24 years.[9]

Marriage still appeals to most adults. Currently, 77% of adults age 18 and older are either married, widowed, or divorced.[9] Thus only about one fifth of today's adults have not married. Within the last decade, the percentage of adults who have decided not to marry has nearly doubled. Singlehood and other alternatives to marriage are discussed later in this chapter. See the Learning from All Cultures box above for a discussion of marriage customs in other cultures.

DIVORCE

Marriages, like many other kinds of interpersonal relationships, can end. Today, marriages—relation-

ships begun with the intent of permanence "until death do us part"—end through divorce nearly as frequently as not ending.

Why should approximately half of marital relationships be so likely to end? Unfortunately, marriage experts cannot provide one clear answer to this question. Rather, they suggest that divorce is a reflection of unfulfilled expectations for marriage on the part of one or both partners, including the following:

- The belief that marriage will ease your need to deal with your own faults and that your failures can be shared by your partner

intimacy
Any close, mutual, verbal or nonverbal behavior within a relationship.

- The belief that marriage will change faults that you know exist in your partner
- The belief that the high level of romance of your dating and courtship period will be continued through marriage
- The belief that marriage can provide you with an arena for the development of your personal power, and that once married, you will not need to compromise with your partner
- The belief that your marital partner will be successful in meeting all of your needs

If these expectations seem to be ones you anticipate through marriage, then you may find that disappointments will abound. To varying degrees, marriage is a partnership that requires much cooperation and compromise. Marriage can be complicated. Because of the high expectations that many people hold for marriage, the termination of marriage can be an emotionally difficult process to undertake (see the Health Action Guide below).

Concern is frequently voiced over the well-being of children whose parents divorce. Different factors, however, influence the extent to which divorce affects children. Included among these factors are the gender and age of the children, custody arrangements, financial support, and the remarriage of one or both parents. For many children, adjustments must be made to accept their new status as a member of a blended family.

ALTERNATIVES TO MARRIAGE

Although the great majority of you have experienced or will experience marriage, alternatives to marriage certainly exist. This section briefly explores singlehood, cohabitation, and single parenthood.

Singlehood

An alternative to marriage for adults is *singlehood.* For many people, being single is a lifestyle that affords the potential for pursuing intimacy, if desired, and provides an uncluttered path for independence and self-directedness. Other people, however, are single because of divorce, separation, death, or the absence of an opportunity to establish a partnership. The U.S. Bureau of the Census indicates that 41% of women and 37% of men over the age of 18 are currently single.[9] If you are single, complete the Personal Assessment on p. 335 to find out whether you are enjoying the single life to the fullest.

Many different living arrangements are seen among singles. Some single people live alone and choose not to share a household. Other arrangements for singles include cohabitation, periodic cohabitation, singlehood during the week and cohabitation on the weekends or during vacations, or the *platonic* sharing of a household with others. For young adults, large

HEALTH
Action Guide

Coping With a Breakup

The end of a marriage or other long-term relationship is always a wrenching and painful experience. The following tips suggest both alternatives to breakup and ways to cope with it.

- *Talk first.* Try to deal effectively and directly with the conflicts. The old theory said that it was good for a couple to fight. However, anger can cause more anger and even lead to violence. Freely venting anger is as likely to damage a relationship as to improve it. Therefore cool off first, then discuss issues fully and freely.
- *Trial separation.* Sometimes only a few weeks apart can convince a couple that it is far better to work together than to go it totally alone. It is generally better to establish the rules of such a trial quite firmly. Will the individuals see others? What are the responsibilities if children are involved? There should also

be a time limit, perhaps a month or two, after which the partners reunite and discuss their situation again.
- *Obtain help.* The services of a *qualified* counselor, psychologist, or psychiatrist may help a couple resolve their problems. Notice the emphasis on the word *qualified.* Some people who have little training or competence represent themselves as counselors. For this reason a couple should insist on verifying the counselor's training and licensing.
- *Allow time for grief and healing.* When a relationship ends, people are often tempted to immediately become as socially and sexually active as possible. This can be a way to express anger and relieve pain. But it can also cause frustration and despair. A better solution for many is to acknowledge the grief the breakup has caused and allow time for healing. Up to a year of continuing one's life and solidifying friendships typically helps the rejected partner establish a new equilibrium.

PERSONAL ASSESSMENT

Are You Enjoying the Single Life?

Is your life on hold just because you are single? Are you living in limbo instead of making a real home for yourself?

To see if you're taking good care of yourself as a single "nester," try this quiz from Janice Harayda, adapted from her book, *The Joy of Being Single.* Total your yes responses, and check the interpretation after the quiz.

	Yes	No
Do you sleep on a real bed rather than a convertible sofa or a mattress on the floor?	___	___
Would you feel comfortable buying such items as monogrammed towels or antiques if you liked them and could afford them?	___	___
Do you have at least one specialty that you can cook with pride for friends?	___	___
Do you already own a condo, co-op, or house? If not, are you saving up for one?	___	___
Do you have family pictures displayed in your home?	___	___
Do you participate in at least one community or neighborhood group, such as a block association, a tennis committee, or the Jaycees?	___	___
Could you invite your boss to your home without feeling embarrassed?	___	___
Do you put up decorations on important holidays?	___	___
Do you occasionally give sit-down dinner parties instead of having the gang over for pizza and beer?	___	___
Do you look forward to coming home from work each night?	___	___

YOUR TOTAL POINTS _____

Interpretation

1-2   Your place probably feels more like a sensory deprivation chamber than a real home.

3-7   You are well on the way to creating a real home and a real life for yourself.

7+   Congratulations. You have a strong sense of who you are and aren't afraid to let your home show it.

To Carry This Further . . .

How does your residence compare with those of your other single friends? Can you learn anything from their arrangements?

---

percentages of single men and women live with their parents (see Table 13-1).

Like habitation arrangements, the sexual intimacy patterns of singles are individually tailored. Some singles practice celibacy, others pursue heterosexual or homosexual intimate relationships in a **monogamous** pattern, and others may have multiple partners. As in all interpersonal relationships, including marriage, the levels of commitment are as variable as the people involved.

Cohabitation

Cohabitation, or the sharing of living quarters by unmarried people, represents yet another alternative to marriage. According to the U.S. Bureau of the Census, the number of unmarried, opposite-gender

Table 13-1 Percentage of Young Adults Living with Their Parents: 1970 and 1994[9]*				
	Age 18–24		Age 25–34	
	1970	1994	1970	1994
Male	54	60	10	16
Female	41	46	7	9
TOTAL	47	53	8	12

*Includes unmarried college students living in dormitories.

monogamous (mo **nog** a mus)
Paired relationship with one partner.

cohabitation
Sharing of a residence by two unrelated, unmarried people; living together.

couples living together doubled between 1980 and 1994, from 1.5 million couples to over 3.5 million couples.[9]

Although cohabitation may seem to imply a vision of sexual intimacy between male and female roommates, several forms of shared living arrangements can be viewed as cohabitation. For some couples, cohabitation is only a part-time arrangement for weekends, during summer vacation, or on a variable schedule. In addition, **platonic** cohabitation can exist when a couple shares living quarters but does so without establishing an intimate relationship. Close friends, people of retirement age, and homosexuals might all be included in a group called *cohabitants*.

The archetype of a cohabitation arrangement is the couple who has drifted into cohabitation as the result of a dating relationship in which sexual intimacy and occasional "overnighting" have already occurred. In the living arrangement that follows, both material possessions and emotional support are generally shared. A contractual relationship is only occasionally established. Monogamy will usually exist. Approximately half of cohabitation relationships will disband, and the people involved will depart with the feeling that they would cohabit again if it appears desirable. Finally, cohabitation is neither more nor less likely to lead to marriage than is a more traditional dating relationship. It is, in fact, only an alternative to marriage.

Single Parenthood

Unmarried young women becoming pregnant and then becoming single parents is a continuing reality in this country. A new and significantly different form of single parenthood is, however, also a reality in this country: the planned entry into a single parenthood by older, better educated people, the vast majority of whom are women.

In contrast to the teenaged girl who becomes a single parent through an unwed pregnancy, the more mature woman who desires single parenting has usually planned carefully for the experience. She has explored several important concerns, including questions regarding how she will become pregnant (with or without the knowledge of a male partner or through artificial insemination), the need for a father figure for the child, the effect of single parenting on her social life, and, of course, its effect on her career development. Once these questions have been resolved, no legal barriers stand in the way of her becoming a single parent.

A very large number of women and a growing number of men are actively participating in single parenthood in conjunction with a divorce settlement or separation agreement involving sole or joint custody of children. In 1994, single women headed up 7.6 million households with children under age 18. In contrast, single men headed up 1.3 million households in 1994 with children under age 18.[9]

A few single parents have been awarded children through adoption. The likelihood of a single person's receiving a child is small, but more people have been successful recently in single-parent adoptions.

SEXUAL ORIENTATION

Sexual orientation refers to the direction in which people focus their sexual interests. People can focus their attention on opposite-gender partners, same-gender partners, or partners of both genders.

Heterosexuality

Heterosexuality (or heterosexual orientation) refers to an attraction to opposite-gender partners. (*Heteros* is a Greek word that means "the other.") Throughout the world, this is the most common sexual orientation. For reasons related to species survival, heterosexuality has its most basic roots in the biological dimension of human sexuality. Beyond its biological roots, heterosexuality has significant cultural and religious support in virtually every country in the world. Most societies expect men to be attracted to women and women to be attracted to men. Worldwide, laws related to marriage, living arrangements, health benefits, child rearing, financial matters, sexual behavior, and inheritance generally support relationships that are heterosexual in nature.

Homosexuality

Homosexuality (or homosexual orientation) refers to an attraction to same-gender partners. The term *homosexuality* comes from the Greek word *homos*, meaning "same." The word *homosexuality* may be used with regard to males or females. Thus we use the terms *homosexual males* and *homosexual females*. Frequently the word *gay* is used to refer to homosexual orientation in both males and females. *Lesbianism* is also used to refer to the sexual attraction between females.

The distinctions among the three categories of sexual orientation are much less clear than their definitions might suggest. Most people probably fall somewhere along a continuum between exclusive heterosexuality and exclusive homosexuality. Kinsey in 1948 presented just such a continuum.[10]

Why does a given individual have a homosexual orientation? There is no simple answer to this question. (College human sexuality textbooks devote entire chapters to this topic.) In the mid-1990s, some research pointed to differences in the sizes of certain brain structures as a possible biological basis for homosexuality.[11] However, for sexual orientation in general, no one theory has emerged that fully explains this developmental process. Regardless of the cause, however, reversal to heterosexuality generally does not occur. Furthermore, most homosexuals report that no one event "triggered" their homosexuality. Many homosexuals also indicate that they knew their orientations were "different" from other children as far back as their prepuberty years.

The extent of homosexuality in our society is a debatable issue. Clearly, gathering valid information of this kind is difficult. The extent of homosexual orientation is probably much greater than many heterosexuals realize. Furthermore, many people refuse to reveal their homosexuality and thus prefer to remain "in the closet."

Although operational definitions of homosexuality may vary from researcher to researcher, Kinsey estimated that about 2% of American females and 4% of American males were exclusively homosexual.[10,12] More recent estimates place the overall combined figure of homosexuals at about 10% of the population.[4] Clearly the expression of same-gender attraction is not uncommon.

Bisexuality

People whose preference for sexual partners includes both genders are referred to as *bisexuals.* Bisexuals may fall into one of three groups: those who are (1) genuinely attracted to both genders, (2) homosexual but also feel the need to behave heterosexually, or (3) aroused physically by the same gender but attracted emotionally to the opposite gender. Some people participate in a bisexual lifestyle for extended periods, whereas others move quickly to a more exclusive orientation. Little research has been conducted on bisexuality, and thus the size of the bisexual population is not accurately known.

A particularly pressing reason for learning more about the bisexual lifestyle is its relationship to the transmission of HIV infection. Next to intravenous drug users, bisexuals hold the greatest potential for extending HIV infection into the heterosexual population. Since the prevalence of bisexuality is unknown, the consistent use of safer sex practices becomes more important than ever.

PARAPHILIAS

A **paraphilia** is a "preference for unusual sexual practices."[3] A paraphilia involves special erotic activities, some of which have the potential to harm nonconsenting individuals. In the interest of brevity the following lists a variety of paraphilias:

- Zoophilia: sexual excitement through contact with animals; also called *bestiality*
- Pedophilia: sexual contact with children
- Incest: marriage or sexual contact with a close relative
- Fetishism: an obsession with a body part or inanimate object as the primary focus of sexual excitement
- Transvestism: sexual excitement gained from cross-dressing, or wearing the clothes of another gender
- Exhibitionism: displaying one's genitals to an involuntary observer
- Voyeurism: observing unsuspecting people removing their clothes or engaging in sexual activity
- Masochism: obtaining sexual excitement from receiving pain
- Sadism: obtaining sexual excitement from causing pain to another person
- Sadomasochism: obtaining sexual excitement by both causing and receiving pain

platonic (pluh ton ick)
Close association between two people that does not include a sexual relationship.

paraphilia
A preference for unusual sexual practices.

Summary

- Biological and psychosocial factors contribute to the complex expression of our sexuality.
- The structural basis of sexuality begins as the male and female reproductive structures develop in the growing embryo and fetus. Structural sexuality changes as one moves through adolescence and later life.
- The psychosocial processes of gender identity, gender preference, and gender adoption form the basis for an initial adult gender identification.

- The male and female reproductive structures are external and internal. The complex functioning of these structures is controlled by hormones.
- The menstrual cycle's primary functions are to produce ova and to develop a supportive environment for the fetus in the uterus.
- The sexual response pattern consists of four stages: excitement, plateau, orgasm, and resolution.
- Many older people remain interested and active in sexual activities. Physiological changes may alter the way in which some older people perform sexually.
- Although most individuals marry at some time in their lives, alternatives to marriage exist, including singlehood, cohabitation, and single parenthood.
- Three sexual orientations are heterosexuality, homosexuality, and bisexuality.

Review Questions

1. Describe the following foundations of our biological sexuality: the genetic basis, the gonadal basis, and structural development.
2. Define and explain the following terms: gender identity, gender preference, gender adoption, initial adult gender identification, and transsexualism.
3. Identify the major components of the male and female reproductive systems. Trace the passageways for sperm and ova.
4. Explain the menstrual cycle. Identify and describe the four main hormones that control the menstrual cycle.
5. What similarities and differences exist between the sexual response patterns of males and females?
6. Approximately what percentage of today's college students report having had sexual intercourse?
7. Explain the differences between heterosexuality, homosexuality, and bisexuality. How common are each of these sexual orientations in our society?

Think About This . . .

- How would you summarize your feelings about the changes in your body that took place during puberty?
- To what extent do you think that knowledge about the menstrual cycle will be pertinent to you as you move through adulthood? (This question is for BOTH men and women.)
- Do you think a celibate lifestyle is possible or practical in the late 1990s? Why or why not?
- What are your estimates of the percentages of men and women at your college or university who have had sexual intercourse?
- In comparison with a decade ago, are heterosexuals generally more comfortable or less comfortable with homosexuals in our society? Support your answer with specific examples.

References

1. Thibodeau GA, Patton KT: *The human body in health and disease*, St Louis, 1992, Mosby.
2. Hyde JS: *Understanding human sexuality*, ed 5, New York, 1994, McGraw-Hill.
3. Haas K, Haas A: *Understanding sexuality*, ed 3, St Louis, 1993, Mosby.
4. Crooks R, Baur K: *Our sexuality*, ed 5, Menlo Park, Calif, 1993, Benjamin-Cummings.
5. Thibodeau GA: *Structure and function of the body*, ed 10, St Louis, 1993, Mosby.
6. Hatcher RA et al: *Contraceptive technology*, ed 16, New York, 1994, Irvington Publishers.
7. Masters W, Johnson V: *Human sexual response*, Boston, 1966, Little, Brown.
8. Rathus SA, Nevid JS, Fichner-Rathus L: *Human sexuality in a world of discovery*, Needham Heights, Mass, 1993, Allyn and Bacon.
9. U.S. Bureau of the Census: *Statistical abstract of the United States: 1995*, ed 115, Washington, DC, 1995, US Government Printing Office.
10. Kinsey A, Pomeroy W, Martin C: *Sexual behavior in the human male*, Philadelphia, 1948, WB Saunders.

11. Allen LS, Gorski RA: Sexual orientation and the size of the anterior commissure in the human brain, *Proc Nat Acad Sci USA* 89(15): 7199-7202, 1992.

12. Kinsey A et al: *Sexual behavior in the human female*, Philadelphia, 1953, WB Saunders.

13. Fletcher R: Mating, the family, and marriage: a sociological view. In Reynolds V, Kellet J, editors: *Mating and marriage*, Oxford, 1991, Oxford University Press.

Suggested Readings

Haas K, Haas A: *Understanding sexuality,* ed 3, St Louis, 1993, Mosby.
A college-level textbook suitable for an introductory human sexuality course, this book presents a comprehensive overview of issues and scientific topics related to sexuality.

Haynes C, Edwards D: *2002 ways to say "I love you,"* Holbrook, Mass, 1994, Adams Media Group.
A 122-page book that lists 2002 different ways to let your partner know of your love. Many of the suggestions are simple and will help the reader discover how easy it is to communicate the feelings of love.

Liautaud MV, editor: *Swatting the mosquitoes of marriage: how to keep little annoyances from becoming a big deal,* Grand Rapids, Mich, 1994, Zonderuan Publishing House.
A collection of articles from *Marriage Partnership* magazine. Articles cover issues related to money, sex, conflict, work, romance, the house, and children. Most articles have checklists and worksheets for couples to use.

Marcus E: *Is it choice?* San Francisco, 1993, HarperCollins.
Provides answers to 300 wide-ranging questions about homosexuality. Questions about relationships, spiritual contexts, sexual behavior, discrimination, and coming out are covered. "Dear Abby" recommends this book as an excellent resource.

Nolan M, Sarrett E: *I'm so tired of other people, I'm dating myself: an insider's guide to being single,* Nashville, Tenn, 1993, Janet Thomas Books.
A humorous look at life in the world of the single person.

Sex on the Internet

It's like a singles bar without the loud music. If you have a computer and a modem, you can gain access to the world's largest "meet market." From the comfort of your home, you can browse the Internet and meet people for conversation, friendship, romance, and even "sex" (such as it is in cyberspace). There is a cover charge, but you won't have to buy drinks to start up a conversation or get your toes smashed on the dance floor. You won't even have to worry about getting diseases (save for the occasional computer virus).

However, there are drawbacks when you enter this hangout. Can you be sure the person you're chatting with is all he or she seems to be? How can you be certain of a person's personality, age, or even his or her gender? And is there a safe way to meet a "cyberfriend" face-to-face? The Internet way of meeting people has its own built-in set of advantages—but inviting the world into your home has its dangers as well.

Today's Internet user can find a variety of potential conversation topics using a Web browser and typing in various keywords. As the Internet grows, so do its various websites and USENET discussion groups. Some people see this expansion as a source of entertainment. They think that the Internet is a fun and interesting way to meet people who share their interests. Others think that the Internet allows pornographers, pedophiles, and other deviants to perpetuate their behavior and prey on innocent children. Both groups are attempting to use the law either to keep the Internet as a haven for free speech or to clean it up and make it safer for children. This clash of ideals is creating a continual battle over the nature and character of the Internet.

Fun and games on the Internet

The Internet is a large group of computer networks, both public and private, that connects millions of computer users in an estimated 150 countries. Over 70,000 private computer bulletin boards exist in the United States alone, and private commercial networks such as Prodigy, America Online, and CompuServe provide nearly 6 million subscribers worldwide with access to the Internet.[1] Although the Internet contains information about all facets of life, the sexually oriented sites are proving to be the most popular areas among the general public. For example, alt.sex, a USENET discussion group where people can chat in real time with other users, is the most often visited site on the Internet.[2] Brian Reid, director of the Network Systems Laboratory at Digital Equipment Corporation, reports that between 180,000 and 500,000 users drop into this discussion group on a monthly basis.[3]

At websites, computer bulletin boards that usually include photographs, interested parties can find almost anything that conforms to their sexual desires. Many pictures of nude men and women that can be found at most adult-oriented video stores and booksellers can be downloaded (placed on a user's computer disk or printed on his or her own printer).[1] However, other types of less common sexual images are also available at websites, including explicit images that many people find objectionable.

The positive side of the Internet

Despite the potentially offensive graphic images available on-line, the Internet does have several good points. One positive aspect is that people who are interested in meeting others can use the Internet as a sort of virtual pick-up bar without many of the unpleasant consequences. It gives people the freedom either to be themselves without fear of repercussions or to adopt a totally new persona. Best of all, cybersex participants don't have to worry about looking their best during a virtual date.[4] Who you are (or who you pretend to be) becomes more important than what you look like in cyberspace chat rooms.

Sexually oriented Internet sites can also be positive in the sense that they sometimes inspire creative impulses and prevent people from engaging in destructive behavior. Some sites house participatory novels in which users can immerse themselves and create new realities for themselves and other participants.[5] In this respect, these sites are similar to fantasy game pages that house activities such as Dungeons & Dragons. People are able to cast off their old identities and create exciting new personas that are able to engage in sexual practices that the users themselves would never attempt in real life. Thus the Internet becomes a harmless outlet for sexual fantasies: the ultimate safe sex.

A third plus to using the Internet to meet people is that occasionally, people who use it do fall in "virtual love," choose to meet face to face, and end up developing a relationship or even getting married.[4] Although this is a rare occurrence, the chance that it could happen is enough to keep some people involved with on-line romances in the hope of finding a perfect cybermate who will be as good in person.

Pitfalls of on-line sex
Although virtual sex has many good points in its favor, there are also several negative aspects. One of the worst possible scenarios of on-line sex is discovering that the person with whom you have been pursuing a virtual relationship is not who he or she claims to be. This pitfall is particularly dangerous when one of the parties in the relationship is a minor. In response to a recent on-line query, 130 female teenagers stated that they had posted erotic stories on a sexually oriented bulletin board and corresponded with adult men. In the stories, the teenagers pretended to be adults. Several of the teenagers also admitted that they had scheduled face to face meetings with these adult men without telling anyone.[6] Although none of the teenagers reported any negative consequences as a result of these meetings, the potential for danger was most certainly present. A recent case in which a female 13-year-old from Kentucky ended up in Los Angeles after being lured there by her adult male Internet correspondent provides evidence to prove this point.[3] Additionally, several cases exist in which pedophiles have used computer bulletin boards to contact children, learned their names and addresses, and set up meetings with them. Several rapes have occurred as a result of this.[7]

A second drawback to on-line sex is the considerable cost. Although chat rooms are sometimes free and websites have "visitor's passes" that allow sneak previews, most of the hard-core sexual activity can be very expensive. Some chat rooms charge as much as $12 an hour for a conversation.[4] To get to the more explicit photographs and participatory novels on the Internet, a member's fee is required, which ranges anywhere from $19.95 for 6 months to $129.95 for a year. These fees are generally paid by credit card on-line. A digital video camera, which is necessary to create real-time pictures to transmit through a personal computer, costs at least $100.[8] Upgrades to computer memory and equipment to handle more technologically advanced transmissions such as video clips can also be costly, running into the thousands of dollars.

A third potential problem is cybersex addiction. Some people become so involved with virtual reality that they find themselves uninterested in the real world. A librarian at a large college recently reported that many college students have to be asked to log off the library's computers that have Internet connections. These students ignore library policy that limits their Internet use to 30 minutes. One student had to be threatened by campus police; he was logged onto a sexually oriented chat room for almost 4 hours. In another case at the same college a library employee was disciplined after he was caught downloading sexually explicit material.[9] As a result of these incidents the college now blocks many sexually explicit sites and has disabled its computers' ability to download any material.

Avoiding sex on the Internet
With all the publicity and notoriety surrounding sexually oriented Internet sites, many concerned parents want to ensure that their children do not have access to sexual material through their personal computers. Other people are offended by cybersex and do not want it coming into their homes for religious or moral reasons. For these people, several options exist. Parents can subscribe to an on-line service that blocks potentially offensive sites. CompuServe, one of the largest on-line providers, recently suspended 200 sex discussion groups in response to German authorities' contention that the groups violated German obscenity laws.[10] Also, America Online and Prodigy have mechanisms available on their services to block access to areas that most parents would consider inappropriate for their children.[3] These mechanisms are available free of charge with subscription to the services.

A second option is to purchase a program that will block out undesirable material. One such program, Surfwatch, will automatically block access to 1000 sites and let you screen all user groups, websites, and other electronic avenues. The cost of this program is $49.95 plus a $5.95 monthly service fee. Other types of blocker programs include NetNanny, which lets parents monitor everything that passes through their computer, and Time's Up, which lets parents set up time limits and appropriate times for their children to use the computer.[8]

A third, decidedly low-tech option is the most obvious and also the most overlooked. Parents should watch what their children are doing while they are on-line and monitor all activities, perhaps by making computer use a family activity.[3] As columnist Michael J. Miller points out, much of the fear that children will accidentally stumble onto a sexually oriented site is unfounded. Unlike broadcast media, on the Internet, you must enter a specific address or follow a specific link to reach a sexually oriented site. Parents who watch their kids will know exactly where the kids go during an on-line jaunt. Additionally, parents should teach their children some basic safety information such as never to give out their real name, address, or telephone number to people they meet on-line. Children should understand that even though they may have on-line friends, these people are really strangers that they know little about.[3–8]

The Telecommunications Competition and Deregulation Act

In February 1996, President Clinton signed into law the Telecommunications Competition and Deregulation Act, a law that contains a provision called the Telecommunications Decency Act to block indecency on-line. Anyone caught transmitting obscene, lewd, or indecent communications by any electronic means could be fined as much as $100,000 and sent to prison for as long as 2 years.[1,10,11] Civil libertarians and users of sexually oriented Internet sites oppose this law, stating that the First Amendment guarantees freedom of speech and that this freedom should include the Internet. They also believe that the law as written is too broad and confusing; it could be interpreted as banning any use of profanity or nudity on-line, including news reports, legal documents, literature, and even the Bible.[11]

Some parents and religious groups, on the other hand, are applauding this new act. They feel it gives them more control over what kinds of material are coming into their homes. They believe that this legislation is necessary to protect children from being exposed to pornography on-line. They also believe the law is good because it specifically targets material that is patently offensive and depicts graphic sexual activity.[11]

A line has been drawn in the sand regarding sex on the Internet. Supporters of the new law are joining organizations such as Enough is Enough, the National Coalition against Pornography, and the American Family Association Law Center.[7] These groups work to defend traditional values and fight against increased pornography. Meanwhile, web search engines such as Yahoo protested the legislation by turning their Web pages to black with white lettering for 48 hours to demonstrate "virtual mourning," and the American Civil Liberties Union filed a federal court complaint to block enforcement of the law.[11]

Using the Internet for sexual purposes can have both positive and negative consequences; therefore people who do so should weigh all factors involved before they decide to enter the world of cybersex. Parents should be especially careful about what they allow to come into their homes via the personal computer. Although blocking methods and the new federal laws provide some protection from sexually oriented material, it is ultimately the individual's responsibility to choose and to monitor what type of information comes up while surfing the Internet.

For Discussion . . .
Have you or someone you know ever explored sexually oriented Websites on the Internet? If so, was it a positive or a negative experience? Would you be willing to meet a virtual friend face-to-face? Why or why not? Do you support the new Telecommunications Indecency Act? Why or why not?

References
1. Lewis PH: Despite a new plan for cooling it off, cybersex stays hot, *New York Times*, p A1, March 26, 1995.
2. Nashawatz C: Where the wild things are: anonymous sex is back, *Entertainment Weekly*, September 23, 1994.
3. Levy S, Stone B: No place for kids: a parents' guide to sex on the Net, *Newsweek*, July 3, 1995.
4. Van der Leur G: Twilight zone of the id, *Time*, (45)2, 1995.
5. Machure B: MUDs and MUSHes and MOOs, *PC Magazine*, p10, April 30, 1995.
6. Bennahan DS: Lolitas on-line, *Harper's Bazaar*, p 3406, Sept 1995.
7. Zipperer J: The naked city, *Christianity Today*, Sept 12, 1994.
8. Miller MJ: Cybersex shock, *PC Magazine*, Oct 10, 1995.
9. Anonymous: Personal communication, March 23, 1996.
10. Mezer M: A bad dream comes true in cyberspace, *Newsweek*, p 2, Jan 8, 1996.
11. Wagner M: Tempers flare over web censorship, *Computerworld*, Feb 12, 1996.

Managing Your Fertility

Healthy People 2000 Objectives

The Healthy People 2000 document set forth many important objectives in the areas of family planning fertility control, pregnancy, and childbirth. Unfortunately, tracking data for many of the family planning objectives are not available. The information that *is* available focuses mainly on adolescents and teenagers. The objectives for these age-groups included reducing pregnancy rates among adolescents, reducing the proportion of young people who have sexual intercourse, increasing the rate of abstinence among those who have already had sexual intercourse, and increasing contraceptive use by sexually active adolescents and teens.

Progress toward achieving these objectives has been mixed. The proportion of young people initiating sexual activity by age 15 and by age 17 has increased. Some headway has been made in promoting abstinence from sexual activity in girls who have already engaged in sexual intercourse. The only objective for which gains can be reported is the increased use of contraceptives among teenagers.

We are generally moving toward achieving our national objectives related to pregnancy and childbirth. The rate of severe pregnancy complications is down significantly, and the infant mortality rate in the United States is lower than it has ever been. More women are receiving prenatal care during the first trimester of pregnancy, breastfeeding rates are slightly higher, and cesarean delivery rates have fallen.

How you decide to control your **fertility** will have an important effect on your future. Your understanding of information and issues related to fertility control will help you make responsible decisions in this complex area.

For traditional-age students, these decisions may be fast approaching. Frequently, nontraditional students are parents who have had experiences that make them useful resources for other students in the class.

BIRTH CONTROL VS. CONTRACEPTION

Any discussion about the control of your fertility should start with an explanation of the subtle differences between the terms **birth control** and **contraception.** Although many people use the words interchangeably, they reflect different perspectives about fertility control. *Birth control* is an umbrella term that refers to all of the procedures you might use to prevent the birth of a child. Birth control includes all available contraceptive measures, as well as sterilization, use of the intrauterine device (IUD), and abortion procedures.

Contraception is a much more specific term for any procedure used to prevent the fertilization of an ovum. Contraceptive measures vary widely in the mechanisms they use to accomplish this task. They also vary considerably in their method of use and their rate of success in preventing conception. A few examples of contraceptive methods are the use of condoms, oral contraceptives, spermicides, and diaphragms.

Beyond the numerous methods mentioned, certain forms of sexual behavior not involving intercourse could be considered forms of contraception. For example, mutual masturbation by couples eliminates the possibility of pregnancy. This practice, as well as additional forms of sexual expression other than intercourse (such as kissing, touching, and massage), have been given the generic term **outercourse.** Not only does outercourse protect against unplanned pregnancy, it may also significantly reduce the transmission of sexually transmitted diseases, including HIV infection.

REASONS FOR CHOOSING TO USE BIRTH CONTROL

People choose to use birth control for many reasons. Many career-minded individuals carefully plan the timing and spacing of children so that they can best provide for their children's financial support without sacrificing their job status. Others choose methods of birth control to ensure that they will never have children. Some use birth control methods to permit safe participation in a wide variety of sexual behaviors. Fear of contracting a sexually transmitted disease prompts some people to use specific forms of birth control.

Financial and legal considerations can be significant factors in the choice of certain birth control methods. Many people must by necessity take the cost of a method into account when selecting appropriate birth control. The cost of sterilization and abortion can prohibit some low-income people from choosing these alternatives, especially since federal funds do not support such procedures. A number of states have established statutes and policies that make contraceptive information and medical services relatively difficult to obtain.

Another important consideration in the use of birth control methods is the availability of professional services. An example of the effect of this factor may be the selection of birth control methods by college students. Some colleges and universities provide contraceptive services through their student health centers. Students enrolled in these schools have easy access to low-cost, comprehensive contraceptive services. Students enrolled in colleges that do not provide such complete services may find that access to accurate information and clinical services is difficult to obtain and that private professional services are expensive.

For many people, religious doctrine will be a factor in their selection of a birth control method. This influence can be seen in the Roman Catholic Church's ban on the use of all forms of contraception other than natural family planning and in the condemnation of abortion by certain religious groups.

THEORETICAL EFFECTIVENESS VS. USE EFFECTIVENESS

People considering the use of a contraceptive method need to understand the difference between the two effectiveness rates given for each form of contraception. *Theoretical effectiveness* is a measure of a contraceptive method's ability to prevent a pregnancy when the method is used precisely as directed during every act of intercourse. *Use effectiveness*, however, refers to the effectiveness of a method in preventing conception when used by the general public. Use effectiveness rates take into account factors that lower effectiveness below that based on "perfect" use. Failure to follow proper instructions, illness of the user, forgetfulness, physician (or pharmacist) error, and a subconscious desire to experience risk or even pregnancy are a few of the factors that can lower the effectiveness of even the most theoretically effective contraceptive technique.

Effectiveness rates are often expressed in terms of the percentage of women users of childbearing age who do not become pregnant while using the method for 1 year. For some methods the theoretical- and use-effectiveness rates are vastly different; the theoretical rate is always higher than the use rate. Table 14-1 presents data concerning effectiveness rates, advantages, and disadvantages of many birth control methods.

SELECTING YOUR CONTRACEPTIVE METHOD

In this section, we discuss some of the many factors that should be important to you as you consider selecting a contraceptive method. Remember that no method possesses equally high marks in all of the following areas. It is important that you and your partner select a contraceptive method that is both acceptable and effective, as determined by your unique needs and expectations. Completing the Personal Assessment on p. 348 will help you make this decision.

For a contraceptive method to be acceptable to those who wish to exercise a large measure of control over their fertility, the following should be given careful consideration:

- *It should be safe.* The contraceptive approach you select should not pose a significant health risk for you or your partner.
- *It should be effective.* Your approach must have a high success rate in preventing pregnancy.
- *It should be reliable.* The form you select must be able to be used over and over again with consistent success.
- *It should be reversible.* Couples who eventually want to have a family should select a method that can be reversed.
- *It should be affordable.* The cost of a particular method must fit comfortably into a couple's budget.
- *It should be easy to use.* Complicated instructions or procedures can make a method difficult to use effectively.
- *It should not interfere with sexual expression.* An ideal contraceptive fits in comfortably with a couple's intimate sexual behavior.

CURRENT BIRTH CONTROL METHODS
Withdrawal

Withdrawal, or **coitus interruptus,** is the contraceptive practice in which the erect penis is removed from the vagina just before ejaculation of semen. Theoretically this procedure prevents sperm from entering the deeper structures of the female reproductive system. The use effectiveness of this method, however, reflects how unsuccessful this method is in practice (see Table 14-1).

There is strong evidence to suggest that the clear preejaculate fluid that helps neutralize and lubricate the male urethra can contain *viable* (capable of fertilization) sperm.[1] This sperm can be deposited near the cervical opening before withdrawal of the penis. This phenomenon may in part explain the relatively low effectiveness of this method. Furthermore, withdrawal does not protect users from the transmission of STDs.

Periodic Abstinence

There are four approaches included in the birth control strategy called **periodic abstinence:** (1) the

fertility
The ability to reproduce.

birth control
All of the methods and procedures that can prevent the birth of a child.

contraception
Any method or procedure that prevents fertilization.

outercourse
Sexual activity that does not involve intercourse.

coitus interruptus (withdrawal) (**co ih tus in ter rup tus**)
A contraceptive practice in which the erect penis is removed from the vagina before ejaculation.

periodic abstinence
Birth control methods that rely on a couple's avoidance of intercourse during the ovulatory phase of a woman's menstrual cycle; also called *fertility awareness* or *natural family planning.*

Table 14-1 Effectiveness Rates of Birth Control for 100 Women during 1 Year of Use

| Method | Estimated Effectiveness | | Advantages | Disadvantages |
	Theoretical	Use		
No method (chance)	15%	15%	Inexpensive	Totally ineffective
Withdrawal	85%	75%-80%	No supplies or advance preparation needed; no side effects; men share responsibility for family planning	Interferes with coitus; may be difficult to use effectively; women must trust men to withdraw as orgasm approaches

Periodic abstinence
  Calendar
  Basal body
    temperature
  Cervical mucus
    method
  Symptothermal
	90%-98%	75%-85%	No supplies needed; no side effects; men share responsibility for family planning; women learn about their bodies	Difficult to use, especially if menstrual cycles are irregular, as is common in young women; abstinence may be necessary for long periods; lengthy instruction and ongoing counseling may be needed

Cervical cap	94%	82%	No health risks; helps protect against some STDs and cervical cancer	Limited availability
Spermicide	97%-98%	75%-85%	No health risks; helps protect against some STDs; can be used with condoms to increase effectiveness considerably	Must be inserted 5 to 30 minutes before coitus; effective for only 30 to 60 minutes; some women may find them awkward or embarrassing to use
Diaphragm with spermicide	97%-98%	80%-90%	No health risks; helps protect against some STDs and cervical cancer	Must be inserted with jelly or foam before every act of coitus and left in place for at least 6 hours after coitus; must be fitted by health care personnel; some women may find it awkward or embarrassing to use; may be inconvenient to clean, store, and carry
Male condom and male condom with spermicide	98% 99%	80%-90% 95%	Easy to use; inexpensive and easy to obtain; no health risks; very effective protection against some STDs; men share responsibility for family planning	Must be put on just before coitus; some men and women complain of decreased sensation
Female condom	90%+	74%-79%	Relatively easy to use; no prescription required; polyurethane is stronger than latex; provides some STD protection; silicone-based lubrication provided; useful when male will not use a condom	Contraceptive effectiveness and STD protection not as high as with male condom; couples may be unfamiliar with a device that extends outside the vagina; more expensive than male condoms
IUD	99%	95%-98%	Easy to use; highly effective in preventing pregnancy; does not interfere with coitus; repeated action not needed	May increase risk of pelvic inflammatory disease (PID) and infertility in women with more than one sexual partner; not usually recommended for women who have never had a child; must be inserted by health care personnel; may cause heavy bleeding and pain in some women

Table 14-1, cont'd

| Method | Estimated Effectiveness | | Advantages | Disadvantages |
	Theoretical	Use		
Combined pill (Estrogen-progestin) Triphasic pill	99%	97%-98%	Easy to use; highly effective in preventing pregnancy; does not interfere with coitus; regulates menstrual cycle; reduces heavy bleeding and menstrual pain; helps protect against ovarian and endometrial cancer	Must be taken every day; requires medical examination and prescription; minor side effects such as nausea or menstrual spotting; possibility of circulatory problems, such as blood clotting, strokes, and hypertension, in a small percentage of users
Minipill (progestin only)	99%	96%-97%		
Depo-Provera	99%+	99%+	Easy to use; highly effective for 3-month period; continued use prevents menstruation	Requires supervision by a physician; administered by injection; some women experience irregular menstrual spotting in early months of use
Subdermal implants (progestin only)	99%+	99%+	Highly effective for 5-year period; helps prevent anemia and regulates menstrual cycle	Requires minor surgery; some women experience irregular menstrual spotting
Tubal ligation	99%+	99%+	Permanent; removes fear of pregnancy	Surgery-related risks; generally considered irreversible
Vasectomy	99%+	99%+	Permanent; removes fear of pregnancy	Generally considered irreversible

calendar method, (2) the basal body temperature (BBT) method, (3) the Billings cervical mucus method, and (4) the symptothermal method.[2] All four methods attempt to determine the time a woman ovulates. Figure 14-1 (p. 349) shows a day-to-day fertility calendar used to calculate fertile periods. Most research indicates that an ovum is viable for only about 24 to 36 hours after its release from the ovary. (Once inside the female reproductive tract, some sperm can survive up to a week.) When a woman can accurately determine when she ovulates, she must refrain from intercourse long enough for the ovum to begin to disintegrate. Fertility awareness, rhythm, natural birth control, and natural family planning are terms interchangeable with periodic abstinence. Remember that periodic abstinence methods *do not* provide protection against the spread of sexually transmitted diseases, including HIV infection.

Periodic abstinence is the only acceptable method endorsed by the Roman Catholic Church. For some people who have deep concerns for the spiritual dimensions of their health, the selection of a contraceptive method other than periodic abstinence may indicate a serious compromise of beliefs.

The **calendar method** requires close examination of a woman's menstrual cycle for at least eight cycles. Records are kept of the length (in days) of each cycle.

A *cycle* is defined as the number of days from the first day of bleeding of one cycle to the first day of bleeding of the next cycle.

To determine the days she should abstain from intercourse, a woman should subtract 18 from her shortest cycle; this is the first day she should abstain from intercourse. Then she should subtract 11 from her longest cycle; this is the last day she must abstain from intercourse (see the Health Action Guide on p. 350).[2]

The *basal body temperature method* requires a woman (for about 3 or 4 successive months) to take her body temperature every morning before she rises from bed. A finely calibrated thermometer, available in many drugstores, is used for this purpose. The theory behind this method is that a distinct correlation exists between body temperature and the process of ovulation. Just before ovulation, the body temperature supposedly dips and then rises about 0.5° to 1.0° F for the

calendar method
A form of periodic abstinence in which the variable lengths of a woman's menstrual cycle are used to calculate her fertile period.

PERSONAL ASSESSMENT

Which Birth Control Method Is Best for You?

To assess which birth control method would be best for you, answer the following questions, and check the interpretation below.

Do I:

	Yes	No
1. Need a contraceptive right away?	___	___
2. Want a contraceptive that can be used completely independent of sexual relations?	___	___
3. Need a contraceptive only once in a great while?	___	___
4. Want something with no harmful side effects?	___	___
5. Want to avoid going to the doctor?	___	___
6. Want something that will help protect against sexually transmitted diseases?	___	___
7. Have to be concerned about affordability?	___	___
8. Need to be virtually certain that pregnancy will not result?	___	___
9. Want to avoid pregnancy now but want to have a child sometime in the future?	___	___
10. Have any medical condition or lifestyle that may rule out some form of contraception?	___	___

Interpretation

If you have checked *Yes* to number:

1. Condoms and spermicides may be easily purchased without prescription in any pharmacy.
2. Sterilization, oral contraceptives, hormone implants or injections, cervical caps, and periodic abstinence techniques do not require that anything be done just before sexual relations.
3. Diaphragms, condoms, or spermicides can be used by people who have coitus only once in a while. Peri-

odic abstinence techniques may also be appropriate but require a high degree of skill and motivation.

4. IUDs should be carefully discussed with your physician. Sometimes the use of oral contraceptives or hormone products results in some minor discomfort and may have harmful side effects.
5. Condoms and spermicides do not require a prescription from a physician.
6. Condoms and, to a lesser extent, spermicides and the other barrier methods may help protect against some sexually transmitted diseases. No method (except abstinence) can guarantee complete protection.
7. Be a wise consumer: check prices, ask pharmacists and physicians. The cost of sterilization is high, but there is no additional expense for a lifetime.
8. Sterilization provides near certainty. Oral contraceptives, hormone implants or injections, or a diaphragm-condom-spermicide combination also give a high measure of reliable protection. Periodic abstinence, withdrawal, and douche methods should be avoided. Outercourse may be a good alternative.
9. Although it is sometimes possible to reverse sterilization, it requires surgery and is more complex than simply stopping use of any of the other methods.
10. Smokers and people with a history of blood clots should probably not use oral contraceptives or other hormone approaches. Some people have an allergic reaction to a specific spermicide and should experiment with another brand. Some women cannot be fitted with a diaphragm or cervical cap because of the position of the uterus. The woman and her health care provider will then need to select another suitable means of contraception.

To Carry This Further . . .

There may be more than one method of birth control suitable for you. Always consider how a method you select can also help you avoid an STD. Study the methods suggested above, and consult Table 14-1 to determine what techniques may be most appropriate.

---

rest of the cycle. The woman is instructed to refrain from intercourse during the interval when the temperature change takes place.

Drawbacks of this procedure include the need for consistent, accurate readings and the realization that all women's bodies are different. Some women may not fit the temperature pattern projection because of biochemical differences in their bodies. Also, body

temperatures can fluctuate because of a wide variety of illnesses and physical stressors.

The *Billings cervical mucus method* is another periodic abstinence technique. Generally used with other periodic abstinence techniques, this method requires a woman to evaluate the daily mucous discharge from her cervix. Users of this method become familiar with the changes in both appearance (from clear to cloudy)

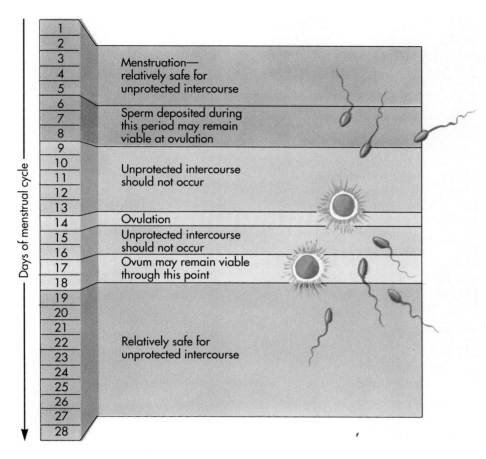

Figure 14-1   Periodic abstinence (fertility awareness or natural family planning) can combine use of the calendar, basal body temperature measurements, and Billings mucus techniques to identify the fertile period. Remember that most women's cycles are not consistently perfect 28-day cycles as shown in most illustrations.

and consistency (from watery to thick) of their cervical mucus throughout their cycles. Women are taught that the unsafe days are when the mucus becomes clear and is the consistency of raw egg whites. Such a technique of ovulation determination must be learned from a physician or family planning professional.

The *symptothermal method* of periodic abstinence combines the use of the BBT method and the cervical mucus method.[2] Of course, couples using the symptothermal method are already using a calendar to chart the woman's body changes. Thus some family planning professionals consider the symptothermal method a combination of all of the periodic abstinence approaches.

Vaginal Spermicides

Although they are not recommended as the primary form of fertility control, spermicidal agents are often recommended to be used with other forms of birth control. Alone, **spermicides** offer a reasonable amount of contraceptive protection for the woman

who is sexually active on an *infrequent* basis. Spermicides containing nonoxynol 9 provide some protection (but *not full* protection) against STDs and HIV infection.

Vaginal spermicide.

spermicides
Chemicals capable of killing sperm.

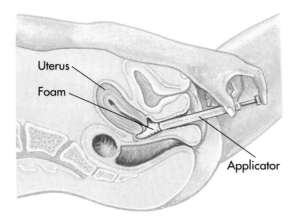

HEALTH
Action Guide

Determining Your Cycle

Even if you are not sexually active or are not planning to use periodic abstinence, you will find it helpful to use the calendar method of calculations to find the days in your cycle on which you are most fertile. (Hopefully, you are already keeping a record of your cycles on a calendar. This is a good addition to your health history.)

*   Subtract 18 from your shortest cycle. Subtract 11 from your longest cycle. The days in between are your unsafe days. Record your results.
*   What is your first unsafe day? What is your last unsafe day?
*   Can you identify the approximate time during your unsafe days that ovulation actually takes place?

Figure 14-2 Spermicidal foams and suppositories are placed deep into the vagina in the region of the cervix no longer than 30 minutes before intercourse.

Modern spermicides are safe, reasonably effective, reversible forms of contraception that can be obtained without a physician's prescription; they can be purchased in most drugstores and in many supermarkets. Like condoms, spermicides are relatively inexpensive. When used together, spermicides and condoms provide a high degree of contraceptive protection and disease prevention.

Spermicides, which are available in foam, cream, paste, or film form, are made of water-soluble bases with a spermicidal chemical incorporated in the base. The base material is designed to liquefy at body temperature and distribute the spermicidal component in an even layer over the tissues of the upper vagina (Figure 14-2). The Star Box at right describes a unique film type of spermicide.

Spermicides are not specific to sperm cells; they also attack other cells and thus may provide the woman with some additional protection against many sexually transmitted diseases and **pelvic inflammatory disease (PID).** However, when used alone, spermicides do not provide sufficient protection against most pathogens, including the virus that causes AIDS.

Condoms

Colored or natural, smooth or textured, straight or shaped, plain or reservoir-tipped, dry or lubricated—

Vaginal Contraceptive Film

A unique spermicide delivery system developed in England is vaginal contraceptive film (VCF). Vaginal contraceptive film is a sheet containing nonoxynol 9 that is inserted over the cervical opening. Shortly after insertion of the VCF, it dissolves into a gel-like material that clings to the cervical opening. The VCF can be inserted up to an hour before intercourse. Over the course of several hours, the material will be washed from the vagina in the normal vaginal secretions.

This spermicide is a nonprescription form of contraception that is as effective as other spermicidal foams and jellies. A box of 12 sheets costs about $7. Like other spermicidal agents, VCF may also help in minimizing the risk of some STDs and PID.

Condoms.

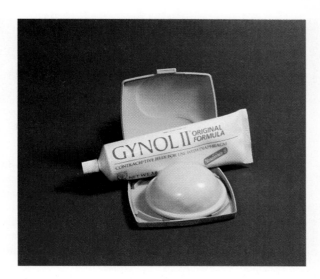

Diaphragm and contraceptive jelly.

the condom is approaching an art form. This is perhaps an exaggeration. Nevertheless, the familiar **condom** remains a safe, effective, reversible contraceptive device. All condoms manufactured in the United States must be approved by the FDA.

For couples who are highly motivated in their desire to prevent a pregnancy, the effectiveness of a condom can approach that of an oral contraceptive—especially if condom use is combined with a spermicide. (Some lubricated condoms now also contain a spermicide.) For couples who are less motivated or who use condoms on an irregular basis, the condom can be considerably less effective. This readily available and inexpensive method of contraception requires responsible use if it is to achieve a high level of effectiveness (see the Health Action Guide on p. 352).

The condom offers a measure of protection against sexually transmitted diseases. For both the man and the woman, chlamydial infections, gonorrhea, HIV infection, and other STDs are less likely to be acquired when the condom is used. When combined with a spermicide containing nonoxynol 9, condoms may become even more effective against the spread of STDs. Although advertisements suggest that condoms provide protection against the transmission of genital herpes, users of condoms must remember that this protection is limited to the penis and vagina—not to the surrounding genital region, where significant numbers of lesions are found. Like other barrier methods of contraception, the condom is a reasonable choice for couples who are motivated in their desire to prevent a pregnancy and who are willing to assume the level of responsibility required. See the Star Box on p. 353 for a discussion of the female condom.

Diaphragm

The **diaphragm** is a soft rubber cup with a spring-like metal rim that, when properly fitted and properly inserted by the user, rests in the top of the vagina. In its proper position the diaphragm covers the cervical opening (Figure 14-4 on p. 354). During intercourse the diaphragm stays in place quite well and cannot usually be felt by either the man or the woman.

The diaphragm is always used with a spermicidal cream or jelly. The diaphragm should be covered with an adequate amount of spermicide inside the cup and around the rim. When used properly with a spermicide, the diaphragm is a relatively effective contraceptive, and when combined with the man's use of a condom, its effectiveness is even greater.

Diaphragms must always be fitted and prescribed by a physician. The cost of obtaining a diaphragm and keeping a supply of spermicide may be higher than that of other methods. Also, a high level of motivation to follow the instructions *exactly* is important.

Diaphragms and other vaginal barrier methods (such as the cervical cap) provide some protection against sexually transmitted diseases, including gonorrhea and chlamydia, PID, and cervical cancer. However, the ability of diaphragms and other vaginal bar-

pelvic inflammatory disease (PID)
A generalized infection of the pelvic cavity that results from the spread of an infection through a woman's reproductive structures.

condom
A latex shield designed to cover the erect penis and retain semen on ejaculation; "rubber."

diaphragm
A soft rubber cup designed to cover the cervix.

HEALTH Action Guide

Maximizing the Effectiveness of Condoms

These simple directions for using condoms correctly, in combination with your motivation and commitment to regular use, should provide you with reasonable protection:

- Keep a supply of condoms at hand. Condoms should be stored in a cool, dry place so that they are readily available at the time of intercourse. Condoms that are stored in wallets or automobile glove compartments may not be in satisfactory condition when they are used. Temperature extremes are to be avoided. Check the condom package for the expiration date.
- Do not test a condom by inflating or stretching it. Handle it gently, and keep it away from sharp fingernails.
- For maximum effectiveness, put the condom on before genital contact. Either the man or the woman can put the condom in place. Early application is particularly important in the prevention of STDs. Early application also lessens the possibility of the release of preejaculate fluid into the vagina.
- Unroll the condom on the erect penis. For those using a condom without a reservoir tip, a $\frac{1}{2}$-inch space should be left to catch the ejaculate. To leave this space, pinch the tip of the condom as you roll it on the erect penis. Do not leave any air in the tip of the condom (Figure 14-3).
- Lubricate the condom if this has not already been done by the manufacturer. When doing this, be certain to use a water-soluble lubricant and not a petroleum-based product such as petroleum jelly. Petroleum can deteriorate the latex material. Other oil-based lubricants, such as mineral oil, baby oil, vegetable oil, shortening, and certain hand lotions, can quickly damage a condom. Use water-based lubricants only!
- After ejaculation, be certain that the condom does

Figure 14-3 Pinch the end of the condom to leave $\frac{1}{2}$ inch of space at the tip.

not become dislodged from the penis. Hold the rim of the condom firmly against the base of the penis during withdrawal. Do not allow the penis to become flaccid (soft) while still in the vagina.
- Inspect the condom for tears before throwing it away. If the condom is damaged in some way, immediately insert a spermicidal agent into the vagina.

rier methods to provide protection against HIV infection for either partner is not known. If you are concerned about possible HIV infection, either avoid sexual activity or use a latex condom and spermicide in combination.[3]

Cervical Cap

The **cervical cap** is a small, thimble-shaped device that fits over the entire cervix. Resembling a small diaphragm, the cervical cap is placed deeper than the diaphragm. The cap is held in place by suction rather than by pushing against anatomical structures (Figure 14-5 on p. 355). As with the diaphragm, a spermicide

is used with the cervical cap. Thus it requires many of the same skills for insertion and care as does the diaphragm. The use effectiveness of the cervical cap appears to be approximately equal to that of the diaphragm. These devices are distributed in the United States through physician prescription.

Intrauterine Device

The **intrauterine device (IUD)** is a method of birth control that works by reducing the chances that a fertilized ovum will be able to implant itself into the uterus. Most health professionals believe that the IUD

REALITY—the Female Condom

In April 1993, the Wisconsin Pharmacal Company finally gained approval to market a female condom called REALITY. This device consists of a soft, loose-fitting polyurethane sheath and two flexible rings (see photo). REALITY is inserted like a tampon and lines the inner contours of the vagina. The device extends outside the vagina and covers the labia. REALITY will sell in three-packs for about $6.50.

REALITY does not require a physician's prescription. This device is prelubricated and is intended for one-time use. Manufacturer's studies have shown that female condoms have fewer leaks and less slippage and dislodgement and provide less risk of exposure to semen than do male condoms. The polyurethane used is stronger and more resistant to oils than the latex membrane used for male condoms. Despite these claims, the FDA contends that male latex condoms provide greater contraceptive protection and protection from STDs than female condoms.[3]

Cervical cap.

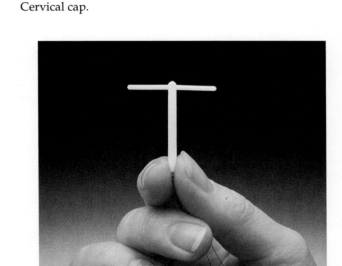

Progestasert IUD.

does not prevent conception; thus in a technical sense, the IUD is not a contraceptive device but rather a birth control device.

Two types of IUDs are available in the United States: the Progestasert (a T-shaped IUD containing progestin) and the Copper T 380-A (ParaGard), a T-shaped IUD wrapped with copper wire. The Progestasert must be replaced every year, but the Copper T 380-A can remain in place for up to 4 years. Only a skilled physician can prescribe and insert an IUD. As with many other forms of contraception, IUDs do not offer protection against STDs, including the AIDS virus.

As Table 14-1 indicates, IUDs are very effective birth control devices, surpassed in effectiveness only by abstinence, sterilization, and oral (or implanted, or injected) contraceptives. Some women using IUDs experience increased menstrual bleeding and cramping. Two un-

common but potentially serious side effects of IUD use are uterine perforation (in which the IUD imbeds itself into the uterine wall) and PID (which is a life-threatening infection of the abdominal cavity). However, a study by the World Health Organization indicates that today's IUDs do not increase the risk of pelvic infection except in the early weeks after insertion.[4]

cervical cap
A small, thimble-shaped device designed to fit over the cervix.

intrauterine device (IUD)
A small, plastic, medicated or unmedicated device that prevents continued pregnancy when inserted in the uterus.

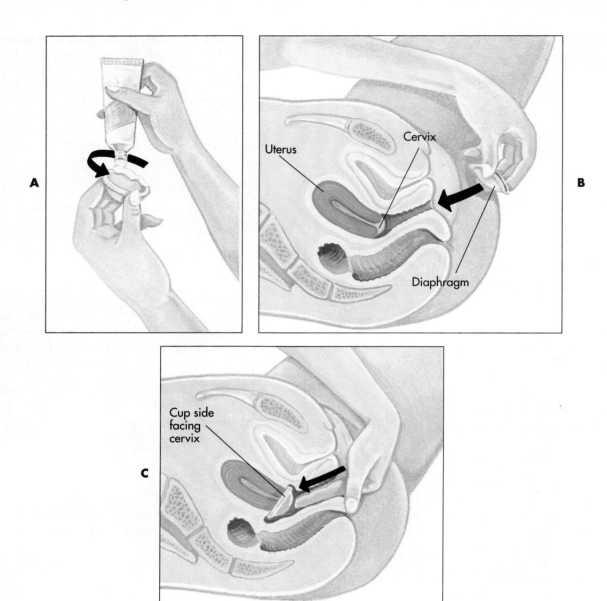

Figure 14-4   **A,** Spermicidal cream or jelly is placed into the diaphragm. **B,** The diaphragm is folded lengthwise and inserted into the vagina. **C,** The diaphragm is then placed against the cervix so that the cup portion with the spermicide is facing the cervix. The outline of the cervix should be felt through the central part of the diaphragm.

A woman deciding whether to use an IUD must discuss any concerns openly with her physician. The IUD can be a very acceptable form of contraception, especially for women who are in their middle to late reproductive years, unable to take birth control pills, in a stable monogamous relationship, and not at risk for STDs.

Oral Contraceptives

Developed in the 1950s, the **oral contraceptive pill** provides the highest effectiveness rate of any single reversible contraceptive method used today. "The pill" is the method of choice for nearly 17 million users in the United States.[5]

Use of the pill requires a physician's examination and prescription. Since oral contraceptives are available in a wide range of formulas, follow-up examinations are important to ensure that a woman is receiving an effective dosage with as few side effects as possible. Matching the right prescription with the woman may require a few consultations.

All oral contraceptives contain synthetic (laboratory-made) hormones. The *combined pill* uses both

Figure 14-5   After the spermicidal cream or jelly is placed in the cervical cap, the cap is inserted into the vagina and placed against the cervix.

synthetic estrogen and synthetic progesterone in each of 21 pills. In 1984, *triphasic pills* were introduced in the United States. In these pills the level of synthetic progesterone varies every 7 days during the cycle.[2] Estrogen levels remain constant during the cycle. As with many forms of contraception, it must be emphatically stated that *oral contraceptives do not provide protection from the transmission of STDs, including HIV infection.* Furthermore, the use of antibiotics lowers the pill's contraceptive effectiveness.

Oral contraceptives function in several ways. The estrogen in the pill tends to reduce ova development and ovulation. The progesterone in the pill helps reduce ovulation (by lowering the release of luteinizing hormone). The progesterone in the pill also causes the uterine wall to develop inadequately and helps thicken cervical mucus, thus making it difficult for sperm to enter the uterus. (For a discussion of the "morning after" pill, see the Star Box on p. 356.)

The physical changes produced by the oral contraceptive provide some beneficial side effects in women. Since the synthetic hormones are taken for 21 days and then are followed by **placebo pills** or no pills for 7 days, the menstrual cycle becomes regulated. Even women who have irregular cycles immediately become "regular." Since the uterine lining is not developed to the extent seen in a non–pill-taking woman, the uterus is not forced to contract with the same amount of vigor. Thus menstrual cramping is reduced, and the resultant menstrual flow is diminished. Research indicates that oral contraceptive use may provide protection against anemia, PID, noncancerous breast tumors, recurrent ovarian cysts, ectopic pregnancy, endometrial cancer, and cancer of the ovaries.[2] No conclusive evidence has been found that links oral contraceptive use to breast cancer. However, oral contraceptive use may be linked to a slight increase in cervical cancer risk.[2]

The negative side effects of the oral contraceptive pill can be divided into two general categories: (1) unpleasant and (2) potentially dangerous. The unpleasant side effects generally subside within 2 or 3 months for most women. A number of women report some or many of the following symptoms:

- Tenderness in breast tissue
- Nausea
- Mild headaches
- Slight, irregular spotting
- Weight gain
- Fluctuations in sex drive
- Mild depression
- More frequent vaginal infections

The potentially dangerous side effects of the oral contraceptive pill are most often seen in the cardiovascular system. Blood clotting, strokes, hypertension, and heart attack all seem to be associated with the estrogen component of the combined pill. When compared with nonusers, the risk of dying from cardiovascular complications is only slightly increased among healthy young oral contraceptive users. Nevertheless, the risks associated with pregnancy and childbirth are still much greater than those associated with oral contraceptive use (see the Learning from All Cultures box on p. 356).

Oral contraceptives.

oral contraceptive pill
A pill taken orally, composed of synthetic female hormones that prevent ovulation or implantation; "the pill."

placebo pills (pla **see** bo)
Pills that contain no active ingredients.

The Morning–After Pill

A "morning-after pill" is an oral contraceptive a woman can take to reduce the possibility of pregnancy after unprotected intercourse. The FDA has not officially approved any oral contraceptive that could be used in this fashion. Formerly, the drug DES (diethylstilbestrol) was used as a type of morning-after pill, although it was primarily for women who were victims of rape. Because of its potentially dangerous side effects, DES was removed from the market. A relatively high-dose combined oral contraceptive (Ovral) is now unofficially the drug of choice as a morning-after pill.

Physicians, who have the right to prescribe drugs for purposes other than those specifically indicated by the FDA, are now prescribing Ovral for patients who have unprotected midcycle intercourse. Some physicians prefer not to use Ovral in this fashion. In taking this drug a woman must take two Ovral pills within 3 days of unprotected intercourse (preferably within 12 to 24 hours). Then she must take two more Ovral pills 12 hours after her first dose of pills. The use of Ovral will start menstrual flow within a few weeks.[2]

The use of a morning-after pill in cases of rape or contraceptive failure is understandable. However, frequent use in cases of unprotected intercourse seems to many people to be a reflection of irresponsibility. What do you think?

There are some **contraindications** for the use of oral contraceptives. If you have a history of blood clotting, migraine headaches, liver disease, a heart condition, high blood pressure, obesity, diabetes, epilepsy, or anemia, or if you have not established regular menstrual cycles, the pill probably should not be your contraceptive choice. A thorough health history is important before a woman starts to take the pill.

Two additional contraindications are receiving considerable attention by the medical community. Cigarette smoking and advancing age are highly associated with an increased risk of potentially serious side effects. Increasing numbers of physicians are not prescribing oral contraceptives for their patients who smoke. The risk of cardiovascular-related deaths is greatly enhanced in women over age 35. The risk is even higher in female smokers over 35. The data are quite convincing.[2]

For the vast majority of women, however, the pill, when properly prescribed, is safe and effective. Careful scrutiny of one's health history and careful follow-

LEARNING from ALL CULTURES

Maternal Deaths during Pregnancy and Childbirth

Throughout the world, one woman dies every minute because of pregnancy-related complications. Most of these deaths take place in developing countries among poor women who have little access to health care services. In developing countries, pregnancy-related complications account for one fourth to one half of the deaths among women of reproductive age. Worldwide, approximately 500,000 women die each year because of pregnancy or childbirth complications.[10]

With the exception of women in China, a typical woman in the developing world has a 1 in 33 chance of dying from pregnancy or childbirth. In contrast, typical women in the developed world have only a 1 in 1500 chance of dying during pregnancy or childbirth.[10]

What makes pregnancy and childbirth so risky in developing countries? The most significant direct causes of death are (1) hemorrhage (severe bleeding after childbirth, abortion, prolonged labor, or ectopic pregnancy), (2) infection (after childbirth or abortion, or related to STDs and resultant PID), and (3) eclampsia (high blood pressure during pregnancy).

What do you think are some of the obstacles that women face in developing countries that make them so vulnerable to this tragedy? Among these, consider issues such as the status of women, the health care delivery system, the age of marriage, prenatal care, and nutrition and health education efforts in developing countries? Do we face some of these same issues in North America?

up examinations when a problem is suspected are essential elements that can provide a margin of safety. The ease of administration, the relatively low cost, and the effectiveness of the pill make it a sound choice for many women.

Minipills

Some women prefer not to use the combined oral contraceptive pill. Thus to avoid some of the potentially serious side effects of the combined pill, some physicians are prescribing **minipills.** These oral contraceptives contain no estrogen—only low-dose progesterone. The minipill seems to work by making an unsuitable environment for the transportation and implantation of the fertilized ovum. The effectiveness of the minipill is slightly lower than that of the combined pill. *Breakthrough bleeding* and **ectopic pregnancy** are more common in minipill users than in combined-pill users.

Injectable Contraceptives

In late 1992 the FDA approved a form of synthetic progesterone called *Depo-Provera.* This contraceptive is injectable and provides an extremely high degree of effectiveness for a 3-month period. The success rate for Depo-Provera is higher than 99%. For women who prefer not to take daily birth control pills or use the Norplant implants described below, Depo-Provera may be a good alternative.

New users of Depo-Provera report occasional breakthrough bleeding as the most common unpleasant side effect.[2] Once the woman's body becomes adjusted to the presence of this drug, breakthrough bleeding is reduced considerably. After this time, the most commonly reported side effect is amenorrhea (the absence of periods), which is understandable, since the drug inhibits ovulation. Many women consider amenorrhea to be a desirable effect of Depo-Provera use. Unlike users of oral contraceptives and subdermal implants, who return to fertility a few months after stopping their use, women who stop using Depo-Provera may experience infertility for a period of up to 1 year.[2]

Subdermal Implants

In late 1990, subdermal implants (Norplant) were approved for use in the United States. This form of contraception uses six silicone rods filled with synthetic progesterone. Using a local anesthetic, the physician implants these rods just beneath the skin of the woman's upper or lower arm. The rods release low levels of the hormone for 5 years. An extremely

The Norplant subdermal implant.

effective contraceptive, subdermal implants appear to produce minimal side effects. Irregular patterns of menstrual bleeding are the most common side effect. Norplant implants cost approximately $600 to $800 for a 5-year supply.

Sterilization

All of the contraceptive mechanisms or methods already discussed have one quality in common: they are reversible. Although microsurgical techniques are providing medical breakthroughs, **sterilization** should still be considered an irreversible procedure.[6] When you decide to use sterilization, you no longer control your own fertility because you no longer will be able to produce offspring. For this reason, couples considering sterilization procedures usually must undergo extensive discussions with a physician or

---

contraindications
Factors that make the use of a drug inappropriate or dangerous for a particular person.

minipills
Low-dose progesterone oral contraceptives.

ectopic pregnancy
A pregnancy in which the fertilized ovum implants at a site other than the uterus, typically in the fallopian tubes.

sterilization
Generally permanent birth control techniques that surgically disrupt the normal passage of ova or sperm.

family planning counselor to identify their true feelings about this finality. People must be aware of the possible changes in self-concept they might have after sterilization. If you are a man who equates fertility with masculinity, you may have trouble accepting your new status as a sterile man. If you are a woman who equates motherhood with femininity, you might have adjustment problems after sterilization.

The male sterilization procedure is called a *vasectomy.* Accomplished with a local anesthetic in a physician's office, this 20- to 30-minute procedure consists of the surgical removal of a section of each vas deferens. After a small incision is made through the scrotum, the vas deferens is located and a small section removed. The remaining ends are either tied or *cauterized* (Figure 14-6, *A*).

Immediately after a vasectomy, sperm may still be present in the vas deferens. A backup contraceptive is recommended until a physician microscopically examines a semen specimen. This examination usually occurs about 6 weeks after the surgery. After a vasectomy, men can still produce male sex hormones, get erections, have orgasms, and ejaculate. (Recall that sperm account for only a small portion of the semen.)

Some men even report increased interest in sexual activity, since their chances of impregnating a woman are virtually nonexistent.

What happens to the process of spermatogenesis within each testicle? Sperm cells are still being produced, but they are destroyed by specialized white blood cells called *phagocytic leukocytes.*

The most common method of female sterilization is *tubal ligation.* During this procedure, the fallopian tubes are cut and the ends tied back. Some physicians cauterize the tube ends to ensure complete sealing (Figure 14-6, *B*). The fallopian tubes are usually reached through the abdominal wall. In a *minilaparotomy,* a small incision is made through the abdominal wall just below the navel. The resultant scar is quite small and is the basis for the term *band-aid surgery.*

Female sterilization requires about 20 to 30 minutes, with the patient under a local or general anesthetic. The use of a *laparoscope* has made female sterilization much simpler than in the past. The laparoscope is a small tube equipped with mirrors and lights. Inserted through a single incision, the laparoscope locates the fallopian tubes before they are cut, tied, or cauterized. When a laparoscope is used

A

Vas deferens cut and tied on each side

Fallopian tubes cut and tied

B

Ovary

Uterus

Fallopian tube is cauterized

Figure 14-6   The most frequently used forms of male and female sterilization. **A,** Vasectomy. **B,** Tubal ligation.

through an abdominal incision, the procedure is called a *laparoscopy.*

Women who are sterilized still produce female hormones, ovulate, and menstruate. However, the ovum cannot move down the fallopian tube. Within a day of its release, the ovum will start to disintegrate and be absorbed by the body. Freed of the possibility of becoming pregnant, many sterilized women report an increase in sex drive and activity.

Two other procedures produce sterilization in women. *Ovariectomy* (the surgical removal of the ovaries) and *hysterectomy* (the surgical removal of the uterus) accomplish sterilization. However, these procedures are used to remove diseased (cancerous, cystic, or hemorrhaging) organs and are not primarily considered sterilization techniques.

Abortion

Regardless of the circumstances under which pregnancy occurs, women may now choose to terminate their pregnancies. No longer must women who do not want to be pregnant seek potentially dangerous, illegal abortions. On the basis of current technology and legality, women need never experience childbirth. The decision will be theirs to make.

Abortion should never be considered a first-line, preferred form of fertility control. Rather, abortion is a final, last-chance undertaking. It should be used only when responsible control of one's fertility could not be achieved. The decision to abort a fetus is a highly controversial, personal one—one that needs serious consideration by each woman.

On the basis of the landmark 1973 U.S. Supreme Court case *Roe v. Wade,* the United States joined many of the world's most populated countries in legalizing abortions within the following guidelines:

1. For the first 3 months of pregnancy (first trimester), the decision to abort lies with the woman and her doctor.
2. For the next 3 months of pregnancy (second trimester), state law may regulate the abortion procedure in ways that are reasonably related to maternal health.
3. For the last weeks of pregnancy (third trimester) when the fetus is judged capable of surviving if born, any state may regulate or even prohibit abortion except where abortion is necessary to preserve the life or health of the mother. If a pregnancy is terminated during the third trimester, a viable fetus would be considered a live birth and would not be allowed to die.

Each year, approximately 1.5 million women make the decision to terminate a pregnancy in the United States.[5] Thousands of additional women probably consider abortion but elect to continue their pregnancies.

Clearly, abortion is a political issue. It will be interesting to see how future abortion-related decisions will unfold. Special interest groups on both sides of the issues, the Supreme Court, state legislatures, federal agencies (such as the FDA and the Department of Health and Human Services), the Congress, and the President all have a say in the abortion debate in this country. Regardless of the eventual outcomes of this debate, here are the present abortion procedures available in the United States.

First–trimester abortion procedures

Menstrual extraction. Also referred to as *menstrual regulation, menstrual induction,* and *preemptive abortion,* menstrual extraction is a process carried out between the fourth and sixth week after the last menstrual period (or in the days immediately after the first missed menstrual period). Generally performed in a physician's office under a local anesthetic or *paracervical anesthetic,* a small plastic *cannula* is inserted through the undilated cervical canal into the cavity of the uterus. Once the cannula is in position, a small amount of suction is applied by a hand-held syringe. By rotating and moving the cannula across the uterine wall, the physician can withdraw the endometrial tissue.

Vacuum aspiration. Induced abortions undertaken during the sixth through ninth weeks of pregnancy are generally done through *vacuum aspiration* of the uterine contents. Vacuum aspiration is the most commonly performed abortion procedure. This procedure is similar in nature to menstrual extraction. Unlike menstrual extraction, however, vacuum aspiration may require **dilation** of the cervical canal and the use of a local anesthetic. In this more advanced stage of pregnancy, a larger cannula must be inserted into the uterine cavity. This process can be accomplished by using metal dilators of increasingly larger sizes to open the canal. After aspiration by an electric vacuum pump, the uterine wall may also be scraped to confirm complete removal of the uterine contents.

abortion
Induced premature termination of a pregnancy.

dilation
Gradual expansion of an opening or passageway, such as the cervix.

Dilation and curettage (D & C). When a pregnancy is to be terminated during the ninth through fourteenth weeks, vacuum aspiration gives way to a somewhat similar procedure labeled **dilation and curettage,** or more familiarly, **D & C.** D & C usually requires a general anesthetic, not a local anesthetic.[2]

Like vacuum aspiration, the D & C involves the gradual enlargement of the cervical canal through the insertion of increasingly larger metal dilators. When the cervix has been dilated to a size sufficient to allow for the passage of a *curette,* the removal of the endometrial tissue can begin. The curette is a metal instrument resembling a spoon, with a cup-shaped cutting surface on its end. As the curette is drawn across the uterine wall, the soft endometrial tissue and fetal parts are scraped from the wall of the uterus. (The D & C is also used in the medical management of certain health conditions of the uterine wall, such as irregular bleeding or the buildup of endometrial tissue.)

As in the case of menstrual extraction, both vacuum aspiration and D & C are very safe procedures for the woman. The need to dilate the cervix more fully in a D & C increases the risk of cervical trauma and the possibility of perforation, but these risks are reported to be low. Bleeding, cramping, spotting, and infections present minimal controllable risks when procedures are done by experienced clinicians under clinical conditions.

The abortion pill. The Roussel-Uclaf company in Paris, France, has produced a very controversial form of birth control, RU 486 (mifepristone). RU 486 is controversial because it is designed to produce an abortion. This drug is a pill that blocks the action of progesterone. When three 200-mg RU 486 pills are taken and followed 48 hours later by an injection (or vaginal suppository) of prostaglandin, menstruation begins, usually within 5 hours. In May 1994, Roussel-Uclaf agreed to give its patent rights to RU 486 to the Population Council, a New York–based international, nonprofit contraceptive research organization. This action paved the way for the Population Council to test this drug on U.S. women in the fall of 1994. If the testing indicates that RU 486 is as safe and effective as that found in the 150,000 women who have used the drug in Europe, then the FDA is likely to approve RU 486 as a prescription drug.

Second-trimester abortion procedures

When a woman's pregnancy continues beyond the fourteenth week of gestation, termination becomes a more difficult matter. The procedures at this stage become more complicated and take longer to be completed, and complications become more common.

Dilation and evacuation. Vacuum aspiration and D & C can be combined in a procedure called *dilation and evacuation (D & E)* during the earliest weeks of the second trimester (Figure 14-7). The use of D & E increases the likelihood of trauma and postprocedural complications, since larger instruments and greater dilation are required. After about 16 weeks, more intensive procedures will be required to terminate the late second trimester pregnancy.

Hypertonic saline procedure. From the sixteenth week of gestation to the end of the second trimester, intrauterine injection of a strong salt solution into the amniotic sac is the procedure most frequently used. The administration of intrauterine **hypertonic saline solution** requires a skilled operator so that the needle used to introduce the salt solution enters the amniotic sac. Once the needle is in place, some amniotic fluid is withdrawn, allowing the saline solution to be injected.

Some physicians support the saline procedure by dilating the cervix with *laminaria* or another dilatory product and administering the hormone oxytocin to stimulate uterine contractions. The onset of uterine contractions will expel the dehydrated uterine contents within 24 to 36 hours.

Prostaglandin procedure. The use of prostaglandin is the third type of abortion procedure used during the second trimester. Prostaglandins are hormonelike chemicals that have a variety of useful effects on human tissue. Produced naturally within the body, these substances influence the contractions of smooth

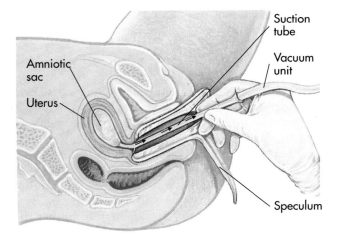

Figure 14-7 During dilation and evacuation, the cervix is dilated and the contents of the uterus are aspirated. This procedure is used to perform abortions up to 16 weeks' gestation.

muscle. Since the uterine wall is composed entirely of smooth muscle, it is particularly sensitive to the presence of prostaglandins. When prostaglandin is administered in sufficient quantity (through either a uterine intramuscular injection or a vaginal suppository), uterine contractions become strong enough to expel the fetal contents.

Third-trimester abortion procedures

Should termination of a pregnancy be required in the latter weeks of the gestational period, a surgical procedure in which the fetus will be removed (*hysterotomy*) or a procedure in which the entire uterus is removed (*hysterectomy*) can be undertaken. As you can imagine, these procedures are more complicated and involve longer hospitalization, major abdominal surgery, and an extended period of recovery.

The U.S. House of Representatives recently voted to ban a rarely used third trimester abortion procedure referred to as *dilation and extraction.* Lawmakers felt this procedure, also called *partial-birth abortion,* was too gruesome to be permitted. Do you know whether the U.S. Senate also passed this ban and whether the legislation is now in effect?

BECOMING PARENTS

Although birth control is especially important for many young couples, most couples eventually want to have children and raise a family. In the past, couples had their children very quickly after either high school or college. Now the trend seems to be to wait longer before having children. Most likely, educational, economic, contraceptive, and occupational factors have laid the groundwork for this trend. To the relief of many people, medical research indicates that women above the age of 30 or 35 are quite capable of having healthy babies.

Parenting Issues for Couples

Before deciding to have children, couples should have frank discussions about the effect that pregnancy and a newborn child will have on their lives. For those students contemplating single parenthood, we ask that you consider these issues as they relate to your particular situation and to excuse our consistent use of plural pronouns. In any event, some or all of the following basic considerations should be discussed:

- What effect will pregnancy have on us individually and collectively?
- Why do we want to have a child?

- What effect will a child have on the images we have constructed for ourselves as adults?
- Can we afford to have a child and provide for its needs?
- How will the responsibilities related to raising a child be divided?
- How will our professional careers be affected by the addition of a child?
- Are we ready now to accept the extended responsibilities that can come with a new child?
- How will we rear our child in terms of religious training, discipline, and participation in activities?
- Are we ready to part with much of the freedom associated with late adolescence and the early young adult years?
- How will we handle the possibility of being awakened by 6 AM each morning for the next few years?
- What plans have been made if we discover that our baby (or fetus) has a serious birth defect?
- Are we capable of handling the additional responsibilities associated with having a disabled child?
- Are we comfortable with the thought of bringing another child into an already overcrowded, violent, bigoted, and polluted world?

If these questions seem strikingly negative in tone, there is indeed a reason for this. We believe that all too frequently the "nuts and bolts" issues related to childbearing and parenting are ignored or at least are placed on the back burner. Although it is important for future parents to consider how cute and cuddly a new baby will be, how holidays will be enhanced with a new child, and how pleased the grandparents will be, we consider these issues secondary to the serious realities of having a child enter your lives. For a more detailed discussion of this topic, see "Focus on . . . The Consequences of Unintended Pregnancy" at the end of this chapter.

---

dilation and curettage (D & C) (kyoo re **tahzh**)
A surgical procedure in which the cervical canal is dilated to allow the uterine wall to be scraped.

hypertonic saline solution
A salt solution with a concentration higher than that found in human fluids.

A Parenting Prescription for the Early Years

Dr. T. Berry Brazelton, internationally known pediatrician and child development specialist, realizes how difficult it is to raise children in the 1990s. Brazelton knows that trying to juggle employment, college work, and family life is especially difficult and can at times seem overwhelming. Firm in his belief that parents can be successful at coping with busy schedules and raising well-adjusted children, Brazelton has identified 14 key parenting points for families with young children.[7]

1. *Separate your home and work environments.* Try to keep the two separate as much as possible.
2. *Plan your daily separation from your children.* Don't just separate without a warm exchange.
3. *Realize that it is okay to feel sad about leaving your child.* This will encourage you to get the best child care available.
4. *Allow yourself to feel a measure of guilt.* In this case, guilt can be a powerful source for solving problems.
5. *Share your stress with friends or support groups.* Interacting with others can provide much-needed support.
6. *Always include your spouse in family activities.* Let him or her have a significant role in important decisions.
7. *Do not feel that you must be a "superparent" or that you must raise "superkids."* Don't hold yourself up to standards that are virtually impossible to reach. It's not fair to you or your kids.
8. *While at work, conserve some energy for your home life.* Plan your day so that you are ready to do more than collapse in front of the television when you get home.
9. *Be sure you understand all the parenting options available at your workplace.* Know the policies related to day care, flexible time schedules, job-sharing possibilities, and sick leave if your child becomes ill.
10. *Prepare yourself for a bit of chaos when you return home after work.* Children often save some of their energy and feelings until they are back with their family.
11. *Hug or hold your young children for at least a few moments when you return from work.* Don't just come home and start your chores or housework without first making close contact with your children.
12. *Encourage your children to help you with your chores.* Most young children want to help. Be patient; encourage and praise their efforts.
13. *Make sure each child has some special time alone with each parent at least once every week.* This shows children that each child is important and deserves attention.
14. *Learn that stress is normal and that you can cope.* Solving problems together as a family can build warm and lasting relationships.

PREGNANCY: AN EXTENSION OF THE PARTNERSHIP

Pregnancy is a condition that requires a series of complex yet coordinated changes to occur in the female body. This chapter follows pregnancy from its beginning, at fertilization, to its conclusion, with labor and childbirth.

Physiological Obstacles and Aids to Fertilization

Many sexually active young people believe that they will become pregnant (or impregnate someone) only when they want to, despite their haphazard contraceptive practices. Because of this mistaken belief, many young people are not sold on the use of contraceptives. It is important for young adults to remember that from a species survival standpoint, our bodies were designed to promote pregnancy. It is estimated that about 85% of sexually active women of childbearing age will become pregnant within 1 year if they do not use some form of contraception.[2]

With regard to pregnancy, each act of intercourse can be considered a game of physiological odds. There are obstacles that may reduce a couple's chance of pregnancy, including the following:

Obstacles to fertilization

1. *The acidic level of the vagina is destructive to sperm.* The low pH of the vagina will kill sperm that fail to enter the uterus quickly.
2. *The cervical mucus is thick during most of the menstrual cycle.* Sperm movement into the uterus is more difficult, except during the few days surrounding ovulation.
3. *The sperm must locate the cervical opening.* The cervical opening is small compared with the rest of the surface area where sperm are deposited.
4. *Half of the sperm travel through the wrong fallopian tube.* Most commonly, only one ovum is released at ovulation. The two ovaries generally "take turns" each month. The sperm have no way of "knowing" which tube they should enter. Thus

it is probable that half will travel through the wrong tube.

5. *The distance sperm must travel is relatively long compared with the tiny size of the sperm cells.* Microscopic sperm must travel about 7 or 8 inches once they are inside the female.

6. *The sperm's travel is relatively "upstream."* The anatomical positioning of the female reproductive structures necessitates an "uphill" movement by the sperm.

7. *The contoured folds of the tubal walls trap many sperm.* These folds make it difficult for sperm to locate the egg. Many sperm are trapped in this maze.

There are also a variety of aids that tend to help sperm and egg cells join. Some of these are listed below.

Aids to fertilization

1. *An astounding number of sperm are deposited during ejaculation.* Each ejaculation contains about a teaspoon of semen.[8] Within this quantity are between 200 and 500 million sperm cells. Even with large numbers of sperm killed in the vagina, millions are able to move to the deeper structures.

2. *Sperm are deposited near the cervical opening.* Penetration into the vagina by the penis allows for the sperm to be placed near the cervical opening.

3. *The male accessory glands help make the semen nonacidic.* The seminal vesicles, prostate gland, and Cowper's glands secrete fluids that pro-vide an alkaline environment for the sperm. This environment helps sperm be better protected in the vagina until they can move into the deeper, more alkaline uterus and fallopian tubes.

4. *Uterine contractions aid sperm movement.* The rhythmic muscular contractions of the uterus tend to cause the sperm to move in the direction of the fallopian tubes.

5. *Sperm cells move rather quickly.* Despite their tiny size, sperm cells can move relatively quickly— just about 1 inch per hour. Powered by sugar solutions from the male accessory glands and the whiplike movements of their tails, sperm can reach the distant third of the fallopian tubes in less than 8 hours as they swim in the direction of the descending ovum.

6. *Once inside the fallopian tubes, sperm can live for days.* Some sperm may be viable for up to a week after reaching the comfortable, nonacidic environment of the fallopian tubes. Most sperm, however, will survive an average of 48 to 72 hours. Thus they can "wait in the wings" for the moment an ovum is released from the ovary (Figure 14-8).

7. *The cervical mucus is thin and watery at the time of ovulation.* This mucus allows for better passage of sperm through the cervical opening when the ovum is most capable of being fertilized.

Signs of Pregnancy

Aside from pregnancy tests done in a professional laboratory, a woman can sometimes recognize early signs and symptoms. The signs of pregnancy have been divided into three categories:

Presumptive signs of pregnancy

Missed period after unprotected intercourse the previous month

Nausea on awakening (morning sickness)

Increase in size and tenderness of breasts

Darkening of the areolar tissue surrounding the nipples

Probable signs of pregnancy

Increase in the frequency of urination (the growing uterus presses against the bladder)

Increase in the size of the abdomen

Cervix becomes softer by the sixth week (detected by a pelvic examination by clinician)

Positive pregnancy test (see the Star Box on p. 364)

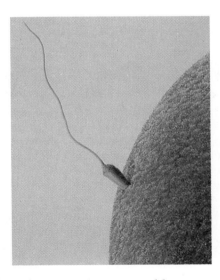

The surface of an ovum is penetrated by sperm at fertilization.

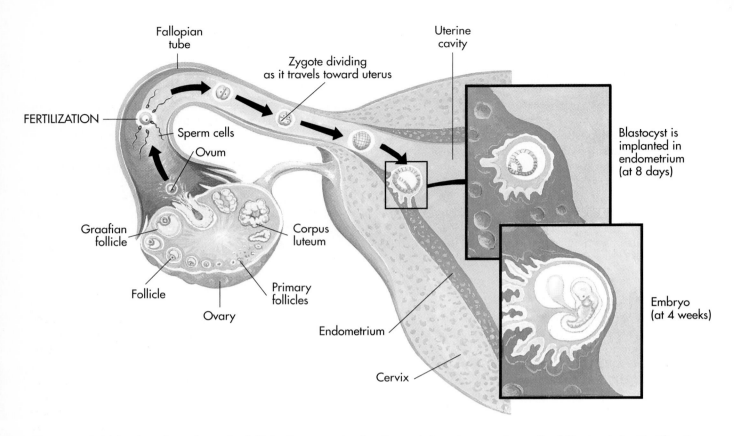

Figure 14-8   After its release from the follicle, the ovum begins its week-long journey down the fallopian tube. Fertilization generally occurs in the outermost third of the tube. Now fertilized, the ovum progresses toward the uterus, where it embeds itself in the endometrium. A pregnancy is established.

Positive signs of pregnancy

Determination of a fetal heartbeat

Feeling of the fetus moving (quickening)

Observation of fetus by ultrasound or optical viewers

Agents That Can Damage a Fetus

A large number of agents that come into contact with a pregnant woman can affect fetal development (see the Star Box on p. 365). Many of these (rubella

---

Home Pregnancy Tests

Home pregnancy test kits have been available for many years. Using technology similar to that in the laboratory-based immune response tests, these pregnancy tests can be conducted in the privacy of one's home. Home pregnancy tests use a urine sample to identify the hormone HCG. The low cost and convenience make these tests attractive to many people.

Despite these advantages, home pregnancy tests are not nearly as accurate as laboratory-based ones. Manufacturers claim that tests are 90% accurate, but research studies have found lower accuracy rates. Inaccuracies result not so much from the test itself but from the diffi-

culties some people have in following directions and interpreting the results. The most common error stems from using the test kit too early in pregnancy, before the HCG can be detected.[2] Such an error (in this case, a false negative) could delay important prenatal care.

Most physicians will immediately order a more accurate test when a woman indicates she had a positive result on her home pregnancy test. This raises questions about duplication of health care costs. Nevertheless, the convenience and privacy provided by home tests continue to make them popular items for sexually active couples.

The fetus at 16 weeks' gestation within the amniotic sac.

Warning: Acne, Accutane, and Birth Defects
Accutane, manufactured by Roche Laboratories, may be the most effective prescription drug for severe cystic acne, a type of acne that often causes deep scarring. In the spring of 1988 the FDA reissued an earlier warning that pregnant women should not use this drug, since it is capable of causing severe birth defects such as brain, skull, facial, and cardiac abnormalities. Women who use Accutane and are planning a pregnancy are encouraged to stop using the drug for two menstrual cycles before becoming pregnant. This gives the body time to clear Accutane from its system before conception. Some physicians recommend that women take a pregnancy test before beginning use of Accutane because of its severe effects on fetuses.

and herpes viruses, tobacco smoke, alcohol, and virtually all other drugs) are discussed in other chapters of this text. The best advice for a pregnant woman is to maintain close contact with her obstetrician during pregnancy and to consider carefully the ingestion of any OTC drug (including aspirin, caffeine, and antacids) that could harm the fetus.

It is also important for any woman to avoid exposure to radiation during the pregnancy. Such exposure, most commonly through excessive x-rays or radiation fallout from nuclear testing, can irreversibly damage fetal genetic structures.

CHILDBIRTH: THE LABOR OF DELIVERY

Childbirth, or *parturition*, is one of the true peak life experiences for both men and women. Most of the time, childbirth is a wonderfully exciting venture into the unknown. For the parents, this intriguing experience can provide a stage for personal growth, maturity, and insight into a dynamic, complex world.

During the last few weeks of the third **trimester,** most fetuses will move deeper into the pelvic cavity in a process called *lightening*. During this movement, the fetus's body will rotate and the head will begin to engage more deeply into the mother's pelvic girdle. Many women will report that their babies have "dropped."

Another indication that parturition may be relatively near is the increased reporting of *Braxton Hicks contractions*. These uterine contractions, which are of mild intensity and often occur at irregular intervals, may be felt throughout a pregnancy. During the last

few weeks of pregnancy *(gestation)*, these mild contractions can occur more frequently and cause a woman to feel as if she is going into labor **(false labor).**

Labor begins when uterine contractions become more intense and occur at regular intervals. The birth of a child can be divided into three stages: (1) *effacement* and dilation of the cervix, (2) delivery of the fetus, and (3) expulsion of the placenta (Figure 14-9). For a woman having her first child, the birth process lasts an average of 12 to 16 hours. The average length of labor for subsequent births is much shorter—from 4 to 10 hours on the average. Labor is very unpredictable: labors that last between 1 and 24 hours occur daily at most hospitals.

Stage One: Effacement and Dilation of the Cervix

In the first stage of labor the uterine contractions attempt to thin (efface) the normally thick cervical walls and to enlarge (dilate) the cervical opening. These contractions are directed by the release of

trimester
A 3-month period; human pregnancies encompass three trimesters.

false labor
Conditions that resemble the start of true labor; may include irregular uterine contractions, pressure, and discomfort in the lower abdomen.

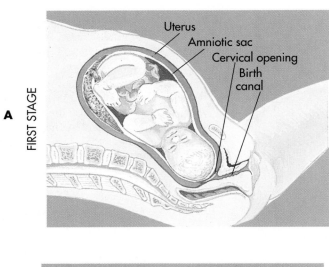

A

FIRST STAGE

Uterus
Amniotic sac
Cervical opening
Birth canal

Uterine contractions thin the cervix and enlarge the cervical opening

B

SECOND STAGE

Uterine contractions are aided by mother's voluntary contractions of abdominal muscles

Fetus moves through dilated cervical opening and birth canal

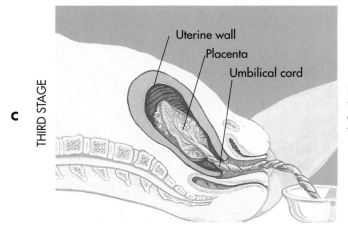

C

THIRD STAGE

Uterine wall
Placenta
Umbilical cord

Placenta detaches from uterine wall and is delivered through the vagina

Figure 14-9   Labor, or childbirth, is a three-stage process. During effacement and dilation, the first stage, the cervical canal is gradually opened by contractions of the uterine wall. The second stage, delivery of the baby, encompasses the actual delivery of the fetus from the uterus and through the birth canal. The delivery of the placenta, the third stage, empties the uterus, thus completing the process of childbirth.

prostaglandins and the hormone oxytocin into the circulating bloodstream. In women delivering their first babies, effacement will occur before dilation. In subsequent deliveries, effacement and dilation usually occur at the same time.

The first stage of labor is often the longest. The cervical opening must thin and dilate to a diameter of 10 cm before the first stage of labor is considered complete.[6] Often this stage begins with the dislodging of the cervical mucous plug. The subsequent *bloody show* (mucous plug and a small amount of blood) at the vaginal opening may indicate that effacement and dilation have begun. Another indication of labor's onset may be the bursting or tearing of the fetal amniotic sac. "Breaking the bag of waters" refers to this phenomenon, which happens in various measures in expectant women.

The pain of the uterine contractions becomes more intense as the woman moves through this first stage of labor. As the cervical opening effaces and dilates from 0 to 3 cm, many women report feeling happy, exhilarated, and confident. In the early phase of the first stage of labor, the contractions are relatively short (lasting from 15 to 60 seconds) and the intervals between contractions range from 20 minutes to 5 minutes as labor progresses. However, these rest intervals will become shorter and the contractions more forceful when the woman's uterus contracts to dilate 4 to 7 cm.

In this second phase of the first stage of labor, the contractions usually last about 1 minute each and the rest intervals drop from about 5 minutes to 1 minute over a period of 5 to 9 hours.

The third phase of the first stage of labor is called *transition*. During transition, the uterus contracts to dilate the cervical opening to the full 10 cm required for safe passage of the fetus out of the uterus and into the vagina (birth canal). This period of labor is often the most painful part of the entire birth process. Fortunately, it is also the shortest phase of most labors. Lasting between 15 and 30 minutes, transition contractions often last 60 to 90 seconds each. The rest intervals between contractions are short and vary from 30 to 60 seconds.

An examination of the cervix by a nurse or physician will reveal whether full dilation of 10 cm has occurred. Until the full 10-cm dilation, women are cautioned not to "push" the fetus during the contractions. Special breathing and concentration techniques help many women cope with the first stage of labor.

Stage Two: Delivery of the Fetus

Once the mother's cervix is fully dilated, she enters the second stage of labor, the delivery of the fetus through the birth canal. Now the mother is encouraged to help push the baby out (with her abdominal muscles) during each contraction. In this second stage the uterine contractions are less forceful than during the transition phase of the first stage and may last 60 seconds each, with a 1- to 3-minute rest interval.

This second stage may last up to 2 hours in first births.[8] For subsequent births, this stage will usually be much shorter. When the baby's head is first seen at the vaginal opening, *crowning* is said to have taken place. Generally the back of the baby's head appears first. (Infants whose feet or buttocks are presented first are said to be delivered in a *breech position*.) Once the head is delivered, the baby's body rotates upward to let the shoulders come through. The rest of the body follows quite quickly. The second stage of labor ends when the fetus is fully expelled from the vagina.

Newly delivered babies often look far different from the babies seen on television commercials. Their heads are often cone-shaped as a result of the compression of cranial bones that occurs during the delivery through the birth canal. Within a few days after birth, the newborn's head will assume a much more normal shape. Most babies (of all races) appear bluish at first until they begin regular breathing. All babies are covered with a coating of *vernix,* a white, cheese-like substance that protects the skin.

Stage Three: Delivery of the Placenta

Usually within 30 minutes after the fetus is delivered, the uterus will again initiate a series of contractions to expel the placenta (or *afterbirth*). The placenta is examined by the attending physician to ensure that it was completely expelled. Torn remnants of the placenta could lead to dangerous *hemorrhaging* by the mother. Often the physician will perform a manual examination of the uterus after the placenta has been delivered.

Once the placenta has been delivered, the uterus will continue with mild contractions to help control bleeding and start the gradual reduction of the uterus to its normal, nonpregnant size. This final aspect of the birth process is called **postpartum.** External abdominal massage of the lower abdomen seems to help the uterus contract, as does an infant's nursing at the mother's breast.

---

postpartum
The period after the birth of a baby during which the uterus returns to its prepregnancy size.

Cesarean Deliveries

A **cesarean delivery** (cesarean birth, C-section) is a procedure in which the fetus is surgically removed from the mother's uterus through the abdominal wall. This type of delivery, which is completed in up to an hour, can be performed with the mother having a regional or a general anesthetic.

Currently, 23% of all deliveries are by cesarean section.[5] The use of cesarean deliveries is questioned by some medical experts, although others point to the need for this kind of delivery when one or more of the following factors are present:

- The fetus is improperly positioned.
- The mother's pelvis is too small.
- The fetus is especially large.
- The fetus shows signs of respiratory or cardiac distress.
- The umbilical cord is compressed.
- The placenta is being delivered before the fetus.
- The mother's health is at risk.

Although a cesarean delivery is considered major surgery, most mothers cope well with the delivery and postsurgical and postpartum discomfort. The hospital stay is usually a few days longer than for a vaginal delivery. The mother can still nurse her child and may still be able to have vaginal deliveries with later children. More and more hospitals are allowing the father to be in the operating room during cesarean deliveries. Fortunately, research indicates that early **bonding** between child, mother, and father can still occur with cesarean deliveries. Cesarean deliveries are much more expensive than vaginal deliveries.

INFERTILITY

Most traditional-age college students are interested in preventing pregnancy. However, increasing numbers of other people are trying to do just the opposite: they are trying to become pregnant. It is estimated that about one in six couples has a problem with *infertility*. These couples wish to become pregnant but are unsuccessful.

Why are couples infertile? These reasons are about evenly balanced between men and women. About 10% of infertility cases have no detectable cause. The most frequent male complication is insufficient sperm production and delivery. A number of approaches can be used to increase sperm counts. Among the simple approaches are the application of periodic cold packs on the scrotum and the replacement of tight underwear with boxer shorts. When a structural problem reduces sperm production, surgery can be helpful. Opinion is divided concerning whether increased fre-

quency of intercourse improves fertility. Most experts (fertility endocrinologists) suggest that couples have intercourse at least a couple of times in the week preceding ovulation.

Men can also collect (through masturbation) and save samples of their sperm to use in a procedure called *artificial insemination by partner*. Near the time of ovulation, the collected samples of sperm are then deposited near the woman's cervical opening. In the related procedure called *artificial insemination by donor*, the sperm of a donor are used. Donor semen is screened for the presence of pathogens, including the AIDS virus.

Causes of infertility in women center mostly on obstructions in the reproductive tract and the inability to ovulate. The obstructions frequently result from tissue damage (scarring) caused by infections. Chlamydial and gonorrheal infections often produce fertility problems. In certain women the use of IUDs has produced infections and PID; both of these increase the chances of infertility. Other possible causes of structural abnormalities include scar tissue from previous surgery, fibroid tumors, polyps, and endometriosis. A variety of microsurgical techniques may correct some of these complications.

One of the most recent innovative procedures involves the use of **transcervical balloon tuboplasty.** In this procedure a series of balloon-tipped catheters are inserted through the uterus into the blocked fallopian tubes. Once inflated, these balloon catheters help open the scarred passageways.

When a woman has ovulation difficulties, pinpointing the specific cause can be very difficult. Increasing age produces hormone fluctuations associated with lack of ovulation. Being significantly overweight or underweight also has a serious effect on fertility. However, in women of normal weight who are not approaching menopause, it appears that ovulation difficulties are caused by failure of synchronization between the hormones governing the menstrual cycle. Fertility drugs can help alter the menstrual cycle to produce ovulation. Clomiphene citrate (Clomid), in oral pill form, and injections of a mixture of LH and FSH taken from the urine of menopausal women (Pergonal) are the most common fertility drugs available. Both are capable of producing multiple ova at ovulation.

For couples who are unable to conceive after drug therapy, surgery, and artificial insemination, the use of *in vitro fertilization and embryo transfer (IVF-ET)* is another option. This method is sometimes referred to as the "test tube" procedure. Costing up to $10,000 per attempt, IVF-ET consists of surgically retrieving fertilizable ova from the woman and combining them in a glass dish with sperm. After several days, the fertilized ova are transferred into the uterus. The pregnancy success rate for a single treatment cycle is 19%.[9]

A newer test tube procedure is called *gamete intrafallopian transfer (GIFT)*. Similar to IVF-ET, this procedure deposits a mixture of retrieved eggs and sperm directly into the fallopian tubes. The pregnancy success rate for a single treatment cycle is 29%.[9]

Fertilized ova (zygotes) can also be transferred from a laboratory dish into the fallopian tubes in a procedure called *zygote intrafallopian transfer (ZIFT)*. One advantage of this procedure is that the clinicians are certain that ova have been fertilized before the transfer to the fallopian tubes.

Surrogate parenting is another option that has been explored in the last decade, although the legal and ethical issues surrounding this method of conception have not been fully resolved. Surrogate parenting exists in a number of forms. Typically, an infertile couple will make a contract with a woman (the surrogate parent), who will then be artificially inseminated with semen from the expectant father. In some instances the surrogate will receive an embryo from the donor parents. In some cases, women have served as surrogates for their close relatives. The surrogate will carry the fetus to term and return the newborn to the parents. Because of the concerns about true "ownership" of the baby, surrogate parenting may not be a particularly viable or legal option for many couples. The Star Box at right points out some serious questions raised by surrogate parenting.

The process of coping with infertility problems can be an emotionally stressful experience for a couple. Hours of waiting in physicians' offices, having numerous examinations, scheduling intercourse, producing sperm samples, and undergoing surgical or drug treatments place multiple burdens on a couple. Knowing that other couples are able to conceive so effortlessly adds to the mental strain. Fortunately, support groups exist to assist couples with infertility problems. Some of these groups are listed in the Star Box on p. 370.

What can you do to reduce the chances of developing infertility problems? Certainly avoiding infections of the reproductive organs is one crucial factor. Barrier methods of contraception (condom, diaphragm) with a spermicide reportedly cut the risk of developing infertility in half. The use of an IUD should be carefully considered, and the risk from multiple partners should encourage responsible sexual activity. Men and women should be aware of the dangers from

Surrogate Parenting: Unresolved Questions

Many important questions regarding surrogate parenting have been raised during the last 5 years. Among these are the following:

- Does the surrogate mother sell a service or a product?
- If a surrogate mother charges and is paid a fee, is this different from giving her service free of charge? Do her rights to the baby change?
- Do the people who receive the services of a surrogate mother have the right to reject the baby if it is handicapped or otherwise unacceptable?
- Does the surrogate mother have a right to keep the child?
- Does the surrogate mother have visitation rights to the child?
- Can the infertile couple require the surrogate mother not to consume alcohol, tobacco, or other dangerous products during the pregnancy?
- How can the infertile couple monitor the pregnancy?
- Who pays for long-term health care if the surrogate mother's health status is harmed by the pregnancy or delivery?

working around hazardous chemicals or consuming psychoactive drugs. Maintaining overall good health and having regular medical (and, for women, gynecological) checkups are also good ideas. Finally, since infertility is linked with advancing age, couples may not want to indefinitely delay having children.

cesarean delivery (si **zare** ee an)
Surgical removal of a fetus through the abdominal wall.

bonding
Important initial recognition established between the newborn and those adults on whom the newborn will be dependent.

transcervical balloon tuboplasty
The use of inflatable balloon catheters to open blocked fallopian tubes; a procedure used for some women with fertility problems.

Where to Find Help for Infertility
These agencies can provide you with information about infertility and give referrals to specialists in your area:

American Fertility Society
The Society for Reproductive Medicine
1209 Montgomery Highway
Birmingham, AL 35216-2809
(205) 978-5000

Planned Parenthood Federation of America
810 Seventh Avenue
New York, NY 10019
(212) 541-7800
(800) 829-7732

These agencies can provide help to prospective adoptive parents:
The National Adoption Center
1500 Walnut Street
Suite 701
Philadelphia, PA 19102
(215) 735-9988

The National Committee for Adoption
1930 17th Street, N.W.
Washington, DC 20009
(212) 328-8072

The North American Council on Adoptable Children
1821 University Avenue
Room N-498
St. Paul, MN 55104
(612) 644-3036

Adoptive Families of America, Inc.
3333 Highway 100 North
Minneapolis, MN 55422
(612) 535-4829
Publishes *OURS* Magazine (Organization for United Response)

Summary

- *Birth control* refers to all of the procedures that can prevent the birth of a child.
- *Contraception* refers to any procedure that prevents fertilization.
- Each birth control method has both a theoretical effectiveness rate and a use effectiveness rate. For some contraceptive approaches, these rates are similar (such as hormonal methods), and for others the rates are very different (such as condoms, diaphragms, and periodic abstinence).
- Many factors should be considered when deciding which contraceptive is best for you.
- Sterilization (vasectomy and tubal ligation) is usually considered an irreversible procedure.

- Currently, abortion remains a woman's choice under the guidelines of the 1973 *Roe v. Wade* decision and various state restrictions.
- Abortion procedures vary according to the stage of the pregnancy.
- There are many important issues for couples to discuss before deciding to have children.
- Childbirth takes place in three distinct stages: effacement and dilation of the cervix, delivery of the fetus, and delivery of the placenta.
- Infertility is an important concern for some couples. Various technologies are improving infertile couples' chances of having children.

Review Questions

1. Explain the difference between the terms *birth control* and *contraception*. Give examples of each.
2. Explain the difference between theoretical and use effectiveness rates. Which one is always higher? Why is it important to know the difference between these two rates?

3. Identify some of the factors that should be given careful consideration when selecting a contraceptive method. Explain each factor.
4. For each of the methods of birth control, explain how it works and its advantages and disadvantages.

5. How do minipills differ from the combined oral contraceptive? What is a morning-after pill? How do subdermal implants (Norplant) differ from Depo-Provera?
6. Identify and describe the different abortion procedures that are used during each trimester of pregnancy. When is the safest time for an abortion?

7. What are some obstacles and aids to fertilization presented in this chapter? Can you think of others?
8. Identify and describe the events that occur during each of the three stages of childbirth. Approximately how long is each stage?
9. What can be done to reduce chances of infertility? Explain IVF-ET, GIFT, and ZIFT procedures.

 Think About This . . .

- What factors would be most important to you in selecting an appropriate contraceptive method?
- How well do you think college students understand that oral contraceptives do not protect against STDs, including HIV infection?
- Under what circumstances, if any, do you believe abortion is acceptable? Unacceptable?
- Will you or your partner someday undergo sterilization? If so, which of you will have the surgery?
- Can you identify locations at or near your college where professional family-planning services are available?

- What effects do you think starting parenthood at a later age has on the parent and on the child?
- How do you feel about a couple's choice not to have children?
- If a woman should not smoke, drink, or use other drugs during pregnancy, should these limitations also be placed on the father? Why or why not?
- To what extent should fathers participate in the birth experience?
- Do you plan to become a parent? If so, when?

References

1. Masters WH, Johnson VE, Kolodny RC: *Human sexuality,* ed 5, New York, 1995, HarperCollins.
2. Hatcher RA et al: *Contraceptive technology,* ed 16, New York, 1994, Irvington.
3. Goldberg MS: Choosing a contraceptive, *FDA Consumer* 27(7):18-25, 1993.
4. Farley TMM et al: Intrauterine devices and pelvic inflammatory disease: an international study, *Lancet* 339(8796):785-788, 1992.
5. US Bureau of the Census: *Statistical abstract of the United States: 1995,* ed 115, Washington, DC, 1995, US Government Printing Office.
6. Haas K, Haas A: *Understanding sexuality,* ed 3, St Louis, 1993, Mosby.
7. Brazelton TB: Bringing up baby: a doctor's prescription for busy parents, *Newsweek* p 68, Feb 13, 1989.
8. Hyde JS: *Understanding human sexuality,* ed 5, New York, 1994, McGraw-Hill.
9. Medical Research International, Society for Assisted Reproductive Technology, The American Fertility Society: In-vitro fertilization-embryo transfer (IVF-ET) in the United States: 1990 results from the IVF-ET registry, *Fertil Steril* (57)1:15, 1992.
10. Population Information Program: Mothers' lives matter: maternal health in the community, *Population Reports* 16:2, 1988; Series L: No 7, Center for Communications Programs; Johns Hopkins University.

Suggested Readings

Jones C: *Breastfeeding your baby: a guide for the contemporary family,* New York, 1993, Collins Books.

A certified childbirth educator covers practical advice on all aspects of breastfeeding. Topics include preventing and solving problems, how to combine breastfeeding and bottle-feeding, and how family and friends can help. Clear illustrations and straightforward advice.

Rosenberg HS, Epstein YM: *Getting pregnant when you thought you couldn't: the interactive guide that helps you up the odds,* New York, 1993, Warner Books.

A useful resource for infertile couples, written by a nationally recognized married couple who have themselves struggled to conceive a child. Presents lots of information in a sensitive, thorough manner.

Sears W, Sears M: *The birth book: everything you need to know to have a safe and satisfying birth,* Boston, 1994, Little, Brown.

The authors are parents of eight children and are nationally renowned pediatric specialists. Gives expectant parents practical advice about every aspect of birthing, including preparing for birth, labor, and delivery. Issues of using technology, defining the father's role, and turning the surgical birth into a rewarding experience are discussed.

Walker M: *Sexual nutrition,* Garden City Park, NY, 1994, Avery Publishing Group.

An examination of factors related to fertility: nutrients and their relation to improved sex drive, stamina, and performance. A guide to enhancing relationships through healthful changes in diet.

The Consequences of Unintended Pregnancy

"It can't happen to me."

This thought is often used to justify risky actions. Sometimes we even get away with it. We write a bad check but manage to get money to the bank in time to cover it. We leave the seat belt off for a short trip down the block. Sometimes we have sex without protection. It's not the right time in the cycle to get pregnant. Only one pill was missed. Nothing will happen, we tell ourselves. It can't happen to me.

Each day, thousands of single women receive the news that they are pregnant.[1] For those who have been trying to have a child, this news is welcomed. For others, however, the news may not be so joyous. Even in ideal situations, an unintended pregnancy can cause emotional and financial strain for the woman, the potential father, and their families.

Important People in the Decision-Making Process

If the father-to-be or the potential grandparents were not there to hear the news with her, the woman faces the task of telling them she's pregnant. This is often a time of fear and uncertainty for the woman, and the way these people ultimately handle the news can be of critical importance to her.[2] A supportive family and father-to-be make later decision processes easier to deal with, whereas lack of support is sure to cause problems down the road.

The decisions of the potential father concerning the woman and an unplanned pregnancy are extremely important. He may abandon the woman altogether, which will make support from the woman's family even more critical. If he chooses to stay, more decisions must be made. He may want to marry her. He may not want marriage but may still want to play an active role in supporting and rearing the child. He may want to play only a limited role. Whatever his decision, his role is a determining factor for decisions to be made later.

The families of both parents-to-be also play an important role in determining the outcome of the situation, especially when the potential parents are young. In many situations the families may be the primary source of financial support, and lack of this support may prove devastating. The type of emotional support that the potential grandparents provide to the young couple may also be crucial to their decisions regarding the unexpected pregnancy.

Marriage

Traditionally, marriage has been the most socially acceptable alternative for pregnant women and their partners.

In recent years, however, unwed motherhood has become more common and less stigmatized. Currently 30% of births in the United States are to unmarried women, and only 33% of teenage mothers are married.[1,3] Economic factors may play a role in determining whether or not a couple should get married when an unexpected pregnancy occurs. If the woman is financially secure or is receiving financial support from her family, she may find that single parenthood is the most desirable option. If income from both parents is necessary to support the child, marriage may prove to be the logical choice.

Cultural norms may also be considered in the marriage decision. In some segments of American culture, marriage is not considered a necessary consequence of an unplanned pregnancy. Common-law marriages (a relationship where both partners consent to live as a married couple without the formal exchange of vows) are more accepted in Hispanic-American culture.[3] In African-American culture the family is often more matriarchal (female-centered) in structure, reducing the role of the father.[4] In white culture, marriage is more often considered to be the most acceptable choice, but marriage is not always an inevitable step after pregnancy. The belief systems within different cultures are often very strong determining factors in the decisions made by potential parents.

Abortion

Eventually a decision must be reached concerning the fate of the child. The woman must decide to become a parent, put the child up for adoption, or terminate her pregnancy. Some women may consider abortion as an option. This decision is often a complicated and difficult one. The viability of choosing abortion may strongly depend on where a woman lives, her financial situation, and who is involved in the decision-making process with her. A woman is also faced with moral, religious, and legal questions when making such a decision. If her religious and moral beliefs are not compatible with those of her family or the father-to-be, these relationships may become greatly strained. The woman may also struggle with her own belief system and religious upbringing when making such a decision. For younger girls, the decision may be further complicated by the law. Many states require parental consent before an abortion is performed for girls below a certain age. This may eliminate the abortion option for those girls who do not want their parents to know about their pregnancies or for girls whose parents refuse to give consent.[5]

Although an abortion eliminates many long-term financial obligations, this option can be quite expensive in the short term. Because of restricted federal funding for abortion providers, the procedure usually costs several hundred dollars, and the price can run into the thousands for late-term abortions. Elective abortion is not normally covered by insurance, so the cost is strictly out-of-pocket. In many states the low availability of abortion providers is also an obstacle; a day's drive or an overnight stay is sometimes needed. The time involved may make a "secret" trip to a clinic difficult to pull off without deception of family, friends, or employers.[5]

Adoption

Putting the baby up for adoption may be an acceptable alternative for those women who reject abortion but do not wish to take on the responsibilities of childbearing. Many women may choose this option if they are not able to financially support a baby but also cannot consider aborting the child because of moral convictions. This option may eliminate the lifetime financial commitment but may be very difficult to deal with emotionally. The act of giving up a baby after carrying it to term can be heart-rending. The mother may have misgivings about the adoption for many years afterward. Many women who initially choose adoption for their child wind up changing their minds along the way, sometimes even after the baby is born. In recent years, several bitter court battles have been waged over such situations.

Parenthood

If the mother chooses the parenthood option, carrying the baby to term requires selfless devotion to its care. This often requires budgeting for the baby's needs well before it is born.[6] Most first-time parents do not realize the enormous costs that having a baby entails. The cost of giving birth varies widely among states. In 1993 the average total cost of hospital and physician charges for an uncomplicated vaginal delivery was $8840 in New York, but less than half that amount in Arkansas. New York was the most expensive state in which to have a cesarean delivery, with an average cost of $13,700, whereas a cesarean birth in Oklahoma cost about $7730.[7] Pediatrician bills during the first year of a child's life average $600 (assuming the child is healthy), and other necessities for the baby are even more expensive. For example, diapers can run between $500 and $700 a year during the pre–potty training days.[8] Clothes can cost as much as $1000 the first year because the child grows so quickly. Feeding can cost as much as $2000, depending on whether the mother is willing or able to breastfeed.[8]

Because of the large amount of money involved, immediate gratification must be put on hold to save money for later use. For many new parents, this is a problem, especially if they are suddenly being forced to take care of their own finances with little or no help from family. The mother may have to make major changes in lifestyle as well to keep the unborn child healthy. Drinking and smoking should be avoided, which may be quite difficult for those women who are used to participating in these activities. Abstaining from tobacco and alcohol use while out with friends may be difficult for some, and staying home from such outings may strain relationships with friends. As with family, the support of friends can go a long way toward easing the strain of an unintended pregnancy.[6]

Prenatal Care, Day Care, and Insurance

Prenatal care is necessary but can be costly and difficult to find. For a typical, uncomplicated pregnancy, the average cost for adequate prenatal care is $500.[8] Finding a doctor who will supervise care of the baby through birth is becoming more difficult because of the increasing number of lawsuits filed against doctors for malpractice. Such suits have driven many physicians out of obstetrics and caused others to raise prices. To lessen the risk of such suits, doctors who are willing to provide prenatal care are often requiring that expectant women stick to a strict set of behavioral guidelines. A woman is often asked to reveal and document intimate details about her sexual activity, menstrual history, and personal habits. Free clinics are available in some areas for those who cannot afford care otherwise, but the same behavioral restrictions and intense questioning can be expected there as well.[6]

Women who decide to become parents must take steps to ensure that the baby will be taken care of after it is born. The mother must arrange for day care if she hopes to work or continue with school. This can be a problem if there is no spouse or family member able or willing to take care of the baby during times when the mother is gone. Many day care facilities do not take care of newborns, and some require that the child be potty-trained before enrolling. Day care facilities can be quite expensive and often have waiting lists for admission. U.S. Census Bureau data place the average cost of day care for a family with a preschool child and working mother at $79 per week in 1993.[9] These costs tend to be higher in the West and Northeast and in urban environments.[9,10] Preschool day care in urban areas averaged about $400 per month in 1992, care in the urban Northeast averaged $500 per month, and the average for the rural South was $300 per month.[10] More workplaces and schools are now offering free or inexpensive day care services, but such programs are not found everywhere, and waiting lists cause delays as well. Some women are forced to take time off from school because of unintended pregnancy, and some leave altogether resulting from the financial hardships and physical strain of balancing school and parenthood. About half of all teenage mothers drop out of school.[1] Recent legislation has made it easier for new parents to take leave from work without penalty, but the law does not apply to all employers. As a result, some women are forced to leave jobs to care for their children.

Insurance can also be difficult to obtain for the baby. Some providers have waiting periods before insuring an individual.[6] A woman covered under her parents' policies may find that her own child cannot be covered, requiring the woman to obtain a separate policy for the baby. Some companies may not offer coverage of individuals.[6] Obtaining a new policy for mother and unborn child may be difficult as well. Some companies may treat pregnancy as a preexisting condition that may not be covered.[6] Making a budget and sticking to it is therefore crucial to cover medical costs until insurance can be obtained.

In the heat of passion, people often fail to think rationally about the potential outcomes of unprotected sex. Therefore the time to prepare for the romantic moment is *before* you are in a position where you don't want to think about the possibility of an unintended result. If you choose to be sexually active, find a form of contraception that works for you and use it consistently.

For Discussion . . .
What would you do if you (or your partner) became pregnant unintentionally? What decisions would you make regarding the pregnancy? If you are a parent, how would you react if one of your children was involved in an unintended pregnancy? Would your personal decisions be different?

References
1. Book bags and baby bottles, *Scholastic Update* 127(11), March 1995.
2. Bezduch-Moore SL: I was pregnant at sixteen, *Teen Magazine* 39(3), March 1995.
3. Russell C: Why teen births boom, *American Demographics* September 1995.
4. Freeman EW, Rickels K: *Early childbearing: perspectives of black adolescents on pregnancy, abortion, and contraception,* Newbury Park, Calif, 1993, Sage Publications.
5. Thompson S: *Going all the way: teenage girls' tales of sex, romance and pregnancy,* New York, 1995, Hill and Wang.
6. Foglino A: Single, pregnant, and struggling to stay in college, *Glamour* November 1995.
7. Winthrop A: How much does it cost to give birth? *American Baby,* p 14, May 1995.
8. What price parenthood, *Town and Country Monthly* 148(5169), June 1994.
9. Census data on child care, *Children Today* 23(4), Fall/Winter 1995.
10. Mitchell A: Day care in the '90s, *Good Housekeeping* 215(3), Sept 1992.

PART 6

CONSUMERISM AND ENVIRONMENT

Making Consumer and Health Care Choices

Healthy People 2000 Objectives

Access to primary medical services by virtually every member of the community is a cornerstone of health consumerism and is an important Healthy People 2000 objective. The Midcourse Review reports that limited progress has been made toward achieving this goal. At the current rate, the objective will not be fully met by the year 2000.

One glance at today's newspaper will demonstrate that our nation has a long way to go in making primary and preventive health care affordable to every person, which was another Healthy People 2000 objective. The Midcourse Review does not assess progress toward this goal. Perhaps by the end of the decade, we will have a more comprehensive approach to meeting this critical need.

Another objective was for pharmacies and other dispensers of medications to become electronically linked so that information about potentially harmful drug interactions and drug/condition interactions could be shared with consumers of these medications. The Midcourse Review does not address this objective. However, we can assume that the consolidation of pharmacies into national chains and the development of computer software are contributing to the rapid development of this system.

Health care providers often evaluate you by criteria pertaining to their area of expertise. The nutritionist knows you by the food you eat. The physical fitness professional knows you by your body type and activity level. In the eyes of the expert in health-related consumerism, you are the product of the health information you believe, the health-influencing services you use, and the products you consume. When your decisions about health information, services, and products are made after careful study and consideration, your health will probably be improved. However, when your decisions lack insight, your health, as well as your pocketbook, may suffer.

HEALTH INFORMATION
The Informed Consumer

To be an informed consumer, people must learn about services and products that can influence health. Practitioners, manufacturers, advertisers, and sales personnel use a variety of approaches in an attempt to get individuals to buy these products or use these services. Because health is potentially at stake when people "buy" into these messages, informed consumerism is important. Complete the Personal Assessment on p. 380 to rate your own skills as a health care consumer.

Sources of Information

The sources of information on a particular health topic to which you have access are as diverse as the number of people you know, the number of publications you read, and the number of experts you see or hear. At present, no single agency or profession regulates the quantity or quality of the health-related information you receive. In the section that follows, we look at many different sources of information. Readers will quickly recognize that all are familiar sources and that some provide more accurate and honest information than others.

Family and friends
From a health consumerism point of view, the accuracy of information provided by a friend or family member may be questionable. Too often the information provided by family and friends is based on common knowledge that is wrong. In addition, family members or friends may provide information they believe is in your best interests rather than providing factual information that may have a more negative effect on you.

Beyond simply wanting to help, today more than ever, family and friends may provide health-related information as a part of their involvement in the pyramid sales of health products. Strong encouragement toward the use of a particular line of food supplements or vitamins could lead to a forceful sales pitch or even the offer of an opportunity to be a part of their sales team.

Advertisements and commercials
Many people spend a good portion of every day watching television, listening to the radio, and reading newspapers or magazines. Since many advertisements are health oriented, you should not be surprised to learn that these are significant sources of information. You should also remember that the primary purpose of advertising is to sell products or services. Perhaps no single combination of these factors is more evident than in the currently popular "infomercials" in which a compensated studio audience watches a skillfully produced program designed to inform them about the benefits of a particular product or service.

In contrast to advertisements and commercials, the mass media routinely supplies public service messages that give valuable health-related information.

Labels and directions
Federal law requires that many consumer product labels, including many kinds of food (see Chapter 5) and all medications, contain specific information. For example, when a prescription medication is dispensed by a pharmacist, a detailed information sheet describing the drug should be given along with the medication (Figure 15-1).

Many health care providers and agencies provide consumers with detailed directions about their health problem. Generally, information from these sources is accurate, current, and provided with the health of the consumer in mind.

Folklore
Because it is often passed down from generation to generation, folklore about health is the primary source of health-related information for some people.

The truthfulness of health-related information obtained from family members, neighbors, and co-workers is difficult to evaluate. As a general rule, however, we would recommend caution concerning its scientific soundness. A blanket criticism is not warranted, however, since folk wisdom is on occasion supported by scientific evidence. Also, the emotional support provided by the suppliers of this information could be the best medicine some people need.

PERSONAL ASSESSMENT

Are You a Skilled Health Consumer?

Circle the selection that best describes your practice. Then total your points for an interpretation of your health consumer skills.

    1   Never
    2   Occasionally
    3   Most of the time
    4   All of the time

1. I read all warranties and then file them for safekeeping.   1 2 3 4
2. I read labels for information pertaining to the nutritional quality of food.   1 2 3 4
3. I practice comparative shopping and use unit pricing, when available.   1 2 3 4
4. I read health-related advertisements in a critical and careful manner.   1 2 3 4
5. I challenge all claims pertaining to secret cures or revolutionary new health devices.   1 2 3 4
6. I engage in appropriate medical self-care screening procedures.   1 2 3 4
7. I maintain a patient-provider relationship with a variety of health care providers.   1 2 3 4
8. I inquire about the fees charged before using a health care provider's services.   1 2 3 4
9. I maintain adequate health insurance coverage.   1 2 3 4
10. I consult reputable medical self-care books before seeing a physician.   1 2 3 4
11. I ask pertinent questions of health care providers when I am uncertain about the information I have received.   1 2 3 4
12. I seek second opinions when the diagnosis of a condition or the recommended treatment seems questionable.   1 2 3 4
13. I follow directions pertaining to the use of prescription drugs, including continuing their use for the entire period prescribed.   1 2 3 4
14. I buy generic drugs when they are available.   1 2 3 4
15. I follow directions pertaining to the use of OTC drugs.   1 2 3 4
16. I maintain a well-supplied medicine cabinet.   1 2 3 4

YOUR TOTAL POINTS _____

Interpretation

16-24 points   A very poorly skilled health consumer
25-40 points   An inadequately skilled health consumer
41-56 points   An adequately skilled health consumer
57-64 points   A highly skilled health consumer

To Carry This Further . . .

Could you ever have been the victim of consumer fraud? What will you need to do to be a skilled consumer?

Testimonials

People feel strongly about sharing information that has been beneficial to them. The recommendations made by other people concerning a particular practitioner or health-related product may at first appear to be nothing more than testimonials. Since they are frequently the basis for decision-making by others, we assign a small measure of importance to them as sources of health-related information. However, the exaggerated testimonials that accompany the sales pitches of the medical quack or the "satisfied" customers appearing in advertisements and on commercials and infomercials should never be interpreted as valid endorsements.

Mass media

Health programming on cable television stations, lifestyle sections in newspapers, health care correspondents appearing on national network news shows, and a growing number of health-oriented magazines are four examples of health-related information in the mass media.

Although in general, health-related information is presented well, it is sometimes presented with such

Prozac 20 Mg Pulvule
Fluoxetine—Oral

USES: This medication is used to treat mental depression, obsessive-compulsive symptoms associated with Tourette's disorder, and in the treatments of obesity and bulimia nervosa.

This medication has also been used to treat PMS (premenstrual syndrome).

HOW TO TAKE THIS MEDICATION: May be taken with food to prevent stomach upset.

Take this as prescribed. Try to take each dose at the same time(s) each day so you remember to routinely take it.

SIDE EFFECTS: May cause drowsiness or dizziness. Use caution performing tasks that require alertness.

Other side effects include heartburn, loss of appetite, headache, anxiety, flushing or sweating, change in sexual desire or ability. If these symptoms persist or become bothersome, inform your doctor.

Notify your doctor if you develop a rapid heart rate., difficulty breathing, difficulty urinating, a rash or hives while taking this medication.

PRECAUTIONS: Tell doctor if you had a recent heart attack or if you have a history of seizures; heart, liver, or kidney disease; or diabetes.

Fluoxetine may affect the amount of glucose (sugar) in your blood, so your dosage of diabetes medication may need to be adjusted when fluoxetine is started or discontinued.

Women who are pregnant, plan to become pregnant, or are breast-feeding should inform their doctors.

Avoid alcohol while taking this medication.

DRUG INTERACTIONS: Before taking fluoxetine, tell your doctor what prescription and nonprescription medications you are taking (or have taken in the last two weeks), especially tranquilizers, antidepressants (Buspar), MAO inhibitors (isocarboxazid or Marplan, phenelzine or Nardil, tranylcypromine or Parnate), lithium, tryptophan, medication for anxiety (tranquilizers like Valium), and medication for diabetes.

Do not take any nonprescription medication without consulting your doctor.

NOTES: Do not allow anyone else to take this medication.

MISSED DOSE: It is not necessary to make up the missed does. Skip the missed dose and resume your usual dosing shedule. Do not "double up " the dose to catch up.

STORAGE: Store at room temperature between 59 and 86 degrees F (between 15 and 30 degrees C) away from moisture and sunlight. Do not store in the bathroom.

The information in this leaflet may be used as an educational aid. This information does not cover all possible uses. actions, precautions, side effects, or interactions of this medicine. This information is not intended as medical advice for individual problems.

Copyright First Databank—The Hearst Corporation

Figure 15-1   Prozac, a serotonin-specific antidepressant, is one of today's most frequently prescribed medications. Note that it has several "off-label" uses beyond depression. Pharmacies provide patient information sheets like this one with each prescription dispensed.

quickness or superficiality that it is of limited use. However, the consumer who desires more complete coverage of a health-related topic can obtain it by combining sources. This is particularly possible with information sources related to the coverage given to nutrition, AIDS, heart disease, and cancer.

Practitioners

The health care consumer also receives much information from individual health practitioners and their professional associations. In fact, patient education is so clearly provided by today's health care practitioner that finding one who does not exchange some information with a patient would be unusual. Education enhances patient **compliance** with health care directives, which is important to the practitioner and the consumer.

An important development in the area of practitioner-provided information and patient education has been the evolution of the hospital as an educational institution. Wellness centers, chemical dependence programs, sports medicine centers, and commu-

nity-based outreach centers have become more common. It is noted, however, that some chemical dependence programs are being closed as health insurance companies become less willing to cover these services.

On-line computer services

With the expansion of computer technology in the last decade, new avenues for accessing health-related information have developed. Today over 7 million home computer users who subscribe to an on-line service can access the Internet for electronic mail, listserv, and "chat" rooms devoted to health-oriented topics. In addition, computer-based access to health-related sources of information is available. Telnet and Gopher services, as well as World Wide Web pages, open expansive collections of information, including text

compliance
Willingness to follow the directions provided by another person.

and video, to people interested in health-related information.

Health reference publications

It is now believed that a substantial portion of all households own or subscribe to a health reference publication, such as the *The Johns Hopkins Medical Handbook*[1] or the *Physicians' Desk Reference (PDR)*,[2] or a newsletter such as *The Harvard Medical School Health Letter* or *The Johns Hopkins Medical Letter: Health After 50*.

Personal computer programs and videocassettes featuring health-related information are important sources of information for some consumers.

Reference libraries

Even though a large percentage of households possess health-related reference material and health care professionals are dispensing more and more information to the consumer, public and university libraries continue to be much-used sources of health-related information. Reference librarians can be consulted, and audiovisual collections and printed materials can be checked out. With increasing frequency, more and more of these holdings are becoming available through home computer–based on-line services.

Consumer advocacy groups

A variety of nonprofit consumer advocacy groups patrol the health care marketplace, particularly in relation to services and products (see the Star Box below). These groups produce and send out information designed to aid the consumer in recognizing questionable services and products. Large, well-organized groups, such as The National Consumers' League and Consumers' Union, and smaller groups at the state and local levels champion the right of the consumer to receive valid and reliable information about health care products and services.

Consumer Protection Agencies and Organizations

Federal Agencies
Office of Consumer Affairs, Food and Drug Administration
U.S. Department of Health and Human Services
5600 Fishers Lane
Rockville, MD 20857
(301) 443-5006

Federal Trade Commission
Consumer Inquiries
Public Reference Branch
6th Street and Pennsylvania Avenue
Washington, DC 20580
(202) 326-2222

Fraud Division
Chief Postal Inspector
U.S. Postal Service
475 L'Enfant Plaza
Washington, DC 20260
(202) 268-4299

Consumer Information Center
Department SC
Pueblo, CO 81009
(719) 948-3334

U.S. Consumer Product Safety Commission Hotline
Washington, DC
(800) 638-CPSC

Consumer Organizations
Consumers Union of the U.S., Inc.
101 Truman Avenue
Yonkers, NY 10703
(914) 378-2000

The National Consumers' League
1522 K Street, N.W.
Suite 406
Washington, DC 20005
(202) 639-8140

Professional Organizations
American Medical Association
535 N. Dearborn
Chicago, IL 60610
(312) 464-5000

American Hospital Association
840 N. Lake Shore Dr.
Chicago, IL 60611
(312) 280-6000

American Pharmaceutical Association
Health Education Center Service
2215 Constitution Avenue, NW
Washington, DC 20037
(202) 628-4410

Voluntary health agencies

Volunteerism and the traditional approach to health care and health promotion are virtually inseparable. Few countries besides the United States boast so many national voluntary organizations, with state and local affiliates, dedicated to the enhancement of health through research, service, and public education. The American Cancer Society, the American Red Cross, and the American Heart Association are all voluntary (not-for-profit) health agencies. Consumers can, in fact, anticipate finding a voluntary health agency for virtually every health problem.

Government agencies

Government agencies are effective providers of information to the public. Through meetings and the release of information to the media, agencies such as the Food and Drug Administration, Federal Trade Commission, United States Postal Service, and Environmental Protection Agency contribute to public awareness of health issues. Particularly in terms of labeling, advertising, and the distribution of information through the mail, government agencies also control the quality of information sent out to the buying public. The various divisions of the National Institutes of Health regularly release research findings and recommendations pertaining to clinical practices, which in turn reach the consumer through clinical practitioners.

Despite their best intentions, federal health agencies are often less effective than what the public deserves. A variety of factors, including inadequate staff, poor administration, and lobbying by special interest groups, prevent these federal agencies from enforcing the consumer protection legislation that exists. As a result, the public is left with a sense of false confidence regarding the consumer protection provided by the federal government.

State government also provides the public with health-related information. State agencies are primary sources of information, particularly in the areas of public health and environmental protection.

Qualified health educators

Health educators work in a variety of settings and provide their services to diverse groups of individuals. Community health educators work with virtually all of the agencies mentioned in this section; patient educators function in primary care settings; and school health educators are found at all educational levels. Increasingly, health educators are being employed in a wide range of wellness-based programs in community, hospital, corporate, and school settings.

HEALTH CARE PROVIDERS

The types and sources of health information just discussed can contribute greatly to the decisions we make as informed consumers. The choices we make about physicians, health services, and medical payment plans will reflect our commitment to remain healthy and our trust in specific people who are trained in keeping us healthy. Refer to the Health Action Guides on pp. 384 and 385 for tips on choosing a physician and a hospital.

Physicians and Their Training

In every city and many smaller communities, the local telephone directory will attest to the many types of physicians engaged in the practice of medicine. These health care providers hold the academic degree of Doctor of Medicine (MD) or Doctor of Osteopathy (DO).

At one time, **allopathy** and **osteopathy** were clearly different health care professions in terms of their healing philosophies and modes of practice. Today, however, MDs and DOs receive similar educations and engage in very similar forms of practice. Both can function as **primary care physicians** or as board-certified specialists. The differences that exist are in terms of the osteopathic physician's greater tendency to use manipulation in treating health problems. Additionally, DOs perceive themselves as being more holistically oriented than MDs.

The training of medical and osteopathic physicians is a long process. Usually, 4 years of initial undergraduate preparation is required. There is heavy emphasis on the sciences—biology, chemistry, mathematics,

---

allopathy (ah **lop** ah thee)
System of medical practice in which specific remedies (often pharmaceutical agents) are used to produce effects different from those produced by a disease or injury.

osteopathy (os tee **op** ah thee)
System of medical practice that combines allopathic principles with specific attention to postural mechanics of the body.

primary care physician
The physician who sees a patient on a regular basis, rather than a specialist who sees the patient only for a specific condition or procedure.

HEALTH
Action Guide - - - - ➤

Choosing a Physician

When choosing a physician, plan to obtain answers to the following questions *during* your initial visit:

- Obtain a description of the physician's medical background, such as education, residencies, and specialty areas.
- How does the physician keep up with new developments in the medical profession? Does the physician attend seminars and conferences, take courses, read medical journals, write articles, participate in professional organizations, or teach at a medical school?
- What are the normal office hours? What should be done if help is needed outside of normal office hours?
- What is included in a comprehensive physical examination?
- How does the physician feel about second and third opinions?
- Which hospitals is the physician affiliated with in your area?
- With which specialists is the physician associated?
- What is the physician's fee schedule?

Ask yourself the following questions *after* your visit:
- Was I comfortable with the physician's age, gender, race, and national origin?
- Was I comfortable with the physician's demeanor?

- Did I find communication with the physician to be understandable and reassuring? Were all my questions answered?
- Did the physician seem interested in having me as a patient?
- Are the physician's training and practice speciality in an area most closely associated with my present needs and concerns?
- Does the physician have staff privileges at a hospital of my preference?
- Does the physician's fee-for-service policy in any way exclude or limit my ability to receive necessary services?
- Did the physician take a complete medical history as a part of my initial visit? Was prevention, health promotion, or wellness addressed by the physician at any point during my visit?
- Did I at any point during my visit sense that the physician was unusually reluctant or anxious to try new medical procedures or medications?
- When the physician is unavailable, are any colleagues on call for 24 hours? Did I feel that telephone calls from me would be welcomed and responded to in a reasonable period?

If you have answered yes to most of these questions, you have found a physician with whom you should feel comfortable. If you have been using the services of a particular physician but are becoming dissatisfied, how could you resolve this dissatisfaction?   ◄ - - - - - -

anatomy, and physiology. Most undergraduate schools have preprofessional courses of study for students interested in medical or osteopathic schools.

Once accepted into professional schools, students generally spend 4 or more years in intensive training that includes advanced study in the preclinical medical sciences and clinical practice. On completion of this phase of training, the students are awarded the MD or DO degree and then take the state medical license examination. Most newly licensed physicians complete an internship and residency at a hospital. During this period, physicians gain experience in various clinical areas or begin residency programs. Residency programs vary in length from 3 to 4 years. At the conclusion of residency programs, board-eligible or board-certified status is granted. The Star Box on p. 386 describes several of the more familiar areas of specialization.

Nonallopathic Practitioners

In addition to medical and osteopathic physicians, several forms of alternative health care exist within the large health care market. Included within this group is **chiropractic, acupuncture,** homeopathy, massage, **reflexology,** and **ayurveda.** Although long scoffed at by the traditional medical community as being ineffective and unscientific, many people use these forms of health care and feel strongly that they are as effective (or more effective) than allopathic and osteopathic medicine.

At the urging of many people in both the medical and alternative health care fields, the National Institutes of Health agreed to fund an initial study of the effectiveness of alternative health care procedures. The first fruits of this study, a 1995 report titled *Alternative Medicine: Expanding Medical Horizons,*[4] draws together our current understanding of alternative

HEALTH
Action Guide - - - - ➡

Choosing a Hospital

Despite efforts in self-care and health promotion, most people will experience hospitalization at some time in their lives. Serious threatening illnesses and rarer diseases are best treated in large research-oriented hospitals at major medical centers or regional teaching hospitals. Less serious illness or elective procedures can be accommodated in community hospitals. Regardless of the type of hospital, however, these characteristics should be looked for[3]:

- The hospital building should be neat, clean, and well maintained.
- There should be recreational relaxation areas for patients to use, including outside areas.
- The public areas of the hospital (lobbies, snackbars, parking structures, and business areas) should be comfortable and clean.
- Visiting hours should be liberal, and children should be allowed some access.
- Accommodations should be available for family and friends to stay overnight.
- Patients' meals should be carefully selected, attractively prepared, and efficiently served.
- Special meals should be provided when medically appropriate, and families should be assisted in post-discharge meal planning.
- Hospital rooms should be attractive, comfortable, and well situated for nursing services.
- Smoking by patients, staff, and visitors should be carefully controlled. ◄ - - - - -

approaches and provides a framework for well-controlled research into the effectiveness of each approach. Double-blind studies, so called because neither the participants nor the researchers know which treatment each participant is receiving, will be conducted. It is hoped that the use of this method with the careful selection of participants will produce a clearer picture of alternative health care approaches. To date, however, the federal government has not endorsed any alternative health care practices.

Restricted-Practice Health Care Providers

We receive much of our health care from medical physicians. However, most of us also use the services of various health care specialists who also have advanced graduate level training. Among these professionals are dentists, psychologists, podiatrists, and optometrists.

Dentists (Doctor of Dental Surgery, DDS) are trained to deal with a wide range of diseases and impairments of the teeth and oral cavity. Dentists undergo undergraduate predental programs that emphasize the sciences, followed by 4 additional years of graduate study in dental school and, with increasing frequency, an internship program. State licensure examinations are required. As with medical physicians, dentists can also specialize by completing a postdoctoral master's degree in fields such as oral surgery, **orthodontics,** and **prosthodontics.** Dentists

chiropractic
Manipulation of the vertebral column to relieve pressure and cure illness.

acupuncture
Insertion of fine needles into the body to alter electroenergy fields and cure disease.

reflexology
Massage applied to specific areas of the feet to treat illness and disease in other areas of the body.

ayurveda (ai yur **vey** da)
Traditional Indian medicine based on herbal remedies.

orthodontics
Dental specialty that focuses on the proper alignment of the teeth.

prosthodontics
Dental specialty that focuses on the construction and fitting of artificial appliances to replace missing teeth.

Medical Specialties

The American Board of Medical Specialties is a nonprofit organization that represents 23 medical specialty boards.* Each board is composed of expert physicians already qualified in a particular field. These specialty boards evaluate physicians who wish to practice in a specific area of medicine. Some of the more common specialty areas consumers might encounter are listed below.

Specialty	Scope of Practice
• Allergy	Treatment of sensitivity disorders
• Anesthesiology	Use of drugs to sedate or anesthetize
• Cardiovascular surgery	Various forms of heart surgery
• Dermatology	Skin diseases and disorders
• Emergency medicine	Care of accident victims
• Family practice	Broad-based family medical care
• Geriatrics	Diseases and disorders of the elderly
• Gynecology	Female reproductive health care
• Internal medicine	Nonsurgical treatment of internal organ systems
• Neurology	Diseases and disorders of the nervous system
• Nephrology	Kidney diseases and disorders
• Obstetrics	Prenatal care and child delivery
• Oncology	Treatment of unusual growths and tumors
• Ophthalmology	Disorders of the eye
• Orthopedic surgery	Surgery for structural disorders of the bones and joints
• Otorhinolaryngology	Ear, nose, and throat problems
• Pathology	Diagnosis of disease through the examination of body tissues
• Pediatrics	Childhood health concerns
• Psychiatry	Mental and emotional diseases or disorders
• Radiology	Use of radiation to diagnose and treat diseases and injuries
• Urological surgery	Surgery for urinary tract diseases and male reproductive dysfunctions

*Governed by these 23 medical boards are 85 practice specialties.

are also permitted to prescribe therapy programs (such as appliances for the treatment of temporomandibular joint dysfunction) and drugs that pertain to their practices (primarily analgesics and antibiotics).

Psychologists provide services related to an understanding of behavior patterns or perceptions. Over 40 states have certification or licensing laws that prohibit unqualified people from using the term *psychologist.* The consumer should examine the credentials of a psychologist. Legitimate psychologists have received advanced graduate training (often leading to a PhD or EdD degree) in clinical, counseling, industrial, or educational psychology. Furthermore, these practitioners will have passed state certification examinations and, in many states, will have met further requirements that allow them to offer health services to the public. Psychologists may have special interests and credentials from professional societies in individual, group, family, or marriage counseling. Some are certified as sex therapists.

Unlike *psychiatrists,* who are medical physicians, psychologists cannot prescribe or dispense drugs. They may refer to or consult with medical physicians about clients who might benefit from drug therapy.

Podiatrists are highly trained clinicians who practice podiatric medicine, or care of the feet (and ankles). Although not MDs or DOs, doctors of podiatric medicine (DPM) treat a wide variety of conditions related to the feet, including corns, bunions, warts, bone spurs, hammertoes, fractures, diabetes-related conditions, athletic injuries, and structural abnormalities. Podiatrists perform surgery, prescribe medications, and apply orthotics (supports or braces), splints, and corrective shoes for structural abnormalities of the feet.

Doctors of podiatric medicine follow an educational path similar to that taken by MDs and DOs, consisting of a 4-year undergraduate preprofessional curriculum, 4 additional years of study in a podiatric medical school, and an optional residency of 1 or 2 years. Board-certified areas of specialization include surgery, orthopedics, and podiatric sports medicine. Hospital affiliation generally requires board certification in a specialized area.

Optometrists are eye specialists who deal primarily with vision problems associated with **refractory errors.** They examine the eyes and prescribe glasses or contact lenses to correct visual disorders. Sometimes optometrists also attempt to correct certain ocular muscle imbalances with specific exercise regimens. Optometrists must complete undergraduate training and additional years of coursework at one of 16 accredited colleges of optometry in the United States or two Canadian colleges before taking a state licensing examination.[5]

Opticians are technicians who manufacture and fit eyeglasses or contact lenses. Although they are rarely licensed by a state agency, they perform the important function of grinding lenses to the precise prescription designated by an optometrist or *ophthalmologist* (physicians who have specialized in vision care). To save money and time, many consumers take an optometrist's or ophthalmologist's prescription for glasses or contact lenses to optician-staffed retail stores that deal exclusively with eyewear products.

Nurse Professionals

Nurses constitute a large group of health professionals who practice in a variety of settings. Frequently, the responsibilities of nurses vary according to their academic preparation. Registered nurses (RNs) are academically prepared at two levels: (1) the technical nurse, and (2) the professional nurse. The technical nurse is educated in a 2-year associate degree program. The professional nurse receives 4 years of education and earns a bachelor's degree. Both technical and professional nurses must successfully complete state licensing examinations before they can practice as RNs.

Many professional nurses continue their education and earn master's and doctoral degrees in nursing or other health-related fields. Some professional nurses specialize in a clinical area (such as pediatrics, gerontology, public health, or school health) and become certified as nurse practitioners. Working under the supervision of physicians, nurse practitioners perform many of the diagnostic and treatment procedures performed by physicians. The ability of these highly trained nurses to function at this level provides communities with additional primary care providers, as well as freeing physicians to deal with more complex cases. Many college health centers employ nurse practitioners because of their ability to deliver high-quality care at a low cost to the institution.

Licensed practical nurses (LPNs) are trained in hospital-based programs ranging from 12 to 18 months. Because of their brief training, LPNs' scope of practice is limited. Most LPN training programs are gradually being phased out.

Allied Health Care Professionals

Our primary health care providers are supported by a large group of allied health care professionals, who often take the responsibility for highly technical services and procedures. Such professionals include respiratory and inhalation therapists, radiological technologists, nuclear medicine technologists, pathology technicians, general medical technologists, operating room technicians, emergency medical technicians, registered nurse midwives, physical therapists, occupational therapists, cardiac rehabilitation therapists, dental technicians, physician assistants, and dental hygienists. Depending on the particular field, the training for these specialty support areas can take from 1 to 5 years of post–high school study. Programs include hospital-based training leading to a diploma through associate, bachelor's, and master's degrees. Most allied health care professionals must also pass state or national licensing examinations.

SELF–CARE

The emergence of the **self-care movement** suggests that many people are becoming more responsible for the maintenance of their health. They are developing the expertise to prevent or manage numerous types of illness, injuries, and conditions. They are learning to assess their health status and treat, monitor, and reha-

---

refractory errors
Incorrect patterns of light wave transmissions through the structures of the eye.

self-care movement
Trend toward individuals taking increased responsibility for prevention or management of certain health conditions.

bilitate themselves in a manner that was once thought possible only with the direct help of a physician or some other health care specialist.

The benefits of this movement are that self-care can (1) lower health care costs, (2) be effective care for particular conditions, (3) free physicians and other health care specialists to spend time with other patients, and (4) enhance interest in health-related activities.

Self-care is an appropriate alternative to professional care in three areas. First, self-care may be appropriate for certain acute conditions that have familiar symptoms and are of limited duration and seriousness. Common colds and flu, many home injuries, sore throats, and nonallergic insect bites are often easily managed with self-care.

A second area in which self-care might be appropriate is therapy. For example, many people are now administering injections for allergies and migraine shots and continuing physical therapy programs in their homes. Asthma, diabetes, and hypertension are also conditions that can be managed or monitored with self-care.

A third area in which self-care has appropriate application is health promotion. Weight loss programs, physical conditioning activities, and stress reduction programs are particularly well suited to self-care.

People interested in practicing more self-care must be skilled consumers. The self-care marketplace is growing very rapidly and is expected to be a multibillion-dollar industry by the end of the decade. Equipment such as blood pressure–measuring instruments, stethoscopes, and screening kits for cholesterol and pregnancy, as well as OTC drugs, can represent significant investments. Clearly, your money, time, and willingness to develop expertise are important components in this growing area of health care consumerism.

HEALTH CARE COSTS AND REIMBURSEMENT

As depicted in Figure 15-2, there are many avenues for receiving health care. However, being able to afford quality health care is among the most important concerns of the American public. Today over 38.9 million Americans lack health insurance to pay health care costs,[6] including over 10 million dependent children. Furthermore, Americans are less optimistic today about their ability to have adequate health insurance coverage, find reasonably priced health care, and afford long-term home-bound or nursing

home care than ever before.[7] Unfortunately, the word *crisis* is appropriate to use when talking about our ability to continue to afford high-quality health care today.

Central to our concern with health care is its cost. As a nation, Americans are now spending over $1 trillion a year on health care, and by the year 2000 the amount is expected to exceed $1.5 trillion.[8] At today's rates, annual health care costs per person will approach $5500 by the year 2000.[8] For the country as a whole, 13.3% of our gross domestic product was devoted to health care costs in 1993.[9] Table 15-1 provides a breakdown of annual health care expenditures in the United States.

In light of factors such as the high cost of modern medical technology, an emphasis on long life at any cost, the growing number of older people with chronic conditions that require expensive extended care, and the AIDS epidemic, controlling the cost of medical care is one of the most complex problems facing the nation. Nevertheless, well over 40 different plans have been advanced since 1990 in response to this problem. These range from only modest changes to the current system to tax credit strategies and mandatory employment-based insurance to a federally controlled national health plan.[10] However, no single plan has yet caught the favor of the American public or their policy makers in Washington.

Health Insurance

Health insurance is a financial agreement between an insurance company and an individual or group for the payment of health costs. After paying a premium to an insurance company, the policyholder is covered for specific benefits. The Star Box on p. 390, left, summarizes the types of policies that are available. Each policy is different in terms of coverage for illnesses and injuries. Merely having an insurance policy does not mean that all health care expenses will be covered. Most health insurance policies require various forms of payments on the part of the policyholder, which include provisions for deductible amounts, fixed indemnity benefits, coinsurance, and exclusions. For most Americans, participation in the health care system is possible if they have adequate health insurance. In 1993, 34% of all health care bills were paid for by private health insurance.[11]

A *deductible* amount is an established amount that the insuree must pay before the insurer reimburses for services. For example, if a person has been billed for $500 worth of services, their policy might require a

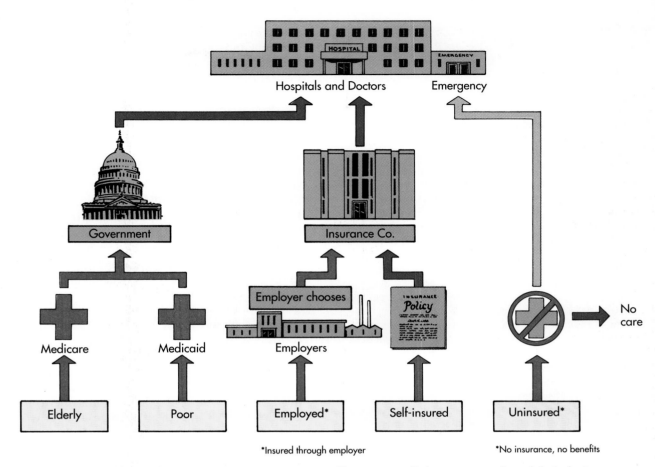

Figure 15-2   In the current U.S. health care system, many layers of bureaucracy lie between people and their doctors.

payment to the provider of $200 before the insurance company will pay the remaining $300. Usually, the lower the deductible amount is, the higher the premium will be.

A policy with *fixed indemnity* benefits will pay only a specified amount for a particular procedure or service. If the policy pays only $1000 for an appendectomy and the actual cost of the appendectomy was $1500, then the policy owner will owe the health care provider $500. A policy with *full-service* benefits, which pays the entire cost of a particular procedure or service, may be worth the extra cost.

Policies that have *coinsurance* features require that the policy owner and the insurance company share the costs of certain covered services, usually on a percentage basis. One standard coinsurance plan requires that the policyholder pay 20% of the costs above a deductible amount, and the company pays the remaining 80%.

An *exclusion* refers to a service or expense that is not covered by the policy. Elective or cosmetic surgery procedures, unusual treatment protocols, prescription drugs, and certain kinds of consultations are common exclusions in many policies. Illness and injuries that already exist at the time of purchase (preexisting conditions) are often excluded. Also, injuries incurred during high-risk activities (ice hockey, hang gliding, mountain climbing, intramural sports) might not be covered by a policy.

Health insurance can be obtained through individ-

Table 15-1 Household Health Care Expenditures	
Commodity	Amount (in billions)
Hospitals	$256.0
Physicians	$125.7
Nursing homes	$ 53.1
Drugs/supplies	$ 54.6
Dental care	$ 34.0
Other	$120.0

Types of Health Insurance Coverage

When considering a health insurance policy, you should evaluate the following types of coverage.

Hospital. Hospital coverage refers to insurance that covers inpatient hospital expenses. With hospital expenses approaching $800 per day, you want to be certain that your policy provides for this expense.

Surgical. Surgical coverage provides for the fees surgeons charge for specific surgical care.

Regular medical. Regular medical covers physicians' fees for nonsurgical care. Often maximum benefits are specified for certain types of nonsurgical procedures.

Major medical. Major medical coverage is for unusually large, often unpredictable medical expenses. Major medical coverage is designed to extend beyond a health insurance policy's regular medical coverage. Although major medical benefits have very high maximum benefit limits (often hundreds of thousands of dollars), these benefits are often paid on a coinsurance basis. Thus you may pay a portion of the medical expense.

Dental. Initial coverage provides for various types of dental care.

Disability. Disability insurance (also called *income protection insurance*) provides for income lost because of your inability to work after an illness or injury.

ual policies or group plans. Group health insurance plans usually offer the widest range of coverage at the least expensive price and are often purchased cooperatively by companies and their employees. In 1993 the average employee's portion of health insurance (family plan) was $107 per month.[12] Fortunately, no employee is refused entry into a group insurance program. However, when employees leave the company, they often lose their group health insurance coverage. Today, as many large American companies downsize, tens of thousands of employees can lose this important group health insurance, virtually without warning.

Individual policies can be purchased by one person (or a family) from an insurance company. These policies are often much more expensive than group plans and may provide much less coverage. People who do not have access to a group plan should still attempt to secure individual policies, since the financial burdens resulting from a severe accident or illness that is not covered by some form of health insurance can be devastating. Many colleges and universities offer annually renewable health insurance policies that students

can purchase (see the Star Box below). The Health Action Guide on p. 391 gives the consumer some questions to consider before purchasing a health insurance policy.

Health Maintenance Organizations

Health maintenance organizations (HMOs) are health care delivery plans under which health care providers agree to meet the covered medical needs of subscribers for a prepaid amount of money. For a fixed monthly fee, enrollees are given comprehensive health care with an emphasis on preventive health care. Enrollees receive their care from physicians, specialists, allied health professionals, and educators who are hired or contractually retained by the HMO. In theory, HMOs were to be the ideal blend of medical care and health promotion, offering the advantages described below. Today, however, there is growing concern that too many HMOs are being too tightly controlled by a profit motive in which physicians are being paid to not refer patients to specialists or are prevented (gag rules) from discussing certain treatment options with patients because of their costs to the HMOs.[13,14] In 1995, 56 million Americans were enrolled in HMOs, with an average cost per worker of $3485 versus $3850 for workers having a more traditional group health plan.[15]

When operated in the manner consistent with how most members believe they should be operated, one of the potential advantages offered by HMOs is cost

Health Insurance for College Students

The days when students could leave for college confident that their health needs would be met by the family health insurance plans held by their parents are nearly gone. Today many young adults 18 years of age and older need to provide their own health care coverage, regardless of whether they are students. Accordingly, colleges and universities are likely to offer health care insurance packages for students to purchase on an annual basis. The annual premium for a typical student health insurance program may range from $300 for a single student up to $1400 for a student with a spouse and dependent children. When considering your health insurance coverage, it is important to learn whether more affordable health insurance of equal or better coverage than that sold by your school could be purchased from an insurance agent.

HEALTH
Action Guide

Selecting a Health Insurance Policy

Before you purchase a health insurance policy, ask yourself the following questions. The more questions you can answer with a "yes," the better you should feel that the policy you select is right for you.

General Questions
- Do I really need an individual insurance policy?
- Am I already covered by a group insurance policy?
- Is the insurance company I'm considering rated favorably by *Best's Insurance Reports* or my state insurance department?
- Have I compared health insurance policies from at least two other companies?
- Does this company have a "return rate" of 50% or more?
- Can I afford this insurance policy?

- Do I understand the factors that might raise the cost of this policy?

Specific Questions
- Do I clearly understand which health conditions are covered and which are not?
- Do I clearly understand whether I have fixed indemnity benefits or full-service benefits?
- Do I clearly understand the deductible amounts of this policy?
- Do I clearly understand when the major medical portion of this policy starts?
- Do I clearly understand all information in this policy that refers to exclusions and preexisting conditions?
- Do I clearly understand any disability provisions of this policy?
- Do I clearly understand all information concerning both cancellation and renewal of this policy?

containment. Since most of the medical services with an HMO are centralized, there is little duplication of facilities, equipment, or support staff. Central filing of records allows several HMO physicians to have access to a single client's record file. This saves time, administrative costs, and the overlapping of care. HMOs also routinely use health promotion activities to encourage clients to practice illness prevention.[16] All of these approaches could help lower health care costs.

Additional new approaches to reducing health costs involve the formation of *independent practice associations* (IPAs) and *preferred provider organizations* (PPOs). An IPA is a modified form of an HMO that uses a group of doctors who offer prepaid services out of their own offices and not in a central HMO facility. IPAs are viewed as "HMOs without walls." A PPO is a group of private practitioners who sell their services at reduced rates to insurance companies. When policyholders choose a physician who is in that company's PPO, the insurance company will pay the entire physician's fee. When a policyholder selects a non-PPO physician, the insurance company will pay only a portion of that physician's fee. Today, in excess of 63% of all employees are in some form of managed care program (HMOs, IPAs, or PPOs).[15]

Government Insurance Plans

Created in 1965 by amendments to the Social Security Act, **Medicare** and **Medicaid** represent governmental types of health insurance. Medicare provides health care reimbursements primarily for people aged 65 years or older. Medicare is a contributory program—that is, through their working years, all employed citizens contribute a portion of their salaries (through Social Security taxes) to the Medicare fund. At present, that amount is 1.45% of the Social Security taxes (FICA) paid on annual earnings.[17] When they reach age 65, some of their health care expenses are covered by Medicare. Regardless of their age, people who require kidney dialysis or transplants are covered by Medicare.

Medicare
Contributory governmental health insurance, primarily for people 65 years of age or older.

Medicaid
Noncontributory governmental health insurance for people receiving other types of public assistance.

Medicare is actually composed of two parts. Medicare A is essentially a hospital insurance program. Part A will pay for necessary hospital care (semiprivate room) after payment of the required deductible, for medically necessary inpatient care in a nursing home (skilled level care), and hospice care. In addition, it will pay 80% of the cost of approved durable medical equipment, such as walkers, and for all units of blood used by an inpatient, after the first three units.[18] Medicare B is a voluntary program (for which the subscriber must pay a monthly fee, currently $46.10/month) that supplements Medicare A. Medicare B provides regular medical insurance that covers a broad range of physicians' fees and other health care services. Physicians who "accept assignment" from Medicare agree to charge their elderly patients only the amount that Medicare will cover. Those who do not accept assignment may charge an amount up to 115% of the Medicare amount.[18] However, by doing so, they will be asking their elderly patients not only to pay the 20% copayment but an additional 15% as well. Consequently, many elderly will go only to physicians who accept assignment. Both Medicare plans are subject to yearly changes in coverages and administrative procedures.

One of the most recent attempts by Medicare at cost containment in the area of health care is the prospective pricing system established in 1984 by the federal government. Under this system, Medicare reimbursements to hospitals are based on 467 diagnosis-related groups (DRGs) rather than on the costs accrued by the hospitals. Each hospital stay is now assigned a DRG classification, and reimbursement to the hospital is based on that classification. This system encourages hospitals to deliver services at or below the DRG payment schedule.

Currently, a principal focus of American political thought is to balance the federal budget before or only shortly after the end of the decade. Regardless of the particular plan advanced, changes in various aspects of Medicare are a certainty. Regardless of the specific agenda advanced by one group or another, it is hoped that the "new Medicare" will offer older Americans a broader range of choices of health care providers, reduce the amount of fraud and waste associated with current operations, and stimulate greater cooperation among physicians, hospitals, drug manufacturers, and recipients in cost containment.[19]

Medicaid is a noncontributory program for citizens who are receiving other types of public welfare assistance. It is designed to provide both a variety of types of health-related coverage, including hospital, nursing home, physicians, and home care, and Medicare deductibles. Unlike Medicare, Medicaid has no age requirements and is administered cooperatively through federal and state agencies. Medicaid is particularly important to older adults, since it will cover nursing home care once eligibility has been established. In 1995, 20% of the entire Medicaid budget of $155 billion ($31 billion) was spent for nursing home care, principally for the elderly.[20]

Because of the bureaucracy currently surrounding these two governmental insurance programs, a number of private physicians and voluntary hospitals are reluctant to accept Medicaid and Medicare clients. An important concern now seems to be how the United States can provide proper health care for all of its citizens, including the aged, economically disadvantaged, and those whose life savings can be quickly depleted by a catastrophic illness (see the Learning from All Cultures box on p. 393).

Medicare Supplement Policies (Medigap)

Because Medicare A and Medicare B require deductibles and copayment to be made by patients before they will begin payment, insurance to cover these gaps in coverage has been developed. In the most basic "medigap" policies (policy version A), often sold via television, reimbursement is made to the patient for the deductible and copayment portions of the approved charges, as determined by the DRG (Medicare A) and approved physician fee (Medicare B). More expensive and more comprehensive Medicare supplement policies (policy versions B through J) are also available that pay for hospital care and equipment not covered by Medicare A and for physician fees that exceed the approved amount of coverage for Medicare B. The difference in costs between the basic medigap policies and the more comprehensive policies that literally pay for everything that is not covered by Medicare is substantial.

Extended Care Insurance

With the aging of the population and the greater likelihood that nursing home care will be required (at about $32,000 per year), extended care policies have been developed and are being sold. When purchased at an early age (by mid-50s), these policies are much more affordable than if purchased when it is apparent that a spouse or family member will require institutional care. However, not all older adults will need extensive nursing home care, so an extended care policy could be an unnecessary expenditure.

LEARNING *from* ALL CULTURES

Health Care in the United States and Canada

Approximately 14% of the United States population does not have access to health care. This amounts to approximately 37 million people, primarily among the poor.[21] A substantial number of people lacking medical coverage are people who work full time at very low-paying jobs without health-care benefits. This population may suffer more than the very poor or unemployed because they may not be poor enough to qualify for Medicaid.[22]

Usually people who need emergency or immediate care will not be turned away at a hospital. However, people without health coverage lack primary care—preventive measures like checkups, screenings, and prenatal care. Because of this lack of preventive attention, they eventually may need more extensive and costly care.[22]

Other countries, such as Canada, have addressed the issue of universal health care. Since 1972, Canadian residents have been guaranteed health insurance coverage through a system funded by the federal government and the ten provincial and two territorial governments. Of the total health care cost, 30% to 40% is paid by the federal government, about 25% comes from private sources, and the rest is contributed by the provinces, usually through taxes.[23]

Each individual is guaranteed health care in Canada, but the system is not socialized medicine. Physicians do not work for the government but are independent providers. Providers must, however, accept the provincial plan's reimbursement as total payment if a province is to continue to receive federal support.[23]

Would the Canadian system work in the United States? From where in the federal and state budgets would the funding come? Some argue that there are too many groups of people who would not benefit from a system like the Canadian one. Why would certain groups oppose such a system?

HEALTH-RELATED PRODUCTS

As you might imagine, prescription and OTC drugs constitute an important part of any discussion of health-related products.

Prescription Drugs

Caution: Federal law prohibits dispensing without prescription.

This FDA warning appears on the labels of approximately three fourths of all medications. Prescription drugs must be ordered for patients by a licensed practitioner. Because these compounds are legally controlled and may require special skills in their administration, our access to these drugs is limited.

Although over 2500 compounds listed in the current edition of the *PDR* represent the drugs that can be prescribed by a physician, only 200 drugs make up the bulk of the 2,140,799 new prescriptions and refills dispensed by 34,000 pharmacies in 1994.[24] The most frequently prescribed drugs, by units dispensed, are Zantac (ulcers), Procardia (high blood pressure), Mevacor (high cholesterol), Vasotec (high blood pressure), and Prozac (depression). Working through physicians and pharmacists, pharmaceutical companies contribute to the improvement of health while generating sales in excess of $25.6 billion per year.[25] Health care dollars spent for prescription drugs account for 13% of the total health care costs accrued by Americans.

Research and development of new drugs

As consumers of prescription drugs, you may be curious about the process by which drugs gain FDA approval for marketing. The rigor of this process may be why fewer than 15 to 20 new drugs are added to the list of approved drugs each year.

On a continuous basis, the nation's pharmaceutical companies are exploring the molecular structure of various chemical compounds in an attempt to discover important new compounds with desired types and levels of biological activity. Once these new compounds are identified, extensive in-house research with computer simulations and animal testing is required to determine whether clinical trials with humans are warranted. Of the 125,000 or more compounds under study each year, only a few thousand receive such extensive preclinical evaluation. Even fewer of these are then taken to the FDA to begin the evaluation process necessary to gain approval for further research with humans. Once a drug is approved for clinical trials, the pharmaceutical companies can secure a patent, which prevents the drug from being manufactured by other companies for the next 17 years.

The $125 million price tag for bringing a new drug into the marketplace reflects this slow, careful process. If this 7-year process goes well, a pharmaceutical company will enjoy 10 years of legally protected retail sales before generic versions of the drug can be offered by other companies.

Generic versus brand name drugs

When a new drug comes into the marketplace, it carries with it three names: its **chemical name,** its **generic name,** and its **brand name.** During the time the 17-year patent is in effect, no other drug with the same chemical formulation can be sold. When the patent expires, other companies can manufacture a drug of equivalent chemical composition and market it under the brand name drug's original generic name. Because extensive research and development are not necessary at this point, the production of generic drugs is far less costly than the initial development of the brand name drug. Nearly all states allow pharmacists to substitute generic drugs for brand name drugs, as long as the prescribing physician approves.

In 1995 a new publication, the *Physicians' Desk Reference—Generics,* became available.[26] Like its companion publications for prescription and OTC drugs, *PDR—Generics* should be well received by both clinicians and the public.

Over-the-Counter Drugs

When people are asked when they last took some form of medication, for many the answer might be, "I took aspirin, or a cold pill, or a laxative this morning." In making this decision, people engaged in self-diagnosis, determined a course for their own treatment, self-administered their treatment, and freed a physician to serve people whose illnesses are more serious than theirs. None of this would have been possible without readily available, inexpensive, and effective OTC drugs (see Table 15-2 for a comparison of OTC pain relievers).

In comparison with the 2500 prescription drugs available, there are perhaps as many as 300,000 different OTC products, routinely classified into 26 different families (see the Star Box on p. 395). Like prescription drugs, nonprescription drugs are regulated by

Table 15-2   A Comparison of Common Over-the-Counter Pain Relievers

Aspirin (Bayer, Bufferin)	Acetaminophen (Tylenol)	Ibuprofen (Advil, Nuprin)
How they work		
Suppresses the body's pain- and inflammation-promoting chemicals at site of pain or injury	Apparently blocks pain-promoting chemicals in brain; no antiinflammatory effect	Works similarly to aspirin
Additional benefits		
In small daily doses, aspirin's blood-thinning properties help reduce the likelihood of heart attack or stroke in those at risk	Easier on stomach than aspirin	Easier on stomach than aspirin
Relatively inexpensive	Virtually no side effects when used according to product guidelines	Requires lower dose to produce same painkilling effect as aspirin
Disadvantages		
Stomach irritation	May not work as effectively against swelling or arthritis-related pain as aspirin or ibuprofen	Does not offer heart protection benefits
Risks		
Possibility of gastrointestinal bleeding	Prolonged or intensive use may result in liver damage	High doses may lead to kidney damage

Whether or not prolonged use of any of these OTC pain relievers is good or bad for you is something you must decide with your physician. Your age, weight, family, and personal medical histories all play a role in determining how and at what dosage you will benefit from these products. See Appendix 1 for information about naproxen (Aleve) and ketoprofen (Orudis, Actron).

Categories of Over-the-Counter (OTC) Products
- Antacids
- Antimicrobials
- Sedatives and sleep aids
- Analgesics
- Cold remedies and antitussives
- Antihistamines and allergy products
- Mouthwashes
- Topical analgesics
- Antirheumatics
- Hematinics
- Vitamins and minerals
- Antiperspirants
- Laxatives
- Dentrifices and dental products
- Sunburn treatments and preventives
- Contraceptive and vaginal products
- Stimulants
- Hemorrhoidals
- Antidiarrheals
- Dandruff and athlete's foot preparations

the FDA. However, for OTC drugs the marketplace is a more powerful determinant of success.

The regulation of OTC drugs is based on a provision in a 1972 amendment to the 1938 Food, Drug, and Cosmetic Act. As a result of that action, OTC drugs were placed in three categories (I, II, and III) on the basis of the safety and effectiveness of their active ingredient(s). Today, only category I OTC drugs that are safe, effective, and truthfully labeled are to be sold. The FDA's drug classification process also allows some OTC drugs to be made stronger and some prescription drugs to become nonprescription drugs by reducing their strength through reformulation. In the latter case, 1995 marked the arrival in the OTC market of highly advertised heartburn remedies that were previously available only as prescription drugs. An evening of television was hardly complete without at least one commercial for either Tagamet HB or Pepcid AC, both of which are hydrogen ion blockers that reduce the production of stomach acid. In 1996, Rogaine, the only FDA-approved treatment for male pattern baldness, will be sold for the first time without a prescription (see Appendix 1).

The current labeling of OTC drugs also reflects the regulatory process described. The labels must clearly state the type and quantity of active ingredients, alcohol content, side effects, instructions for appropriate use, warnings against inappropriate use, and the risks

of using the product with other drugs (polydrug use). Unsubstantiated claims must be carefully avoided in advertisements for these products.

Cosmetics

Concern over the safety of cosmetics has existed for more than 50 years. Hyperallergic reactions, bacterial infections, and the presence of carcinogens (agents that cause cancer) and teratogens (agents that cause birth defects) remain at the center of this concern. Because cosmetics are not generally classified as drugs, their regulation is limited in terms of FDA involvement. Legislation is regularly proposed that would increase the ability of the FDA to better control this important segment of the personal care retail trade.

HEALTH CARE QUACKERY AND CONSUMER FRAUD

A person who earns money by marketing inaccurate health information, unreliable health care, or ineffective health products is called a fraud, quack, or charlatan. **Consumer fraud** flourished with the old-fashioned medicine shows of the late 1880s. Unfortunately, consumer fraud still flourishes (see the article on melatonin at the end of this chapter). You need look no further than large city newspapers to see questionable advertisements for disease cures and weight loss products. Quacks have found in health and illness the perfect avenues to realize maximum gain with minimum effort.

chemical name
Name used to describe the molecular structure of a drug.

generic name
Common or nonproprietary name of a drug.

brand name
Specific patented name assigned to a drug by its manufacturer.

consumer fraud
Marketing of unreliable and ineffective services, products, or information under the guise of curing disease or improving health; quackery.

HEALTH
Action Guide

Recognizing Quackery

"Duck" when you encounter these!

- Makes promises of quick, dramatic, simple, painless, or drugless treatment or cures
- Uses anecdotes, case histories, or testimonials to support claims
- Displays credentials or uses titles that might be confused with those of the scientific or medical community, such as Stan Smith, Ph.D. (in result)
- Claims a product or service provides treatment or cure for multiple or all illnesses and conditions
- States that this treatment or cure is either secret or not yet available in the United States

- States that medical doctors should not be trusted because they do more harm than good with their approaches to diagnosis and treatment
- Reports that most disease is due to a faulty diet and can be treated with nutritional supplements
- Promotes the use of hair analysis to diagnose illnesses or deficiencies
- Claims that "natural" products are superior to those sold in drugstores or dispensed by physicians
- Supports the "freedom of choice" concept that should allow you to try something even though it has not been proved safe and effective

When people are in poor health, they may be afraid of dying. So powerful are their desires to live and be free of suffering that people are vulnerable to promises of health improvement and life extension. Even though many people have great faith in their physicians, they also would like to have access to experimental treatments or products touted as being superior to currently available therapies. When tempted with the promise of real help, people are sometimes willing to set aside traditional medical care. Of course, quacks recognize this vulnerability and present a variety of "reasons" to move in their direction (see the Health Action Guide above).[27] Gullibility, blind faith, impatience, superstition, ignorance, or hostility toward professional expertise eventually carry the day. In spite of the best efforts of agencies at all levels, no branch of government can protect consumers from their own errors of judgement that so easily play into the hands of quacks and charlatans.

Regardless of the specific motivation that leads people into consumer fraud, the outcome is frequently the same. First, the consumer suffers financial loss. The services or products provided are grossly overpriced, and the consumers have little recourse to help them recover their money. Second, the consumers often feel disappointed, guilty, and angered by their own carelessness as consumers. Far too frequently, consumer fraud may lead to unnecessary suffering.

Summary

- Sources of health information include family, friends, commercials, labels, and information supplied by health professionals.
- Physicians can be either Doctors of Medicine (MDs) or Doctors of Osteopathy (DOs). They receive similar training and engage in similar forms of practice.
- Although alternative health care providers, including chiropractors, naturopaths, and acupuncturists, meet the health care needs of many people,

systematic study of these forms of health care is only now under way.
- Restricted-practice health care providers play important roles in meeting the health and wellness needs of the public.
- Nursing at all levels is a critical health care profession.
- Self-care is often a viable approach to preventing illness and reducing the use of health care providers.

- Our growing inability to afford health care services has reached crisis proportions in this country.
- Health insurance is critical in our ability to afford modern health care services.
- HMOs provide an alternative way to receive health care services, although there is concern about the influence of the profit motive in their operation.
- Medicare and Medicaid are governmental plans for paying for health care services that could be significantly altered in our current quest for a balanced budget.
- The development of prescription medication is a long and expensive process for pharmaceutical manufacturers.
- Critical health consumerism, including the avoidance of health quackery, requires careful use of health-related information, products, and services.

Review Questions

1. Determine how you would test the accuracy of the health-related information you have received in your lifetime.
2. Identify and describe some sources of health-related information presented in this chapter. What factors should you consider when using these sources?
3. Point out the similarities between allopathic and osteopathic physicians. What is a nonallopathic health care practitioner? Give examples of each type of nonallopathic practitioner.
4. Describe the services that are provided by the following limited health care providers: dentists, psychologists, podiatrists, optometrists, and opticians. Identify several allied health care professionals.
5. In what ways is the trend toward self-care evident? What are some reasons for the popularity of this movement?
6. What is health insurance? Explain the following terms relating to health insurance: deductible amount, fixed indemnity benefits, full-service benefits, coinsurance, exclusion, and preexisting illness.
7. What is a health maintenance organization? How do HMO plans reduce the costs of health care? What are IPAs and PPOs?
8. What do the chemical name, brand name, and generic name of a prescription drug represent? OTC drugs are categorized according to what two factors?
9. What is health care quackery? What responsibilities have been given to the FDA? What can a consumer do to avoid consumer fraud?

Think About This . . .

- How do you rate yourself as an informed consumer of health information, services, and products?
- Are there any types of providers mentioned in this chapter whom you would not choose to consult? Explain your answer.
- To what extent and in what ways have you engaged in self-care?
- Many insurance companies exclude certain kinds of illness (such as AIDS) from coverage and will not pay for the needed drugs. Who then should cover the cost? Under what circumstances do you think that expensive medications should be prescribed for terminally ill patients?
- Is life insurance more important than health insurance for young adults? Explain your answer.
- Why do you think it is difficult to get people to seek help for preventive care even though it is usually less expensive than treatment services?
- When you read a newspaper or magazine, do some health-rated advertisements seem questionable to you?

References

1. Mee C, editor: *The Johns Hopkins medical handbook,* New York, 1992, Medletter Associates.
2. *Physicians' desk reference,* ed 48, Oradel, NJ, 1995, Medical Economics.
3. Inlander C: *Take this book to the hospital with you: a consumer guide to surviving your hospital stay,* New York, 1991, Pantheon Books.
4. *Alternative Medicine: Expanding Medical Horizons—A*

Report to the National Institutes of Health on Alternative Medical Systems in the United States, NIH Pub No 94-066, December 1994.

5. American Optometric Association, Office of the Executive Director, personal communication, March 7, 1996.
6. Employee Benefit Research Institute, Foster-Higgins National Survey of Employer-Sponsored Plans/1993, US Census Bureau, *USA Today,* p 8A, Aug 9, 1994.
7. Carlson E: AARP submits health-care reform proposal to members for their review, *AARP Bulletin* 33(3):1, 1992.
8. Federal budget estimates for 1991-1996, Department of Health and Human Services estimate for 1991, Department of Commerce estimates for 1991-1996, *USA Today,* p 3B, May 6, 1991.
9. Human Development Report 1994 (United Nations), *USA Today,* p 1A, June 16, 1994.
10. Aaron H: *Serious and unstable condition: financing America's health care,* Washington, DC, 1991, Brookings Institute.
11. Health Care Financing Administration (1993), *USA Today,* p 1A, Jan 13, 1995.
12. Bureau of Labor Statistics bi-annual survey, *USA Today,* p 1A, Nov 17, 1994.
13. Kelly K: HMOs dogged by issue of cost versus care, *USA Today,* p 1D, Oct 17, 1995.
14. Gray P: Gagging the doctors, *Time,* p 50, January 8, 1996.
15. US Department of Health and Human Services, Group Health Association of America, CareData Reports, Foster Higgins, *USA Today,* p 1D, Oct 17, 1995.
16. McKenzie JF, Pinger RR: *Introduction to community health,* New York, 1995, HarperCollins College Publishing.
17. US Department of Health and Human Services, Social Security Administration: *Medicare,* SSA Pub No 06-10043, May 1993.
18. Detlefs D, Myers R: *1993 Medicare: What you need to know about Medicare in simple, practical terms,* 1992, William M Mercer.
19. Medicare under attack in Congress, *AARP Voter* 9(1):1-2, Spring 1995.
20. Health Care Financing Administration, *USA Today,* p 6A, Sept 25, 1995.
21. Ries P: Characteristics of persons with and without health care coverage: United States, 1989, *Advance data from vital and health statistics, No. 201,* Hyattsville, Md, 1991, National Center for Health Statistics, Centers for Disease Control.
22. Butler PA: *Too poor to be sick: access to medical care for the uninsured,* Washington, DC, 1988, American Public Health Association.
23. Fuchs BC, Skolovsky J: *CRS report for Congress: the Canadian health care system,* Washington, DC, 1990, Congressional Research Service, The Library of Congress.
24. Top 200 drugs, *American Druggist,* Feb 4, 1996.
25. Annual Rx review: Nicotine patches lead Rx activity to new heights, *Drug Topics* 137(7):72, 1993.
26. *Physicians' Desk Reference—Generics,* Montvale, NJ, 1995, Medical Economics Data Production.
27. Cornacchia HJ, Barrett S: *Consumer health: a guide to intelligent decisions,* ed 5, St Louis, 1993, Mosby.

Suggested Readings

Simon G, Silverman H: *The pill book,* New York, 1995, Bantam Books.

A reader-friendly publication designed to provide the general public with a dependable guide to prescription medication. Information related to drug interactions and side effects is also presented, as well as an illustrated guide to the most prescribed medications.

Inlander C: *Take this book to the hospital with you: a consumer guide to surviving your hospital stay,* New York, 1991, Pantheon Books.

Because most of us will experience hospitalization, the author provides a checklist for evaluating the "patient friendliness" of hospitals. Provides additional hints for making hospital stays more pleasant.

Taylor RL: *Health fact, health fiction—getting through the media maze,* Dallas, 1990, Taylor Publishing.

A physician writes about the problem of health hype through the media, which causes too many people to act on health information that is not credible. Encourages a sound approach for evaluation of health messages and health risks.

Physicians' Desk Reference—Generics, Montvale, NJ, 1995, Medical Economics Data Production.

Similar to *PDRs* related to prescription and OTC medication, this new version details the growing list of generic drugs. Today these once "doctor-only" publications can be found in most bookstores.

ON...

Evaluating Health Hype: A Look at Melatonin

It acts as a sleep aid. It helps prevent jet lag. It can act as a contraceptive and may help improve your sex life. It may slow the aging process and ward off heart disease. It acts as an antioxidant to help prevent cancer. It may slow the growth of tumors and cataracts. A month's supply costs about 10 dollars. It's perfectly legal.

And you've been under its influence all your life.

This "wonder drug" is melatonin, a hormone produced by the brain. Its normal role is to regulate the sleep cycle. The pineal gland, a pea-sized structure deep within the brain, releases melatonin naturally in the evenings in response to darkness.[1] Melatonin prepares the body for a natural stage of sleep, which ends with the return of daylight.[2] However, recent research suggests that melatonin may have practical uses beyond its hormonal functions, and as a result it's a hot commodity.

Consumer hype in action

Through the first half of the 1990s, melatonin has undergone a surge in popularity as a nutritional supplement. It had been used for a number of years by travelers to reduce the effects of jet lag,[2] but it has now gained public acceptance outside of the frequent flyer crowd. It is found in drugstores, nutrition centers, supermarkets, and service stations. Sales of melatonin increased twentyfold from 1993 to 1995.[1] Melatonin has been the focus of dozens of articles and several books in recent years as well.

Melatonin is the most recent in a long line of nutritional supplements and compounds touted as "cure-alls" by the advertising hype machine. You have probably heard of the virtues of such compounds as beta-carotene, ginseng root, ginkgo, and other such products from television, radio, print, and store advertisements. Often such products are introduced very quickly to the public through massive advertising campaigns. The average consumer can find it hard to make an informed choice between brands of a product or whether to use the product at all. Sometimes performance and safety information on a product is lacking, especially with some nutritional supplements that do not fall under regulation of the FDA. This raises several questions: Is this product safe? Does it do what the ads say it does? Is all of this attention warranted for the product?

Research data—pros and cons

At face value, preliminary melatonin research sounds very promising. One of the leading researchers on melatonin is Dr. Russel J. Reiter at the University of Texas Health Science Center in San Antonio. Reiter has studied this hormone for 30 years. He believes melatonin may help him "die young as late in life as possible" and takes 1 milligram or less of it each night.[3] Reiter has demonstrated that melatonin helps prevent free radical damage to cells. Free radicals, which are produced normally by our bodies, are chemicals that can destroy molecules within living systems by oxidizing (removing particles from) them. Free radicals can degrade cells and, when exposed to DNA, can create mutations that may in turn cause cells to become cancerous. In studies on rats, Reiter showed that doses of melatonin reduced DNA damage by 41% to 99% in specimens treated with free radical–forming compounds.[4] Thus melatonin, like the much-ballyhooed beta-carotene, may be valuable as an antioxidant. This characteristic of melatonin may make it useful in treating such maladies as Parkinson's disease and Alzheimer's disease.[4]

Other research has been just as intriguing. When the pineal glands of young rats were transplanted into older rats (and vice versa), the older rats had a significant increase in their normal life spans, had a regeneration of their thymus glands (an important immune system organ), and gained a new shine to their coats. The thymus glands of the younger rats degenerated at a rate much faster than normal, and the young rats died earlier than normal. Other studies involving rats have demonstrated that melatonin helps protect rats from the effects of ionizing radiation and protected their lungs against the deadly herbicide paraquat.[3] Although this research on rodents looks promising, the data may not be applicable to people, since rodents do not always respond to hormones in the same way that humans do.[1] Claims on improving one's sex life may simply be derived from the sleep-inducing effects of melatonin; a good night's sleep may help sexual performance and may make one feel more amorous in the morning.[1] However, research on hamsters suggests that melatonin may even be harmful to the sex drive. One study showed that high doses of melatonin administered to male hamsters resulted in shrinkage of the testicles.[1] More long-term studies on humans may have to be performed to determine whether melatonin indeed has an antiaging effect on human physiology.

In humans, it has been shown that high doses of melatonin in combination with certain other chemicals can prevent ovulation, and thus it has been suggested as

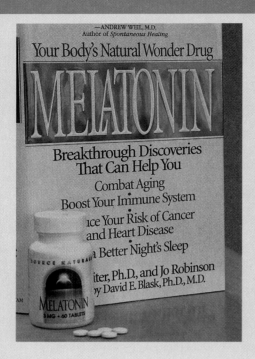

an alternative to the more common estrogen-based birth control pill. Since melatonin has been shown to reduce the risk of cancer, it may prove to be safer than the estrogen-based pills.[1] However, no such pill has been approved for use in the United States, and data are lacking on the effects of melatonin on the female reproductive system as a whole. It is not known if these experimental compounds will prove to be safe over the long run, and it has been speculated that the high doses of melatonin in these compounds may be unsafe for younger women. Whereas data on the long-term effects of melatonin use are lacking, the short-term side effects discovered to date appear to be fairly minimal. Very high doses of melatonin (over 5000 mg) have been found to cause stomach discomfort and residual sleepiness in people.[3] More long-term studies may help clear up questions concerning the high-dose effects of melatonin on humans.

Why the popularity may not last

The "cure-all" and "wonder drug" labels recently given to melatonin are not unprecedented for a nutritional supplement. Vitamin C, a necessary component of the body's metabolic pathways, has been used to treat such afflictions as colds, sore throats, rheumatoid arthritis, high cholesterol, and premenstrual syndrome, just to name a few.[5] Vitamin C can be obtained in tablet form or within such foods as citrus fruits, tomatoes, and spinach.

However, high doses (over 3000 mg/day) of vitamin C have been known to cause kidney stones in some people, so high-potency supplements can put one at risk for this side effect.[5] Otherwise, vitamin C has seemingly lived up to its press clippings.

The hype surrounding melatonin may prove difficult to live up to, however. If all of these claims sound too good to be true, perhaps they are. Since melatonin is a nutritional supplement, it is not classified as a drug by the FDA unless the manufacturer or supplier makes medical claims for it.[6] Also, since melatonin is a hormone produced naturally within humans, it can be patented only under specific circumstances. As a result, melatonin can be manufactured and sold by anyone with the proper resources and with less governmental regulation or intervention than drug manufacturers experience. Correct dosages for melatonin have therefore not been established, and there are little data on the potential reactions of melatonin with other nutritional supplements or with drugs.[3]

Nutritional supplements have not always proved to be as safe as advertised. Take the case of L-tryptophan, an amino acid supplement that became popular in the late 1980s. Amino acids are the "building blocks" of proteins, and tryptophan is one of the 20 amino acids used for this purpose in humans. This form of tryptophan was recalled by the FDA in 1990 after it was linked to hundreds of cases of eosinophilia-myalgia syndrome (EMS). This condition is marked by muscular pain, an increased number of eosinophils (a type of white cell) in the blood, rashes, and stomach ache.[7] Over 1500 cases of EMS (and 38 deaths) were linked to consumption of L-tryptophan produced by a single manufacturing company. Although the EMS cases were most likely the result of an irregularity within the product caused during processing, the FDA pulled all L-tryptophan off the shelves for fear of such an error happening again.[6]

Using common sense with nutritional supplements

As of this writing, no severe side effects such as those that occurred with L-tryptophan have been reported to the FDA regarding melatonin; however, this does not mean that unpleasant or even life-threatening side effects will never occur as a result of using melatonin. So what's a smart, health-conscious consumer to do? Before choosing to use melatonin or any type of supplement, keep in mind the following tips:

- Remember that just because dietary supplements are advertised as "natural" and are sold over the counter doesn't mean that they're harmless or completely safe. Amino acids and herbs that are found in many supplements are chemical compounds that can be just as dangerous as prescription drugs.

- Before you begin taking any dietary supplement, check with your doctor. Supplements may interact with prescription drugs you are taking and cause negative side effects or render your prescription medications useless. This tip is especially important for senior citizens or other individuals who may take more than one type of prescription drug.
- Be extra careful about taking supplements if you are prone to allergies or have any other type of immune disorder, such as asthma. Some types of supplements (including melatonin) may act as stimulants to the immune system and cause you to have an attack.
- Be very cautious about supplement dosages. Whereas some supplements, such as vitamins, have a recommended dietary allowance established by nutrition experts, most other types of supplements do not have an official RDA. Never assume that if one tablet works well, two tablets will work even better.
- Keep in mind that for many supplements, no scientific studies have been completed that establish effectiveness or that measure side effects of long-term usage.
- Never take any kind of dietary supplement while you are pregnant or nursing without the advice and consent of your doctor. Some supplements can be harmful to the developing fetus or to a nursing infant.
- Don't give supplements to children without checking with your pediatrician. Some supplements that are not harmful to adults in recommended dosages can cause severe side effects in children.
- Don't rely on the advice of sales clerks in health food or supplement stores. Although they can give you examples of individual cases in which a supplement appeared to help someone's condition, they cannot legally prescribe any type of supplement for a condition. Remember that although these people may be well-intentioned, they are not health care professionals.
- Above all, if you have a serious physical condition such as heart disease or arthritis, never attempt to self-medicate with supplements. Seek out competent medical advice from a licensed physician. Many serious illnesses are treatable with prescription drugs or surgery if they are caught early, but trying to treat yourself with supplements alone can be dangerous or even fatal.

When making choices about your health, it always pays to be a smart consumer. Taking a supplement such as melatonin once in a while for insomnia might not hurt, but overreliance on dietary supplements to create miracle cures is a potentially dangerous practice. Before you begin taking any type of supplement, talk with your doctor, read up on the subject, and make an informed choice. Your good health depends on your conscientious efforts.

For Discussion . . .
Do you feel that nutritional supplements should be regulated more strictly by the government? What types of safety precautions, if any, should be taken by the FDA before a nutritional supplement is allowed onto store shelves?

References
1. Podolsky D: A natural wonder drug? *US News and World Report* 119(15), Oct 16, 1995.
2. How to beat jet lag, *Newsweek,* Nov 6, 1995.
3. Cowley, Geoffrey: Melatonin (hormone that allegedly curbs the aging process), *Newsweek* 126(6), Aug 7, 1995.
4. But quenched by ubiquitous hormone, *Science News* 144(7), Aug 14, 1993.
5. *The Doctor's Book of Home Remedies,* 1990, Emmaus, Penn, Rodale Press.
6. Casey B: Bitter pill, *In Health* 5(1), Jan 2, 1991.
7. Nightingale SL: Update on EMS and L-tryptophan, *JAMA* 268(14), 1992.

Protecting Your Safety

Healthy People 2000 Objectives

The Healthy People 2000 Midcourse Review assesses progress toward target goals in the two broad areas of violent and abusive behavior and unintentional injuries. Unfortunately, the review indicates that we are making headway on only three of the 18 objectives in the area of violence. First, suicide rates have remained stable for the entire population, although rates among young men seem to be on the rise. Second, the incidence of rape and reported rape has declined. Third, the number of adolescents ages 14 to 17 who carry weapons has dropped.

The nation is losing ground in the areas of homicides, firearm-related deaths, assault injuries, and suicide attempts by adolescents. The Midcourse Review warns that if present trends continue, the death rate from firearms will exceed the death rate from automobile accidents by the year 2003.

The review highlights progress toward meeting 14 of the nation's 16 safety objectives. We have moved farther away from our goals of reducing hip fractures among older adults and increasing the number of residences with smoke detectors. Seven of the remaining safety objectives have been reached or surpassed, and three others have almost been achieved.

As recently as 15 years ago, the suspicious disappearance of a school-aged child or the death of a bystander during a drive-by shooting was virtually unheard of. In the mid-1990s, violent crimes are committed so frequently in the United States that they rarely make front-page headlines. However, in June 1994 the brutal deaths of Nicole Brown Simpson, former wife of football Hall of Famer O.J. Simpson, and her friend Ronald Goldman put one form of violence—domestic violence—back on the front page.[1]

Domestic violence directed at women and children seems to be increasing, and many people fear being a random victim of a homicide, robbery, or carjacking. Law enforcement officials contend that gang activities and hard-core drug involvement are significant factors that have increased violent behavior in our society.

Although violence may seem to be focused in urban areas, no community is completely safe. Even people who live in small towns and rural areas now must lock their doors and remain vigilant about protecting their safety. Crime on college campuses is on the rise,[2] much of which is a direct result of alcohol use.

For some students the content in this chapter may be the most important information in this textbook. Becoming a victim of violent behavior or sustaining an unintentional injury can harm your health as much (or more) than any of your own unhealthy behavior. The goal of this chapter is to help you understand the scope of violence in our society and learn what you can do to avoid becoming a victim. Complete the Personal Assessment on p. 404 to see whether you are adequately protecting your own safety.

INTENTIONAL INJURIES

Intentional injuries are injuries that are committed on purpose. With the exception of suicide (which is self-directed), intentional injuries reflect violence committed by one person acting against another person. Categories of intentional injuries include homicide, robbery, rape, suicide, assault, child abuse, spouse abuse, and elder abuse. Each year in the United States, intentional injuries cause about 50,000 deaths and another 2 million nonfatal injuries.[3]

The U.S. Department of Justice reported that 6.4 million violent crimes (excluding homicide) were committed in 1991.[4] In other words, there were 31 violent crimes for every 1000 people age 12 and older. Although this rate of violent crime may sound high, it is lower than the record of 35 crimes per 1000 people in 1981. Let's look at some of these violent crimes in more detail.

Homicide

Homicide, or murder, is the intentional killing of one person by another. Sadly, the United States leads the industrialized world in homicide rates. In 1993 a total of 24,526 people were murdered in the United States.[4] Fortunately, homicides may have reached a peak. Preliminary data gathered at the time of this writing indicate that the homicide rate is now actually dropping in the United States.[5]

Criminal justice experts are trying to pinpoint why U.S. homicide rates are dropping. No one answer has emerged, but speculation centers on better community policing efforts; the 1994 passage of the sweeping Federal Crime Bill; recent legislation, such as the Brady law; and a variety of tough state laws, such as the "three strikes and you're out" provisions that mandate life sentences without parole for repeat violent offenders.

There are some clear trends when it comes to the people involved in homicides. The most vulnerable group of homicide victims are African-Americans, especially young male African-Americans. Homicide is the leading cause of death for male African-American ages 15 to 44. African-American men have a 1 in 21 lifetime chance of becoming a victim of homicide.[6]

Another clear trend related to homicide is the extent to which illegal drug activity is related to homicide. A variety of research studies from large cities indicate that 25% to 50% of all homicides are drug related.[7] Most of these murders are related to activities involved in drug trafficking, including disputed drug transactions. Additionally, high percentages of both homicide assailants and victims have drugs in their systems at the time of the homicide.[7]

Finally, another clear trend is that handguns are the weapon of choice for homicides. In 1993, handguns were used in 57% of the homicides in the United States.[4] This is not surprising because handgun use among most categories of violent crime reached record levels in 1992. In 1992, 13% of all violent crimes were committed with offenders using handguns.[8] The proliferation of handguns and their use in violent crimes led to the passage of the so-called Brady law (see the Star Box on p. 405).

intentional injuries
Injuries that are purposely committed by a person.

homicide
The intentional killing of one person by another person.

PERSONAL ASSESSMENT

How Well Do You Protect Your Safety?

This quiz will help you measure how well you manage your personal safety. For each item below, circle the number that reflects the frequency with which you do the safety activity. Then, add up your individual scores and check the interpretation at the end.

3   I regularly do this
2   I sometimes do this
1   I rarely do this

1. I am aware of my surroundings and do not get lost.   3 2 1
2. I avoid locations in which my personal safety could be compromised.   3 2 1
3. I intentionally vary my daily routine (such as walking patterns to and from class, parking places, and jogging or biking routes) so that my whereabouts are not always predictable.   3 2 1
4. I walk across campus at night with other people.   3 2 1
5. I am careful about disclosing personal information (address, phone number, social security number, my daily schedule, etc.) to people I do not know.   3 2 1
6. I carefully monitor my alcohol intake at parties.   3 2 1
7. I watch carefully for dangerous weather conditions and know how to respond if necessary.   3 2 1
8. I do not keep a loaded gun in my home.   3 2 1
9. I know how I would handle myself if I were to be assaulted.   3 2 1
10. I maintain adequate insurance for my health and my property.   3 2 1
11. I keep emergency information numbers near my phone.   3 2 1
12. I keep my first aid skills up-to-date.   3 2 1
13. I use deadbolt locks on the doors of my home.   3 2 1
14. I use the safety locks on the windows at home.   3 2 1
15. I check the batteries used in my home smoke detector.   3 2 1
16. I have installed a carbon monoxide detector in my home.   3 2 1
17. I use adequate lighting in areas around my home and garage.   3 2 1
18. I have the electrical, heating, and cooling equipment in my home inspected regularly for safety and efficiency.   3 2 1
19. I use my car seat belt.   3 2 1
20. I drive my car safely and defensively.   3 2 1
21. I keep my car in good mechanical order.   3 2 1
22. I keep my car doors locked.   3 2 1
23. I have a plan of action if my car should break down while I am driving it.   3 2 1
24. I use appropriate safety equipment, such as flotation devices, helmets, and elbow pads, in my recreational activities.   3 2 1
25. I can swim well enough to save myself in most situations.   3 2 1
26. I use suggestions for personal safety each day.   3 2 1

TOTAL POINTS _____

Interpretation

Your total may mean that:

72-78 points	You appear to carefully protect your personal safety.
65-71 points	You adequately protect many aspects of your personal safety.
58-64 points	You should consider improving some of your safety-related behaviors.
Below 58 points	You must consider improving some of your safety-related behaviors.

To Carry This Further . . .

Although no one can be completely safe from personal injury or possible random violence, there are ways to minimize the risks to your safety. Scoring high on this assessment will not guarantee your safety, but your likelihood for injury should remain relatively low. Scoring low on this assessment should encourage you to consider ways to make your life more safe. Refer to the text and this assessment to provide you with useful suggestions to enhance your personal safety. Which safety tips will you use today?

The Brady Law

On November 31, 1993, President Bill Clinton signed into law the most sweeping handgun-control bill since 1968 (when Congress banned mail-order purchases of rifles, shotguns, handguns, and ammunition shortly after the assassinations of Robert Kennedy and Dr. Martin Luther King, Jr.). This bill was named after James Brady, the former White House press secretary who was seriously wounded in the 1981 assassination attempt on President Ronald Reagan.[10]

The signing of the Brady Bill into law was the culmination of a 7-year crusade by Brady and his wife, Sarah. This gun control bill was endorsed by virtually every major law enforcement organization in the country. The Brady Bill was opposed by the National Rifle Association, which was convinced that the bill endangered the constitutional right to bear arms and would not deter violent crime to any significant degree.

The law requires a 5-day waiting period and a background check on handgun buyers. The purpose of the background check is to prevent people with certain criminal records from purchasing handguns from licensed dealers.

Domestic Violence

Family life in the 1990s is a far cry from that portrayed in the popular 1950s and 1960s television shows like the *Donna Reed Show, Father Knows Best,* and *Ozzie and Harriet.* The composition of families has changed considerably. In the 1950s a common family pattern included children being raised by both parents. Generally, the father was the income earner and the mother stayed at home and managed the growing family.

Today, family patterns are much more complex. Children are more frequently being raised in blended families or in families headed by single parents. In fact, since 1970, single-parent households have increased 112%, from 4 to 8.9 million homes.[9] A much higher percentage of women are employed outside the home. Because of pressing family economic concerns, many children take care of themselves during after-school hours. Sociologists indicate that families, and the individuals in those families, are under more stress than ever.

Add to this precarious nature of the American family the additional factors of increased societal drug use, increased presence of handguns, and increased crime and violence. What emerges is no surprise—increased domestic violence.

Partner abuse

Partner abuse refers to violence committed against a domestic partner. Most often the victims are women, and a significant percentage of these women are spouses or former spouses of the assailant. Figures from the U.S. Department of Justice[11] are frightening and make it difficult to believe that the United States can achieve its Healthy People 2000 objective in this area. More than 2.5 million women are victims of some form of violence every year. Nearly two in three female victims of violent crimes are related to or know their attacker. About three out of four female victims resist the actions of their offenders either physically or verbally.

The most vulnerable female victims are African-American and Hispanic, live in large cities, are young and unmarried, and are from lower socioeconomic groups.[11] However, these trends do not mean that only women from these classifications are vulnerable to violent behavior. Women across all economic, racial, and age categories are potential victims. For example, in the aftermath of the tragic murder of Nicole Brown Simpson, the picture of an affluent woman who had been a victim of domestic violence emerged.

One of the real difficulties related to domestic violence is the vast underreporting of this crime to law enforcement authorities. The U.S. Department of Justice estimates that about half of the victims of domestic violence do not report the crime to police. Too many victims view their violent situations as private or personal matters and not actual crimes. Despite painful injuries, many victims view the offenses against them as minor.[11]

Of course, it is easy to criticize the victims of domestic violence for not reporting the crimes committed against them, but this may be unfair. Why do women stay in these relationships? Many women who are injured may fear being killed if they report the crime. Women may also fear for the safety of their children. Women who receive economic support from an abuser may fear being left with no financial resources.

However, help is available for victims of partner abuse. Most communities have family support or domestic violence hotlines that abused people can call for help. Communities are establishing shelters where abused women and their children can seek safety

partner abuse
Violence committed against a domestic partner.

Denise Brown speaks out against domestic violence.

while their cases are being handled by the police or court officials. If you are being abused or know of someone who is the victim of domestic violence, do not hesitate to use the services of these local hotlines or shelters. Also, check the resources listed in the Health Reference Guide at the back of this text.

Child abuse

Like many cases of partner abuse, **child abuse** tends to be a silent crime. It is estimated that about 1 million children are victims of child abuse and neglect each year.[12] Of course, some children are victims of repeated crimes, and since many victims do not report their crimes, the actual incidence of child abuse is difficult to determine.

Children are abused in various ways.[13] Physical abuse reflects physical injury, such as bruises, burns, abrasions, cuts, and fractures of the bones and skull. Sexual abuse includes acts that lead to sexual gratification of the abuser. Examples include fondling,

touching, and various acts involved in rape, sodomy, and incest. Child neglect is also a form of child abuse and includes an extreme failure to provide children with adequate clothing, food, shelter, and medical attention. A strong case can also be made for psychological abuse as a form of child abuse. Certainly, children are scarred by family members and others who routinely damage their psychological development. Unfortunately, this form of abuse is especially difficult to identify and measure.

The most frequent form of child abuse is neglect.[13] The incidence of child neglect is approximately three times the incidence of physical abuse and about seven times the incidence of child sexual abuse. Each form of abuse can have devastating short- and long-term consequences for the child.

Research studies in the various areas of child abuse reveal some interesting trends. Abused children are much more likely than nonabused children to grow up to be child abusers themselves. It is also now understood that abused children are more likely to suffer from poor educational performance, increased health problems, and low levels of overall achievement. Recent research also points out that abused children are significantly more likely than nonabused children to become involved in adult crime and violent criminal behavior.[13]

It is beyond the scope of this book to discuss in detail how to reduce child abuse. However, the violence directed against children can likely be lessened through a combination of early identification measures and violence prevention programs. Teachers, friends, relatives, social workers, counselors, psychologists, police, and the court system must not hesitate to intervene early in cases of suspected child abuse. The later the intervention, the more likely that the abuse will have worsened. Once abuse has occurred, it is likely to happen again.

Violence prevention programs can help parents and caregivers learn how to resolve conflicts, improve communication, cope with anger, improve parenting skills, and challenge the view of violence presented in movies and television.[14] In these programs, it may be possible to stop violence before it begins to damage the lives of young children. Figure 16-1 provides simple alternatives parents can choose to avoid hitting a child.[15]

Elder abuse

Among the nation's 31 million elderly people, 1.5 million are the victims of neglect and abuse. Particularly vulnerable are elderly women over the age of 75 years. More often than not, the abusers are the adult children of the victims.

Figure 16-1   Alternatives to hitting your child.

Many elderly people are hit, kicked, attacked with knives, denied food and medical care, and have their Social Security checks and automobiles stolen. It is likely that this reflects a combination of factors, particularly the stress of caring for failing older people by middle-aged children who are also faced with the additional demands of dependent children and careers. In many cases, the middle-aged children were themselves abused, or there may be a chemical dependence problem. The alternative, institutionalization, is so expensive that it is often not an option for either the abused or the abusers.

Although protective services are available in most communities through welfare departments, elder abuse is frequently unseen and unreported. In many cases, the elderly people themselves are afraid to report their children's behavior because of the fear of embarrassment that they were not good parents to their children. Regardless of the cause, however, elder abuse must be reported to the appropriate protective service so that intervention can occur.

Gangs and Youth Violence

In the last 15 years, gangs and gang activities have been increasingly responsible for escalating violence and criminal activity. Before that time, gangs used fists, tire irons, and occasionally, cheap handguns ("Saturday night specials") as tools of enforcement. Now, gang members do not hesitate to use AK-47s (semiautomatic military assault weapons) that have the potential to kill large groups of people in a few seconds.

Most, but not all, gangs arise from big city environments where many socially alienated, economically disadvantaged young people live. Convinced that society has no significant role for them, gang members can receive support from an association of peers that has well-defined lines of authority. Rituals and membership initiation rites are important in gang socialization. Gangs often control particular territories within a city.[16] Frequently, gangs are involved in criminal activities, the most common of which are illicit drug trafficking and robberies. In the mid-1990s, gang-related murders and drive-by shootings are contributing to the rising death toll among young people.

It is not only older male teenagers and young adults who are members of today's gangs. Increasingly, law enforcement officials see younger people (ages 12, 13, and 14) joining gangs. Some gangs have recently included young women as members, and some cities report a growing number of all-female gangs. Some female gangs are reported to be every bit as ruthless as the male gangs.[17]

Youth violence is also spreading from the inner cities to the suburbs. Public health officials and law enforcement personnel claim that youth violence is growing in epidemic proportions. Attorney General Janet Reno[18] has stated that youth violence is "the greatest single crime problem in America today."

Attempting to control gang and youth violence is particularly expensive for communities. When you consider that for every gang-related homicide, there are about 100 nonfatal gang-related intentional injuries, it becomes obvious that gang violence is an

child abuse
Harm that is committed against a child; usually referring to physical abuse, sexual abuse, or child neglect.

expensive health care proposition. Furthermore, gang and youth violence takes an enormous financial and human toll on law enforcement, judicial, and corrections departments. Reducing gang and youth violence will be a daunting task for the nation as it approaches the year 2000.

Gun Violence

The tragic effect of gun violence has already been touched on in a few sections of this chapter. Guns are being used more than ever in our society and in other parts of the world (see the Learning from All Cultures box below). In 1992, people armed with handguns committed a record 931,000 violent crimes.[8] More than 60% of the homicides and 55% of the suicides committed each year in the United States involve the use of guns. As previously mentioned, gun violence is a leading killer of teenagers and young men, especially African-American men, and the use of semiautomatic assault weapons by individuals and gang members is increasing. Accidental deaths of toddlers and young children from loaded handguns is another dimension of the violence attributable to guns in our

society. In addition, guns are often used in **carjackings** (see the Health Action Guide on p. 409).

The proliferation of firearm use has prompted serious discussions concerning the enactment of gun control laws. For years, gun control activists have been in direct battle with the National Rifle Association (NRA) and its congressional supporters. Gun control activists want fewer guns manufactured and greater controls over the sale and possession of handguns. Gun supporters believe that such controls are not necessary and that people (the criminals) are responsible for gun deaths, not simply the guns. This debate will certainly continue.

Bias and Hate Crimes

One sad aspect of any society is how some segments of the majority treat certain people in the minority. Nowhere is this more violently pronounced than in **bias and hate crimes.** These crimes are directed at individuals or groups of people solely because of a racial, ethnic, religious, or other difference attributed to the victims. Victims are often verbally and physically attacked, their houses are spray

LEARNING
from ALL CULTURES

Violence Exists in All Cultures

As this edition of *Focus on Health* goes to press, the people of the United States are coming to grips with legal aspects related to three well-known cases of American violence. The trial of the confessed killer of young Polly Klaas, the arraignment of the suspected Unabomber, and the trial of the two suspects in the bombing of the federal building in Oklahoma City are front-page news stories. It is impossible to follow national news reports without daily reminders that we live in a violent society.

Unfortunately, Americans are not alone in their sharing of grief over violent acts. Violence occurs on a daily basis in all corners of the world. Among the continuing acts of violence are the bombings in the Middle East, factional fighting in Bosnia, and bloody uprisings in politically fragile African countries. To these tragedies, we must add the terrorist acts in the United Kingdom and the fighting between Russia and certain ethnic enclaves of the former Soviet Union. Violent deaths take their toll on people in all cultures.

Two especially tragic events took place in the spring

of 1996. These events shocked the world because they involved horrible massacres of innocent people. The first occurred in the small, peaceful town of Dunblane, Scotland. A heavily armed middle-aged man entered an elementary school and killed 16 kindergartners and their teacher. The man, a suspected pedophile, also wounded 12 children before killing himself.

The second tragedy took place halfway around the world in Tasmania, an island state off the southern coast of Australia. In this instance, a 29-year-old man with a history of mental problems started shooting tourists in the resort city of Port Arthur. Before he was finally captured, the suspect had killed over 30 people, including a number of small children. Videotaped footage of this rampage was seen worldwide.

These mass murders remind us that violent acts can take place anywhere. This is a sad reminder, but perhaps there is a message amid these tragedies: we should never take our lives (or those of our loved ones) for granted. Perhaps we should better appreciate the time we have to share our affection and support with those who mean so much to us. 🌐

HEALTH
Action Guide

Preventing Carjacking

In the last 5 years a new form of violence has reached the streets of America. This crime is commonly called *carjacking*. Unlike auto theft, in which a car thief attempts to steal an unattended parked car, carjacking involves a thief's attempt to steal a car with a driver still behind the wheel.

Most carjacking attempts begin when a car is stopped at an intersection, usually at a traffic light. A carjacker will approach the driver and force him or her to give up the car. Resisting an armed carjacker can be extremely dangerous. Law enforcement officials offer the following tips to prevent carjacking[19]:

- Drive only on well-lit and well-traveled streets, if possible.
- Always keep your doors locked when driving your car.
- Observe traffic that may be following you. If you think that something suspicious is happening, try to locate a police officer or a busy, populated area to seek help.
- If someone approaches your car and you cannot safely drive away, roll the window down only slightly and leave the car running and in gear. If the situation turns bad, use your wits and quickly flee the scene, either in the car or on foot. Remember: your life is worth more than your car.
- If another car taps the rear bumper of your car (a common carjacking maneuver to get you to exit your car) and you feel uncomfortable about getting out of your car, tell the other driver that you are driving to the police station to complete the accident report.

painted with various slurs, and many are forced to move from one neighborhood or community to another. According to Federal Bureau of Investigation (FBI) 1993 statistics, there were 7587 hate crime incidents in the United States, involving 9372 victims.[9]

Typically, the offenders in bias or hate crimes are fringe elements of the larger society who believe that the mere presence of someone with a racial, ethnic, or religious difference is inherently bad for the community, state, or country. Examples of groups commonly known to commit bias and hate crimes in the United States are skinheads, the Ku Klux Klan, and other white supremacist groups. Increasingly, state and fed-

eral laws have been enacted to make bias and hate crimes serious offenses.

With a small but growing presence of neo-Nazi groups in Europe and clear evidence of ethnic cleansing in Bosnia, Serbia, Croatia, and the former Soviet Union, bias and hate crimes are a worldwide problem. It is hoped that the recent push on college campuses to promote multicultural education and the celebration of diversity will make today's generation of college graduates well aware of the importance of tolerance and inclusion rather than bigotry and exclusion.

Stalking

In recent years the crime of stalking has received considerable attention. **Stalking** refers to an assailant's planned efforts at pursuing an intended victim. Most stalkers are male. (One notable exception is the convicted female stalker of talk show host David Letterman.) Many of these stalkers are excessively possessive or jealous and pursue people with whom they formerly had a relationship. Some stalkers pursue people with whom they have had only an imaginary relationship.

Some stalkers have served time in prison and have waited for years to "get back" at their victims. In some cases, stalkers go to great lengths to locate their intended victims and frequently know their daily whereabouts. Although not all stalkers plan to batter or kill their victims, their presence and potential for violence are enough to create an extremely frightening environment for the intended victim and family.

Fortunately, since 1990, virtually all states have enacted or tightened their laws related to stalking and have created stiff penalties for stalkers (see the Star

carjacking
A crime that involves a thief's attempt to steal a car while the owner is behind the wheel; carjackings are usually random, unpredictable, and frequently involve handguns.

bias and hate crimes
Criminal acts directed at a person or group solely because of a specific characteristic, such as race, religion, ethnic background, or political belief.

stalking
A crime involving an assailant's planned efforts to pursue an intended victim.

Box below). In many areas the criminal justice system is proactive in letting possible victims of stalking know, for example, when a particular prison inmate is going to be released. In other areas, citizens are banding together to provide support and protection for people who may be victims of stalkers.

If you think you are or someone you know is being stalked, contact the police (or a local crisis intervention hotline number) to report your case and use their guidance. You might sense that you are a potential stalking victim either through the circumstances of a past relationship or through the unusual behavior of someone who seems to be irrationally jealous of you or overly obsessed with you. Report a person who continues to pester or intimidate you with phone calls, written notes or letters, or unwanted gifts. Report people who make persistent efforts to be with you after you have told them you do not want to see them. Until the situation is resolved, be alert for potentially threatening situations and keep in close touch with friends.

SEXUAL VICTIMIZATION

Ideally, sexual intimacy is a mutual, enjoyable form of communication between two people. Far too often, however, relationships are approached in an aggressive, hostile manner. These sexual aggressors always

Must Victims Face Their Stalkers?
U.S. constitutional law dictates that criminals have the right to face their accusers in court. In early 1996, this court procedure came under attack from stalking victims and their attorneys. One celebrated case involved rock star and actress Madonna and a man accused of trespassing on her property in a purported attempt to establish a relationship with her.

Madonna did not want to face this man directly in court. Such a face-to-face meeting in court would have accomplished exactly what her accused may have wanted in the first place: an opportunity to be near his victim.

However, the judge in the case mandated that Madonna appear in court to face the accused rather than to testify on videotape. (In some cases, child abuse victims are permitted to testify on videotape because of the psychological trauma that could result from face-to-face confrontations with alleged perpetrators.) What do you think? Should this courtesy be extended to adult victims of stalking crimes? Are there cases in which the rights of the victim supersede the rights of the accused?

have a victim—someone who is physically or psychologically traumatized. *Sexual victimization* occurs in many forms and in a variety of settings. In this section we briefly look at sexual victimization as it occurs in rape and sexual assault, sexual abuse of children, sexual harassment, and the commercialization of sex.

Rape and Sexual Assault

As violence in our society increases, the incidence of *rape* and *sexual assault* correspondingly rises. The victims of these crimes fall into no single category. Victims of rape and sexual assault include young and old, male and female. They can be the mentally retarded, prisoners, hospital patients, and college students. We all are potential victims, and self-protection is critical. Read the Star Box below concerning myths about rape.

Sometimes a personal assault begins as a physical assault that may turn into a rape situation. Rape is generally considered a crime of sexual aggression in which the victim is forced to have sexual intercourse.

Myths about Rape
Despite the fact that we are all potential victims, many of us do not fully understand how vulnerable we are. Rape in particular has associated with it a number of myths (false assumptions), including the following:

- *Women are raped by strangers.* In approximately half of all reported rapes, the victim has some prior acquaintance with the rapist. Increasingly, women are being raped by husbands, dating partners, and relatives.
- *Rapes almost always occur in dark alleys or deserted places.* The opposite is true. Most rapes occur in or very near the victim's residence.
- *Rapists are easily identified by their demeanor or psychological profile.* Most experts indicate that rapists do not differ significantly from nonrapists.
- *The incidence of rape is overreported.* Estimates are that only one in five rapes is reported.
- *Rape happens only to people in low socioeconomic classes.* Rape occurs in all socioeconomic classes. Each person, male or female, young or old, is a potential victim.
- *There is a standard way to escape from a potential rape situation.* Each rape situation is different. No one method to avoid rape can work in every potential rape situation. Because of this, we encourage personal health classes to invite speakers from a local rape prevention services bureau to discuss approaches to rape prevention.

Current thought concerning rape characterizes this behavior as a violent act that happens to be carried out through sexual contact. (See the Health Action Guides on rape prevention guidelines and help for the rape victim.)

Acquaintance and date rape

In recent years, closer attention has been paid to the sexual victimization that occurs during relationships. *Acquaintance rape* refers to forced sexual intercourse between individuals who know each other. *Date rape* is a form of acquaintance rape that involves forced sexual intercourse by a dating partner. Studies on a number of campuses suggest that about 20% of college women reported having experienced date rape. An even higher percentage of women report being kissed and touched against their will. Alcohol is frequently a significant contributing factor in these rape situations. (See Chapter 8 concerning alcohol's role in campus crime.) Some men have reported being psychologically coerced into intercourse by their female dating partners. In many cases the aggressive partner will display certain behaviors that can be categorized (see the Health Action Guide on p. 413).

Psychologists believe that aside from the physical harm of date rape, a greater amount of emotional damage may occur. Such damage stems from the concept of broken trust. Date rape victims feel particularly violated because the perpetrator was not a stranger: it was someone they initially trusted, at least to some degree. Once that trust is broken, developing new relationships with other people becomes much more difficult for the date rape victim.

Nearly all victims of date rape seem to suffer from *posttraumatic stress syndrome.* They can have anxiety, sleeplessness, eating disorders, and nightmares. Guilt concerning their own behavior, self-esteem, and judgment of other people can be overwhelming, and the individual may require professional counseling. Because of the seriousness of these consequences, all students should be aware of the existence of date rape.

Sexual abuse of children

One of the most tragic forms of sexual victimization is the sexual abuse of children. Children are especially vulnerable to sexual abuse because of their dependent relationships with parents, relatives, and caregivers (such as babysitters, teachers, and neighbors). Often, children are unable to readily understand the difference between appropriate and inappropriate physical contact. Abuse may range from blatant physical manipulation, including fondling, to oral sex, sodomy, and intercourse.

HEALTH Action Guide

Rape Prevention Guidelines

To prevent rape from occurring:

- Never forget that you could be a candidate for personal assault.
- Use approved campus security or escort services, especially at night.
- Think carefully about your patterns of movement to and from class or work. Alter your routes frequently.
- Walk briskly with a sense of purpose. Try not to walk alone at night.
- Dress so that the clothes you wear do not unnecessarily restrict your movement or make you more vulnerable.
- Always be aware of your surroundings. Look over your shoulder occasionally. Know where you are so that you won't get lost.
- Avoid getting into a car if you do not know the driver well.
- If you think you are being followed, look for a safe retreat. This might be a store, a fire or police station, or a group of people.
- Be especially cautious of first dates, blind dates, or people you meet at a party or bar who push to be alone with you.
- Let trusted friends know where you are and when you plan to return.
- Keep your car in good working order. Think beforehand how you would handle the situation should your car break down.
- Limit, and even avoid, alcohol to minimize the risk of rape.
- Trust your best instincts if you are assaulted. Each situation is different. Do what you can to protect your life.

Because of the subordinate role of children in relationships involving adults, sexually abusive practices often go unreported. Sexual abuse can leave emotional scars that make it difficult to establish meaningful relationships later in life. For this reason, it is especially important for people to pay close attention to any information shared by children that could indicate a potentially abusive situation. Most states require that information concerning child abuse be reported to law enforcement officials.

HEALTH
Action Guide ----→

Help for the Rape Victim

If you have been raped, seek help as soon as possible. The following procedures may be helpful.

- *Call the police immediately to report the assault.* Police can take you to the hospital and start gathering information that may help them apprehend the rapist. Fortunately, many police departments now use specially trained officers (many of whom are female) to work closely with rape victims during all stages of the investigation.
- If you would rather not contact the police immediately, *call a local rape crisis center.* Operated generally on a 24-hour hotline basis, these centers have trained counselors to help you evaluate your options, contact the police, escort you to the hospital, and provide aftercare counseling.
- *Do not alter any potential evidence related to the rape.* Do not change your clothes, douche, take a bath, or rearrange the scene of the crime. Wait until all the evidence has been gathered.
- *Report all bruises, cuts, and scratches, even if they seem insignificant.* Report any information about the attack as completely and accurately as possible.
- *You will probably be given a thorough pelvic examination.* You may have to ask for STD tests and pregnancy tests.
- Although it is unusual for a rape victim's name to appear in the media, you might *request that the police withhold your name* as long as is legally possible.

◄-----➔

Sexual harassment

Sexual harassment consists of "unwanted attention of a sexual nature that creates embarrassment or stress."[20] Examples of sexual harassment include unwanted physical contact, excessive pressure for dates, sexually explicit humor, sexual innuendos or remarks, offers of job advancement based on sexual favors, and overt sexual assault. Unlike more overt forms of sexual victimization, sexual harassment may be applied in a subtle manner and can, in some cases, go unnoticed by co-workers and fellow students. Nevertheless, sexual harassment produces stress that cannot be resolved until the harasser is identified and forced to stop. Both men and women can be victims of sexual harassment.

Sexual harassment can occur in many settings, including employment and academic settings. On the college campus, harassment may be primarily in terms of the offer of sex for grades. If this occurs to you, think carefully about the situation and document the specific times, events, and places where the harassment took place. Consult your college's policy concerning harassment. Next, you could report these events to the appropriate administrative officer (perhaps the affirmative action officer, dean of academic affairs, or dean of students). You may also want to

HEALTH
Action Guide

Avoiding Date Rape

The first step in avoiding date rape is to consider your partner's behaviors. Many, but not all, date rapists show one or more of the following behaviors: a disrespectful attitude toward you and others, lack of concern for your feelings, violence and hostility, obsessive jealousy, extreme competitiveness, a desire to dominate, and unnecessary physical roughness. Consider these behaviors as warning signs for possible problems in the future. Reevaluate your participation in the relationship.

Below are some specific ways both men and women can avoid a date rape situation:

Men
- *Know your sexual desires and limits.* Communicate them clearly. Be aware of social pressures. It's OK not to score.
- *Being turned down when you ask for sex is not a rejection of you personally.* Women who say no to sex are not rejecting the person; they are expressing their desire not to participate in a single act. Your desires may be beyond control, but your actions are within your control.
- *Accept the woman's decision.* "No" means "No." Don't read other meanings into the answer. Don't continue after you are told "No!"
- *Don't assume that just because a woman dresses in a sexy manner and flirts that she wants to have sexual intercourse.*

- *Don't assume that previous permission for sexual contact applies to the current situation.*
- *Avoid excessive use of alcohol and drugs.* Alcohol and other drugs interfere with clear thinking and effective communication.

Women
- *Know your sexual desires and limits.* Believe in your right to set those limits. If you are not sure, STOP and talk about it.
- *Communicate your limits clearly.* If someone starts to offend you, tell him so firmly and immediately. Polite approaches may be misunderstood or ignored. Say "No" when you mean "No."
- *Be assertive.* Often men interpret passivity as permission. Be direct and firm with someone who is sexually pressuring you.
- *Be aware that your nonverbal actions send a message.* If you dress in a sexy manner and flirt, some men may assume you want to have sex. This does not make your dress or behavior wrong, but it is important to be aware of a possible misunderstanding.
- *Pay attention to what is happening around you.* Watch the nonverbal clues. Do not put yourself into vulnerable situations.
- *Trust your intuitions.* If you feel you are being pressured into unwanted sex, you probably are.
- *Avoid excessive use of alcohol and drugs.* Alcohol and other drugs interfere with clear thinking and effective communication.

discuss the situation with a staff member of the university counseling center.

If harassment occurs in the work environment, the victim should document the occurrences and report them to the appropriate management or personnel official. Reporting procedures will vary from setting to setting. Sexual harassment is a form of illegal sex discrimination and violates Title VII of the Civil Rights Act of 1964.

In 1986 the U.S. Supreme Court ruled that the creation of a "hostile environment" in a work setting was sufficient evidence to support the claim of sexual harassment. This action served as an impetus for thousands of women to step forward with sexual harassment allegations. Additionally, some men are also filing sexual harassment lawsuits against female supervisors.

Not surprisingly, this rising number of complaints

has served as a wake-up call for employers. From university settings to factory production lines to corporate board rooms, employers are scrambling to make certain that employees are fully aware of actions that could lead to a sexual harassment lawsuit. Sexual harassment workshops and educational seminars on harassment are now common and serve to educate both men and women about this complex problem.

Violence and the Commercialization of Sex

It is beyond the scope of this book to explore whether sexual violence can be related to society's exploitation or commercialization of sex. However, sexually related products and messages are intentionally placed before the public to try to sway consumer decisions. Do you believe that there could be a connection between commercial products, such as violent pornography in films and magazines, and violence against women? Does prostitution lead directly to violence? Do sexually explicit "900" phone numbers cause an increase in violent acts? Can the sexual messages in beer commercials lead to acquaintance rape? What do you think?

UNINTENTIONAL INJURIES

Unintentional injuries are injuries that have occurred without anyone intending that any harm be done. Common examples include injuries resulting from car crashes, falls, fires, drownings, firearm accidents, recreational accidents, and residential accidents. Each year, unintentional injuries account for over 150,000 deaths and millions of nonfatal injuries.

Unintentional injuries are very expensive for our society, both from a financial standpoint and from a personal and family standpoint. Fortunately, to a large extent it is possible to avoid becoming a victim of an unintentional injury. By carefully considering the tips presented in the safety categories that follow, you will be protecting yourself from many preventable injuries.

Since this section of the chapter focuses on a selected number of safety categories, we encourage readers to consider some additional, related activities. For further information in the area of safety, consult a safety textbook (one of which is listed in the references for this chapter).[21] To review important points in the area of first aid skills, consult Appendix 2 in this text. Finally, we encourage you to take a first aid course from the American Red Cross. American Red Cross first aid courses incorporate a significant amount of safety prevention information along with the teaching of specific first aid skills.

Residential Safety

Many serious accidents and personal assaults occur in dorm rooms, apartments, and houses. As a responsible adult, you should make every reasonable effort to prevent these tragedies from happening. One good idea is to discuss some of the following points with your family or roommates and see what cooperative strategies you can implement:

- Fireproof your residence. Are all electrical appliances and heating and cooling systems in safe working order? Are flammable materials safely stored?
- Prepare a fire escape plan. Install smoke or heat detectors.

- Do not give personal information over the phone to a stranger.
- Use initials for first names on mailboxes and in phone books.
- Install a peephole and deadbolt locks on outside doors.
- If possible, avoid living in first floor apartments. Change locks when moving to a new apartment or home.
- Put locks on all windows.
- Require repair people or delivery people to show valid identification.
- Do not use an elevator if it is occupied by someone who makes you feel uneasy.
- Be cautious around garages, laundry rooms, and driveways (especially at night). Use lighting for prevention of assault.

Recreational Safety

The thrills we get from risk-taking are an essential part of our recreational endeavors. Sometimes we can get into serious accidents because we fail to consider important recreational safety information. Do some of the following recommendations apply to you?

- Seek appropriate instruction for your intended activity. Few skill activities are as easy as they look.
- Always wear your automobile seat belt.
- Make certain that your equipment is in excellent working order.
- Involve yourself gradually in an activity before attempting more complicated, dangerous skills.
- Enroll in an American Red Cross first aid course to enable you to cope with unexpected injuries.
- Remember that alcohol use greatly increases the likelihood that people will get hurt.
- Protect your eyes from serious injury.
- Learn to swim. Drowning occurs most frequently to people who never intended to be in the water.
- Obey the laws related to your recreational pursuits. Many laws are directly related to the safety of the participants.
- Be aware of weather conditions. Many outdoor activities turn to tragedy with sudden shifts in the weather. Always prepare yourself for the worst possible weather.

Firearm Safety

Each year about 13,000 Americans are murdered with guns and another 2000 die in gun-related accidents. Most murders are committed with handguns. (Shotguns and rifles tend to be more cumbersome than handguns and thus are not as frequently used in murders, accidents, or suicides.) Over half of all murders result from quarrels and arguments between acquaintances or relatives. With many homeowners arming themselves with handguns for protection against intruders, it is not surprising that over half of all gun accidents occur in the home. Children are frequently involved in gun accidents, often after they discover a gun they think is unloaded. Handgun owners are reminded to adhere to the following safety reminders:

- Make certain that you follow the gun possession laws in your state. Special permits may be required to carry a handgun.
- Make certain that your gun is in good mechanical order.
- If you are a novice, enroll in a gun safety course.
- Consider every gun to be a loaded gun, even if someone tells you it is unloaded.
- Never point a gun at an unintended target.
- Keep your finger off the trigger until you are ready to shoot.
- When moving with a handgun, keep the barrel pointed down.
- Load and unload your gun carefully.
- Store your gun and ammunition safely in a locked container. Use a trigger lock on your gun when not in use.
- Take target practice only at approved ranges.
- Never play with guns at parties. Never handle a gun when intoxicated.
- Educate children about gun safety and the potential dangers of gun use. Children must never believe that a gun is a toy.

Motor Vehicle Safety

The greatest number of accidental deaths in the United States take place on highways and streets. Young people are most likely to die from a motor vehicle accident. According to Bever,[21] the following is a description of a prime candidate for such a death:

a male, 15 to 24 years of age, driving on a two-lane, rural road between the hours of 10 pm and 2 am on a Saturday night. If he has been drinking and is driving a subcompact car or motorcycle, the likelihood that he and his passengers will have a fatal accident is even more pronounced.

Motor vehicle accidents also cause disabling injuries. With nearly 2 million such injuries each year, concern for the prevention of motor vehicle accidents should be important for all college students, regardless of age. With this thought in mind, we offer some important safety tips for motor vehicle operators:

- Make certain that you are familiar with the traffic laws in your state.
- Do not operate an automobile or motorcycle unless it is in good mechanical order. Regularly inspect your brakes, lights, and exhaust system.
- Do not exceed the speed limit. Observe all traffic signs.
- Always wear safety belts, even on short trips. Require your passengers to buckle up. Always keep small children in child restraints.
- Never drink and drive. Avoid horseplay inside a car.
- Be certain that you can hear the traffic outside your car. Keep the car's music system at a reasonable decibel level.
- Give pedestrians the right-of-way.
- Drive defensively at all times. Do not challenge other drivers. Refrain from drag racing.
- Look carefully before changing lanes.
- Be especially careful at intersections and railroad crossings.
- Carry a well-maintained first aid kit that includes flares or other signal devices.
- Alter your driving behavior during bad weather.
- Do not drive when you have not had enough sleep (see "Focus on Drowsy Driving," pp. 420-421).

Home Accident Prevention for Children and the Elderly

Approximately 1 person in 10 is injured each year in a home accident. Children and the elderly spend significantly more hours each day in a home setting than do young adults and midlife people. It is especially important that accident prevention be given primary consideration for these groups (see the Health Action Guide on p. 416). Here are some important tips to remember. Can you think of others?

For everyone
- Be certain that you have adequate insurance protection.
- Install smoke detectors appropriately.
- Keep stairways clear of toys and debris. Install railings.
- Maintain electrical and heating equipment.
- Make certain that inhabitants know how to get emergency help.

unintentional injuries
Injuries that have occurred without anyone intending that harm be done.

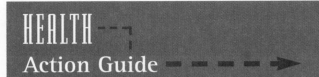

HEALTH Action Guide

Making Your Home Safe, Comfortable, and Secure

Entry
- Install a deadbolt lock on the front door and locks or bars on the windows.
- Add a peephole or small window in the front door.
- Trim bushes so burglars have no place to hide.
- Add lighting to the walkway and next to the front door.
- Get a large dog.

Bedroom and nursery
- Install a smoke alarm and a carbon monoxide detector.
- Remove high threshold at doorway to avoid tripping.
- Humidifiers can be breeding grounds for bacteria; use them sparingly and follow the manufacturer's cleaning instructions.
- In the nursery, install pull-down shades or curtains instead of blinds with strings that could strangle a child.

Living room
- Secure loose throw rugs or use ones with nonskid backing.
- Remove trailing wires where people walk.
- Cover unused electrical outlets if there are small children in the home.
- Provide additional lighting for reading, and install adjustable blinds to regulate glare.

Kitchen
- To avoid burns, move objects stored above the stove to another location.
- Install ceiling lighting and additional task lighting where food is prepared.
- Keep heavy objects on bottom shelves or countertops; store lightweight or seldom-used objects on top shelves.
- Promptly clean and store knives.
- Keep hot liquids such as coffee out of children's reach, and provide close supervision when the stove or other appliances are in use.
- To avoid food-borne illness, thoroughly clean surfaces that have come into contact with raw meat.

Bathroom
- A child can drown in standing water; keep the toilet lid down and the tub empty.
- Clean the shower, tub, sink, and toilet regularly to remove mold, mildew, and bacteria that can contribute to illness.
- Store medications in their original containers in a cool, dry place out of the reach of children.
- Add a bath mat or nonskid strips to the bottom of the tub.
- Add grab bars near the tub or shower and toilet, especially if there are elderly adults in the home.
- Keep a first-aid kit stocked with bandages, first-aid ointment, gauze, pain relievers, syrup of Ipecac, and isotonic eyewash; include your physician's and a nearby emergency center's phone numbers.

Stairway
- Add a handrail for support.
- Remove all obstacles or stored items from stairs and landing.
- Repair or replace flooring material that is in poor condition.
- Add a light switch at the top of the stairs.
- If there is an elderly person in the home, add a contrasting color strip to the first and last steps to identify the change of level.

Fire prevention tips
- Install smoke detectors on every level of your home.
- Keep fire extinguishers handy in the kitchen, basement, and bedrooms.
- Have the chimney and fireplace cleaned by a professional when there is more than ¼ inch of soot accumulation.
- Place space heaters at least 3 feet from beds, curtains, and other flammable objects.
- Don't overload electrical outlets, and position drapes so that they don't touch cords or outlets.
- Recycle or toss combustibles, such as newspapers, rags, old furniture, and chemicals.
- If you smoke, use caution with cigarettes and matches; never light up in bed.
- Plan escape routes and practice using them with your family.

For children

- Know all the ways to prevent accidental poisoning.
- Use toys that are appropriate for the age of the child.
- Never leave young children unattended, especially infants.
- Keep any hazardous items (guns, poisons, etc.) locked up.
- Keep small children away from kitchen stoves.

For the elderly

- Protect from falls.
- Be certain that elderly people have a good understanding of the medications they may be taking. Know the side effects.
- Encourage elderly people to seek assistance when it comes to home repairs.
- Make certain that all door locks, lights, and safety equipment are in good working order.

Refer to pp. 406-407 for additional information related to the protection of older adults.

CAMPUS SAFETY AND VIOLENCE PREVENTION

Although many of the topics in this chapter are quite unsettling, students and faculty must continue to lead normal lives in the campus environment despite potential threats to our health. The first step in being able to function adequately is knowing about these potential threats. You have read about these threats in this chapter; now you must think about how this information applies to your campus situation.

The campus environment is no longer immune to many of the social ills that plague our society. At one time the university campus was thought to be a safe haven from the real world. Now there is plenty of evidence to indicate that significant intentional and unintentional injuries can happen to anyone at any time on the college campus.

For this reason, you must make it a habit to think constructively about protecting your safety. In addition to the personal safety tips presented earlier in this chapter, remember to use the safety assistance resources available on your campus. One of these might be your use of university-approved escort services, especially in the evenings as you move from one campus location to another. Another resource is the campus security department (campus police). Typically, campus police have a 24-hour emergency phone number. If you think you need help, do not hesitate to call this number. Campus security departments frequently offer short seminars on safety topics to student organizations or residence hall groups. Your counseling center on campus might also offer programs on rape prevention and personal protection.

If you are motivated to make your campus environment safer, you might wish to contact two organizations that specifically focus on campus crime.[2] The first is Safe Campuses Now, a nonprofit student group that tracks legislation, provides educational seminars, and monitors community incidents involving students. For information about Safe Campuses Now, including how to start a chapter on your campus, call (706) 354-1115. Another nonprofit organization, Security on Campus, Inc., aims at preventing campus violence and crime, but it also helps victims enforce their legal rights. This group can be reached at (215) 768-9330. We encourage you to become active in making your campus a safer place to live.

Summary

- Everyone is a potential victim of violent crime.
- Each year in the United States, intentional injuries cause about 50,000 deaths and another 2 million nonfatal injuries.
- Homicide is the leading cause of death for young male African-Americans. Handguns are the weapon of choice for homicides.
- Because of factors related to family structure, increased drug use and crime, and the inability of people to resolve conflicts peacefully, domestic violence is on the rise.
- Forms of child abuse include physical abuse, sexual abuse, and child neglect. Child neglect is the most common form.

- Youth violence is skyrocketing, and much of the violence is related to gang activities.
- Bias and hate crimes, as well as the crime of stalking, are increasingly recognized as serious violent acts.
- Rape and sexual assault, acquaintance rape, date rape, and sexual harassment are forms of sexual victimization in which victims often are both physically and psychologically traumatized.
- Unintentional injuries are injuries that occur accidentally. The numbers of fatal and nonfatal unintentional injuries are exceedingly high.

Review Questions

1. Identify some of the categories of intentional injuries. How many people are affected each year by intentional injuries?
2. What are some of the most important facts concerning homicide in the United States? How are most homicides committed?
3. Identify changes in the traditional family structure that may be related to increased family stress and domestic violence. What additional factors also may be related to increased domestic violence?
4. What reasons might explain why so many women do not report domestic violence?
5. Aside from the immediate consequences of child abuse, what additional problems do many abused children face in the future?
6. Explain why gangs and gang activities have increased tremendously over the last 15 years. What effect do gangs have on a community?
7. List some examples of groups that are known to have committed bias or hate crimes.
8. Identify some general characteristics of a typical stalker.
9. Explain some of the myths associated with rape. How can date rape be prevented?
10. Identify some examples of behaviors that could be considered sexual harassment. Why are employers especially concerned about educating their employees about sexual harassment?
11. Identify some common examples of unintentional injuries. Point out three safety tips from each of the safety areas listed at the end of this chapter.

Think About This . . .

- To what extent are you concerned about your personal safety? Are you comfortable with your level of concern? Or do you think you should be more or less concerned?
- According to published reports, after the tragic deaths of Nicole Brown Simpson and her friend Ronald Goldman, phone calls to domestic violence hotlines increased tremendously. What were some of your feelings about domestic violence as you watched the news coverage of this story?
- Has there been any gun violence at your college?

Are you aware of any students carrying guns or other concealed weapons on your campus?
- Do you know of educational programs on your campus that have dealt with rape prevention or sexual harassment? Where can you go on your campus to seek help for crises related to these issues?
- Is there a particular place on your campus where you believe that your personal safety is threatened? If so, how do you cope with this threat?

References

1. Turque B et al: He could run . . . but he couldn't hide, *Newsweek*, p 16, June 27, 1994.
2. Cohen G: Campus crime: a false sense of security, *U. Magazine*, p 18, May 1994.
3. Bureau of Justice Statistics: *Injuries from crime: special report*, US Department of Justice, Washington, DC, 1989, US Government Printing Office.
4. Bureau of Justice Statistics: *Sourcebook of criminal justice statistics—1994*, US Department of Justice, Washington, DC, 1995, US Government Printing Office.
5. Marshall S: Killings rise 3%, despite overall drop in crime rate, *USA Today*, p 3A, May 2, 1994.
6. Swanson JM, Albrecht M: *Community health nursing: promoting the health of aggregates*, Philadelphia, 1993, WB Saunders.
7. Bureau of Justice Statistics: *Drugs, crime, and the justice system: a national report*, US Department of Justice, Washington, DC, December, 1992, US Government Printing Office.
8. Bureau of Justice Statistics: *Guns and crime: handgun victimization, firearm self-defense, and firearm theft*, US Department of Justice, Washington, DC, April 1994, US Government Printing Office.
9. US Bureau of the Census: *Statistical abstract of the United*

States: 1995, ed 115, Washington, DC, 1995, US Government Printing Office.

10. Hunt T: Brady Bill becomes law, *The Muncie Star,* Dec 1, p 1, 1993.

11. Bachman R: *Violence against women: a national crime victimization survey report,* US Department of Justice, Washington, DC, January 1994, US Government Printing Office.

12. DeWitt CB: From the director, *Research in Brief,* National Institute of Justice, US Department of Justice, Washington, DC, October 1992, US Government Printing Office.

13. Widom CS: The cycle of violence, *Research in Brief,* National Institute of Justice, US Department of Justice, Washington, DC, October 1992, US Government Printing Office.

14. Prothrow-Smith D: Stop violence before it begins, *USA Today,* p 11A, Feb 24, 1994.

15. National Committee for Prevention of Child Abuse: *12 alternatives to whacking your kid,* Chicago, undated pamphlet.

16. Covey HC, Menard S, Franzese RJ: *Juvenile gangs,* Springfield, Ill, 1992, Charles C Thomas.

17. Leslie C et al: Girls will be girls, *Newsweek,* p 44, Aug 2, 1993.

18. Kantrowitz B: Wild in the streets, *Newsweek,* p 40, Aug 2, 1993.

19. Maynard G: The start of a trend: second carjacking attempt reported, *The Muncie Star,* p 1, Oct 21, 1993.

20. Haas K, Haas A: *Understanding sexuality,* ed 3, St Louis, 1993, Mosby.

21. Bever DL: *Safety: a personal focus,* ed 3, St Louis, 1992, Mosby.

Suggested Readings

American Red Cross: *First aid: responding to emergencies,* St Louis, 1996, Mosby Lifeline.
A comprehensive guide for handling first aid emergencies and a workbook used by many colleges and universities in their introductory first aid courses. Well illustrated and easy to follow; a considerable amount of safety and prevention information is included.

Petrocelli W, Repa K: *Sexual harassment on the job: what it is and how to stop it,* Berkeley, Calif, 1992, Nolo Press.

A guide to identifying, handling, and preventing instances of sexual harassment for both women and men. An important focus is on the legal issues involving harassment, including resource lists and various state laws.

Scott K: *Sexual assault: will I ever feel okay again?* Minneapolis, 1993, Bethany House Publishers.
A survivor of rape tells about what it takes to rebound from the pain, fear, and shame. A good resource for victims or those who know or work with victims.

 AS WE GO TO PRESS . . .

One of the most notorious hate crimes in recent memory has finally gotten the full attention of the federal government. Since early 1995, 33 Southern black churches have been burned to the ground. A task force of over 100 federal agents is now coordinating an intense investigation to identify the arsonists and to discover any possible coordinated efforts in these violent crimes. Congress is also attempting to strengthen laws that increase the federal government's power to prosecute church-burning crimes.

FOCUS ON...

Drowsy Driving

Dean was driving home from college late on a moonlit Friday night. His on-campus job kept him working until 9 PM after a day of classes. He had stopped to shoot pool with some friends after work and started his hour-long trek home at about 11:30. Just after midnight, Dean turned onto a 15-mile stretch of perfectly straight highway that cut through pastures and fields. The summer night was crystal clear. The radio was playing loudly, there were few oncoming cars, and visibility was good.

"I felt fine," Dean recalled later. "I was a little run down, but I wasn't sleepy at all. I was cruising along listening to tunes, and the next thing I knew I was surrounded by corn. The sound of the stalks hitting the car must have woken me up. It scared the hell out of me. I guess I fell asleep for a few seconds, but I don't know how it could have happened."

The Danger of Driving While Sleepy
Dean experienced a phenomenon that is too often ignored. Falling asleep at the wheel is something that no one thinks will happen to them, yet drowsy driving is estimated to cause up to 200,000 accidents per year on American roads.[1,2] Dean was lucky. His car veered right where a dirt tractor path connected with the road, and he missed a deep ditch by only a few feet. He avoided power poles, trees, and oncoming traffic as well. "Since then, I've put off several late-night trips when I thought I might be too tired. I even took a nap once on an overnight drive when I felt myself drifting," Dean said. "If I hadn't fallen asleep at the wheel before, I probably would have kept driving."

Sleepiness is a significant cause of traffic fatalities. Up to 3% of all yearly vehicular deaths in the United States can be attributed to driving while drowsy, yet Americans remain woefully uneducated to this problem.[1]

Sleepiness undermines a person's ability to make sound decisions and reduces attention span considerably.[2] Any condition that impairs the judgment of drivers should be taken seriously. It has been estimated that 100 million Americans fail to get enough sleep and that up to 50% of *all* accident-related fatalities (not just driving fatalities) can be attributed to sleep deprivation.[3]

Early Warning Signs
Drivers are often not aware that they are in need of sleep until after they get behind the wheel, or they ignore the signs of sleep deprivation and drive anyway. When drowsiness sets in, drivers are often caught by surprise,

and they can fall asleep without realizing it. Being able to recognize the signs of sleep deprivation before we fall victim to it is therefore important. Some of the symptoms of sleep deprivation you should watch out for are[1,2]:

- Struggling against fatigue throughout the day
- Needing caffeine to stay alert, especially on a daily basis
- Falling asleep quickly (within 5 minutes) after stopping to rest
- Having an irritable or argumentative attitude without knowing why
- Needing an alarm clock to wake up in the morning (well-rested people wake up on time naturally)

Tips to Avoid Drowsy Driving
Because of the stealthy manner in which sleep can overtake you, it is important to evaluate your condition before getting behind the wheel and also while you are on the road. It is also important to prevent regular sleep deprivation. We must reduce the risk of falling asleep while driving by using common sense. The following suggestions should help reduce your chances of driving while drowsy[1]:

- Get plenty of sleep. About 8 hours of sleep per night is desirable. If this is not practical, try to catch up on sleep when possible (take naps, sleep more on weekends, etc.).
- Take breaks while driving. Stop at least every 2 hours on long trips. If possible, avoid driving alone so the driving duties can be split. Don't eat heavy meals, and avoid too much caffeine.
- Stay alert. Talk, listen to the radio, sing, or do whatever you can to keep from drifting off. Don't let all of the passengers in the car sleep; having someone to converse with can help keep the driver alert.
- Don't get too comfortable. Getting too relaxed can promote dozing off. Avoid using cruise control. Reduce use of the heater, and keep the windows open when possible.
- Don't drink and drive. This is true anytime, but even a small amount of alcohol in the system can intensify the effects of fatigue on the body.
- If you feel yourself drifting off or you think you may be in danger of falling asleep, stop driving. Dozing off for a few seconds (a phenomenon known as *microsleep*) is a significant warning sign of fatigue. Don't try to fight through fatigue while driving. Pull off the road at a safe place and take a nap if you need to.

Take time to heed the warning signs of fatigue. Remember that dozing off at the wheel creates a potentially dangerous situation for both yourself and others on or near the road. Being able to recognize when you are at risk of falling asleep and taking steps to avoid driving while drowsy are more than just common sense; they're a necessity for your own and others' personal safety. Getting a few extra winks of sleep and taking the time to ensure you are alert before you get into the driver's seat could save lives.

For Discussion . . .
How much sleep do you get each night on average? Do you regularly experience any of the signs of fatigue mentioned in this article? Do you experience fatigue more often during certain times of the day or week? If so, can you think of ways to increase the amount of sleep you get? What would you have to give up to accomplish this goal?

References
1. Matson M: Forgotten menace on our highways, *Reader's Digest*, 144(86), June 1994.
2. Toufexis A: Drowsy America, *Time*, 136(26), Dec 17, 1990.
3. Bennett G: Why you must get more sleep, *McCall's*, 122(3), Dec 1994.

Chapter

17

Controlling Environmental Influences

Healthy People 2000 Objectives

Progress has been inconsistent in meeting the environmental objectives set forth in the Healthy People 2000 document. We have made substantial headway in promoting cleaner air. Fewer counties in the United States now exceed air pollution limits, and the national objectives in this area are likely to be met or surpassed.

Another objective was to reduce human exposure to solid waste contamination of water, air, and soil. The Midcourse Review does not assess progress in this area, probably because not enough data are available to track gains or losses. However, the review reports that the average production of solid waste (measured in pounds per person per day) has increased substantially. This trend makes it less likely that exposure to solid waste can be reduced.

On a positive note, efforts are under way to collect and recycle these wastes so that we can meet our goal of establishing effective recycled materials programs by the year 2000. In addition, the levels of most environmental carcinogens have fallen, and our production of 200 specific environmental toxins, such as lead, has dropped.

Efforts to increase the number of states in which indoor radon levels could be reduced through construction and monitoring standards have been relatively unsuccessful. Perhaps this lack of progress reflects our limited awareness of radon and its role as an environmental toxin.

Throughout this book we have read about areas of health over which people have significant control. For example, people select the foods they eat, how much alcohol they consume, and how they manage the stressors in their lives.

The study of the environment and its effect on health provides an interesting contrast to the daily control people have over their own health. Perhaps because of the natural processes of life and death and the vital function of the environment, we are inclined to think that we cannot make personal decisions concerning it. This is, however, changing.

In comparison with the 1980s, when concerns about the environment focused on problems over which we had little direct responsibility or control (such as the ozone layer and nuclear accidents), the 1990s have been characterized by a focus on the individual and the home. Issues such as the disposal of municipal waste, the recycling of glass, plastic, and aluminum, the venting of radon gas from basements, and the reduction of water use reflect the fact that people can act to support the environment (see the Star Box at right).

Environmental concerns also extend to developing countries as well. With the world population at 5.67 billion in 1994 and moving toward 10.8 billion in 2060 (with the greatest rate of increase in Third World countries), the demands made on the environment are already substantial. As the continuing destruction of the tropical rain forests shows, the search for living space and natural resources continues unabated despite our knowing the experiences of those who damaged the environment in earlier decades. Complete the Personal Assessment on p. 424 to see how well you are helping protect the environment.

10 Things You Can Do to Improve the Environment

1. Visit and help support our national parks.
2. Recycle newspapers, glass, plastic, and aluminum.
3. Conserve energy and use energy-efficient lighting.
4. Keep tires properly inflated to improve gas mileage and extend tire life.
5. Plant trees.
6. Organize a Christmas tree recycling program in your community.
7. Find an alternative to chemical pesticides for your lawn.
8. Purchase only those brands of tuna marked "dolphin safe."
9. Organize a community group to clean up a local stream, highway, park, or beach.
10. Become a member of an environmental action group, such as the Environmental Defense Fund, the Nature Conservancy, or the Sierra Club.

WORLD POPULATION GROWTH

Population growth affects the environment beyond our own homes and communities to include the entire planet. Each year the population of the world grows by 90 million people. By the middle of the next century, there could be 50% more people than there are today (Figure 17-1 on p. 425). By the year 2060, it is projected that 10.8 billion people will be alive. By the year 2000, more than half of the developing countries in the world may not be able to feed their populations from food grown on their own land.[1] As seen in Somalia, the consequences of overpopulation, combined with nonenvironmental factors such as limited agriculture and governmental instability, can lead to human suffering of the highest magnitude. However, as the Earth's population increases by 1 million peo-

ple every 4 years, we struggle to make family planning available to everyone, to encourage later marriage and childbearing, to encourage breastfeeding not only for the health of infants but also to lengthen the interval between pregnancies, and to improve the status and well-being of women so that they have new roles for themselves and their families. Failing to control population growth, crowding, water pollution and scarcity, hazardous waste accumulation, and air pollution will move us closer yet to ecological disaster.

AIR POLLUTION

If you think that air pollution is a modern concern reflecting technology that has gone astray, keep in mind that the air is routinely polluted by nature. Sea salt, soil particles, ash, dust, soot, microbes, assorted trace elements, and plant pollens are consistently found in the air.

Pollution caused in part by humans also has a long history. From the fires that filled our ancestors' caves with choking smoke, through the "killer fogs" of nineteenth-century London, to the dust storms of the Great Depression, humans have contributed to air pollution. Today, its effects can be seen in countries throughout the world. The five countries that produce the most airborne gases that contribute to global

PERSONAL ASSESSMENT

Are You Helping the Environment?

How many ways can you help the environment? Give yourself two points for each of the following that you do on a regular basis, one point for each that you do occasionally, and a zero for those that you do not do. Total your points and compare your score with those that follow the assessment.

_____ 1. Promptly repair leaky faucets.

_____ 2. Use the microwave as often as possible rather than the stove or the oven.

_____ 3. Buy brands that come in minimal amounts of packaging.

_____ 4. Do not run excess water while washing dishes.

_____ 5. Use paper bags rather than plastic.

_____ 6. Use sponges or dishcloths for spills rather than paper towels.

_____ 7. Recycle newspapers rather than throw them out.

_____ 8. Snip six-pack rings.

_____ 9. Walk or bicycle rather than drive.

_____ 10. Purchase products in the larger sizes.

_____ 11. Preheat your oven for the minimal amount of time necessary.

_____ 12. Turn off water while brushing your teeth.

_____ 13. Do not use a trash compactor.

_____ 14. Serve fresh fruits and vegetables rather than processed foods.

_____ 15. Pull weeds by hand rather than spraying.

_____ 16. Carpool to work.

_____ 17. Limit garbage disposal use as much as possible.

_____ 18. Use canvas or cloth bags for shopping.

_____ 19. Sweep driveways and sidewalks rather than use a hose.

_____ 20. Recycle bottles and jars.

_____ 21. Pick up litter when you see it.

_____ 22. Make note pads out of used office stationery and paper.

_____ 23. Wear clothing that is right for the weather.

_____ 24. Use rechargeable batteries.

_____ 25. Clean the lint screen in the dryer after each load.

_____ 26. Put trash in only one bag (or the fewest needed).

_____ 27. Use refillable containers for household products (such as liquid hand soap).

_____ 28. Keep the water heater at the lowest level needed.

_____ 29. Open blinds and curtains during daylight periods during winter months.

_____ 30. Close blinds and curtains during periods of bright sunshine during summer months.

_____ 31. Turn off lights when you leave a room.

_____ 32. Take quick showers rather than leisurely baths.

_____ 33. Turn off stereos, radios, and televisions when leaving the house.

_____ 34. Turn off the water when washing the car and use a bucket when possible.

_____ 35. Place a brick or a plastic bottle of water inside the toilet storage tank.

_____ 36. Buy laundry detergents that are phosphate-free when there are other options available.

_____ 37. Drink "ice water" from the refrigerator rather than run tap water to get it cooler.

_____ 38. Run the dishwasher only when full.

_____ 39. Use hairspray in nonaerosol bottles.

_____ 40. Clean and change filters on the furnace and air conditioner on a regular basis.

_____ 41. Keep a reusable mug or cup at home or the office.

_____ 42. Purchase clothing that can be washed rather than only dry cleaned.

_____ 43. Wash clothing only when dirty.

_____ 44. Close the refrigerator door promptly.

_____ 45. Keep the car properly tuned.

_____ 46. Collect rain water for use in plants and gardens.

_____ 47. Donate outgrown clothing to nonprofit organizations.

_____ 48. Participate in organized cleanup days when they are held in your community.

_____ 49. Replace conventional shower head with a water-conserving model.

_____ 50. Write elected officials to support environmental legislation.

_____ YOUR TOTAL POINTS

Interpretation

90-100 points: Your conservation efforts are in the superior range. Keep up the excellent work!

80-89 points: You are clearly above average and should also be congratulated!

70-79 points: Although your score is average, your efforts at conserving the environment are important contributions to the total effort. Keep up the good work and look for additional ways to conserve.

60-69 points: Your score is passing but below average. Try to find more ways to help the environment. You have room for improvement.

59 and below: Time has not run out! You can still earn a passing grade but you need to follow the suggestions in this assessment and chapter to help the environment.

To Carry This Further...
Share these suggestions, or any others that you find useful, with family, friends, classmates, and other associates as a means of further helping our environment.

warming (the United States, the former USSR, Japan, China, and Brazil) are located in North America, Europe, Asia, and South America (see pp. 426-427).[2] The most devastating episode of pollution in history was the Kuwait oil well fires that were set during the Gulf War (see the Star Box on p. 426).

Sources of Air Pollution

The sources of modern air pollutants should be familiar to you. A leading source is the internal combustion engine. Automobiles, trucks, and buses contribute a variety of materials to the air, including carbon monoxide and hydrocarbons. Industrial

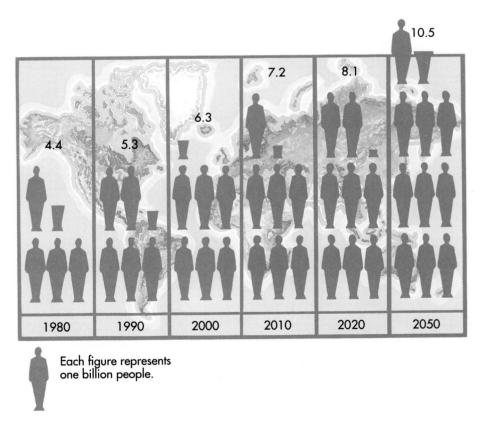

Figure 17-1   At its current rate of growth, the world's population will reach 10 billion about 25 years sooner than predicted a decade ago.

Environmental Terrorism

In terms of air pollution, no single episode of contamination has ever surpassed that of the oil well fires in Kuwait. The 727 wells set on fire by retreating Iraqi troops in January 1991 burned 5,000,000 barrels of crude oil per day. The oil was converted into thick oily pollutants and noxious gases that were released into the atmosphere. The last of these fires was not extinguished until November 1991. Today children and adults with allergies, bronchial asthma, and pneumonia are commonly seen in Kuwaiti hospitals. Long-term influences may include lung cancer.

processes, domestic heating, refuse burning, and the use of pesticides and herbicides also contribute to our air pollution problem. In recent years the massive deforestation of the tropical rain forest in the Amazon River basin of South America has contributed significant amounts of gaseous and particulate pollutants to the air.

Gaseous pollutants

The pollutants dispersed into the air by the sources just identified are generally in the form of gases, including carbon dioxide and carbon monoxide. Carbon dioxide is the natural by-product of combustion and is produced whenever fuels are burned. Electricity production, car and truck emissions, and industry are the principal producers of carbon dioxide.

As first predicted well over a decade ago, the progressive increase in carbon dioxide appears to have resulted in a **greenhouse effect** (Figure 17-2). This effect has caused a slight but progressive warming of the earth's surface. An increase of only 1.5 degrees since 1860, resulting from increased trapping of industrial gases, has resulted in a shift of the world's hydrologic cycles.[3] Today the atmosphere is more

greenhouse effect
Warming of the Earth's surface that is produced when solar heat becomes trapped by layers of carbon dioxide and other gases.

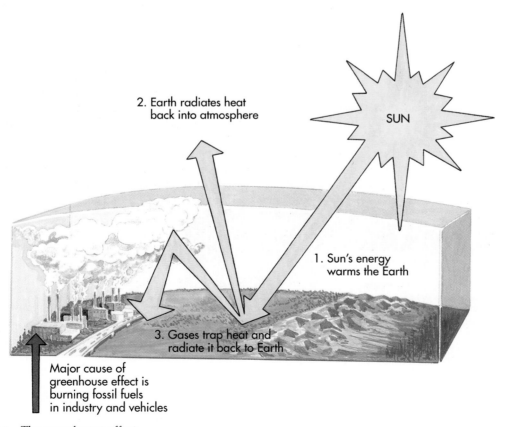

Figure 17-2   The greenhouse effect.

laden with moisture, and air circulation patterns have shifted, leading to greater extremes in all aspects of weather. Weather events in 1995 offered clear examples of these extremes, including:

- Heavy March rains in California
- The second most active tornado season in the Midwest
- A heat wave that killed more than 800 people during July in the Northeast and Midwest
- 11 hurricanes in the Caribbean
- Extensive flooding in France and the Netherlands
- The worst drought of the century in Brazil
- Massive June monsoons in India and neighboring countries
- A 5-degree increase over Siberia's average temperature

Whether these trends will continue into the next century is, of course, uncertain. Current attempts to reduce hydrocarbon emissions could be effective enough to begin moderating the temperature increase noted during this century.

Carbon monoxide, the colorless and odorless gas produced when fuels are burned incompletely, has already been discussed in conjunction with cardiovascular disease (see Chapter 10). Also occurring in gaseous form are methane, from decaying vegetation; the terpenes, produced by trees; and benzene and benzopyrene, which may cause cancer when taken into the respiratory system.[4]

Nitrogen and sulfur compounds are pollutants produced by a variety of industrial processes, including the burning of high–sulfur content fuels, especially coal. When nitrogen and sulfur oxides combine with moisture in the atmosphere, they are converted to nitric and sulfuric acid. The resulting **acid rain,** acid snow, and acid fog are responsible, for example, for the destruction of aquatic life and vegetation in the eastern United States and Canada.[5]

In urban areas located in cooler climates (or other cities during the winter months), sulfur oxides and particulate matter (from heating systems) combine with moisture to form a grayish haze, or **smog.** This *gray-air smog* contributes to respiratory problems that are common in these areas during the winter months. In warmer areas, or during the summer months in other areas, brown-air smog develops when hydrocarbons and particulate matter from automobile exhaust interact in the presence of sunlight.[5] This photochemical smog produces ozone. Ozone is highly reactive to the human respiratory system, plants, and materials such as rubber.

An environmental concern currently being studied is the destruction of the ultraviolet light-absorbing ozone layer.[6] Nitrous oxides and materials containing **chlorofluorocarbons (CFCs)** can destroy this protective ozone layer within the stratosphere. Nitrous oxides come from the burning of fossil fuels like coal and gasoline. CFCs are used in air conditioners, many fast-food containers, insulation materials, and solvents.

Although changes in the ozone layer have been recognized for over a decade, the progress of deterioration is advancing in spite of international efforts to slow its place. In a recent study, German researchers reported significant holes in the protective layer over both the North and South poles during the winter of 1991-1992.[7] If deterioration of the ozone layer continues, health dangers such as skin cancer, cataracts, snowblindness, and premature wrinkling of skin will continue to increase.

Particulate pollutants

There are many particulate pollutants, including both naturally occurring materials and particles derived from industrial processes, mining, agriculture, and, of course, tobacco smoke. Inhalation of particulate matter can cause potentially fatal respiratory diseases, including those caused by quartz dust, asbestos fibers, and cotton fibers. Because of its widespread presence, asbestos is of particular concern. In 1989 the **Environmental Protection Agency (EPA)** ordered asbestos use to be stopped by the year 1997 and current sources of asbestos to be removed from public buildings. In the latter regard, some people question whether the expense involved ($10 billion in school removal alone) can be justified on the basis of the less than clearly defined asbestos safety standards.[8]

Trace mineral elements, including lead, nickel, iron, zinc, copper, and magnesium, are also among the particles polluting the air. Chronic **lead toxicity** is among the most serious health problems associated with this form of air pollution, although significant progress has been made because of legislation requiring the use of nonleaded gasoline. However, even today, lead toxicity is disproportionately seen in children of low-income families, principally because of the lead-based paints found in older houses, heavy motor vehicle traffic on city streets, and the use of lead soldering in older plumbing systems. For these children, lower IQs, attention disorders, and long-term learning disabilities may result.

Temperature Inversions

On a normal sunny day, radiant energy from the sun warms the ground and the air immediately above it. As this warmed air rises, it carries pollutants upward and disperses them into a larger, cooler air mass above. Cool air sinking to replace the rising warmed air minimizes the concentration of pollutants.

On those occasions when high pressure settles over an area, warm air can be trapped immediately above the ground. Unable to rise, this trapped, warm, polluted air layer stagnates and produces a potentially health-threatening *subsidence inversion*.[5] (This is the inversion layer that meteorologists talk about on the evening news.)

A second form of thermal inversion, *radiation inversion,* is frequently seen during winter.[5] At this time of year, late afternoon cooling of the ground causes a layer of cool air to develop under a higher, warmer layer of air. With the inability of the cool layer of air to rise, pollutants begin to accumulate near the ground and remain there until the next morning. Warming of the ground later in the morning restores the heating of the lower-level air and reestablishes the normal dispersal of pollutants.

Indoor Air Pollution

Not all air pollution occurs outside. Concern is growing over the health risks associated with indoor air pollution. Toxic materials, including cigarette smoke (see Chapter 9), asbestos, radon, formaldehyde, vinyl chloride, and cooking gases, can be found in buildings ranging from houses and apartments to huge office complexes and manufacturing plants.

Of all of the indoor air pollutants, none is of greater concern than *tobacco smoke.* In December 1992 the EPA identified environmental tobacco smoke to be a Group A (known human) carcinogen.[9] It now is believed that 3000 lung cancer deaths occur annually because of this pollutant. Between 150,000 and 300,000 illnesses in infants and young children occur annually as a result of exposure to environmental tobacco smoke.[9]

Radon gas is a form of indoor air pollution whose role as a serious health risk is currently under investigation.[10] This radioactive gas enters buildings through a variety of routes (the water supply, block walls, slab joints, drains, even cracks in the floor) from underlying rock formations and stone building materials where it is found. Because radon gas can concentrate when air is stagnant, energy-efficient airtight homes, schoolrooms, and buildings are most affected. Tests conducted on homes in various areas of the country suggest that 20% of all homes have higher than normal levels and 10% have dangerously high levels. Radon buildup is a concern because of the relation-

ship of radon exposure to the development of lung cancer.

Those who are concerned about the level of radon gas in their homes can purchase test kits (manufactured by some 200 companies at a cost of $10 to $50) or have their homes tested by radon testing laboratories. Opponents of the "radon myth," however, suggest that these tests may generate false-positive rates in excess of 90%.[10] Further, the repair of homes with high radon levels can be expensive, with some costing as much as $30,000. One form of repair, the installation of a home ventilation system, may cost from $300 to $500.

Environmental tobacco smoke and radon gas join formaldehyde (from building material), vinyl chloride (from PVC plumbing), and other pollutants (including asbestos from insulation) to form the basis of the *sick building syndrome.*[11] For people with respiratory illnesses and immune system hypersensitivies, as well as the elderly, home or work sites could be less

---

acid rain
Rain that has a lower pH (more acidic) than that normally associated with rain.

smog
Air pollution made up of a combination of smoke, photochemical compounds, and fog.

ozone layer
Layer of triatomic oxygen that surrounds the Earth and filters much of the sun's radiation before it can reach the Earth's surface.

chlorofluorocarbons (CFCs)
Gaseous chemical compounds that contain chlorine and fluorine.

Environmental Protection Agency (EPA)
Federal agency charged with the protection of natural resources and the quality of the environment.

lead toxicity
Blood lead level above 25 micrograms/deciliter. (If adopted, the new standard will be 10 micrograms/deciliter.)

radon gas
A naturally occurring radioactive gas produced by the decay of uranium.

healthy than was once thought. The Health Action Guide below describes ways of preventing indoor air pollution.

Health Implications

Because of the complex nature of many health problems, it is difficult to clearly assess the effects of air pollution on health. Age, gender, genetic predisposition, occupation, residency, and personal health practices complicate this assessment. Nevertheless, air pollution may severely affect health problems for elderly people, people who smoke or have respiratory conditions such as asthma, and people who must work in polluted air.

WATER POLLUTION

Although water is the most abundant chemical compound on the Earth's surface, we are finding it increasingly difficult to maintain a plentiful and usable supply. Pollution, excessive use, and misuse are depriving people of the water they need to meet their typical needs (see Table 17-1). As recently as 1994, it was estimated that fully 40% of the freshwater in the United States was unusable.[12]

Yesterday's Pollution Problem

Like air pollution, water pollution is not solely a phenomenon of twentieth century overpopulation or

Table 17-1 Home Water Use	
Use	Gallons
Washing car	100
Taking a bath	36
Washing clothes	35 to 60
Washing dishes	10 to 30
Brushing teeth	10 to 20
Shaving	10 to 20
Watering lawn	8/min
Taking a shower	7/min
Flushing toilet	5 to 7
Leaky faucet	2/day

unchecked technology. Nature has, in fact, routinely polluted our surface and ground water with minerals leached from the soil, acids produced by decaying vegetation, and the decay of animal products. Also, people have polluted their own water supplies. As recently as one generation ago, people living in rural areas occasionally found that their feed lots, chicken coops, and septic tank systems polluted their water supplies.

Today's Pollution Problem

Today, water sources are most often damaged by pollutants from agricultural, urban, and industrial sources. Most of these pollutants are either biological or chemical products, and many can be either removed from the water or brought within acceptable

---

HEALTH
Action Guide ------▶

Preventing Indoor Air Pollution

To minimize the level of indoor pollution in your home, follow these simple steps. How easy or difficult would it be to improve your current level of prevention?

- Hang dry-cleaned clothing outside to air out before hanging it in the closet.
- Clean humidifiers, and replace belts on a regular basis.
- Limit use of aerosol personal care products to the bare minimum.
- Store fuel for mowers, snow blowers, trimmers, and other gasoline-powered tools in an approved container in a well-ventilated area.

- Do not run the engine of a car in an attached garage or closed carport.
- Properly close containers of household cleaning products that are capable of emitting toxic fumes.
- Ventilate rooms in which new carpet and drapes have been installed as often as possible.
- Have fireplaces cleaned and inspected regularly.
- Eliminate smoking of cigarettes within the home.
- Discard unused paint, hobby supplies, herbicides, and pesticides on a regular basis.
- Inspect gas appliances for proper ventilation.
- Use products that are as free as possible from asbestos and formaldehyde when remodeling.

◀------

safety limits. For some pollutants, however, management technology has been only partially successful or is still being developed.

Sources of Water Pollution

Water pollution is not the result of only one type of pollutant. In fact, many sources of water pollution exist.

Pathogens

Pathogenic agents, in the form of bacteria, viruses, and protozoa, enter the water supply through human and animal wastes. Communities with sewage treatment systems designed around a combined sanitary and storm system can, during heavy rain or snow melt, allow untreated sewage to rush through the processing plant. In addition, pathogenic organisms can enter the water supply when sewage is flushed from boats. Pathogenic agents are also introduced into the water supply from animal wastes at feed lots and at meat processing facilities.

Sewage treatment plants and public health laboratories routinely test for the presence of pathogenic agents. Unfortunately, however, *undertreated* water is consumed by nearly one fifth of the U.S. population (50 million people).[13] The presence of **coliform bacteria** indicates human or animal feces.

Biological imbalances

Aquatic plants tend to thrive in water rich in nitrates and phosphates. This overabundance leads to **eutrophication,** which can render a stream, pond, or lake unusable.[14]

During hot, dry summers, aquatic plants die in large numbers. Since the decay of vegetation requires aerobic bacterial action, the biochemical oxygen demand will be high.[15] To satisfy the biochemical oxygen demand, much of the water's oxygen is used. When such a condition exits, fish may be killed in great numbers. **Putrefaction** of the dead fish not only further pollutes the water but also fouls the air.

Toxic substances

Of the pollutants found in today's surface water and groundwater supply, perhaps none are of greater concern than toxic chemical substances. These chemical toxins, including metals and hydrocarbons, are dangerous because when in the surface water, they have the ability to enter the food chain. When they do, their concentration per unit of weight increases with each life form in the chain. By the time humans consume the fish that have fed on the contaminated lower forms of aquatic life, the toxic chemicals have been concentrated to dangerous levels.[15] In ground-water supplies, of course, toxic substances are consumed directly by humans in drinking water.

Among the important toxic substances is mercury in the form of methyl mercury. Derived from industrial wastes, methyl mercury is ingested and concentrated by shellfish and other fish. When humans eat these fish regularly, mercury levels increase to the point that hemoglobin and central nervous system function can be seriously impaired.

A variety of other metals have also been found in North American rivers, lakes, and groundwater sources. In the surface water, arsenic, cadmium, copper, lead, and silver are all capable of entering the food chain. In many cases, only very low levels of these metals need to be taken into the body before damage to health becomes evident.

Of the wide variety of agricultural products currently used on American and Canadian farms, *pesticides* and *herbicides* are among the most toxic. Containing more than 1800 different chemical compounds, these agricultural products deliver a diverse array of chemicals to our water supplies, as well as directly on or in the food that people eat. The level of herbicides in the water supply rises particularly rapidly during the summer months.[16]

Today there is mounting concern regarding pesticides and herbicides and the development of testicular cancer and drop in sperm production in men, leukemia in children, and breast cancer in women.[17] Currently the FDA has more than 85 of these agricultural products under study and has proposed new guidelines regarding their appropriate use and disposal.

Among the most serious of the toxic chemicals found in our water are the chlorinated hydrocarbons, including *DDT* (dichlorodiphenyltrichloroethane), *chlordane,* and *Kepone* (chlordecone). The **mutagenic, carcinogenic,** and **teratogenic** effects of these hydrocarbon products continue to receive careful study.

PCBs (polychlorinated biphenyls) are another group of hydrocarbons causing a great deal of concern because of their presence in the water supply.[15] PCBs are, on the basis of their chemical structure, very stable, heat-resistant compounds that have been used extensively in transformers and electrical capacitors. In many areas of the country, discarded electrical equipment has broken open and released PCBs into the surrounding water supply. Tests are now being conducted at these dump sites to determine the extent of contamination of the underground water supply. In laboratory animals, PCBs produce liver and kidney damage, gastric and reproductive disorders, skin lesions, and tumors.[15] Studies on people who have been exposed to high levels of PCBs in drinking water have been ongoing for several years. It is now known that PCBs can concentrate in the fat that comprises breast tissue and that they have been found in women with breast cancer.[18] Since 1990 the use of PCBs in electrical equipment has been banned.

As suggested above, *chlorine*, one of the most extensively used chemicals in industry, is now recognized as a prevalent pollutant of the country's water supply, particularly for the Great Lakes. Experts believe that elevated levels of chlorine from chlorine-containing chemicals inflict damage on animals and could result in a variety of health problems in humans.[19]

The Clear Water Act (1994) mandated changes in the plastics, organic chemicals, pulp and paper processing, and wastewater management industries to replace chlorine with an acceptable substitute. Progress in meeting various requirements will be closely monitored.

Other sources

Three additional types of pollution that affect our water are important, although their effect on human health is not fully understood. The pollution from these sources is detrimental to aquatic life; alters the aesthetic value of our waterways; and reduces recreational use of our rivers, lakes, and shores.

Oil spills include not only the severe spills resulting from tanker accidents but also spills that occur on inland waters and those that result from the seeping of crude oil from the ground. Any kind of oil spill can foul our water. Fish, aquatic plants, seabirds, and beaches can be damaged by both surface-oil film and tar masses that float below the surface or roll along the ocean bottom. Less noticeable but potentially harmful to human health is the contamination of groundwater by inappropriately disposed of oil-based products or by gasoline leaking from underground storage tanks.

Power plants that use water from lakes and rivers to cool their stream turbines cause *thermal pollution.* When this heated water is returned to its source, temperatures in the water may rise significantly. As temperatures increase, the oxygen-carrying capacity of the water decreases and the balance of aquatic life forms is altered. In water that is raised only 10° C (18° F), entire species of fish can disappear and aquatic plants can proliferate out of control.[5]

Finally, *sediments* in the form of sand, clay, and other soil constituents regularly reach waterway channels. Rivers, lakes, reservoirs, and oceans serve as settling basins for these sediments. If cleared land areas cannot be returned to vegetative cover, then dredging may be required to keep the waterway usable, although this is an expensive and relatively ineffective response.

Oceanic oil spills destroy the habitat of hundreds of wildlife species, such as the sea otter, and remain in the ocean for decades.

Effects on Wetlands

The progressive loss of wetlands resulting from drainage and the dumping of debris is of great concern. With the loss of wetlands, the natural habitat for countless species of fish, shellfish, birds, and marine mammals is lost. By the end of this century, over half of the country's wetlands will have vanished.[20] On a more positive note, concerted efforts to reestablish wetlands are occurring throughout the country, such as in California. Unfortunately, at the same time, continued loss occurs in other areas.

Health implications

When water becomes polluted, its quality falls below acceptable standards for its intended use, and

coliform bacteria
Intestinal tract bacteria whose presence in a water supply suggests contamination by human or animal waste.

eutrophication
Enrichment of a body of water with nutrients, which causes overabundant growth of plants.

putrefaction
Decomposition of organic matter.

mutagenic
Capable of promoting genetic alterations in cells.

some aspects of our health will be harmed (see the Health Action Guide at right). Polluted water is associated with disease and illness, but it also distresses us emotionally, limits our social activities, and challenges us intellectually and spiritually to become more active stewards of our environment.

LAND POLLUTION

Since we live, work, and play on land, it may be difficult to believe that land constitutes only about 30% of the earth's surface. The rest is, of course, water. When we consider the rivers, streams, marshes, and lakes found on our land surfaces, our land surface seems even smaller. Uninhabitable land areas, such as swamps, deserts, and mountain ranges, further reduce the available land on which humans can live. Our land is a precious commodity—one that we have taken for granted.

The effects of our growing population on our limited land resources are becoming more evident. However, the greatest effect on our land comes from the products our society discards: *solid waste* products and *chemical waste* products.

Solid Waste

The trash that is collected from our homes is composed of a wide variety of familiar materials. Each year, Americans dispose of paper, newspaper, cardboard, clothing, yard waste, wood pallets, food waste, cafeteria waste, glass, metal, disposable tableware, plastics, and an endless variety of other types of *municipal solid waste* (MSW). Each individual American produces over 4.3 pounds of MSW each year.[21] Collectively, we have produced 200 million tons of solid waste.

Although it is important, MSW makes up only a small amount of the solid waste discarded in this country. Agricultural, mining, and industrial wastes contribute much more to our solid waste problems. Regardless of the source, solid waste requires some form of disposal. Traditionally, these forms have been taken:

- *Open dumping.* Solid waste is compacted and dumped on a dump site. Open dumps are discouraged or illegal in many urban areas.
- *Sanitary landfill.* Solid waste is compacted and buried in huge open pits. Each day, a layer of soil is pushed over the most recently dumped material to encourage decomposition, reduce unpleasant odors, and contain the material to keep it from being scattered.
- *Incineration.* Solid waste can be incinerated. A

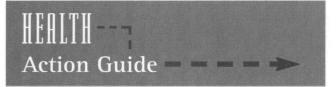

HEALTH Action Guide

Making Drinking Water Safe

When traveling outside of the United States, you should be aware that water supplies in more than 100 countries are considered unsafe. You can avoid waterborne illnesses by following these guidelines:

- Drink bottled water (but be careful of locally bottled water; it can also be unsafe).
- Boil water.
- Use iodine or water-purification tablets.
- Avoid using ice.
- Do not use tap water when brushing teeth.
- Avoid vegetables and fruits washed in unclean water.

To take the above advice further, before traveling be certain that all your immunizations are current, and request medication for diarrhea from your physician.

variety of types of incinerators exist, including cement kilns, boilers and furnaces, and commercial incinerators.
- *Ocean dumping.* When near enough to the ocean, solid waste can also be collected, loaded into barges, and taken to offshore dump sites.

Our ability to solve our solid waste disposal problems may depend on **recycling,** or the ability to convert many of our disposable items into reusable materials (see the Star Box on p. 435). It has been difficult to convince manufacturers and the public that many of our solid waste products should be recycled. Efforts to recycle glass, aluminum, paper, and plastic

carcinogenic
Related to the production of cancerous changes; property of environmental agents, including drugs, that may stimulate the development of cancerous changes within cells.

teratogenic
Capable of promoting birth defects.

recycling
The ability to convert disposable items into reusable materials.

LEARNING *from* ALL CULTURES

Canada's Green Plan

In December 1990, Canada introduced an environmental plan for the 1990s to improve and protect the environment. The Green Plan was designed to create and implement programs to protect and clean up Canada's land, air, water, and resources and to curb waste and use of energy. The plan called for an increase of 50% in spending on the environment over the next 6 years and for more funding for environmental groups not associated with the government.[26]

One particular area of concern included in the Green Plan is the ecosystems of the Arctic region. Some 40% of Canadian land is in the far North; therefore Canada has a history of involvement in Arctic issues. Most of the contaminants present in the Arctic region come from south-ern areas, but these pollutants are deposited in Arctic lakes. These toxins ultimately affect the food chain. Scientists suspect that air toxins recirculate in the atmosphere, and when they get to the Arctic, the temperature is too cold for the toxins to pass off as vapor somewhere else. As a result, the Arctic could become the depository for pollutants. A goal of the Green Plan is to study the problem of contaminants in the Arctic and find solutions to the ongoing accumulation of toxins. Canada is also committed through the plan to clean up hazardous waste sites in the far North.[26]

Pollution of the Arctic region is only one of many environmental concerns of the Green Plan. Considering the sparse population in the region and the harsh environment, should the cleanup and protection of the area be of great importance?

Thousands of sanitary landfills like this one are found throughout the United States. Each of us should ask, "Is this really the best way to dispose of solid waste?" "How much of this garbage am I responsible for?" "How can I reduce the amount I contribute?"

Recycling

Newspapers

Egg cartons, cereal boxes, dry wall, insulation, ceiling tiles, bedding

Glass

Food and beverage containers "Glassphalt"*

Steel

Automobiles, construction materials

"New" aluminum cans†

Aluminum

Plastics

"Plastic lumber"‡ (plastic mixtures)

Coat hangers, flower pots, insulation, toys (polystyrene [styrofoam])

Carpeting, automobile parts, tennis ball felt (soda bottles)

*A combination of glass and asphalt that makes an attractive roadway.
†20 recycled aluminum cans can be made for the same amount of energy required to make one new can from ore.
‡A durable construction material similar to wood that can be made into fence posts, decks, or park benches.

Figure 17-3   Many useful products can be made from recycled materials. The amount of material that is recycled depends on consumer demand for these products. Would you be willing to use an alternative product made from recycled components, such as a deck made of plastic lumber?

have not been fully adopted by society. Cost of recycling and a lack of markets for reclaimed materials often discourage municipalities and industries from practicing more recycling. Lack of time and interest, failure to understand how to recycle, messiness, and the lack of curbside pickup are also frequently mentioned as reasons for not recycling in the home.

Chemical Waste

According to many environmental consumer group leaders, the quality of our lives is deteriorating, in part because of the unsafe disposal of hazardous chemicals from industrial and agricultural sources. In 1993 alone, according to the EPA, 33.5 billion pounds of potentially toxic chemicals were released into the

The Three R's of Controlling Solid Waste Disposal
As consumers and environmentally concerned citizens, we need to do more than control the disposal of solid waste so that it does not adversely influence our health and the health of our environment. We must prevent this waste from occurring in increasing quantities. To accomplish this goal, a commitment to reduce, reuse, and recycle must be made.

The first step in dealing with the problem of solid waste disposal is to find ways to *reduce* the use of materials that eventually pollute our environment. A concerned public willing to make do with less, such as the amount of packaging material used with small consumer products, is a positive step. As concerned citizens, we must all learn to *reuse* as much as possible. Glass milk bottles that can be used again by the dairy, as well as cloth diapers rather than the nondegradable disposable diapers, are examples of reuse at its best.

Finally, we must *recycle* as much material as possible. Recent experience has taught us that Americans will recycle when a system for collecting material is in place. However, recycling will go only as far as the demand and a market for recycled materials exists.

When combined, the three R's of reduction, reuse, and recycling could significantly reduce our need to engage in the more expensive disposal of toxic wastes.

air, water, land, sewers, and into toxic waste dump sites.[22] Currently, it is estimated that there are as many as 31,500 toxic waste dump sites sprinkled across the country.[15] Because it costs much more money to detoxify, recycle, and reuse toxic chemical products than to dump them, too many chemical companies have been more than willing to secretly and unlawfully bury their chemical wastes.

Pesticides

Since Rachel Carson wrote her now-classic book *Silent Spring* in 1962, the public has been aware of the potential dangers associated with the use of some **pesticides.** Although Carson's primary concern was with the pesticide DDT, a number of other hazardous pesticides have since been removed from the marketplace. Tighter controls established by the EPA have restricted the availability of other, less hazardous pesticides. Farmers contend they need to use effective poisons to save their crops from insect destruction. However, equal concern seems to be focused now on the effects of pesticides on food and water supplies,

soil quality, animals, other insects, and humans. Harmful agents such as pesticides can enter an **ecosystem** and affect the entire food chain. The Star Box on p. 437 suggests nontoxic ways to garden and control home insects, thus reducing the need to use pesticides.

Herbicides

Herbicides also contribute to the growing problem of water and soil pollution and to the contamination of the food chain. These weed-killing chemicals are sprayed on plants and incorporated into the soil with plowing but are not totally taken up by the plant tissues they are intended to kill. The extent to which herbicides causes illness in humans is not fully known, although the potential appears to be real.

RADIATION

We have lived in the nuclear age since the end of World War II. Today the hopes for nuclear energy primarily lie in its enormous potential to reduce our dependence on fossil fuels as energy sources. Also, nuclear energy can (and already does) improve our industrial and medical technology, as evidenced by an expanding use of radioactive materials in the diagnosis and treatment of various health disorders.

The two greatest concerns over nuclear energy are (1) the harmful health effects that come from day-to-day exposure to radiation and (2) the potential for a nuclear accident of regional or global consequences. In the opinion of some, a third concern, that of nuclear terrorism, also exists.

Fission, the decay of radioactive materials, produces not only a great amount of energy but also **ionizing radiation** in the form of radioactive particles. We are exposed to various forms of ionizing radiation daily through natural radiation, including ultraviolet

pesticide
Agent used to destroy insects and other pests.

ecosystem
An ecological unit made up of both animal and plant life that interact to produce a stable system.

ionizing radiation
Form of radiation capable of releasing electrons from atoms.

IMPORTANT NOTICE OF PROPOSED SETTLEMENT OF CLASS ACTION AND FAIRNESS HEARING

IN THE UNITED STATES DISTRICT COURT FOR THE SOUTHERN DISTRICT OF ALABAMA SOUTHERN DIVISION

Russell Price, et al vs. Ciba-Geigy Corporation

NO. 94-0647-CB-S

U.S. WORKERS WITH ON-THE-JOB EXPOSURE TO GALECRON®

and Their Spouses, Children, Other Relatives and Legal Representatives:

GALECRON® WAS A COMMERCIAL AGRICULTURAL PESTICIDE WHICH WAS MARKETED IN THE U.S. BY CIBA-GEIGY CORPORATION. IT WAS NOT MARKETED FOR RESIDENTIAL OR HOME GARDENING USE.

U.S. WORKERS WITH ON-THE-JOB EXPOSURE TO GALECRON® MAY BE ELIGIBLE FOR FREE MEDICAL MONITORING AND/OR CASH PAYMENTS UNDER A PROPOSED LEGAL SETTLEMENT.

Health damage associated with job-related exposure to Galecron, a powerful pesticide, was the basis of a recent class-action suit against Ciba-Geigy Corporation.

---

radiation from the sun and natural radioactive mineral deposits, and synthetic radiation, including waste from nuclear reactors, industrial products, and x-ray examinations. Most of the exposures we get on a daily basis produce negligible health risks. Although it is clear that no kind of radiation exposure is good for you, safe levels of exposure are difficult to determine.

Health Effects of Radiation Exposure

The health effects of radiation exposure depend on many factors, including the duration, type, dose of exposure, and individual sensitivity. Clearly, heavy exposure (as in a severe nuclear accident) can produce **radiation sickness** or immediate death. Lesser exposure can be quite harmful as well. Of particular concern are the effects of radiation on egg and sperm production, embryonic development, and dangerous or irreversible changes to the eyes and skin. Cancer, particularly of the blood-forming tissue, is also a concern. From a health perspective, the message is clear: avoid any unnecessary exposure to radioactive materials. Make it a point to question the value of diagnostic x-ray examinations, especially routine dental and chest x-ray studies and mammograms. Routine x-ray stud-

ies have been discouraged by numerous professional societies and consumer groups. Recent studies suggest that the risk is minimal for most people.[23]

Electromagnetic Radiation

What do water bed heaters, electric razors, electric blankets, high-tension electrical transmission lines, and cellular telephones have in common? They all produce electromagnetic fields or electromagnetic waves, even more specifically, electromagnetic fields that come in close proximity to the body or pass very near your home, as in the case of transmission lines.

In recent years, concern has been voiced as to whether the electromagnetic fields generated by these familiar devices could cause cancer. Research using laboratory animals and studies comparing the incidence of cancer in people using these devices with those who do not have been far from conclusive. A recent study of 138,905 utility workers whose exposure to electromagnetic fields was in conjunction with power line sources did, however, show a higher than expected rate of death from brain cancer.[24] Therefore, in light of this study and until more research has been done regarding non–employment-

---

Nontoxic Home Pest Control

Try the following organic solutions to pest control problems:

- **Ants**—boric acid, which is available in a number of different formulations. Use it in a trap.
- **Roaches**—dry things out with a hair dryer. Roaches are attracted to moisture, so seal cracks, fix leaks. Other ideas: Mix equal parts of oatmeal or flour with plaster of Paris—or equal parts of baking soda and sugar—and spread around infested area.
- **Fleas**—before bed, put a light over a shallow pan of soapy water. Turn out all other lights. Empty water every morning and continue for one month. Fleas go for heat and light, and they can't swim.

- **Lawn weeds**—raise the cutting level on your lawn mower so the grass can grow three to four inches tall, giving it a strong root system that will block weeds. Other methods: Pull weeds, spray with soap solution, or douse with fresh human urine (it's very high in nitrogen and will burn the weed).
- **Garden pests**—suck them up with a hand-held vacuum cleaner.
- **Flies, mosquitoes**—fix screens. Vacuum them up. For flies, hang clusters of cloves; make flypaper by spreading honey on yellow (flies' favorite color) paper; scratch an orange peel and leave it out—the citrus oil repels flies.

---

related exposure, some care should be exercised in the use of appliances that generate radiation fields. For example, heaters for water beds should be turned on early to allow the bed to warm and then turned off once in the bed, cellular telephone calls should be kept short, and a morning shave should not last more than a few minutes.

Nuclear Reactor Accidents and Waste Disposal

To generate the nuclear energy to produce electrical energy, more than 100 nuclear power plants have been constructed in North America. Built mostly by utility companies, these nuclear power plants were designed to produce electrical energy in an efficient, economical, and safe manner. Much public criticism has been directed at these power plants, claiming that their safety and efficiency have not been documented.

Concern over the safety of nuclear power plants was heightened in this country and around the world when, on April 26, 1986, a **meltdown** occurred at the Chernobyl nuclear power plant in the Soviet Union. Human error was responsible for creating a situation in which excessive heat was allowed to build up in the core of the nuclear reactor. The resultant explosion killed two people, hospitalized hundreds, and exposed hundreds of thousands of people to nuclear radiation. As a result of the Chernobyl accident, the Russian government had to resettle 200,000 people at an estimated cost of $26 billion. Furthermore, a leading Soviet scientist estimated that 10,000 miners

and soldiers died as a result of exposure to radiation received during cleanup operations after the accident.

The safe disposal of nuclear waste is an additional serious problem that also has not been fully solved. The by-products of nuclear fission remain radioactive for many years. Although the current method of disposing of these wastes is to bury them, eventual leakage into our environment is serious risk.

Proponents of nuclear power maintain that not one person in the United States has died as the result of a power plant accident. They point to a spotless safety record and reiterate that our fossil fuel supply is limited. Supporters of the nuclear industry feel that a public commitment to establishing more nuclear reactors is important for the future of our country. Currently, nearly 20% of our electrical energy is generated by nuclear power.

radiation sickness
Illness characterized by fatigue, nausea, weight loss, fever, bleeding from mouth and gums, hair loss, and immune deficiencies, resulting from overexposure to ionizing radiation.

meltdown
The overheating and eventual melting of the uranium fuel rods in the core of a nuclear reactor.

Radiation Tests

During 1995, attention was called to a potentially dark page in American medical history—the purposeful exposure, between World War II and 1970, of 16,000 American citizens (prisoners, children, mentally retarded people, pregnant women, and patients in public hospitals) to nuclear radiation.[25] In 435 separate projects, of which about 10% are now known to have been excessively dangerous, radiation was used to determine how the human body functions and to develop the procedures that now comprise nuclear medical technology. Today the federal government is establishing methods to compensate the survivors and the families of those who have died.

NOISE POLLUTION

In much the same fashion that a weed is an unwanted plant and can ruin a lawn, noise is an unwanted sound that can be detrimental to our overall health. In some cases a sound that is desirable, such as music, can function like a true noise because of the intensity of the presentation. Regardless, today's world is characterized by sounds whose loudness and unrelenting presence are dangerous to our health. These intense sounds can reduce our hearing acuity, disrupt our emotional tranquility, infringe on our social interactiveness, and interrupt our concentration.

Noise-Induced Hearing Loss

Sound, or a wave of compressed air molecules moving in response to a pressure change, is characterized by two qualities—*frequency* and *intensity*. High intensity is primarily responsible for the loss of hearing experienced by many people living in noise-polluted environments. Intensity of sound exceeding 80 to 85 decibels (1200 to 4800 cycles-per-second frequency range) can cause hearing damage. The Star Box on p. 439 shows sound intensity associated with several common environmental sound sources.

The interpretation of a sound (hearing) is a sophisticated and sensitive physiological process involving the progressive conversion of acoustical energy to mechanical energy, then to hydraulic energy, and, finally, to electrochemical energy. Electrochemical energy is then transmitted by the acoustic nerve to the brain for interpretation. The destructive influence of exposure to sounds of high intensity lies in the destruction of special hair cells in the inner ear that are responsible for converting hydraulic energy into electrochemical energy. Loud music, jet engine noise, vehicular traffic, and a wide range of industrial noises can collapse these sensitive cells. Ironically, the cells that are damaged are those responsible for hearing the high-frequency sounds associated with normal conversation, not those that hear the damaging sound itself. Thus the environmental sources of noise rob you of your ability to hear sound of a far greater value—the sound of the unamplified human voice.

The damage just described is initially reversible. However, with continued exposure, the changes in the sensitive cells of the inner ear become permanent. The Health Action Guide on p. 439 suggests ways to reduce noise pollution.

Noise As a Stressor

In addition to the damaging effects of noise on hearing, the role of noise as a stressor has long been recognized. Indeed, the absence of noise (silence) and prolonged noise are both proven techniques to break the will of prisoners during war. Recently, however, attention has shifted to the role of noise in terms of the stress response, presented in Chapter 3. In people stressed by unrelenting noise, the elevated epinephrine levels contribute to hypertension and other stress-related health problems.

IN SEARCH OF BALANCE

How often have you heard people yearn for a return to the "good old days"? They reminisce about times when people moved more slowly, cared more for their neighbors, and appreciated their natural resources. After listening to these nostalgic impressions, you could believe that our society was once almost idyllic—with little or no pollution, population concerns, or threats of nuclear accidents.

Certainly it is nice to dream, but it is doubtful that our advancing technology and exploding worldwide population will permit us to find such an ideal world. Instead, we need to focus on finding the appropriate balance between technological growth and environmental deterioration. Perhaps some of the organizations listed in the Star Box on p. 440 can help us in our efforts.

We must learn to think beyond the present. Each decision we make for the future should be considered in light of its influence on our environmental systems (see the Star Box on p. 441). If our decisions are based solely on financial gain or personal convenience, we will be committing a monumental disservice to our children and future generations.

Noise Pollution and Its Effects on Hearing

The loudness of sounds is measured in decibels (dB). Sound intensity is determined logarithmically, not arithmetically. Each increase of 10 dB produces a tenfold increase in sound intensity. Thus 30 dB has 10 times the intensity of 20 dB, 40 dB has 100 times the intensity of 20 dB, and 110 dB sounds 10 times as loud as 100 dB. Hearing damage depends on the dB level and the length of exposure. Presented below are dB ranges, common sources, and effects on hearing.

Decibel	Common sources	Effect on hearing
0	Lowest sound audible to human ear	—
30	Quiet library, soft whisper	—
40	Quiet office, study lounge, bedroom away from traffic	—
50	Light traffic at a distance, refrigerator, quiet conversation, gentle breeze	—
60	Air conditioner at 20 feet, normal conversation, sewing machine	—
70	Busy traffic, noisy office or cafeteria	Annoying, and may start to affect hearing if constant
80	Heavy city traffic, alarm clock at 2 feet, typical factory	Starts to affect hearing if exposed more than 8 hours
90	Truck traffic, noisy home appliances, shop tools, lawn mower	Temporary hearing loss can occur in less than 8 hours
100	Chain saw, pneumatic drill (jackhammer), loud motorcycle, or farm equipment	Unprotected exposure for 2 hours can produce serious damage to hearing
120	Rock band concert in front of speakers, sand blasting, loud thunderclap	Immediate danger threat
140	Shotgun blast, jet plane from 50 feet	Immediate pain threat; any length of exposure is dangerous
180	Rocket pad area during launch (without ear protection)	Immediate, irreversible, and inevitable hearing loss

HEALTH Action Guide

Reducing Noise Pollution

Beyond giving your political support to legislation and enforcement policies designed to reduce environmental noise pollution, what can you do to lessen the degree of noise pollution in your life? The following suggestions are only a few of the recommended approaches:

- Limit your exposure to highly amplified music. The damage from occasional exposure to sound intensity between 110 and 120 decibels can be reversible. Daily exposure, however, will result in permanent hearing loss.
- Reduce the volume on your portable headsets. When others can hear the music coming through your headset while you are wearing it, you should probably turn down the volume.
- Wear ear plugs (wax or soft plastic) and sound-absorbing ear muffs when using firearms or operating loud machinery.
- Maintain your automobile, motorcycle, or lawn mower exhaust systems in good working order.
- Furnish your room, apartment, home, and office with sound-absorbing materials. Drapes, carpeting, and cork wall tiles are excellent for reducing both interior and exterior noises.
- Establish noise reduction as a criterion in selecting a site for your residence. An apartment complex near a freeway or airport or property near an interstate highway may prove to be less than desirable.

Since you are a person with a lifetime of hearing ahead, noise pollution reduction deserves your participation and your support.

Organizations Related to Environmental Concerns

Federal Departments, Agencies, and Offices

- Environmental Protection Agency, 401 M St. S.W., Washington, DC 20460; (202) 382-2090
- Council of Environmental Quality, 722 Jackson Pl. N.W., Washington, DC 20503; (202) 395-5750
- Department of Energy, Forrestal Bldg., 1000 Independence Ave. S.W., Washington, DC 20585; (202) 586-6210
- Department of Interior, Interior Bldg., 1849 C St. N.W., Washington, DC 20240; (202) 208-3100
- National Oceanic and Atmospheric Administration, Rockville, MD 20852; (301) 443-8910
- United States Fish and Wildlife Service, 1849 C Street, N.W., Washington, DC 20240; (202) 208-5634

National Organizations

- National Wildlife Federation, 1400 16th St. N.W., Washington, DC 20036; (202) 797-6800 and (800) 432-6564
- Sierra Club, 730 Polk St., San Francisco, CA 94109; (415) 776-2211
- Cousteau Society, Inc., 870 Greenbriar Circle, Suite 402, Chesapeake, VA 23320 (804) 523-9335
- Greenpeace USA, 1436 U Street, N.W., Washington, DC 20009; (202) 462-1177
- The Wilderness Society, 900 17th Street, N.W., Washington, DC 20006; (202) 833-2300
- The Nature Conservancy, 1815 N. Lynn St., Arlington, Va, 22209; (703) 841-5300
- The Environmental Defense Fund, 257 Park Avenue South, New York, NY 10010; (800) 684-3322

Canadian Organizations

- Environment Canada, Ottawa, Ontario K1A OH3; (819) 997-1441)

Summary

- World population is increasing at an alarming rate and with adverse effects on the environment.
- Gases and solid pollutants contribute to air pollution and its associated health concerns.
- Worldwide increases in carbon dioxide production could result in a greenhouse effect, leading to climatic warming and extreme weather conditions.
- Acid rain, acid fog, and acid snow, as well as smog, result from the release of gaseous and particulate pollutants into the air.

- Deterioration of the ozone layer could result in exposure to high levels of ultraviolet radiation and serious health problems.
- Particulate matter, including fibers and trace mineral elements, are found in the air.
- Temperature inversions increase the seriousness of air pollution.
- Indoor air pollution is now recognized as a serious threat to health, particularly from radon gas that can easily accumulate in modern houses.

✫ ✫ ✫ ✫ ✫ ✫   ✫ ✫ ✫ ✫ ✫ ✫

Your Role in Creating a Sustainable Environment

As we search for solutions to complex environmental problems, we may have to make some difficult decisions. For example, will Third World populations be forced to use contraception or sterilization? Will we attempt to feed the world's hungry people? Will we continue to protect endangered species of plants and animals? Will we strive more forcefully for nuclear disarmament? Can we commit ourselves to cleaning up all of our toxic waste sites? Answers to these complex questions about *stewardship* will probably be based not only on our knowledge but also on our moral predispositions.

Answers to these sorts of complex questions can come from recognizing the value of a *sustainable environment*. This environment will be developed only when individuals and groups are willing to do the following:

- Evaluate their environment
- Become environmentally educated
- Choose a simpler, less consumption-oriented lifestyle
- Recognize the limitations of technology in solving problems
- Become involved in environmental protection activities
- Work with people on all sides of environmental issues[2]

These suggestions might sound abstract for a person confronted with a local environmental problem. However, each of these steps can be applied to a local situation with only limited modifications. The PCB soil contamination in Indiana, the nerve gas weapons storage in Kentucky, the toxic waste site cleanup in Missouri, and the transportation of nuclear waste materials in California and other states represent local issues to which these steps can be applied. Are you committed enough to a sustainable environment to practice these steps?

- Water pollution results from a variety of causative agents, including toxic chemicals and pathogens from human and animal wastes.
- Increased levels of pesticides and herbicides can be found in both surface water and groundwater sources.
- Chlorine from a variety of sources, including PCBs, can also be found in both surface water and groundwater sources.
- Municipal solid waste is a small but important component of all solid waste.
- Solid wastes are traditionally buried, dumped, or incinerated.
- Reduction, reuse, and recycling are important aspects of the prevention of environmental pollution.

- Toxic wastes from both industry and agriculture are serious sources of land pollution.
- As with water pollution, pesticides and herbicides have been found to pollute land.
- Radiation, including ultraviolet and ionizing radiation from nuclear power plants, could result in serious health problems.
- Electromagnetic radiation may be associated with severe health problems, including brain cancer.
- Noise pollution can lead to hearing loss, particularly the ability to hear the human voice.
- We must seek a balance between lifestyle and the health of the environment, not only for our generations but for those who will follow.

Review Questions

1. In what direction is the world population changing? What could be the consequences of this change on the environment? How can the rate of this change be moderated?
2. What is the greenhouse effect? How does deforestation influence this process? What is the anticipated consequence of the greenhouse effect?
3. How are acid rain, acid fog, and acid snow produced? What and where is the damage attributed to them?
4. What is causing the deterioration of the ozone layer? What step has been taken to slow this process? What are the consequences of ozone layer deterioration?

5. What are the major particulate pollutants in our air? What is the principal risk associated with lead as a pollutant? What specific diseases are associated with particulate material in our air?
6. How are gray-air smog and brown-air smog formed? When and where is one form more likely to be seen than the other?
7. What air pollutant has recently been classified as a Group A carcinogen? What other pollutants contribute to indoor air pollution? What risks are associated with radon gas?
8. What toxic chemicals are most often the sources of water pollution? What is the consequence of having too little oxygen dissolved in water? What is thermal pollution? How do pesticides and herbicides enter both our water supply and soil? What is the principal source of the chlorine found in water?
9. What are several forms of municipal solid waste?

How much municipal solid waste does the typical person produce per day? How much do Americans produce in a year?
10. How are solid wastes most often disposed of? Why are these techniques less than fully acceptable?
11. What are the three R's of better solid waste prevention?
12. What are the principal sources of radiation that are of concern today? Which are natural sources of radiation, and which are the result of human intervention? What familiar appliances may be sources of electromagnetic fields?
13. How does noise pollution result in hearing loss? What are the most common sources of noise pollution?
14. For whom is a balance between a modern lifestyle and a healthful environment important?

Think About This . . .

- To what extent do your driving habits contribute to air pollution?
- In what ways do your recreational activities contribute to water pollution?
- If land were very affordable, would you build a new house on land reclaimed from a toxic waste dump site?
- How close to a nuclear power plant would you feel comfortable living?
- Is your home protected from the possibility of radon gas?

- The environmental focus of the 1990s has shifted from global concerns, such as the ozone layer, deforestation, and world population, to local concerns, such as recycling and indoor air pollution. Will it now be possible to "think globally while acting locally"?
- Would you be willing to spend more for a lightbulb designed to last 20,000 hours, use little energy, and last several years rather than a much less expensive incandescent bulb to reduce energy costs?

References

1. The environment and population growth: decade for action, *Population Reports* Series M(10):2-3, 1992.
2. Greenhouse gas giants, *USA Today*, June 3, 1992 (based on data supplied by the World Resource Institute).
3. Climatic Research Unit, University of East Anglia, as reported in *Newsweek*, Jan 22, 1996.
4. Arms K: *Environmental science*, ed 2, Fort Worth, Tex, 1994, Saunders College Publishers.
5. Chiras D: *Environmental science: action for a sustainable future*, ed 4, Redwood City, Calif, 1994, Benjamin-Cummings.
6. Kerr JB, McElroy CT: Evidence for large upward trends of ultraviolet-B radiation linked to ozone depletion, *Science* 262:1032-1034, 1993.
7. Gather P et al: Observational evidence for chemical ozone depletion over the Arctic in winter 1991-92, *Nature* 375(6527):131-134, 1995 (letters).
8. Cary P: The asbestos panic attack: how the feds got schools to spend billions on a problem that really didn't amount to much, *U.S. News & World Report* 118(7):61-64, 1995.

9. *Respiratory health effects of passive smoking: lung cancer and other diseases,* Office of Health and Environment, Office of Research and Development, U.S. Environmental Protection Agency, December 1992.
10. Cole L: *Element of risk: the politics of radon,* New York, 1994, Oxford University Press.
11. Menzie R et al: The effect of varying levels of outdoor-air supply on the symptoms of sick building syndrome, *N Engl J Med* 328(12): 821-827, 1993.
12. Kanamine L: EPA: 40% of freshwater is unusable, *USA Today,* p 1A, April 21, 1994.
13. Kanamine L: Under-treated water flows to 50 million, *USA Today,* p 1A, July 28, 1994.
14. Cunningham W, Saigo B: *Environmental science: a global concern,* ed 3, Dubuque, Ia, 1994, William C Brown.
15. Miller GT: *Living in the environment: an introduction to environmental science* ed 7, Belmont, Calif, 1992, International Thomson.
16. Manning A: Tainted water: herbicide levels rise in summer, *USA Today,* p 1D, August 18, 1995.
17. Leiss JK, Savitz DA: Home pesticide use and childhood cancer: a case-control study, *Am J Public Health* 85(2): 249-252, 1995.
18. Falck F et al: Pesticides and polychlorinated biphenyl residues in human breast lipids and their relationship to breast cancer, *Arch Environ Health* 47(2):143-146, 1992.
19. LeMonick MD: Not so fertile ground, *Time* 144(12):68-70, 1994.
20. Cunningham WP: *Understanding our environment,* Dubuque, Ia, 1994, William C Brown.
21. Franklin W, Franklin M: Putting the crusade into perspective: recycling and waste generation both are on the rise, *EPA Journal* 18(3):7, 1992.
22. Toxic buildup, *USA Today,* p 3A, March 28, 1995.
23. Boice J et al: Diagnostic x-ray procedures and risk of leukemia, lymphoma, and multiple myeloma, *JAMA* 265(10):1290, 1991.
24. Savitz DA, Loomis DP: Magnetic field exposure in relation to leukemia and brain cancer mortality among electric utility workers, *Am J Epidemiol* 141(2):123-128, 1995.
25. Hoversten P: Hunting radiation records—and truth, *USA Today,* p 1A, Aug 18, 1995.
26. Hansen P: Canada's Green Plan, *Canada Today/d'aujour'dhui* 22(1):3, 1991.

Suggested Readings

50 simple things you can do to save the earth, 50 simple things kids can do to save the earth, and *The student environmental action guide,* The Earth Works, Berkeley, Calif, 1992, The Earth Works Group. A collection of three of the most practical and comprehensive books written on how we can become stewards of the environment. Each book is intended for a specific group (adults, children, and college students) and offers advice in the context of each group's experiences and environment.

Fisher DE: *Fire and ice—the greenhouse effect, ozone depletion, and nuclear winter,* New York, 1990, Harper & Row. An interesting look at a number of environmental problems facing the world today. Proposed solutions are offered; also contains an appendix listing many citizen environmental groups.

Pedersen A: *The kid's environment book: what's awry and why,* Santa Fe, NM, 1992, John Muir Publishing. Explains serious environmental problems to children without scaring them. Intended for children 8 years of age and older.

Smith AA: *Campus ecology: a guide to assessing environmental quality and creating strategies for change,* Los Angeles, 1993, Living Planet Press. A guidebook for campus groups identifying environmental concerns found on the college campus and suggesting approaches to resolving these concerns. Numerous case studies are included.

MacEachern D: *Enough is enough: the hell-raiser's guide to community activism,* New York, 1994, Avon. This how-to manual is intended for people who want to become more active in shaping public policy, including policy related to the environment. Tips for lobbying, boycotting, and taking an effective role in public meetings are given. A left-leaning viewpoint is noted.

Telecommuting

Technological advances continue to astound and amaze. In recent years, many of the most promising advances have been made in the areas of computer technology and communications technonogy. Computers have improved to the point where processes that used to take hours now can be performed in seconds. Communications now allow contact to be established with virtually anyplace in the world within seconds. Such advances have allowed companies and individual employees to save money and valuable environmental resources by taking advantage of telecommuting.

Loosely defined, telecommuting means working at home by logging into your office computer system from your home computer. This growing trend could transform the way business is performed. Companies and employees could save millions of dollars in transportation costs, and the potential environmental benefits from energy conservation and pollution reduction are very appealing to society as a whole. Plane flights, cab rides, and twice-daily commutes could be replaced by a walk to the computer. But will the environmental benefits of telecommuting outweigh the potential costs? And could changes in the traditional office environment prove to be unmanageable for employees and employers?

How Telecommuting Can Change Everyday Life

Debbie is a stock trader, working for a Wall Street firm. She is on top of the daily trends of the stock market and gets market price updates as they happen. She stays in contact with her clients and buys and sells stock for them on a daily basis.

But you won't find Debbie on the trading floor.

She's in Albuquerque.

Debbie is one of a growing number of employees who have opted to telecommute to work. Debbie's situation demonstrates what is possible with telecommuting using today's technology. It also illustrates the savings that are possible when conventional travel is eliminated from the daily schedule, and it shows the potential social advantages that come from working at home.[1]

When her husband's job required a move to Albuquerque, New Mexico, Debbie tried the traditional commuting route, keeping a regular work-week schedule in New York City and flying to Albuquerque on the weekends. The commute took its toll, and she eventually left her job. Then she got an offer from a Wall Street firm that was willing to help accommodate her in this unusual situation. She now has separate phone lines for a fax machine, voice mail, and a direct link to her New York office. She also obtains up-to-the-minute stock quotes through a real-time stock market quote service. This technology has enabled Debbie to avoid the hassles of commuting and the stress of the trading floor and has allowed her to enjoy life with her family while working.

This all sounds too good to be true. Telecommuting has been hailed as the wave of the future in business, and its potential benefits have been touted in the popular press for several years. However, although it may have its advantages, there are some problems that may occur if telecommuting gains widespread acceptance.

Environmental Advantages and Problems

Telecommuting may have advantages with regard to conservation of natural resources. A 1990 study by the Arthur D. Little environmental consulting firm showed that significant benefits could result if telecommuting and videoconferencing could be substituted for conventional transportation. If such substitutions accounted for 10% to 20% of the time spent working, shopping, conducting meetings, and sending data, a net yearly savings of up to $23 billion could result. We could also conserve 3.5 million gallons of gasoline per year and reduce yearly pollution production by 1.8 million tons.[2]

Telecommuting also reduces vehicular wear and tear and lowers energy requirements and costs incurred by driving.[3] It may also reduce traffic on the roads in general. In an effort to reduce vehicular traffic problems, the Environmental Protection Agency may force California and other heavily populated states to require more telecommuting. California businesses have already been trying to find ways to reduce the number of cars coming to and from work on a weekly basis. Carpooling is already encouraged in California, where multiple-passenger cars are allowed sole access to "carpool only" lanes. But telecommuting has the potential to eliminate many cars altogether from the daily commuting process, which can be painfully slow and time consuming in large metropolitan areas. Businesses in California may also be required to install more fiber-optic networks and advanced teleconferencing equipment to reduce both local and long-range travel by employees.[4]

Home-based employees will also have the ability to make their home offices more environmentally sound than the typical office. Using a personal computer that saves energy (look for the "Energy Star" label) is a start.[5] Plain-paper fax machines eliminate the need to make photocopies of faxed documents, and all waste paper, foam packing materials, and toner cartridges can be recycled as well. Home-based employees can also get an energy audit for their home office to help make it as waste-free as possible.[5]

Although there appear to be many environmental advantages to telecommuting, many potential drawbacks to widespread telecommuting have been noted. As workers find that they do not need to live near urban workplaces, many of these workers may move to more rural areas to enhance their quality of life. This trend is not new, but those people who have moved out of the inner city have at least moved to communities within a moderate drive from the city. Telecommuting allows an employee to live virtually anywhere, and some experts fear that many workers may flee not just the city but the suburbs as well. These rural areas may not have the infrastructure to handle a massive influx of new residents.[6] Urban areas may face decay as citizens (and possibly businesses) leave cities.[3] Forests and open land may be destroyed as population expands in rural areas.[6]

The Social Aspects of Telecommuting
The potential advantages of telecommuting are very appealing for the individual worker. The most obvious advantage is that the employee is freed from the stress of physically commuting to the office, thus being spared the aggravation and wasted time of driving or riding to and from work.[7] Up to 3.1 billion hours of personal time could be gained by substituting telecommuting for general work activities 10% to 20% of the time.[2] Staying at home can also give workers more free time and allow employees (in some cases) to adjust their work schedules to fit their lifestyles.[7] Schedules can be more easily altered to adjust to unexpected occurrences, such as illness of a family member.[8] More time at home can allow workers more quality time with their families and may help employees develop deeper emotional relationships with their families and friends. Having more people at or near home may foster greater community stability as well.[3]

The individual telecommuter may face some problems, however. Being at home more often (and being expected to work in a home setting) may place stress on family relationships.[3] Being away from an office setting may cause workers to feel isolated from other company employees,[3,7] and their social skills may suffer as a result of lack of contact with others. The loss of the office as a community and the sense of support from co-workers

may also be felt. Employees may not be able to judge the importance of their work in relation to the goals of the company.[7-9]

Supervisors may also have difficulty in evaluating the work of their employees. A loss of company loyalty may also develop if workers spend more time networking with other telecommuters than with company people.[9] Because of the increase in technology, employees may find themselves on call at all hours instead of working a normal daily schedule. Employers may begin to expect workers to be available to work anytime and anywhere[7] through the use of pagers, cellular phones, and portable computers.

The Future Is Now
Ready or not, this new era of office employment is here. It is estimated that roughly half of all workers could be telecommuting in some form by the year 2000. Technological advances are also paving the way for increased telecommuting. The advent and growth of fiber-optic systems allow information to be transmitted much more quickly and efficiently than before. Thus high-powered personal computers can communicate with large mainframe computers at high speed with few problems. Differences between computer brands and data types are being overcome as well. The Integrated Services Digital Network can interface with other computers regardless of the type of computer used or the data transmitted.[3] For those employees who do not want to stay tied down to the house, portable laptop computers and fax transmission equipment now make it possible to send and receive information from nearly anywhere.

And, as Debbie will tell you, that includes her back porch.

For Discussion . . .
After weighing the pros and cons, do you think telecommuting is beneficial to the environment? Why? Do you think that you would enjoy a job where telecommuting is a mandatory part of your work schedule? What personal benefits could you get from telecommuting? What are the potential drawbacks?

References
1. Young J: Sand, sun, mutual fund, *Forbes* 152(10), Oct 25, 1993.
2. Raven PH, Berg LR, Johnson GB: Telecommuting: good for the planet (Envirobrief), *Environment*, Philadelphia, 1995, Saunders.
3. Cunningham S: Communication networks: a dozen ways they'll change our lives, *The Futurist* 26(1), Jan-Feb 1992.

4. Keaver M: Technology sows some seeds for environmental protection, *PC Week* 6(17), May 1, 1989.

5. Townsend AK: Setting up your green home office, *E* 5(4), Aug 1994.

6. Information superhighway: an environmental menace, *USA Today Magazine* 124(2604), Sept 1995.

7. Lundquist E: A Labor Day look at PCs; home work, *PC Week* 12(35), Sept 4, 1995.

8. Sullivan N: Double whammy, *Home Office Computing* 12(5), May 1994.

9. Connelly J: Let's hear it for the office, *Fortune* 131, Mar 6, 1995.

PART 7

THE LIFE CYCLE

Chapter

18

Accepting Dying and Death

Healthy People 2000 Objectives

Several Healthy People 2000 objectives focus on increasing the life span and years of healthy life for Americans, reducing death rates from various diseases and health conditions, and reducing infant mortality rates. With a few exceptions, the Midcourse Review indicates that we are progressing steadily toward target goals for many of these objectives.

For the entire American population, life expectancy is increasing at a rapid rate, with the average life span now at nearly 76 years. However, the estimates of years of healthy life are not so encouraging, especially among racial and ethnic minorities. The Midcourse Review reports a decline in health-related quality of life despite the increase in life expectancy.

The year 2000 health objective of reducing the number of deaths caused by unintentional injuries has been achieved. The reduction of traffic fatalities, especially among young people, has been the most important factor in meeting this goal. The number of deaths caused by work-related injuries has been reduced, and we are about halfway toward reaching the target in this area.

The primary goal of this chapter is to help people realize that the reality of death can serve as a focal point for a more enjoyable, productive, and contributive life. Each day in our lives becomes especially meaningful only after we have fully accepted the reality that someday we are going to die. We can then live each day to its fullest, as if it were our last day.

Our mortality provides us with a framework from which to appreciate and conduct our lives. It should help us prioritize our activities so that we can accomplish our goals (in our academic work, our relationships with others, and our recreation) before we die. Quite simply, death gives us our only absolute reason for living.

DYING IN TODAY'S SOCIETY

Since shortly after the turn of the century, the manner in which people experience death in this society has changed significantly. Formerly, most people died in their own homes, surrounded by family and friends. Young children frequently lived in the same home with their aging grandparents and saw them grow older and eventually die. Death was seen as a natural extension of life. Children grew up with a keen sense of what death meant, both to the dying person and to the grieving survivors.

Times have indeed changed. Today approximately 70% of people die in hospitals, nursing homes, and extended care facilities, not in their own homes. The extended family is seldom at the bedside of the dying person.[1] Frequently, frantic efforts are made to keep a dying person from death. Although medical technology has improved our lives, some people believe that it has reduced our ability to die with dignity. Many are convinced that our way of dying has become more artificial and less civilized than it used to be. The trend toward hospice care may be a positive response to this high-tech manner of dying (see p. 454).

DEFINITIONS OF DEATH

Before many of the scientific advancements of the past 30 years, death was relatively easy to define. People were considered dead when a heartbeat could no longer be detected and when breathing ceased. Now, with the technological advancements made in medicine, especially emergency medicine, some patients who give every indication of being dead can be resuscitated. Critically ill people, even those in comas, can now be kept alive for years with many of their bodily functions maintained by medical devices, including feeding tubes and respirators.

Thus death can be a very difficult concept to define. Numerous professional associations and ad hoc interdisciplinary committees have struggled with this problem and have developed criteria by which to establish death. Some of these criteria have been adopted by state legislatures, although there is certainly no consensus definition of death that all states embrace.

Clinical determinants of death refer to measures of bodily functions. Often judged by a physician, who can then sign a legal document called a *medical death certificate*, these clinical criteria include the following:

1. Lack of heartbeat and breathing.
2. Lack of central nervous system function, including all reflex activity and environmental responsiveness. Often this can be confirmed by an **electroencephalograph** reading. If there is no brain wave activity after an initial measurement and a second measurement after 24 hours, the person is said to have undergone *brain death.*
3. The presence of **rigor mortis,** indicating that body tissues and organs are no longer functioning at the cellular level. This is sometimes referred to as *cellular death.*

The *legal determinants* used by government officials are established by state law and often adhere closely to the clinical determinants already listed. A person is not legally dead until a death certificate has been signed by a physician, **coroner,** or health department officer.

EUTHANASIA

There are two types of euthanasia for desperately ill people: they are either intentionally put to death **(direct [active] euthanasia)** or allowed to die without

---

electroencephalograph
An instrument that measures the electrical activity of the brain.

rigor mortis
Rigidity of the body that occurs after death.

coroner
An elected legal official empowered to pronounce death and to determine the official cause of a suspicious or violent death.

direct (active) euthanasia
The process of inducing death, often through the injection of lethal drugs.

being subjected to heroic lifesaving efforts **(indirect [passive] euthanasia).** Direct euthanasia usually involves the administration of large amounts of depressant drugs, which eventually causes all central nervous system functions to stop. Although direct euthanasia is commonly practiced on housepets and laboratory animals, it is illegal for humans in the United States, Canada, and other developed countries. However, in February 1992, the Netherlands became the first developed country to enact legislation that permits euthanasia under strict guidelines. See the Star Box below, which discusses physician-assisted suicide.

Indirect euthanasia is increasingly occurring in a number of hospitals, nursing homes, and medical centers. Physicians who withhold heroic lifesaving techniques or drug therapy treatments or who disconnect life support systems from terminally ill patients are practicing indirect euthanasia. Although some people still consider this form of euthanasia a type of murder, indirect euthanasia seems to be gaining legal and public acceptance for people with certain terminal illnesses—near-death cancer patients, brain-dead accident victims, and hopelessly ill newborn babies. Physicians' orders of *do not resuscitate* (DNR) and *comfort measures only* (CMO) are examples of passive euthanasia that are familiar to hospital personnel.

ADVANCE MEDICAL DIRECTIVES

Because some physicians and families find it difficult to support indirect euthanasia, many people are starting to use legal documents called *advance medical directives.*[2] One of these medical directives is the living will (see the Star Box on p. 451). This is a document that confirms a dying person's desire to be allowed to die peacefully and with a measure of dignity if a time should arise when there is little hope for recovery from a terminal illness or severe injury. Living will statutes exist in all 50 states and the District of Columbia. The living will requires that physicians or family members carry out a person's wishes to die naturally, without receiving life-sustaining treatments.[3] About 20% to 25% of U.S. citizens have signed living wills.[4]

A second important document that can assist ter-

Physician–Assisted Suicide

In early 1996, physician-assisted suicide was the basis for two significant national news stories. The first dealt with Dr. Jack Kevorkian, who was on trial in Michigan for helping two people kill themselves in 1993. Under the provisions of a Michigan law that was in effect in 1993, Kevorkian could face up to 8 years in prison if he is found guilty of intentionally causing the deaths of these patients. The key issue is whether Kevorkian intended to cause death or intended to relieve pain and discomfort. Kevorkian contended in the trial that his intention was to relieve pain and reduce suffering.[13] Do you know how this trial ended? Should physicians be allowed to assist people who wish to die?

The second news story concerned the status of a recent law passed by voters in Oregon. Measure 16 was narrowly passed in November 1994. This law allowed a terminally ill patient to request a lethal dosage of drugs if two or more doctors determined that the patient had less than 6 months to live. In December 1994 a federal judge prevented this law from going into effect. At the time of this writing, this injunction was being appealed at the 9th Circuit Court in San Francisco. If this law were determined to be constitutional, an important legal foundation for physician-assisted suicide will have been established. Do you know the status of this Oregon law?

The Living Will

The living will is a legally binding document in all 50 states and the District of Columbia. This document allows individuals to express their wishes concerning dying with dignity. When such a document has been drawn, families and physicians are better able to deal with the wishes of people who are near death from conditions from which there is no reasonable expectation of recovery. The following is a generic living will. However, people should use a living will that is specific for the state in which they live. For additional information and materials, contact the Choice in Dying organization by using the toll-free number 1 (800) 989-WILL.

INSTRUCTIONS	**Choice In Dying Living Will**
PRINT YOUR NAME	I, _____ being of sound mind, make this statement as a directive to be followed if I become permanently unable to participate in decisions regarding my medical care. These instructions reflect my firm and settled commitment to decline medical treatment under the circumstances indicated below: I direct my attending physician to withhold or withdraw treatment if I should be in an incurable or irreversible mental or physical condition with no reasonable expectation of recovery. These instructions apply if I am a) in a terminal condition; b) permanently unconscious; or c) if I am minimally conscious but have irreversible brain damage and will never regain the ability to make decisions and express my wishes. I direct that treatment be limited to measures to keep me comfortable and to relieve pain, including any pain that might occur by withholding or withdrawing treatment.

**CROSS OUT ANY
STATEMENTS
THAT DO NOT
REFLECT YOUR
WISHES**
	While I understand that I am not legally required to be specific about future treatments, if I am in the condition(s) described above I feel especially strongly about the following forms of treatment:
	    I do not want cardiac resuscitation (CPR).
	    I do not want mechanical respiration.
	    I do not want tube feeding.
	    I do not want antibiotics.
	
	    However, I do want maximum pain relief, even if it may hasten my death.

ADD PERSONAL INSTRUCTIONS (IF ANY)	Other directions (insert personal instructions):

	These directions express my legal right to refuse treatment, under federal and state law. I intend my instructions to be carried out, unless I have rescinded them in a new writing or by clearly indicating that I have changed my mind.
SIGN AND DATE THE DOCUMENT AND PRINT YOUR ADDRESS	Signed: _____ Date: _____ Address: _____
WITNESSING PROCEDURE	I declare that the person who signed this document is personally known to me and appears to be of sound mind and acting of his or her own free will. He or she signed (or asked another to sign for him or her) this document in my presence. Witness: _____
TWO WITNESSES MUST SIGN AND PRINT THEIR ADDRESSES	Address: _____ Witness: _____ Address: _____

© 1994 Choice In Dying, Inc. 1/94
200 Varick Street, New York, NY 10014 1-800-989-WILL   PAGE 2

minally ill or incapacitated patients is the **durable power of attorney for health care** document. This legal document authorizes another person to make specific health care decisions about treatment and care under specified circumstances, most commonly when patients are in long-term vegetative states and cannot communicate their medical wishes. This document helps inform hospitals and physicians which person will help make the critical medical decisions. Usually this person is a loving relative. It is recommended that people complete both a living will and a durable power of attorney for health care document.

> **indirect (passive) euthanasia**
> The process of allowing a person to die by disconnecting life support systems or withholding lifesaving techniques.
>
> **durable power of attorney for health care**
> A legal document that designates who will make health care decisions for people unable to do so for themselves.

EMOTIONAL STAGES OF DYING

A process of self-adjustment has been observed in people who have a terminal illness. The stages in this process have helped form the basis for the modern movement of death education. An awareness of these stages may help you understand how people adjust to other important losses in their lives.

Perhaps the most widely recognized name in the area of death education is Dr. Elisabeth Kübler-Ross. As a psychiatrist working closely with terminally ill patients at the University of Chicago's Billings Hospital, Kübler-Ross was able to observe the emotional reactions of dying people. In her classic book *On Death and Dying*, Kübler-Ross summarized the psychological stages that dying people often experience.[5]

- *Denial.* This is the stage of disbelief. Patients refuse to believe that they actually will die. Denial can serve as a temporary defense mechanism and can allow patients the time to accept their prognosis on their own terms.
- *Anger.* A common emotional reaction after denial is anger. Patients can feel as if they have been cheated. By expressing anger, patients are able to vent some of their fears, jealousies, anxieties, and frustrations. Patients often direct their anger at relatives, physicians and nurses, religious symbols, and normally healthy people.
- *Bargaining.* Terminally ill people follow the anger stage with a stage characterized by bargaining. Patients who desperately want to avoid their inevitable deaths attempt to strike bargains— often with God or a church leader. Some people undergo religious conversions. The goal is to buy time by promising to repent for past sins, to restructure and rededicate their lives, or to make a large financial contribution to a religious cause.
- *Depression.* When patients realize that, at best, bargaining can only postpone their fate, they may begin an unpredictable period of depression. In a sense, terminally ill people are grieving for their own anticipated death. They may become quite withdrawn and refuse to visit with close relatives and friends. Prolonged periods of silence or crying are normal components of this stage and should not be discouraged.
- *Acceptance.* During the acceptance stage, patients fully realize that they are going to die. Acceptance ensures a relative sense of peace for most dying people. Anger, resentment, and depression are usually gone. Kübler-Ross describes this stage as one without much feeling. Patients feel neither happy nor sad. Many are calm and introspective

and prefer to be left either alone or with a few close relatives or friends.

One or two additional points should be made about the psychological stages of dying. Just as each person's life is totally unique, so is each person's death. Unfolding deaths vary as much as do unfolding lives. Some people move through Kübler-Ross's stages of dying very predictably, but others do not. It is not uncommon for some dying people to avoid one or more of these stages entirely.

The second important point to be made about Kübler-Ross's stages of dying is that the family members or friends of dying people often pass through similar stages as they observe their loved ones dying. When informed that a close friend or relative is dying, many people will also experience varying degrees of denial, anger, bargaining, depression, and acceptance. Because of this, as caring people we need to recognize that the emotional needs of the living must be fulfilled in ways that do not differ appreciably from those of the dying.[6]

NEAR–DEATH EXPERIENCES

As Bob lay on the gymnasium floor in apparent cardiac arrest, he watched from above as the team trainer and coaches performed CPR. After observing his own attempted resuscitation, he began walking in the direction of his uncle's voice. The last time he had heard his uncle's voice was a few days before his death 4 years earlier. Suddenly, his uncle instructed Bob to stop and turn back because Bob was not yet ready to join him. Over 24 hours later, Bob regained consciousness in the cardiac intensive care unit of The Ohio State University Hospital.

Death brings an end to our physical existence. Perhaps this is the ultimate connection between death and our physical dimension of health. Many people believe that, in a positive sense, death brings with it a sense of relief and comfort—two qualities that may be most needed when one is dying. The classic work of Raymond Moody,[7] who examined reports of people who had near-death experiences, suggests that we may have less to fear about dying than we have generally thought.

In a comprehensive study of more than 100 people who had near-death experiences, Kenneth Ring[8] reported that these people shared a core experience. This experience was composed of some or all of the following stages:

1. A sense of well-being and peace
2. An out-of-body experience in which the dying person floats above his or her body and is able to witness the activities that are occurring

3. A movement into extreme blackness or darkness
4. A shaft of intense light that generally leads upward or lies in the distance
5. A decision to enter into the light

Central to this experience is the need to make a decision to move toward death or to return to the body that has been temporarily vacated.

Experts are not in agreement as to whether near-death experiences are truly associated with death or more closely associated with the depersonalization that is experienced by some people during particularly frightening situations. In a scientific sense, near-death experiences are impossible to prove. Science can neither verify not deny the existence of out-of-body experiences.[1]

Regardless, for those who have had near-death experiences, simply knowing that death might not be such an unpleasant experience appears to be comforting. Most seem to have formed a new orientation toward living.[1]

INTERACTING WITH DYING PEOPLE

Facing the impending death of a friend, relative, or loved one is a difficult experience. If you have yet to go through this situation, be assured that, as you grow older, your opportunities will increase. This is part of the reality of living.

Most counselors, physicians, nurses, and ministers who spend time with terminally ill people suggest that you display one quality when interacting with dying people: honesty. Just the thought of talking with a dying person may make you feel uncomfortable. (Most of us have had no training in this sort of thing.) Sometimes, to make ourselves feel less anxious or depressed, we may tend to deny that the person we are with is dying. Our words and nonverbal behavior indicate that we prefer not to face the truth. Our words become stilted as we gloss over the facts and merely attempt to cheer up both our dying friend and ourselves. This behavior is rarely beneficial or supportive—for either party.

As much as possible, we should attempt to be genuine and honest. We should not try to avoid crying if we feel the need to cry. At the same time, we can provide emotional support for dying people by allowing them to express their feelings openly. We should resist the temptation of trying to pull someone out of the denial, anger, or depression. We should not feel obliged to talk constantly and to fill long pauses with idle talk. Sometimes nonverbal communication, including touching, may be much more appreciated

than mere talk. Since our interactions with dying people help fulfill our needs, we too should express our emotions and concerns as openly as possible.

TALKING WITH CHILDREN ABOUT DEATH

Because most children are curious about everything, it is not surprising that they are also fascinated about death. From very young ages, children are exposed to death through mass media (cartoons, pictures in newspapers and magazines, and news reports), adult conversations ("Aunt Emily died today," "Uncle George is terminally ill"), and their discoveries (a dead bird, a crushed bug, a dead flower). The manner in which children learn about death will have an important effect on their ability to recognize and accept their own mortality and to cope with the deaths of others.

Psychologists encourage parents and older friends to avoid shielding children from or misleading children about the reality of death. Young children need to realize that death is not temporary and it is not like sleeping. Parents should make certain they understand children's questions about death before they give an answer. Most children want simple, direct answers to their questions, not long, detailed dissertations, which often confuse the issues. For example, when a 4-year-old asks her father, "Why is Tommy's dog dead?" an appropriate answer might be, "Because he got very, very sick and his heart stopped beating." Getting involved in a lengthy discussion about "doggy heaven" or the causes of specific canine diseases may not be necessary or appropriate.

Parents should answer questions when they arise and always respond with openness and honesty. In this way, young children can learn that death is a real part of life and that sad feelings are a normal part of accepting the death of a loved one.

DEATH OF A CHILD

Adults face not only the death of their parents and friends but perhaps also the death of a child. Whether because of sudden infant death syndrome (SIDS), chronic illness, accident, or suicide, children die and adults are forced to grieve the loss of someone who was "too young to die" (see "Focus on . . . Death of an Infant or Unborn Child" at the end of this chapter).

Coping with the death of a child presents adults with a difficult period of adjustment, particularly

Children need support from adults during times of grief.

when the death was unexpected. Experts agree that grieving adults, particularly the parents, should express their grief fully and proceed cautiously on their return to normal routines. Many pitfalls can be avoided. Adults who are grieving for dead children should do the following:

- *Avoid trying to cope by using alcohol or drugs.*
- *Make no important life changes.* Moving to a different home, relocating, or changing jobs usually doesn't help parents deal any better with the grief they are experiencing.
- *Share their feelings with others.* Grieving adults should share their feelings particularly with other adults who have experienced a similar loss. Group support is available in many communities.
- *Avoid trying to erase the death.* Giving away clothing and possessions that belonged to the child cannot erase the memories the adult has of the child.
- *Give themselves the time and space to grieve.* On the anniversary of the child's death or on the child's

birthday, grievers should give themselves special time just for grieving.
- *Don't attempt to replace the child.* Do not quickly have another child or use the deceased child's name for another child.

For most adults, grief over the death of a child will require an extended period. Eventually, however, life can return to normal.

HOSPICE CARE FOR THE TERMINALLY ILL

The thought of dying in a hospital ward, with spotless floors, pay television, and strict visiting hours, leaves many people with a cold feeling. Perhaps this thought alone has helped encourage the concept of **hospice care.** Hospice care provides an alternative approach to dying for terminally ill patients and their families. The goal of hospice care is to maximize the quality of life for dying people and their family members. Popularized in England during the 1960s, yet derived from a concept developed during the Middle Ages (where *hospitable lodges* took care of weary travelers), the hospice helps people die comfortably and with dignity by using one or more of the following strategies:

- *Pain control.* Dying people are not usually treated for their terminal disease; they are provided with appropriate drugs to keep them free from pain, alert, and in control of their faculties. Drug dependence is of little concern, and patients can receive pain medication when they feel they need it.
- *Family involvement.* Family members and friends are trained and encouraged to interact with the dying person and with each other. Family members often care for the dying person at home.[9] If the hospice arrangement includes a hospice ward in a hospital or a separate building (also called a hospice), the family members have no restrictions on visitation.
- *Multidisciplinary approach.* The hospice concept promotes a team approach. Specially trained physicians, nurses, social workers, counselors, and volunteers work with the patient and family to fulfill important needs. The needs of the family receive nearly the same priority as those of the patient.
- *Patient decisions.* Contrary to most hospital approaches, hospice programs encourage patients to make their own decisions. The patient decides when to eat, sleep, go for a walk, and just be alone. By maintaining a personal schedule, the patient is more apt to feel in control of his or her life, even as that life is slipping away.

Another way in which the hospice differs from the hospital approach concerns the care given to the survivors. Even after the death of the patient, the family receives a significant amount of follow-up counseling. Helping families with their grief is an important role for the hospice team.

The number of hospices in the United States has climbed quickly to over 2000.[10] People seem to be convinced that the hospice system does work effectively. Part of this approval may be the cost factor. The cost of caring for a dying person in a hospice is usually less than the cost of full (inpatient) services provided by a hospital. Although insurance companies are delighted to see the lower cost for hospice care, many are still uncertain as to how to define hospice care. Thus not all insurance companies are fully reimbursing patients for their hospice care. Before discussing the possibility of hospice care for members of your family, you should consider the extent of hospice coverage in your health insurance policy.

GRIEF AND THE RESOLUTION OF GRIEF

The emotional feelings that people experience after the death of a friend or relative are collectively called *grief. Mourning* is the process of experiencing these emotional feelings in a culturally defined manner. See the Star Box at right for more information about the grieving process. The expression of grief is seen as a valuable process that gradually permits people to detach themselves from the deceased. Expressing grief, then, is a sign of good health.

Although people experience grief in remarkably different ways, most people have some of the following sensations and emotions:

- *Physical discomfort.* Shortly after the death of a loved one, grieving people display a rather similar pattern of physical discomfort. This discomfort is characterized by "sensations of somatic distress occurring in waves lasting from 20 minutes to an hour at a time, a feeling of tightness in the throat, choking with shortness of breath, need for sighing, and an empty feeling in the abdomen, lack of muscular power, and an intense subjective distress described as a tension or mental pain. The patient soon learns that these waves of discomfort can be precipitated by visits, by mentioning the deceased, and by receiving sympathy."[11]
- *Sense of numbness.* Grieving people may feel as if they are numb or in a state of shock. They may deny the death of their loved one.
- *Feelings of detachment from others.* Grieving people see other people as being distant from them, per-

The Grieving Process

The grieving process consists of four phases, each of which is variable in length and unique in form to the individual. These phases are composed of the following:

1. *Internalization of the deceased person's image.* By forming an idealized mental picture of the dead person, the grieving person is freed from dealing too quickly with the reality of the death.
2. *Intellectualization of the death.* Mental processing of the death and the events leading up to its occurrence move the grieving person to a clear understanding that death has occurred.
3. *Emotional reconciliation.* During this third and often delayed phase, the grieving person allows conflicting feelings and thoughts to be expressed and eventually reconciled with the reality of the death.
4. *Behavioral reconciliation.* Finally, the grieving person is able to comfortably return to a life in which the death has been fully reconciled. Old routines are reestablished and new patterns of living are adopted where necessary. The grieving person has largely recovered.

A mistake that might be made by the friends of a grieving person is encouraging a return to normal behavior too quickly. When friends urge the grieving person to return to work right away, make new friends, or become involved in time-consuming projects, they may be preventing necessary grieving from occurring. It is not easy or desirable to forget about the fact that a spouse, friend, or child has recently died.

haps because the others cannot feel the loss. A person in grief can feel very lonely. This is a common response.

- *Preoccupation with the image of the deceased.* The grieving person may not be able to complete daily tasks without constantly thinking about the deceased.
- *Guilt.* The survivor may be overwhelmed with guilt. Thoughts may center on how the deceased was neglected or ignored. Sensitive survivors feel guilt merely because they are still alive. Indeed, guilt is a common emotion.
- *Hostility.* Survivors may express feelings of loss and remorse through hostility, which they direct

hospice care (**hos** pis)
An approach to caring for terminally ill patients that maximizes the quality of life and allows death with dignity.

at other family members, physicians, lawyers, and others.

- *Disruption in daily schedule.* Grieving people often find it difficult to complete daily routines. They can suffer from an anxious type of depression. Seemingly easy tasks take a great deal of effort. Initiation of new activities and relationships can be difficult. Social interaction skills can be lost.
- *Delayed grief.* In some people, the typical pattern of grief can be delayed for weeks, months, and even years.

The grief process will continue until the bereaved person can establish new relationships, feel comfortable with others, and look back on the life of the deceased person with positive feelings (see the Health Action Guide below). Although the duration of the grief resolution process will vary with the emotional attachments one has to a deceased person, grief usually lasts from a few months to a year. Professional help should be sought when grieving is characterized by unresolved guilt, extreme hostility, physical illness, significant depression, and a lack of other meaningful relationships. Trained counselors, physicians, and hospice workers can all play significant roles in helping people through grief.

RITUALS OF DEATH

Our society has established a number of rituals associated with death that help the survivors accept the reality of death, ease the pain associated with the grief process, and provide a safe disposal of the body (see the Learning from All Cultures box on p. 457). Our rituals give us the chance to formalize our good-byes to a person and to receive emotional support and strength from family members and friends. In recent years, more of our rituals seem to be celebrating the life of the deceased. In doing this, our rituals also reaffirm the value of our own lives.

Most of our funeral rituals take place in funeral homes, churches, and cemeteries. *Funeral homes* (or *mortuaries*) are business establishments that provide a variety of services to the families of dead people. The services are carried out by funeral directors, who are licensed by the state in which they operate. Most funeral directors are responsible for preparing the bodies for viewing, filing death certificates, preparing obituary notices, establishing calling hours, assisting in the preparation and details of the funeral, casket selection, transportation to and from the cemetery, and family counseling. Although licensing procedures vary from state to state, most new funeral directors must complete 1 year of college, 1 year of mortuary school, and 1 year of internship with a funeral home before taking a state licensing examination.

Full Funeral Services

An ethical funeral director will attempt to follow the wishes of the deceased's family and provide only the services requested by the family. Most families want traditional, **full funeral services.** Three signifi-

---

HEALTH
Action Guide - - - - - ➜

Helping the Bereaved

Leming and Dickinson[1] point out that the peak time of grief begins in the week after a loved one's funeral. Realizing that there is no one guaranteed formula for helping the bereaved, friends and caregivers can help by performing some or all of the following:

- Make few demands on the bereaved; allow him or her to grieve.
- Help with the household tasks.
- Recognize that the bereaved person may vent anguish and anger and that some of it may be directed at you.
- Recognize that the bereaved person has painful and

difficult tasks to complete; mourning cannot be rushed or avoided.
- Do not be afraid to talk about the deceased person; this lets the bereaved know that you care for the deceased.
- Express your own genuine feelings of sadness, but avoid pity. Speak from the heart.
- Reassure bereaved people that the intensity of their emotions is very natural.
- Advise the bereaved to get additional help if you suspect continuing severe emotional or physical distress.
- Keep in regular contact with the bereaved; let him or her know you continue to care about them.

◀ - - - - - •

LEARNING *from* ALL CULTURES

Funeral and Burial Rituals

Funeral rituals typically reflect people's religious beliefs and practices. In North America, most people are buried according to Protestant traditions. People pay their respects to the deceased, a minister conducts a service, and in 75% of the cases, the body is buried after a graveside ceremony.

The rest of the human population, however, bury their dead in a variety of ways. The Parsis, a group of people in India, follow an ancient religion called Zoroastrianism. They perform their burial rituals at the seven Towers of Silence, outside of Bombay. The corpse is brought to one of the towers by six individuals dressed in white. The body is left on a tower for vultures to devour, leaving only the skeleton. A few days later the bones are put into a pit. The Parsis believe this method keeps the air, soil, and water from becoming contaminated.[14]

Hindus believe that the physical body must be gone for the soul to continue on to reincarnation. Their ritual consists of washing the dead body and dressing it in a shroud adorned with flowers. The body is carried to a funeral pyre, and the closest male relative lights the fire, walks around the burning body three times, and recites Hindu verses.[14]

Buddhists, who live mostly in China, Japan, Sri Lanka, Myanmar, Vietnam, and Cambodia, also cremate their dead. They believe cremation was favored by Buddha.

Unlike Hindus and Buddhists, Muslims do not believe in cremation. Their ritual is to wash the dead body, dress it in three pieces of white cloth, and put it in a wooden coffin. Burial is within 24 hours of death, since there is no embalming unless dictated by law. The body is taken out of the coffin and buried with the head turned toward Mecca.[14]

Most people do not like to think about their own death or plan for it, but there are some individuals who plan their funerals to to the last detail. What would be your wishes concerning your own funeral and burial?

---

cant components of the full funeral services are as follows.

Embalming

Embalming is the process of using formaldehyde-based fluids to replace the blood components. Embalming helps preserve the body and return it to a natural look. Embalming permits friends and family members to view the body without being subjected to the odors associated with tissue decomposition. Embalming is often an optional procedure, except when death results from specific communicable diseases or when body *disposition* (disposal) is delayed.

Calling hours

Sometimes called a *wake,* this is an established time when friends and family members can gather in a room to share their emotions and common experiences about the dead person. Generally in the same room, the body will be in a casket, with the lid open or closed. Open caskets assist some people to confirm that death truly did occur. Some families prefer not to have any calling hours, sometimes called *visiting hours.*

Funeral service

Funeral services vary according to religious preference and the emotional needs of the survivors. Although some services are held in a church, most funeral services today take place in a funeral home, where a special room might serve as a chapel. Some services are held at the graveside. Families may also choose to have a simple *memorial service* within a few days after the funeral. Completing the Personal Assessment on p. 458 will help you think about what kind of funeral arrangements you would prefer for yourself.

Disposition of the Body

Bodies are disposed of in one of four ways. *Ground burial* is the most common method. About 75% of all bodies are placed in ground burial. The casket is almost always placed in a metal or concrete vault before being buried. The vault serves to further protect the body (a need only of the survivors) and to prevent collapse of ground because of the decaying of caskets. Use of a vault is required by most cemeteries.

full funeral services
All of the professional services provided by funeral directors.

PERSONAL ASSESSMENT

Planning Your Funeral

In line with this chapter's positive theme of the value of personal death awareness, here is a funeral service assessment that we frequently give to our health classes.

This inventory can help you assess your reactions and thoughts about the funeral arrangements you would prefer for yourself.

After answering each of the following questions, you might wish to discuss your responses with a friend or close relative.

1. Have you ever considered how you would like your body to be handled after your death?
   _____ Yes   _____ No

2. Have you already made funeral prearrangements for yourself?
   _____ Yes   _____ No

3. Have you considered a specific funeral home or mortuary to handle your arrangements?
   _____ Yes   _____ No

4. If you were to die today, which of the following would you prefer?
   _____ Embalming   _____ Ground burial
   _____ Cremation   _____ Entombment
   _____ Donation to medical science

5. If you prefer to be cremated, what would you want done with your ashes?
   _____ Buried   _____ Entombed
   _____ Scattered
   _____ Other; please specify _____

6. If your funeral plans involve a casket, which of the following ones would you prefer?
   _____ Plywood (cloth covered)
   _____ Hardwood (oak, cherry, mahogany, maple, etc.)
   _____ Steel (sealer or nonsealer type)
   _____ Stainless steel
   _____ Copper or bronze
   _____ Other; please specify _____

7. How important would a funeral service be for you?
   _____ Very important
   _____ Somewhat important
   _____ Somewhat unimportant
   _____ Very unimportant
   _____ No opinion

8. What kind of funeral service would you want for yourself?
   _____ No service at all
   _____ Visitation (calling hours) the day before the funeral service; funeral held at church or funeral home

   _____ Graveside service only (no visitation)
   _____ Memorial service (after body disposition)
   _____ Other; please specify _____

9. How many people would you want to attend your funeral service or memorial service?
   _____ I do not want a funeral or memorial service
   _____ 1-10 people
   _____ 11-25 people
   _____ 26-50 people
   _____ Over 51 people
   _____ I do not care how many people attend

10. What format would you prefer at your funeral service or memorial service? Select any of the following that you would like.

	Yes	No
Religious music	_____	_____
Nonreligious music	_____	_____
Clergy present	_____	_____
Flower arrangements	_____	_____
Family member eulogy	_____	_____
Eulogy by friend(s)	_____	_____
Open casket	_____	_____
Religious format	_____	_____
Other; please specify		_____

11. Using today's prices, how much would you expect to pay for your total funeral arrangements, including cemetery expenses (if applicable)?
    _____ Less than $4000
    _____ Between $4001 and $5500
    _____ Between $5501 and $7000
    _____ Between $7001 and $8500
    _____ Above $8500

To Carry This Further...
Which items had you not thought about before? Were you surprised at the arrangements you selected? Will you share your responses with anyone else? If so, whom?

Current Organ Donation Issues

Two key issues in current organ donation practices in the United States are: (1) the continued shortage of organ donors and (2) the threat of disease transmission in certain donated tissues or organs.

The shortage of organ donors is life threatening to the thousands of patients waiting for a kidney, heart, lung, liver, pancreas, skin, or bone marrow tissue. Although donor cards are widely available and hospitals are now required by law to ask survivors promptly if they will donate the deceased's organs, only a small percentage of organs and tissues are collected.

Why has the donor system not been more effective? Here are some possible reasons. Many people do not prepare living wills; likewise, most people do not prepare a uniform organ donor card. Many survivors also prefer not to consider organ donation during the stressful aftermath of death. Some physicians and hospital staff workers may feel uncomfortable asking survivors about organ donation.

Beyond the psychological obstacles that surround organ donation are some very real difficulties in the administration of organ donation programs. Regulations at different organ banks may vary, as may state and local laws. These regulations may make it difficult for organ banks to prepare and transport tissues or organs from one location to another. Also, a hospital's ability to instantly recognize a patient as a registered donor requires donor registries across the country to be more compatible with each other. Finally, organ donation networks must find better ways to encourage people to understand the urgent need to provide these "gifts of life."

The second problem facing organ donation reached the public's attention in the spring of 1991. It was discovered that tissues transplanted into multiple people came from a donor who had died from AIDS. This oversight caused considerable public alarm but has resulted in more stringent screening of donor candidates, as well as more careful examination and handling of organs and tissues. These tighter procedures are encouraging news for the public. Clearly, everyone waiting for an organ donation deserves the opportunity to receive a healthy organ.

A second type of disposition is *entombment*. Entombment refers to nonground burial, most often in structures called **mausoleums.** A mausoleum has a series of shelves where caskets can be sealed in vaultlike areas called *niches*. Entombment can also occur in the basements of buildings, especially in old, large churches. The bodies of famous church leaders are sometimes entombed in vaultlike spaces called **crypts.**

Cremation is a third type of body disposition. In the United States, 19% of all bodies are cremated.[12] This practice is increasing. Generally both the body and casket (or cardboard cremation box) are incinerated so that only the bone ash from the body remains. The body of an average adult produces about 5 to 7 pounds of bone ash. These ashes can then be placed in containers called *urns,* and then buried, entombed, or scattered, if permitted by state law. The cost of cremation (from $200 to $500) is much less than ground burial. Some families choose to cremate after having full funeral services.

A fourth method of body disposition is *anatomical donation.* Separate organs (such as corneal tissue, kidneys, or the heart) can be donated to a medical school, research facility, or organ donor network. Certain states permit people to indicate on their driver's licenses that they wish to donate their organs. However, family consent (by next of kin) is also required at the time of death for organ or tissue donation to occur. Recently, hospitals have been required by federal law to inform the family of a deceased person about organ donation at the time of his or her death. The need for donor organs is far greater than the current supply (see the Star Box above). For some, the decision to donate body tissue and organs is rewarding and comforting. Organ donors understand that their small sacrifice can help give life or improve the quality of life for another person. In this sense, their death can mean life for others. To become an organ donor, you must fill out a uniform organ donor card like the one in Figure 18-1.

Some people choose to donate their entire body to medical science. Often this is done through prior arrangements with medical schools. Bodies still require embalming. After they are studied, the remains are often cremated and returned to the family, if requested.

> **mausoleum** (moz oh **lee** um)
> An above-ground structure, which frequently resembles a small stone house, into which caskets can be placed for disposition.
>
> **crypts**
> Burial locations generally underneath churches.

UNIFORM DONOR CARD

of _____
                        (print or type name of donor)

In the hope that I may help others, I hereby make this anatomical gift, if medically acceptable, to take effect upon my death. The words and marks below indicate my wishes:

I give: (a) _____ any needed organs or parts
        (b) _____ only the following organs or parts

_____
         (specify the organ(s), tissue(s), or part(s)

for the purposes of transplantation, therapy, medical research or education;

        (c) _____ my body for anatomical study if needed.

Limitations or special wishes, if any:_____

Signed by the donor and the following two witnesses in the presence of each other:

_____   _____
Signature of Donor   Date of Birth of Donor

_____   _____
Date Signed   City and State

_____   _____
Witness   Witness

This is a legal document under the Anatomical Gift Act or similar laws.
☐ Yes, I have discussed my wishes with my family.
For further information consult your physician or

THE NATIONAL KIDNEY FOUNDATION
30 East 33rd Street   New York, NY 10016

08-21

Figure 18-1   Signing a uniform organ donor card allows you to donate your organs to a research facility, medical school, or organ donor network.

Costs

The full funeral services offered by a funeral home average from $2000 to $2500, and other expenses must be added to this price. Casket prices vary significantly, with the average cost between $1500 and $2500. If the family chooses an especially fancy casket, then the costs could spiral up to $10,000 or more. Costs that extend beyond these expenses include (should one choose them) those shown in the Star Box at right. When all of the expenses associated with a typical funeral are added up, the average cost is between $5000 and $6500.

Regardless of the rituals you select for the handling of your body (or the body of someone in your care), most educators are encouraging people to prearrange their plans. Before you die, you can save your survivors a lot of misery by putting your wishes in writing. *Funeral prearrangements* relieve the survivors of many of the details that must be handled at the time of your death. You can gather much of the information for your obituary notice and your wishes for the disposition of your body. Prearrangements can be made with a funeral director, family member, or attorney. Many individuals also prepay the costs of their funeral. By making arrangements in advance of need, you can enhance your own peace of mind. Currently about 30% to 40% of funerals are preplanned and prepaid. Interestingly, in the 1960s, nearly all funerals were planned by relatives at the time of a person's death.[12]

PERSONAL PREPARATION FOR DEATH

We hope that this chapter helps you discover some new perspectives about death and develop your own personal death awareness. Remember that the ultimate goal of death education is a positive one—to help you best use and enjoy your life. Becoming aware of the reality of your own mortality is a step in the right direction. Reading about the process of dying, grief resolution, and the rituals surrounding death can also help you imagine that someday you too will die.

There are some additional ways in which you can prepare for the reality of your own death. Preparing a will, purchasing a life insurance policy, making funeral prearrangements, preparing a living will, and considering an anatomical or organ donation are measures that help you prepare for your own death (see the Health Action Guide on p. 461). At the appropriate time, you might also wish to talk with family and friends about your own death. You may discover that an upbeat, positive discussion about death can help relieve some of your apprehensions and those of others around you.

Another suggestion to help you emotionally prepare for your own death is to prepare an *obituary*

Estimated Funeral Costs

Cemetery lot	$200-$700
Opening and closing of grave	$200-$700
Vault	$350-$1000
Mausoleum space	$1500-$5000
Honorarium for minister	$75-$100
Organist and vocalists	$50-$75 each
Flowers over casket	$100+
Grave marker	$500-$1500+
Beautician services	$75+

HEALTH Action Guide

Organ Donation

Making an organ donation is one of the most compassionate, responsible acts a person can do. Only a few simple steps are required:

1. You must complete a uniform donor card. Obtain a card from a physician, a local hospital, or the nearest regional transplant or organ bank.
2. Print or type your name on the card.
3. Indicate which organs you wish to donate. You may also indicate your desire to donate all organs and tissues.
4. Sign your name in the presence of two witnesses, preferably your next of kin.
5. Fill in any additional information (for example, date of birth, city and state in which the card is completed, and date the card is signed).
6. Tell others about your decision to donate. Some donor cards have detachable portions to give to your family.
7. Always carry your card with you.
8. If you have any questions, you can call the United Network for Organ Sharing (UNOS) at (800) 24-DONOR, or call (613) 727-1380 in Canada.

notice or **eulogy** for yourself. Include all the things you would like to have said about you and your life. Now compare your obituary notice and eulogy with the current direction your life seems to be taking. Are you doing the kinds of activities for which you want to be known? If so, great! If not, perhaps you will want to consider why your current direction does not reflect how you would like to be remembered. Should you make some changes to restructure your life's agenda in a more personally meaningful fashion?

Another suggestion to help make you aware of your own eventual death is to write your own **epitaph.** Before doing this, you might want to visit a cemetery. (Unfortunately, most of us visit cemeteries only when we are forced to.) Reading the epitaphs of others may help you develop your own epitaph.

Further awareness of your own death might come from attempting to answer these questions in writing (since this pushes you beyond mere thinking): (1) If I had only one day to live, how would I spend it? (2) What one accomplishment would I like to make before I die? (3) Once I am dead, what two or three things will people miss most about me? By answering these questions and accomplishing a few of the tasks suggested in this section, you will have a good start on accepting your own death and the value of life itself.

eulogy
A composition or speech that praises someone; often delivered at a funeral or memorial service.

epitaph
An inscription on a grave marker or monument.

Summary

- Personal death awareness encourages you to live a meaningful life.
- Death denial tends to breed feelings of helplessness and vulnerability.
- Death is determined primarily by clinical and legal factors.
- Euthanasia can be undertaken with either direct or indirect measures.
- The most current advance medical directives are the living will and the durable power of attorney for health care. Both documents permit critically ill people (especially those who cannot communicate) to die with dignity.
- Denial, anger, bargaining, depression, and acceptance are the five classic psychological stages that dying people commonly experience, according to Kübler-Ross. Hospice care provides an alternative approach to dying for terminally ill people and their families.
- The expression of grief is a common experience that can be expected when a friend or relative dies. The grief process can vary in intensity and duration.
- Death in our society is associated with a number of rituals to help survivors cope with the loss of a loved one and to ensure proper disposal of the body.

Review Questions

1. How does the experience of dying today differ from that in the early 1900s?
2. Identify and explain the clinical and legal determinants of death and indicate who establishes each of them.
3. Explain the difference between direct and indirect euthanasia.
4. How does a living will differ from a durable power of attorney for health care document? Why are these advance medical directives becoming increasingly popular?
5. Identify the five psychological stages that dying people tend to experience. Explain each stage.
6. Identify and explain the four strategies that form the basis of hospice care. What are the advantages of hospice care for the patient and the family?
7. Explain what is meant by the term *grief*. Identify and explain the sensations and emotions most people have when they experience grief. When does the grieving process end? How can adults cope with the death of a child? How can we assist grieving people?
8. What purposes do the rituals of death serve? What are the significant components of the full funeral service? What are the four ways in which bodies are disposed?
9. What activities can we undertake to become better aware of our own mortality?

Think About This . . .

- How were issues related to death handled in your family when you were growing up?
- Will hospice care be an option you might choose someday?
- Have you or any of your relatives prepared a living will or a durable power of attorney for health care document?
- At your death, would you want your organs or body tissue donated to help another person? Are there any organs you would prefer not to donate?
- If you found out you were going to die tomorrow, what would you do today?
- If it were determined that you were in a persistent vegetative state, would you want your life support to be disconnected?

References

1. Leming MR, Dickinson GE: *Understanding dying, death, and bereavement,* ed 2, Ft Worth, Tex, 1990, Holt, Rinehart, & Winston.
2. Baer K: Death and dying: the final chapter, *Harvard Health Letter* 20(4): 1-3, 1995.
3. Burnell GM: *Final choices: to live or die in an age of medical technology,* New York, 1993, Plenum Press.
4. Choice in Dying, personal correspondence, March 4, 1996.
5. Kübler-Ross E: *On death and dying,* New York, 1969, Macmillan.
6. Kübler-Ross E: *Death is of vital importance: on life, death, and life after death,* Barrytown, NY, 1995, Station Press.
7. Moody RA: *Life after life,* New York, 1975, Bantam Books.
8. Ring K: *Life at death: a scientific investigation of the near-death experience,* New York, 1980, Coward, McCann & Geoghegan.
9. Sankar A: *Dying at home; a family guide for caregiving,* New York, 1995, Bantam Books.
10. Baer K: Dying with dignity: a guide to hospice care, *Harvard Health Letter* (special supplement), p 9, April 1993.
11. Lindemann E: *Symptomology and management of acute grief.* In Fulton et al, editors: *Death and dying: challenge and change,* Reading, Mass, 1978, Addison-Wesley.
12. Weaver G, Caleca LG: Fading grandeur: the traditional funeral is slowly losing ground, *Indianapolis Star,* p 1A, July 29, 1993.
13. Associated Press: Compassionate face of death: Kevorkian says he tries to stop suicides, *Lexington Herald-Leader,* p A-3, March 2, 1996.
14. Whalen WJ: How different religions pay their funeral respects. In Dickinson G, Leming M, Mermann M, editors: *Dying, death, and bereavement,* Guilford, Conn, 1993, Dushkin Publishing.

Suggested Readings

Caplan S, Lang G: *Grief's courageous journey: a workbook,* Oakland, Calif, 1995, New Harbinger Publications.

Two professionals in a pastoral care department in London, Ontario, Canada, offer their understanding and observations of grief and the grieving-healing process. They discuss their 10-step plan for recovering from the death of a loved one. Readers can use this as a workbook, since many practical activities are presented. A final section explains how to start a grief support group in your own community.

Kübler-Ross E: *Death is of vital importance: on life, death, and life after death,* Barrytown, NY, 1995, Station Hill Press.

Famous physician and world renowned thanatologist Kübler-Ross offers her expertise on a broad range of topics related to dying and death. Contemplative reading for people dealing either professionally or personally with death.

Sankar A: *Dying at home: a family guide for caregiving,* New York, 1995, Bantam Books.

Focusing on aging, dying, and death, a medical anthropologist presents a guide for caregivers of terminally ill people. Sankar prepares caregivers for the important responsibilities that lie ahead. Many accounts from actual caregivers form the basis for introspective reading.

 AS WE GO TO PRESS . . .

Dr. Jack Kevorkian, retired pathologist, was recently present at the thirty-third suicide of a terminally ill person. This death came shortly after another successful acquittal of Kevorkian on charges of murder and assisting in a suicide in the state of Michigan.

Death of an Infant or Unborn Child

Life is fragile at all stages but especially so during the prenatal and early formative years. Indeed, from conception through development, birth, infancy and childhood, humans require an amazing amount of parental care and nurturing. Few other organisms are so dependent on others for their safety and well-being during the early months of life. Thus parents and children are tied together by a physical and emotional bond like no other. When that bond is severed by the tragic death of a young child, the pain and anguish the parents feel can be too much to bear. Getting through such a traumatic experience can be one of life's toughest challenges.

Most pregnancies progress to full term and result in the birth of a healthy child. However, researchers now believe that about one third of pregnancies end in miscarriage. Since the development of accurate home-pregnancy tests, many women are finding out early in the first trimester that they are pregnant. Thus, rather than mistaking the miscarriage for a late heavy menstrual period, more women are now aware that their pregnancy has ended. Most then go through the grieving process discussed here. In addition, other complications occur in a small number of cases. These problems can sometimes cause termination of the pregnancy (miscarriage or elective abortion), death of the baby during birth, or death during infancy. Though most people know that such things can happen, many feel that such tragedies happen only to others. When faced with the death or potential loss of a child, parents often find their belief system shaken and their faith tested.[1]

The Mourning Process

The process of grieving is different for each family. There are no set rules for getting over the loss of a child. There is no right way to mourn and no time limit for the mourning process. The first days, months, and years may seem meaningless, and parents may find themselves living day to day with no real purpose or focus.[2]

Despite the pain each individual in the family feels, care must be taken to preserve family unity. Each person must realize that other family members may grieve in different ways. Wives and husbands may grieve differently, and this can cause strain in their marriage. If one parent seems quiet or preoccupied, the other should not mistake this behavior for a lack of emotion. Parents should also make sure that they do not ignore the feelings of other children in the family. Sometimes the mourning parents become wrapped up in their own grief and forget that the tragedy affects their other children as well. Siblings should be encouraged to discuss their feelings to help with their own grief and to reaffirm their importance within the family.[2]

The way a baby dies can affect the mourning process. Whether the child is lost before birth (miscarriage, abortion), during birth (stillbirth, trauma), or in infancy (sudden infant death syndrome [SIDS], accident, birth defect) can affect how the parents deal with the loss. It can also have an effect on how family and friends provide support for the parents.

Death of an Unborn Child

Miscarriage can be especially difficult to deal with for the woman involved. The baby has been lost within the mother's womb, and she may blame herself for the loss as a result. She may think that something she did (or did not do) has caused the miscarriage.[1,3] "One night just before I found out I was pregnant, I went out with friends and had a few beers," recalls Gabrielle, who had a miscarriage when she was 26.[4] "I didn't know I was pregnant. I was late with my period but didn't suspect I was pregnant until later. I can't help but wonder if the alcohol caused it (the miscarriage)." Consumption of alcohol or over-the-counter medications before a woman knows she is pregnant is a common cause of guilt after a miscarriage. An exact cause of a miscarriage may never be determined, and the woman needs to be reassured that she did not cause any abnormalities in the fetus.[1]

A miscarriage can be painful, embarrassing, and stressful for the woman. Physical symptoms may not occur when the baby dies but may be delayed for some time. Rosalinda became pregnant in the first month after she stopped taking her birth control pills. About 3 weeks into the pregnancy, "I found myself crying uncontrollably while driving home from work," she recalls. "Although I had no visible signs of miscarriage, I was sure something was wrong." Rosalinda had always been successful in other endeavors, but she started to fear that she would fail in her attempts to bring a baby into the world. "At 11 weeks my fears came true. We were on a much-needed vacation in Las Vegas. Two days of cramping turned into uncontrollable hemorrhaging." She and her husband wound up in the hotel lobby trying to get a cab to the hospital. "You can imagine my utter embarrassment as I'm holding a towel in front of me to hide the blood as my husband is haggling with the bellman to let us go to the front of the line."[5]

Sometimes parents find out about a potentially fatal or severely debilitating problem with the fetus before the child is born. In these situations the parents are faced with the choice of continuing the pregnancy or terminating it. Hearing such a diagnosis, taking in all available information, and reaching a decision can be a traumatic experience. Parents must weigh many factors when making this decision, including their spiritual beliefs, potential suffering of the baby (if the long-term prognosis is poor), effects on the family of having a child with special needs, and financial considerations. If a decision is made to terminate the pregnancy (or if a continued pregnancy may result in miscarriage or stillbirth), the couple must be prepared for the sadness and trauma of parting with their baby.[3]

Death during the Birthing Process

In some instances, the parents know beforehand that the baby has a poor chance of surviving through birth, so they have a chance to prepare for this occurrence. For others, however, the baby's death is totally unexpected. Parents who thought they would be bringing home a healthy baby end up dealing with the devastation of losing their child. "The worst part was returning home," recalls Marcus, whose wife delivered a stillborn child after complications during birth. "The nursery was all set up . . . that brought back all of the feelings we had initially experienced after the birth."[6]

In the past, babies with lethal birth defects were often quickly taken away from their mothers, but today many parents are being given the option of spending time holding and saying good-bye to their baby, and medical personnel are encouraged to accommodate the parents and support their wishes in this regard.[3]

Losing a Baby after It Is Born

Even after a baby is delivered, there are health risks. After her miscarriage, Gabrielle gave birth to a seemingly healthy daughter, only to lose her 5 months later. "She just stopped breathing," Gabrielle recalls. "We had all been asleep, and when we went in to check on her she wasn't moving or breathing. We tried to wake her . . . she wasn't face down or anything like that. The doctors had no reason for it. They said it was SIDS."

The loss of a second child was devastating for Gabrielle, and it nearly ruined her marriage. "We were both very tense. We thought about trying again, but we felt jinxed. We fought a lot in the weeks after it happened." Gabrielle and her husband received counseling and eventually began to realize that they were not at fault for their tragic losses. They now have a healthy 3-year-old daughter. "We got up the courage to try one more time, thank God," she says.[4]

Dealing with the Loss of a Baby

Support of family and friends is especially important when trying to recover from the death of a child. Friends and co-workers can help by acknowledging the death of the child and offering support.[2] Often people will not mention the baby because they feel that the parents will become upset by bringing up the subject, but not talking about the baby can cause pain for the parents.[2] Showing up in person (as opposed to just calling or sending a card) to offer support can also help.[7]

While the mother is still in the hospital, medical personnel should be made aware of what the mother has been through. Sometimes a mother who has lost her baby will remain in the maternity wing of the hospital. A discreet notice posted on the door of her room will alert personnel that the room's occupant has lost her child, thus preventing any unfortunate assumptions.[1]

Tactful language can also help prevent unpleasant feelings for the parents. If an unhealthy fetus were miscarried or had to be aborted, sometimes people would try to rationalize the loss for the parents by saying it was "nature's way" of preventing the birth of an imperfect child.[7] Such comments are not only insensitive, but they imply that the parents should be grateful that they lost the baby. Even seemingly innocent comments can cause pain in the wrong context. Rosalinda wondered why she had continued to gain weight for 2 months even though the doctor said the baby had probably died only 3 or 4 weeks into her pregnancy. "'It's probably just pizza,' my husband said. The doctor laughed and agreed." Rosalinda felt that her husband's attempt to lighten the situation was "probably the most insensitive statement I've ever heard him make . . . my opinion of the doctor also dropped dramatically at that point."[5] She later underwent a D & C (dilation and curettage) but was asked to sign a form giving her permission for an abortion even though she had already miscarried. She was "deeply humiliated to have to sign this. Didn't they realize how much I had already been through?"

Often parents will want to hold on to the memory of the child. Such feelings are quite normal and do not mean that the parents are holding on to their grief or are neurotic.[2] Remembering the child can give a sense of meaning to parents' lives. Often parents will do something constructive to help them remember their baby and get over the death. Putting together a scrapbook, donating the baby's clothes and toys to charity, writing memoirs, or setting up a place for remembrance can help the family keep memories of the baby.[2,7,8]

Eventually the grief should lose its intensity. It may flare up again around "anniversaries" (the baby's due date or birthday, the day of the baby's death), but gradually things should become bearable. The family will be forever changed by the experience. The death of a child can cause the value system of the parents to change, and their spiritual beliefs may be shaken as well.[2] But if the parents receive support from medical staff, family, and friends, ultimately the devastation can be overcome. It is hoped that such tragedies, while terribly unfortunate, can make these families stronger and bring them closer together.

For Discussion . . .
What are the differences in dealing with losing a child before, during, or after it is born? If you were faced with the choice of giving birth to a child with severe birth defects or terminating the pregnancy, which would you choose? If you lost a baby, would you try again to have one?

References
1. Hitchcock Pappas DJ, McCoy MC: Grief counseling. In Kuller JA et al, editors: *Prenatal diagnosis and reproductive genetics,* St Louis, 1995, Mosby.
2. Cole D: When a child dies, *Parents' Magazine,* p 3 March 1994.
3. Salmon DK: Coping with miscarriage, *Parents' Magazine,* p 5 May 1991.
4. Anonymous: Personal communication, April 1996.
5. Anonymous: Personal communication, March 1996.
6. Anonymous: Personal communication, Dec 1995.
7. Allison C: For Felicity, *Reader's Digest,* p 199, Jan 1993.
8. Robb DB: Moving on, *Reader's Digest,* p 223, Jan 1995.

Commonly Used Over-the-Counter Products

Pain Relievers

Product	Physiological Function*	Potential Side Effect	Product	Physiological Function	Potential Side Effect
Aspirin (only) Aspirin (with caffeine)	Analgesic (pain relief) Antipyretic (fever reduction) Antirheumatic (inflammation reduction) Anticoagulant (slowed clotting time)	Hypersensitivity Gastrointestinal disturbance Internal bleeding Ototoxicity (toxic action on the ear) Prothrombin depression Overdose potential Reye's syndrome	Acetaminophen (with caffeine) Acetaminophen (with aspirin and caffeine) Ibuprofen	Analgesic (pain relief) Antirheumatic (inflammation reduction)	Gastrointestinal disturbance Headache Nervousness Vision distortion Fluid retention Rash
Acetaminophen (only)	Analgesic (pain relief)	Liver damage	Naproxen	Nonsteroidal anti-inflammatory	Stomach irritation Drowsiness
Acetaminophen (with aspirin)	Antipyretic (fever reduction)	Gastric erosion Kidney failure Irregular heartbeat	Ketoprofen	Nonsteroidal anti-inflammatory	Stomach irritation Drowsiness

*Physiological functions for each form of a product are the same (e.g., for aspirin [only] and aspirin [with caffeine]).

Cold and Cough Products

Active Ingredient*†	Physiological Function	Potential Side Effect	Active Ingredient*†	Physiological Function	Potential Side Effect
Decongestant (sympathomimetic amine) Phenylephrine hydrochloride	Vasoconstriction, which decreases blood flow into nasal tissues, thus decreasing fluid loss	Nervousness, sweating	Cough suppressant Dextromethorphan hydrobromide Codeine	Suppression of sensitivity of the brain's cough control center and reduced CNS activity, thus reducing coughing and facilitating sleep	Mild sedation
Antihistamine Chlorpheniramine maleate	Blockage of histamine's vasodilating effect on capillaries within nasal tissue, thus reducing fluid loss (runny nose)	Drowsiness, drying of the mouth	Alcohol 20% to 25% per unit volume	CNS depression	Reduction in inhibitions when taken in quantity
Analgesic Acetaminophen	Pain relief and fever reduction	Generally few side effects with the amounts found in cold and cough preparations—see p. A1 for additional information on side effects			

*Popular cold and cough medications generally contain an ingredient from each of the five categories listed.
†*Expectorants,* which stimulate respiratory tract secretions, and *bronchodilators,* which increase the diameter of air passages, have also been used in the formulations of cold and cough medications. Their roles are to some degree controversial and are currently under study.

Deodorant and Antiperspirant Products

Two avenues exist for controlling odor resulting from the action of microbes on the organic matter in the perspiration of the apocrine sweat glands.

Function/Product	Active Agents	Adverse Side Effects	Function/Product	Active Agents	Adverse Side Effects
Control or Mask Odor			**Reduce Release of Perspiration**		
Mild deodorant soaps	Hexachlorophene (0.75% or less) Triclocarban (TCC) Tribromosalicylanilide (TBS)	Swelling; blistering on exposure to sun	Antiperspirants	Aluminum chloride Aluminum chlorohydrate Aluminum sulfate	Allergic reactions Should not be used for excessive, offensive, or colored perspiration
Deodorant (toilet water, colognes, perfumes, deodorants)	Alcohol Essential oils Vitamin E	Allergic reactions			

Sun Tanning Products

Sun Protection Factors and Classifications

2   Dark tan for skin that tans easily; minimal protection from sunburn
4   Dark tan for normal skin; minimal to moderate protection from sunburn
6   Golden tan for normal skin; moderate protection from sunburn
8   Gradual tan for normal skin; extra protection from sunburn
15 Gradual tan for sun-sensitive skin; maximal protection from sunburn
25 Protection for sun-sensitive skin; ultraprotection from sunburn
30 Protection for sun-sensitive skin for prolonged exposure

Products with sun protection factors above 30 are available; however, more frequent application of SPF 30 products may be as effective.

Safe and Effective Sunscreens

Aminobenzoic acid
Cinoxate
Diethanolamine *p*-methoxycinnamate
Digalloyl trioleate
Dioxybenzone
Ethyl 4-bis (hydroxypropyl) aminobenzoate

2-Ethylhexyl 2-cyano-3,3 diphylacrylate
Ethylhexyl *p*-methoxycinnamate
2-Ethylhexyl salicylate
Glyceryl aminobenzoate
Homosalate
Lawsone with dihydroxyacetone
Menthyl anthranilate
Oxybenzone

Padimate A
Padimate O
2-Phenylbenzimidazole-5-sulfonic acid
Red petrolatum
Sulisobenzone
Titanium dioxide
Triethanolamine salicylate

Adverse Reactions to Excessive Sun Tanning

Skin cancer   Photosensitivity
Skin aging   Allergies

Dental Hygiene Products

Product	Recommendations for Selection or Use	Product	Recommendations for Selection or Use
Toothbrush	Round, soft bristles in four rows; use 3 to 4 minutes with a proven technique; replace brush every 2 to 3 months, weekly when ill	Dental irrigator	Device using a pressurized stream of water to "pick" food debris lodged between teeth; model with a self-contained pump is considered more effective than one using household water pressure
Disclosing solution	Use periodically to familiarize yourself with the locations in which plaque accumulates and to assess the effectiveness of your brushing and flossing technique; sequence: disclose-brush-inspect-brush-redisclose	Mouthwash	Freshens the breath; capable of effecting some plaque reduction only when used in combination with regular brushing and flossing; fluoridated dental rinses can contribute to the prevention of dental caries when used in combination with brushing and flossing
Dental floss	Waxed or unwaxed cotton fiber thread for use in removing food debris from areas not generally reached by brushing alone; pull thread through adjoining tooth surfaces, gently elevating gingival tissues	Antiplaque dental rinse	Solution whose effervescent action dislodges plaque from dental surfaces; vigorous swishing of the solution should be followed by regular brushing, then a second application of the anti-plaque rinse should follow
Toothpaste	Tartar-control toothpaste is recommended; select a fluoridated product in the midrange of abrasiveness; products designed to "brighten" or "whiten" teeth are generally too abrasive for general use; dentifrice intended for use with the false teeth should not be used on natural teeth		

Acne Products

Active Ingredient	Representative Brands	Effectiveness
Benzoyl peroxide medications	PanOxyl bar Oxy-5 and Oxy-10 Clearasil cream Noxzema Acne 12	The most effective OTC active ingredient, benzoyl peroxide aids in the prevention of new lesion formation
Salicylic acid cleaners	Clearasil Medicated Cleanser Stri-Dex Maximum Strength Pads PROPA pH Cleaning Pads and Lotion	Salicylic acid aids in unseating blackheads; alcohol base helps remove surface oils; no suppression of lesion formation is associated with these products
Sulfur-based medications	Acnomel Cream Fostril Lotion	Does not prevent lesion formation; active ingredient does help dry areas associated with lesions
Alcohol-based cleansers	Sea Breeze Antiseptic for the Skin Noxema Antiseptic Skin Cleanser	Noneffective
Scrubs	Epi-Clear Scrub Cleanser Komix Cleanser	Too abrasive
Medicated soaps	Clearasil Antibacterial Soap Fostex Medicated Cleansing Bar	No more effective than ordinary soap and water

Hair Regrowth Treatment

Product	Physiological Function	Potential Side Effects
Minoxidil (Rogaine)	Vasodilator	Itching, skin irritation; hair loss will recur if use is discontinued

Smoking Cessation

Product	Physiological Function	Potential Side Effects
Nicorette	Nicotine replacement	Jaw ache, difficult breathing, flushing, dry mouth, cough, drug interactions
Nicotrol transdermal patch	Same as Nicorette	Rare (report to your doctor): hives, itching, rash, redness or swelling, irregular heartbeat; more common: rapid heartbeat, mild headache, increased appetite, burning at the site of application

Acid Reducers

Product	Physiological Function	Potential Side Effects
Tagamet HB	Hydrogen ion inhibitor	Drug interactions, mental confusion in the elderly
Pepcid AC	Hydrogen ion inhibitor	Same as Tagamet HB
Zantac 75	Hydrogen ion inhibitor	Same as Tagamet HB
Axid AR	Hydrogen ion inhibitor	Same as Tagamet HB

Appendix

2

First Aid

Accidents are the leading cause of death for people ages 1 to 37. Injuries sustained in accidents can often be tragic. They are grim reminders of our need to learn first aid skills and to practice preventive safety habits.

First aid knowledge and skills allow you to help people who are in need of immediate emergency care. They also can help you save yourself if you should become injured. We recommend that our students enroll in American Red Cross first aid and safety courses, which are available in local communities or through colleges or universities. In this appendix, we briefly present some information about common first

aid emergencies. (Please note that our information is *not* a substitute for comprehensive American Red Cross first aid instruction.)

FIRST AID

- Keep a list of important phone numbers near your phone (your doctor, ambulance service, hospital, poison control center, police and fire departments).
- In case of serious injury or illness, call the appropriate emergency service immediately for help (if uncertain, call "911" or "0").

Specific Problem	What To Do
Asphyxiation Victim stops breathing and skin, lips, tongue, and fingernail beds turn bluish or gray.	Adult: Tip head back with one hand on forehead and other lifting the lower jaw near the chin. Look, listen, and feel for breathing. If not breathing, place your mouth over victim's mouth, pinch the nose, get a tight seal, and give 2 slow breaths. Recheck the breathing; if still not breathing, give breaths once every 5 seconds for an adult, once every 3 seconds for a child, once every 3 seconds for infants (do not exaggerate head tilt for babies).
Bleeding Victim bleeding severely can quickly go into shock and die within 1 or 2 minutes.	With the palm of your hand, apply firm, direct pressure to the wound with a clean dressing or pad. Elevate the body part if possible. Do not remove blood-soaked dressings; use additional layers, continue to apply pressure, and elevate the site. *Continued*

Specific Problem	What To Do
Choking Accidental ingestion or inhalation of food or other objects causes suffocation that can quickly lead to death. There are over 3000 deaths annually, mostly of infants, small children, and the elderly.	The procedure is easy to learn; however, the Heimlich maneuver must be learned from a qualified instructor. The procedure varies somewhat for infants, children, adults, pregnant women, and obese people.
Hyperventilation A situation in which a person breathes too rapidly; often the result of fear or anxiety; may cause confusion, shortness of breath, dizziness, or fainting. Intentional hyperventilation before an underwater swim is especially dangerous, since it may cause a swimmer to pass out in the water and drown.	Have the person relax and rest for a few minutes. Provide reassurance and a calming influence. Having the victim take a few breaths in a paper bag (not plastic) may be helpful. Do not permit swimmers to practice hyperventilation before attempting to swim.
Bee Stings Not especially dangerous except for people who have developed an allergic hypersensitivity to a particular venom. Those who are not hypersensitive will experience swelling, redness, and pain. Hypersensitive people may develop extreme swelling, chest constriction, breathing difficulties, hives, and shock signs.	For nonsensitive people: Scrape stinger from skin and apply cold compresses or over-the-counter topical preparation for insect bites. For sensitive people: Get professional help immediately. Scrape the stinger from skin; position the person so that the stung body part is below the level of the heart; help administer prescribed medication (if available); apply cold compresses.
Poisoning Often poisoning can be prevented with adequate safety awareness. Children are frequent victims.	Call the poison control center immediately; follow the instructions provided. Keep syrup of ipecac on hand.
Shock A life-threatening depression of circulation, respiration, and temperature control, recognizable by a victim's cool, clammy, pale skin; weak and rapid pulse; shallow breathing; weakness; nausea; or unconsciousness.	Provide psychological reassurance. Keep victim calm and in a comfortable, reclining position; loosen tight clothing. Prevent loss of body heat; cover if necessary. Elevate legs 8 to 12 inches (if there are no head, neck, or back injuries, or possible broken bones involving the hips or legs). Do not give food or fluids. Seek further emergency assistance.
Burns Burns can cause severe tissue damage and lead to serious infection and shock.	Minor burns: immerse in cold water and then cover with sterile dressings; do not apply butter or grease to burns. Major burns: seek help immediately; cover affected area with large quantities of clean dressings or bandages; do not try to clean the burn area or break blisters. Chemical burns: flood the area with running water.
Broken Bones Fractures are a common result of car accidents, falls, and recreational accidents.	Do not move the victim unless absolutely necessary to prevent further injury. Immobilize the affected area. Give care for shock while waiting for further emergency assistance.

Epilepsy: Recognition and First Aid

Seizure Type	What It Looks Like	Often Mistaken For	What To Do	What Not To Do
Convulsive Generalized tonic-clonic (also called grand mal)	Sudden cry, fall, rigidity, followed by muscle jerks, frothy saliva on lips, shallow breathing or temporarily suspended breathing, bluish skin, possible loss of bladder or bowel control, usually lasts 2-5 minutes; normal breathing then starts again; there may be some confusion and/or fatigue, followed by return to full consciousness	Heart attack Stroke Unknown but life-threatening emergency	Look for medical identification Protect from nearby hazards Loosen ties or shirt collars Place folded jacket under head Turn on side to keep airway clear; reassure when consciousness returns If single seizure lasted less than 10 minutes, ask if hospital evaluation wanted If multiple seizures, or if one seizure lasts longer than 10 minutes, take to emergency room	Don't put any hard implement in the mouth Don't try to hold tongue; it can't be swallowed Don't try to give liquids during or just after seizure Don't use oxygen unless there are symptoms of heart attack Don't use artificial respiration unless breathing is absent after muscle jerks subside, or unless water has been inhaled Don't restrain
Nonconvulsive	This category includes many different forms of seizures, ranging from temporary unawareness (petit mal) to brief, sudden, massive muscle jerks (myoclonic seizures)	Daydreaming, acting out, clumsiness, poor coordination, intoxication, random activity, mental illness, and many others	Usually no first aid necessary other than to provide reassurance and emotional support. Any nonconvulsive seizure that becomes convulsive should be managed as a convulsive seizure. Medical evaluation is recommended.	Do not shout at, restrain, expect verbal instructions to be obeyed, or grab a person having a nonconvulsive seizure (unless danger threatens)

Mental Disorders

CATEGORIES OF MENTAL DISORDERS

Anxiety Disorders

Anxiety disorders are characterized by a fear that leads to overarousal of heartbeat, muscle tension, and shakiness.

- *Phobic disorder.* Excessive irrational fears. Examples are agoraphobia (fear of open places), claustrophobia (fear of enclosed places), and acrophobia (fear of heights).
- *Panic disorder.* Overwhelming fear of losing control or going crazy. Panic attacks can last from a minute to an hour or more. No clear reason exists as to why panic attacks occur.
- *Generalized anxiety disorder.* Continued, free-floating anxiety that lasts for at least 1 month.
- *Obsessive-compulsive disorder.* Obsessive behavior is characterized by recurring irrational thoughts that remain out of control. Compulsive behavior reflects an irresistible urge to act repeatedly.

Dissociative Disorders

Dissociative disorders are those in which there is a sudden, temporary change in consciousness or self-identity.

- *Psychogenic amnesia.* Inability to recall a stressful event.
- *Psychogenic fugue.* Disorder in which a person loses memory of his or her past, moves to another locale, and takes on a new identity.

- *Multiple personality.* Disorder characterized by sever-al distinct personalities occupying the same person.

Somatoform Disorders

People with somatoform disorders complain of a physical ailment, yet no physical abnormality can be found.

- *Conversion disorder.* Severe, unexplained loss of some physical ability (such as eyesight or use of the legs).
- *Hypochondriasis.* The belief that one is sick, although no medical evidence can be found.

Affective Disorders

In affective disorders a disturbance exists in a person's ability to express emotions.

- *Dysthymic disorder.* Persistent feelings (lasting for at least 2 years) characterized by lack of energy, loss of self-esteem, pessimistic outlook, inability to enjoy other people or pleasurable activities, and thoughts about suicide. The disorder is likely the most common psychological problem in humans.
- *Major depressive disorder.* Depression more severe than dysthymic disorder. Evidenced by poor appetite and significant weight loss, psychomotor symptoms, impaired reality testing, and recurrent thoughts of suicide.

- *Bipolar disorder.* Mood swings from elation to depression (formerly known as manic-depression).

Schizophrenic Disorders

Schizophrenic disorders are largely recognized by a person's verbal behavior. These disorders are characterized by disturbances in thought, perception, and attention. Schizophrenic patients may speak in a meaningless fashion, switch from topic to topic, and convey little important information. They may have delusions of grandeur or persecution, hallucinations, or excited or slowed motor activity. Usually schizophrenic patients do not think that their thoughts and actions are abnormal.

- *Disorganized type.* Characterized by disorganized delusions and frequent hallucinations that may be sexual or religious in nature. Exaggerated social impairment is common.
- *Catatonic type.* Characterized by a marked impairment in motor activity. May hold one body position for hours and not respond to the speech of others.
- *Paranoid type.* Characterized by delusions of persecution, often ones that are complex and systemized. Paranoid schizophrenic patients may experience vivid hallucinations that support their delusions.

THERAPEUTIC APPROACHES TO MENTAL DISORDERS

A variety of approaches can be used to help people who have mental disorders. These approaches involve psychotherapy or the use of biological therapies. A brief outline of the more widely known strategies follows, since a comprehensive presentation on this topic is beyond the scope of this appendix.

Insight-Oriented Therapies

Underlying this category of therapeutic approaches is the belief that the client must gain insight into the experiences that led up to his or her problem or maladaptive behavior. By being able to recognize the underlying motives for one's behavior, a client will be better able to objectively view his or her beliefs, feelings, and thinking patterns. These underlying motives often are beneath the person's level of consciousness. Insight-oriented forms of psychotherapy include cognitive therapy, psychoanalysis, person-centered therapy, transactional analysis, and gestalt therapy.

Behavior Therapy

Discussed briefly in Chapter 6, behavior therapy (also called *behavior modification*) attempts to produce behavior change in a client by using scientifically tested principles of classical and operant conditioning and observational learning. Techniques of behavior therapy include operant conditioning (behavior reinforcement), aversive conditioning, systematic desensitization, assertiveness training, and self-control techniques.

Group Therapy

This form of therapy involves a therapist and several clients who have similar problems. Examples might be group therapy for people with eating disorders, smoking concerns, sexual problems, family problems, or relationship concerns. By meeting together and working to resolve their similar concerns, clients often receive support from other group members. With multiple members, a larger volume of pertinent information exists for clients to share. In a practical sense, group therapy is usually less expensive than individual therapy and the therapist can reach more clients at once.

Biological Therapies

Psychiatrists and other physicians are qualified to approach mental disorders from a medical framework. They are able to use chemotherapy (tranquilizers, antidepressants, lithium), electroconvulsive therapy (ECT or shock therapy), and even psychosurgery (brain surgery). Often these approaches are used with clients who have especially serious psychiatric disorders or who do not respond well to psychotherapy.

Body Systems

THE CIRCULATORY SYSTEM

THE RESPIRATORY SYSTEM

Nasal cavity

Larynx

Trachea

Right main bronchus

Left main bronchus

Right lung

Left lung

Capillary

Alveolar duct

Alveoli

Terminal end of bronchiole

THE MUSCULAR SYSTEM

Sternocleidomastoid

Trapezius

Deltoid

Pectoralis major

Biceps

Triceps

Rectus abdominis

Rectus femoris

Sartorius

Gastrocnemius

Ligaments

THE SKELETAL SYSTEM

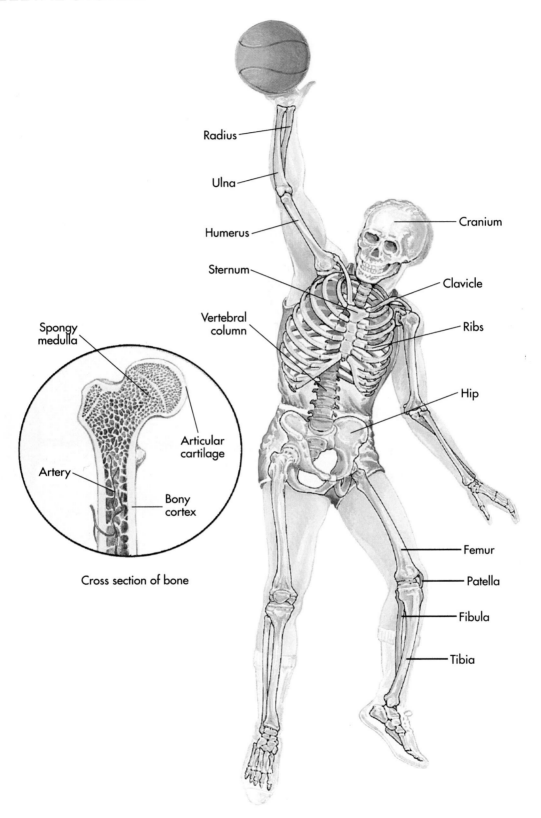

Radius

Ulna

Humerus

Sternum

Vertebral
column

Cranium

Clavicle

Ribs

Hip

Femur

Patella

Fibula

Tibia

Spongy
medulla

Articular
cartilage

Artery

Bony
cortex

Cross section of bone

THE NERVOUS SYSTEM

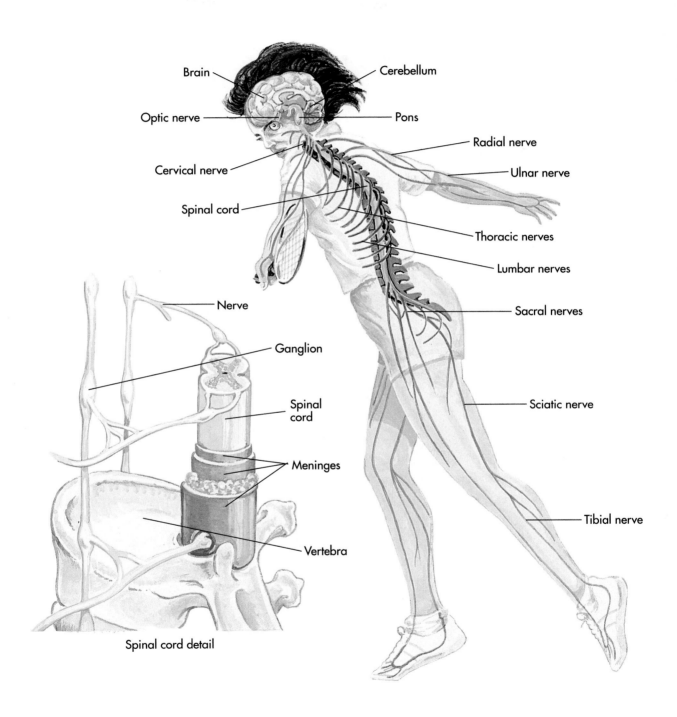

Brain

Cerebellum

Optic nerve

Pons

Radial nerve

Ulnar nerve

Cervical nerve

Spinal cord

Thoracic nerves

Lumbar nerves

Nerve

Sacral nerves

Ganglion

Spinal cord

Meninges

Sciatic nerve

Vertebra

Tibial nerve

Spinal cord detail

THE DIGESTIVE SYSTEM

Teeth

Tongue

Gall-
bladder

Stomach

Duodenum

Small intestine

Large
intestine

Rectum

Villi

Epithelial
fold

Smooth
muscle

Cross section
of intestine wall

THE URINARY SYSTEM

Cortex

Pelvis

Renal
artery

Renal
vein

Ureter

Medulla

Cross section of kidney

Kidney

Ureter

Bladder

Urethra

THE ENDOCRINE SYSTEM

NOTE: Refer to Figures 13-2 and 13-3 for detailed anatomical illustrations of the reproductive systems.

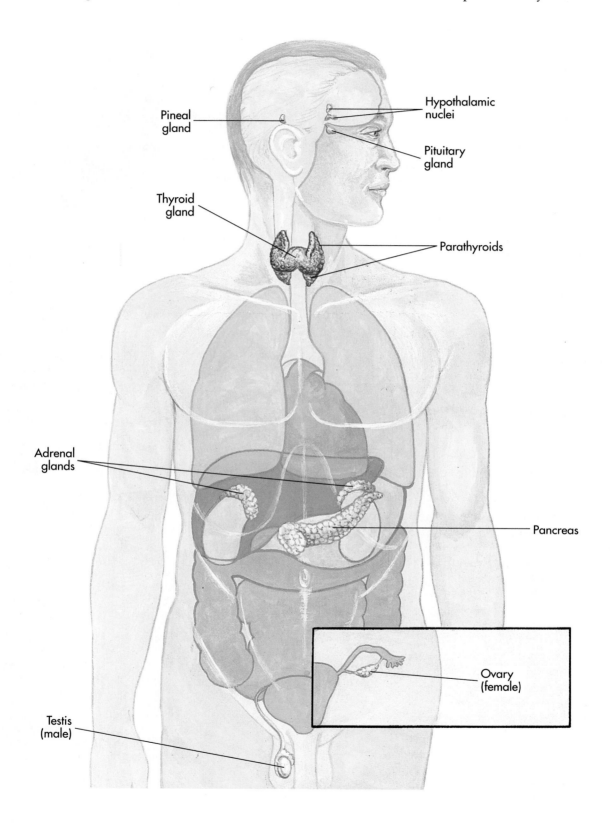

Pineal gland

Hypothalamic nuclei

Pituitary gland

Thyroid gland

Parathyroids

Adrenal glands

Pancreas

Ovary (female)

Testis (male)

Glossary

A

abortion induced premature termination of a pregnancy

absorption passage of nutrients or alcohol through the walls of the stomach or intestinal tract into the bloodstream

abuse any use of a legal or illegal drug that is detrimental to health

acid-base balance acidity-alkalinity of body fluids

acid rain rain that has a lower pH than that normally associated with rain

acquaintance rape forced sexual intercourse between individuals who know each other

acquired immunity significant component of the immune system associated with the formation of antibodies and specialized blood cells that are capable of destroying pathogens

ACTH (adrenocorticotropic hormone) hormone produced in the pituitary gland and transmitted to the cortex of the adrenal glands; stimulates production and release of corticoids

activity requirement calories required for daily physical work

acupuncture insertion of fine needles into the body to alter electroenergy fields and cure disease

acute alcohol intoxication potentially fatal elevation of the blood alcohol concentration, often resulting from rapid consumption of large amounts of alcohol

acute rhinitis the common cold; the sudden onset of nasal inflammation

adaptive thermogenesis physiological response of the body to adjust its metabolic rate to the presence or absence of calories

addiction term used interchangeably with physical dependence

additive effect combined (but not exaggerated) effect produced by the concurrent use of two or more drugs

adrenal cortex outer cell layers of the adrenal glands; cells of the cortex, on stimulation by ACTH, produce corticoid.

adrenal glands paired triangular endocrine glands situated above each kidney; site of epinephrine and corticoid production

adrenaline powerful stress response hormone (*see* epinephrine)

adrenocorticotropic hormone (ACTH) hormone produced in the pituitary gland and transmitted to the cortex of the adrenal glands; stimulates production and release of corticoids

aerobic energy production body's production of energy when the respiratory and circulatory systems are able to process and transport a sufficient amount of oxygen to muscle cells

agent causal pathogen of a particular disease

AIDS acquired immunodeficiency syndrome; viral-based destruction of the immune system, leading to illness and death from opportunistic infections

alcoholism pattern of alcohol use characterized by emotional and physical dependence, as well as a general loss of control over the use of alcohol

allergens environmental substances to which people may be hypersensitive; allergens function as antigens

allopathy system of medical practice in which specific remedies are used to produce effects different from those produced by a disease

alveoli thin, saclike terminal ends of the airways; the sites at which gases are exchanged between the blood and inhaled air

Alzheimer's disease gradual development of memory loss, confusion, and loss of reasoning; can eventually lead to total intellectual incapacitation, brain degeneration, and death

amino acids chief components of protein; synthesized by the body or obtained from dietary sources

amotivational syndrome behavioral pattern characterized by widespread apathy toward productive activities

anabolic steroids drugs that function like testosterone to produce increases in weight and strength

anaerobic energy production body's production of energy when needed amounts of oxygen are not readily available

analgesic drugs drugs that reduce the sensation of pain

anaphylactic shock life-threatening congestion of the airways resulting from hypersensitivity to a foreign protein

androgyny the blending of both masculine and feminine characteristics

anemia condition reflecting abnormally low levels of hemoglobin

aneurysm a ballooning or outpouching on a weakened area of an artery

angina pectoris chest pain that results from impaired blood supply to the heart muscle

angioplasty surgical insertion of a balloon-tipped catheter into the coronary artery to open areas of narrowing

anorexia nervosa emotional disorder in which appetite and hunger are suppressed and marked weight loss occurs

anovulatory not ovulating

antagonistic effect effect produced when one drug nullifies (reduces, offsets) the effects of a second drug

antibodies chemical compounds produced by the immune system to destroy antigens and their toxins

antigens disease-producing microorganisms or foreign substances that on entering the body trigger an immune response

antioncogenes genes whose function is to prevent the activation of oncogenes

ARC AIDS-related complex; condition suggesting some deterioration of the immune system as a result of infection by the HIV agent

arrhythmias irregularities of the heart's normal rhythm or beating pattern

arteriosclerosis calcification of an artery's wall that makes the vessel less elastic, more brittle, and more susceptible to bursting; hardening of the arteries

artificial insemination depositing of sperm in the female reproductive tract in an attempt to impregnate; sperm may be those of the partner or of a donor

artificially acquired immunity type of acquired immunity resulting from the body's response to pathogens introduced into the body through immunizations

asbestos fibrous material found in insulation and many other building materials; causes asbestosis

asphyxiation death resulting from lack of oxygen to the brain

atherosclerosis the buildup of plaque on the inner walls of arteries

attention deficit disorder inability to concentrate well on a specified task; often accompanied by above-normal physical movement; also called *hyperactivity*

audiologists health care professionals trained to assess auditory function

autoimmune immune response against the cells of a person's own body

axon portion of a neuron that conducts electrical impulses to the dendrites of adjacent neurons; neurons typically have one axon

ayurveda traditional Indian medicine based on herbal remedies

AZT (azidothymidine) the first drug approved for use in the treatment of AIDS; capable of reducing symptoms and possibly extending life of a person with AIDS

B

balanced diet diet featuring food selections from each of the five food groups

ballistic stretching a "bouncing" form of stretching in which a muscle group is lengthened repetitively to produce multiply quick, forceful stretches

basal cells foundation cells that underlie the epithelial cells

basal metabolic rate (BMR) the amount of energy (in calories) your body requires to maintain basic functions

behavior modification behavioral therapy designed to change the learned behavior of an individual

benign noncancerous; tumors that do not spread

bestiality alternative term for *zoophilia*

beta blockers drugs that prevent overactivity of the heart, which results in angina pectoris

bias and hate crimes criminal acts directed at a person or group solely because of a specific characteristic, such as race, religion, ethnic background, or political beliefs

binge drinking alcohol use characterized by periods of intense alcohol consumption; for example, drinking heavily on the weekend

bioavailability speed and extent to which a drug becomes biologically active within the body; bioavailability for a drug varies among individuals and within a given individual over time

biochemical oxygen demand index of water pollution based on the rate and extent that organic matter uses dissolved oxygen from a sample of water

biofeedback self-monitoring of physiological processes as they occur within the body

biological sexuality male and female aspects of sexuality

birth control all of the procedures that can prevent the birth of a child

bisexual choosing members of both genders as one's sexual preference

blackout temporary state of amnesia experienced by an alcoholic; an inability to remember events that occur during a period of alcohol use

blood alcohol concentration (BAC) percentage of alcohol in a measured quantity of blood

blood analysis chemical analysis of various substances in the blood; helps determine changes and possible disturbances in the body

body fat analysis determination of the percentage of body tissue composed of fat

body image subjective perception of how one's body appears

bodybuilding sports activity in which the participants train their bodies to reach desired goals of muscular size, symmetry, and proportion

body mass index (BMI) numerical expression of body weight based on height and weight

bonding important initial sense of recognition established between the newborn and those adults on whom the newborn will depend

brain death the absence of brain wave activity after an initial measurement followed by a second measurement 24 hours later

brand name specific name assigned to a patented drug or product by its manufacturer

Braxton Hicks contractions false labor contractions; mild and of irregular spacing

breakthrough bleeding midcycle uterine bleeding; spotting

breech position birth position in which the baby's feet or buttocks are presented first

bulimarexia binge eating followed by purging the body of the food

bulimia emotional disorder in which binge eating patterns are established; usually accompanied by purging

C

calcium channel blockers drugs that prevent arterial spasms; used in the long-term management of angina pectoris

calendar method form of natural family planning in which the variable lengths of a woman's menstrual cycle are used to calculate her fertile period

calipers device to measure the thickness of a skinfold from which percent body fat can be calculated

caloric balance caloric input equals caloric output; weight remains constant

calories units of heat (energy); specifically, 1 calorie equals the heat required to raise 1 kilogram of water 1° C

cannula hollow metal or plastic tube through which materials can be aspirated

carbohydrates chemical compounds comprising sugar or saccharide units; the body's primary source of energy

carbon monoxide chemical compound (CO) that can inactivate red blood cells

carcinogenic related to the production of cancerous changes; property of environmental agents, including drugs, that may

stimulate the development of cancerous changes within cells

carcinoma in situ cancer at its site of origin

cardiac pertaining to the heart

cardiac muscle specialized smooth muscle tissue that forms the middle (muscular) layer of the heart wall

cardiogram reading of heart and lung function from a cardiograph machine

cardiovascular pertaining to the heart (cardio) and blood vessels (vascular)

cardiorespiratory endurance ability of the body to process and transport oxygen required by muscle cells so that these cells can continue to contract

carjacking a crime that involves a thief's attempt to steal a car while the owner is behind the wheel; carjackings are usually random and unpredictable and often involve handguns

CAT scan computerized axial tomography; x-ray procedure designed to visualize structures within the body that would not normally be seen through conventional x-ray procedures

catabolism metabolic process of breaking down tissue for the purpose of converting it to energy

cauterize to apply a small electrical current and permanently close a tube or vessel; to burn

celibacy self-imposed avoidance of sexual intimacy

cell-mediated immunity form of acquired immunity that uses specialized white blood cells to destroy specific antigens that enter the body

central nervous system the brain and spinal cord

cereal germ highly nutritious portions of the cereal grain, often removed during milling

cerebral cortex outer covering of the brain; site of intellect, memory, thought processes, and rationalization

cerebral hemorrhage bleeding from the cerebral arteries within the brain

cerebrovascular accident stroke; brain tissue damage resulting from impaired circulation of blood vessels in the brain

cerebrovascular occlusion blockage to arteries supplying blood to the cerebral cortex of the brain; stroke

cervical cap small, thimble-shaped contraceptive device designed to fit over the cervix

cesarean delivery surgical removal of a fetus through the abdominal wall

chemical name name used to describe the molecular structure of a drug

chemoprevention cancer prevention based on the selection of foods whose nutrient composition is thought to protect the body from certain forms of cancer

child abuse harm committed against a child; usually refers to physical abuse, sexual abuse, or child neglect

chiropractic manipulation of the vertebral column to relieve pressure and cure illness

chlamydia the most prevalent sexually transmitted disease; caused by a nongonococcal bacterium

chlorofluorocarbons (CFCs) gaseous chemical compounds that contain chlorine and fluorine

cholesterol fat-related substance in alcohol form; lipid material manufactured within the body, as well as derived through dietary sources

chronic develops slowly and persists for a long period of time

chronic bronchitis persistent inflammation and infection of the smaller airways within the lungs

chronic fatigue syndrome (CFS) illness that causes severe exhaustion, fatigue, aches, and depression; mostly affects women in their thirties and forties

cilia small, hairlike structures that extend from cells that line the air passage

cirrhosis condition characterized by pathological changes to the liver resulting from chronic heavy alcohol consumption; a frequent cause of death among heavy alcohol users

clitoris small shaft of erectile tissue located in front of the vaginal opening; the female homolog of the male penis

cochlea small, snail-shaped organ of the inner ear in which the energy of sound is converted into electrical energy for transmission to the brain

coenzyme vitamin-based organic compound that assists a particular enzyme in performing its role in regulating biochemical reactions

cohabitation sharing of a residence by two unrelated, unmarried people; living together

coitus penile-vaginal intercourse

coitus interruptus (withdrawal) a contraceptive practice in which the erect penis is removed from the vagina before ejaculation

cold turkey immediate, total discontinuation of use of tobacco or other addictive substances

coliform bacteria intestinal tract bacteria whose presence in a water supply suggests contamination by human or animal waste

collateral circulation ability of nearby blood vessels to enlarge and carry additional blood around a blocked blood vessel

companionate love friendly affection and deep attachment, based on extensive familiarity with another person

compliance willingness to follow the directions provided by another person

condom latex shield designed to cover the erect penis and retain semen on ejaculation

confrontation an approach to convince drug-dependent people to enter treatment

congestive heart failure inability of the heart to pump out all the blood that returns to it; can lead to dangerous fluid accumulations in veins, lungs, and kidneys

consumer fraud marketing of unreliable and ineffective services, products, or information under the guise of curing disease or improving health; quackery

contact inhibition ability of a tissue, on reaching its mature size, to suppress additional growth

contraception any procedure that prevents fertilization

contraindications factors that make the use of a drug inappropriate or dangerous for a particular person

cooldown stretching and walking after exercise

coronary arteries vessels that supply oxygenated blood to heart muscle tissues

coronary artery bypass surgery surgical procedure designed to improve blood flow to the heart by providing alternative routes for blood around points of blockage

coroner an elected legal official empowered to pronounce death and to determine the official cause of a suspicious or violent death

corpus luteum cellular remnant of the graafian follicle after the release of an ovum

corticoids hormones generated by the adrenal cortex; corticoids influence the body's control of glucose, protein, and fat metabolism

CPR cardiopulmonary resuscitation; first aid procedure designed to restore breathing and heart function

crack a crystalline form of cocaine that is smoked; has an instantaneous effect and is highly dependence-producing

creativity innovative ability; insightful capacity to adapt means to ends; to move beyond analytical-logical approaches to experience

cross-tolerance transfer of tolerance from one drug to another within the same general category

crosstraining use of more than one aerobic activity to achieve cardiovascular fitness

crowning first appearance of the fetal head at the vaginal opening

cruciferous vegetables vegetables that have flowers with four leaves in the pattern of a cross

crypts burial locations generally located beneath churches

cunnilingus oral stimulation of the vulva or clitoris

cystitis infection of the urinary bladder

D

date rape a form of acquaintance rape that involves forced sexual intercourse by a dating partner

dehydration abnormal depletion of fluids from the body; severe dehydration can lead to death

delirium tremens (DTs) uncontrollable shaking associated with withdrawal from heavy chronic alcohol use

dendrite portion of a neuron that receives electrical stimuli from adjacent neurons; neurons typically have several such branches or extensions

denial in this case, the failure to acknowledge that alcohol or drug use seriously affects one's life

dependence general term that reflects the need to keep consuming a drug for psychological or physical reasons, or both

depressants the psychoactive drugs that reduce the function of the central nervous system

designated driver a person who abstains from or carefully limits alcohol use to drive others safely

designer drugs drugs that chemically resemble drugs on the FDA Schedule 1

desirable weight weight range deemed appropriate for people of a specific gender, age, and frame size

diaphragm soft rubber vaginal cup designed to cover the cervix

diastolic pressure blood pressure against blood vessel walls when the heart relaxes

dilation gradual expansion of an opening or passageway

dilation and curettage (D & C) surgical procedure in which the cervical canal is dilated to allow the uterine wall to be scraped

dilation and evacuation (D & E) surgical procedure using cervical dilation and vacuum aspiration to remove uterine wall material and fetal parts

direct (active) euthanasia process of inducing death, often through the injection of a lethal drug

distress stress that diminishes the quality of life; commonly associated with disease, illness, and maladaptation

diuresis increased discharge of fluid from the body; frequent urination

diuretic drugs drugs that aid the body in removing excess fluid

drug synergism enhancement of a drug's effect as a result of the presence of additional drugs within the system

durable power of attorney for health care a legal document that designates who will make health care decisions for people unable to do so for themselves

duration   length of time one needs to exercise at the target heart rate to produce the training effect

dynamic   in a state of change; health is dynamic in the sense that it is influenced by factors from both within and outside the individual

.... E ....

ECG   electrocardiograph; an instrument to measure and record the electrical activity within the heart

echocardiography   procedure that uses high-frequency sound waves to visualize the structure and function of the heart

ecosystem   an ecological unit made up of both animal and plant life that interact to produce a stable system

ectopic pregnancy   a pregnancy wherein the fertilized ovum implants at a site other than the uterus, typically in the fallopian tube

effacement   a thinning and pulling back of the cervical opening to allow movement of the fetus from the uterus

electrical impedance   method of testing the percentage of body fat using an electrical current

electroencephalograph   instrument that measures the electrical activity of the brain

embolism   potentially fatal situation in which a circulating blood clot lodges itself in a smaller vessel

enabling   in this case, the inadvertent support that some people provide to alcohol or drug abusers

endometrium   innermost lining of the uterus, broken down and discharged during menstruation

enrichment   process of returning to foods some of the nutritional elements (B vitamins and iron) removed during processing

Environmental Protection Agency (EPA) federal agency charged with the protection of natural resources and the quality of the environment

environmental tobacco smoke   tobacco smoke that is diluted and stays within a common source of air

enzymes   chemical substances that regulate physiological processes

epinephrine   powerful adrenal hormone whose presence in the bloodstream prepares the body for maximal energy production and skeletal muscle response

epitaph   inscription on a grave marker or monument

erection   the engorgement of erectile tissue with blood; characteristic of the penis, clitoris, nipple, labia minora, and scrotum

erotic dreams   dreams whose content elicits a sexual response

essential amino acids   nine amino acids that can be obtained only from dietary sources

essential hypertension   hypertension (high blood pressure) resulting from chronic widespread constriction of arterioles

estrogen   ovarian hormone that initiates the development of the uterine wall

estrogen replacement therapy   medically administered estrogen to replace estrogen lost as the result of menopause

eulogy   a composition or speech that praises someone; often delivered at a funeral or memorial service

eustress   stress that adds a positive, enhancing dimension to the quality of life

eutrophication   enrichment of a body of water with nutrients, which allows for overabundant growth of plants

excitement stage   initial arousal stage of the sexual response pattern

exhibitionism   exposure of one's genitals for the purpose of shocking other people

.... F ....

faith   the purposes and meaning that underlie an individual's hopes and strivings

fallopian tubes   paired tubes that allow passage of ova from the ovaries to the uterus; the oviducts

false labor   conditions that tend to resemble the start of true labor; may include irregular uterine contractions, pressure, and discomfort in the lower abdomen

fast foods   convenience foods; foods featured in a variety of restaurants, including hamburgers, pizza, and tacos

fat density   percent of the total calories in a food item derived from fat

FDA Schedule 1   list comprising drugs that hold a high potential for abuse but have no medical use

fecundity   the ability to produce offspring

fellatio   oral stimulation of the penis

femininity   behavioral expressions traditionally observed in females

fermentation   chemical process whereby plant products are converted into alcohol by the action of yeast cells on carbohydrates

fertility   ability to reproduce

fetal alcohol effects   developmental impairment in a child linked to a mother's use of alcohol during pregnancy

fetal alcohol syndrome   characteristic birth defects noted in the children of some women who consume alcohol during their pregnancies

fetishism   choice of a body part or inanimate object as a source of sexual excitement

fiber   plant material that cannot be digested; found in cereal, fruits, and vegetables

fight-or-flight response   physiological changes in response to a stressor

flaccid   nonerect; the state of erectile tissue when vasocongestion is not occurring

flashback   unpredictable return of a psychedelic trip

flexibility   ability of joints to function through an intended range of motion

follicle-stimulating hormone (FSH)   gonadotropic hormone required for initial development of ova (in the female) and sperm (in the male)

food additives   chemical compounds that are intentionally or unintentionally added to our food supply

foreplay   activities, often involving touching and caressing, that prepare individuals for sexual intercourse

freebase   altered form of cocaine that can be smoked

frequency   number of times per week one should exercise to achieve a training effect

full funeral services   all of the professional services provided by funeral directors

.... G ....

gait   pattern of walking

gamete intrafallopian transfer (GIFT) retrieved ovum and partner's sperm are positioned in the fallopian tube for fertilization and subsequent movement into the uterus for implantation

gaseous phase   portion of tobacco smoke containing carbon monoxide and many other physiologically active gaseous compounds

gateway drugs   easily obtained legal or illegal drugs (alcohol, tobacco, marijuana) whose use may precede the use of less common illegal drugs

gender   general term reflecting a biological basis of sexuality; the male gender or the female gender

gender adoption   lengthy process of learning the behaviors that are traditional for one's gender

gender identification   achievement of a personally satisfying interpretation of one's masculinity or feminity

gender identity   recognition of one's gender

gender preference   emotional and intellectual acceptance of one's gender

gender schema   mental image of the cognitive, affective, and performance characteristics appropriate to a particular gender; a mental picture of being a man or a woman

general adaptation syndrome   sequenced physiological response to the presence of a stressor; the alarm, resistance, and exhaustion stages of the stress response

generativity   midlife developmental task; repaying society for its support through contributions associated with parenting, creativity, and occupation

generic name common or nonproprietary name of a drug

genetic counseling medical counseling regarding the transmission and management of inherited conditions

genetic predisposition inherited tendency to develop a disease process if necessary environmental factors exist

glucose blood sugar; the body's primary source of energy

goblet cells cells within the epithelial lining of the airways that produce the mucus required for cleaning the airways

gonads male or female sex glands; testes produce sperm and ovaries produce eggs

greenhouse effect warming of the Earth's surface that is produced when solar heat becomes trapped by layers of carbon dioxide and other gases

H

habituation term used interchangeably with *psychological dependence*

hallucinogens psychoactive drugs capable of producing hallucinations (distortions of reality)

hashish resins collected from the flowering tops of marijuana plants

health maintenance organizations (HMOs) groups that supply prepaid comprehensive health care with an emphasis on prevention

health promotion movement in which knowledge, practices, and values are transmitted to people for their use in lengthening their lives, reducing the incidence of illness, and feeling better

healthy body weight weight range based on waist and hip measurements and reflecting an acceptable, healthy amount of fat within the central body cavity

heart catheterization procedure wherein a thin catheter is introduced through an arm or leg artery into the coronary circulation to visualize areas of blockage

heart-lung machine device that oxygenates and circulates blood during bypass surgery

hemorrhaging bleeding; often implies profuse bleeding

heterosexual having a sexual preference for a member of the opposite gender

high-density lipoprotein (HDL) the type of lipoprotein that transports cholesterol from the bloodstream to the liver where it is eventually removed from the body; high levels of HDL are related to a reduction in heart disease

HIV human immunodeficiency virus

holistic health views health in terms of its physical, emotional, social, intellectual, spiritual, and occupational makeup

homicide the intentional killing of one person by another

homosexual choosing a member of one's own gender as one's sexual preference

hospice care approach to caring for terminally ill patients that maximizes the quality of life and allows death with dignity

host negligence a legal term that reflects the failure of a host to provide reasonable care and safety for people visiting the host's residence or business

hot flashes temporary feelings of warmth experienced by women during and after menopause; caused by blood vessel dilation

Human Genome Project international quest by geneticists to identify the location and composition of every gene within the human cell

human papillomavirus sexually transmitted virus capable of causing precancerous changes in the cervix; causative agent for genital warts

humoral immunity form of acquired immunity that uses antibodies to counter specific antigens that enter the body

hypercellular obesity form of obesity seen in individuals who possess an abnormally large number of fat cells

hyperglycemia elevated blood glucose levels; an important indicator of diabetes mellitus

hyperparathyroidism condition reflecting the overactive production of parathyroid hormone by the parathyroid glands

hypertonic saline solution salt solution with a concentration higher than that found in human fluids

hypertrophic obesity form of obesity in which fat cells are enlarged

hypochondriasis neurotic conviction that one is ill or afflicted with a particular disease

hypothalamus portion of the midbrain that provides a connection between the cerebral cortex and pituitary gland

hysterectomy surgical removal of the uterus

I

immune system system of biochemical and cellular elements that protect the body from invading pathogens and foreign materials

immunizations laboratory-prepared pathogens that are introduced into the body for the purpose of stimulating the body's immune system

introspective looking inward to examine one's feelings and beliefs

in vitro fertilization and embryo transfer (IVF-ET) laboratory fertilization of an ovum taken from the woman with subsequent return of the developing embryo into the woman's uterus

incest marriage or coitus (sexual intercourse) between closely related individuals

incomplete protein food that lacks one or more of the essential amino acids

incubation stage time required for a pathogen to multiply significantly enough for signs and symptoms to appear

independent practice association (IPA) a modified HMO in which a group of physicians provides prepaid health care but not from a central location within an HMO

indirect (passive) euthanasia process of allowing a person to die by disconnecting life support systems or withholding life-saving techniques

infatuation an often shallow, intense attraction to another person

infertility inability of a male to impregnate or of a female to become pregnant

inhalants psychoactive drugs that enter the body through inhalation

inhibitions inner controls that prevent a person's engaging in certain types of behavior

insulin pancreatic hormone required by the body for the effective metabolism of carbohydrates

insulin-dependent (type 1) diabetes mellitus form of diabetes generally seen for the first time in childhood or adolescence; juvenile onset diabetes

intensity level of effort one puts into an activity

intentional injuries injuries that are purposely inflicted on one person by another person

interstitial cell stimulating hormone (ICSH) a gonadotropic hormone of the male required for the production of testosterone

interstitial cells specialized cells within the testicles that on stimulation by ICSH produce the male sex hormone testosterone

intimacy any close, mutual verbal or nonverbal behavior within a relationship

intrauterine device (IUD) small plastic medicated or unmedicated device that when inserted in the uterus prevents continued pregnancy

ionizing radiation form of radiation capable of releasing electrons from atoms

isokinetic exercises muscular strength training exercises that use machines to provide variable resistances throughout the full range of motion

isometric exercises muscular strength training exercises that use a resistance so great that the resistance object cannot be moved

L

labia majora larger, more external skin folds that surround the vaginal opening

labia minora small, liplike folds of skin immediately adjacent to the vaginal opening

lactating breastfeeding; nursing

lactovegetarian diet vegetarian diet that allows for the consumption of milk and dairy products

laminaria plugs made of seaweed that on exposure to moisture expand and dilate the canal into which they have been placed

lead toxicity blood lead level above 25 micrograms/deciliter (if adopted, the new standard will be 10 micrograms/deciliter)

legumes peas and beans; plant sources high in the essential amino acids

lesbianism female homosexuality

lightening movement of fetus deeper into the pelvic cavity before the onset of the birth process

lipoprotein proteinlike structure in the bloodstream to which circulating fatty materials attach; associated with cardiovascular disease

living will document confirming a person's desire to be allowed to die peacefully and with a measure of dignity in case of terminal illness or major injury

low-density lipoprotein (LDL) the type of lipoprotein that transports the largest amount of cholesterol in the bloodstream; high levels of LDL are related to heart disease

luteinizing hormone (LH) female gonadotropic hormone required for fullest development and release of ova; ovulating hormone

Lyme disease systemic bacterial infection transmitted by deer ticks

M

macrobiotic diet vegetarian diet composed almost entirely of brown rice

mainstream smoke the smoke inhaled and then exhaled by a smoker

mammogram x-ray examination of the breast

masculinity behavioral expressions traditionally observed in males

masochism sexual excitement while being injured or humiliated

mastectomy removal of breast tissue

masturbation self-stimulation of the genitals

maternal supportive tissues general term referring to the development of the placenta and other tissues specifically associated with pregnancy

mausoleum above-ground structure into which caskets can be placed for disposition and that frequently resembles a small stone house

maximum heart rate maximum number of times the heart can beat per minute

Medicaid noncontributory governmental health insurance for people receiving other types of public assistance

Medicare contributory governmental health insurance, primarily for people 65 years of age or older

meltdown the overheating and eventual melting of the uranium fuel rods in the core of a nuclear reactor

menarche time of a female's first menstrual cycle

menopause decline and eventual cessation of hormone production by the reproductive system

menstrual extraction procedure using vacuum aspiration to remove uterine wall material within 2 weeks after a missed menstrual period

menstrual phase phase of the menstrual cycle during which the broken-down lining of the uterus (endometrium) is discharged from the body

menstruation the cyclic buildup and destruction of the uterine wall

metabolic rate rate or intensity at which the body uses energy

metastasis spread of cancerous cells from their site of origin to other areas of the body

midlife period between 45 and 64 years of age

midlife crisis period of emotional upheaval noted among some midlife people as they struggle with the finality of death and the nature of their past and future accomplishments

migraine headaches severe, recurrent headaches, usually affecting one side of the head

minerals chemical elements that serve as structural elements within body tissue or participate in physiological processes

minipills low-dose progesterone oral contraceptives

misuse inappropriate use of legal drugs intended to be medications

monogamous paired relationship with one partner

mononuclear leukocytes large white blood cells that have only one nucleus

mononucleosis ("mono") viral infection characterized by weakness, fatigue, swollen glands, and low-grade fever

monounsaturated fats fats made of compounds in which one hydrogen-bonding position remains to be filled; semisolid at room temperature; derived primarily from peanut and olive oils

morning-after pill high-dose combination oral contraceptive used to terminate a possible pregnancy

motorized scraper a motor-driven cutter that shaves off plaque deposits from inside artery walls

mucus clear, sticky material produced by specialized cells within the mucous membranes of the body; mucus traps much of the suspended particulate matter from tobacco smoke

MRI scan magnetic resonance imaging; an imaging procedure that uses a giant magnet to generate an image of body tissue

multiorgasmic capacity potential to have several orgasms within a single period of sexual arousal

murmur an atypical heart sound that suggests a backwashing of blood into a chamber of the heart from which it has just left

muscular endurance ability of a muscle or muscle group to function over time; depends on well-developed respiratory and circulatory systems

muscular strength ability to contract skeletal muscles to engage in work

mutagenic capable of promoting genetic alterations in cells

myelin white, fatty insulating material that surrounds the axons of many nerve cells

myocardial infarction heart attack; the death of heart muscle as a result of a blockage in one of the coronary arteries

myotonia buildup of neuromuscular tonus within a particular tissue

N

narcolepsy sleep-related disorder in which a person has a recurrent, overwhelming, and uncontrollable desire to sleep

narcotics psychoactive drugs derived from the oriental poppy plant; narcotics relieve pain and induce sleep

naturally acquired immunity type of acquired immunity resulting from the body's response to pathogens introduced into the body through immunizations

nerve blockers drugs that can stop the flow of electrical impulses through the nerves into which they have been injected

neuromuscular tonus level of nervous tension within the muscle

neuron nerve cell; the structural unit of the nervous system

neurophysiological nervous system function; processes through which the body senses and responds to its internal and external environments

neurotransmitters chemical messengers released by neurons that permit electrical impulses to be transferred from one nerve cell to another

nicotine physiologically active, dependence-producing drug found in tobacco

nitroglycerin a blood vessel dilator used by some cardiac patients to relieve angina

nocturnal emission ejaculation that occurs during sleep; "wet dream"

nodes in this case, the electrical centers found in cardiac muscle

nomogram graphic means of finding an unknown value

non–insulin-dependent (type 2) diabetes mellitus form of diabetes generally seen for the first time in people 35 years of age and older; adult-onset diabetes

nonoxynol 9 a spermicide commonly used with contraceptive devices

nontraditional students administrative term used by colleges and universities for students who, for whatever reason, are pursuing undergraduate work at an age other than that associated with traditional college years (18-24)

norepinephrine adrenaline-like neurotransmitter produced within the nervous system

nurse practitioners registered nurses who have taken specialized training in one or more clinical areas and are able to engage in limited diagnosis and treatment of illnesses

nutrients elements in foods that are required for the growth, repair, and regulation of body processes

O

obesity condition in which overweight is the result of excess body fat

oncogenes genes that are believed to activate the development of cancer

oogenesis production of ova in a biologically mature female

oral contraceptive pill pill taken orally, composed of synthetic female hormones that prevent ovulation or implantation; "the pill"

orgasmic platform expanded outer third of the vagina that during the plateau phase of the sexual response grips the penis

orgasmic stage third stage of the sexual response pattern; the stage during which neuromuscular tension is released

orthodontics dental specialty that focuses on the proper alignment of the teeth

osteoarthritis arthritis that develops with age

osteopathy a form of allopathic medicine whose historical beginnings were centered in the manipulation of the musculoskeletal system

osteoporosis resorption of calcium from the bone caused by the inability of the body to use dietary calcium; seen primarily in postmenopausal women

outercourse sexual activity that does not involve intercourse

ovary female reproductive structure that produces ova and the female gonadal sex hormones estrogen and progesterone

overload principle principle whereby a person gradually increases the resistance load that must be moved or lifted

overweight condition in which body weight is above desirable weight

ovolactovegetarian diet diet that excludes the use of all meat but does allow the consumption of eggs and dairy products

ovulation the release of a mature egg from the ovary

oxidation in this case, the process that removes alcohol from the bloodstream

oxygen debt physical state that occurs when the body can no longer process and transport sufficient amounts of oxygen for continued muscle contraction

ozone layer layer of triatomic oxygen that surrounds the Earth and filters much of the sun's radiation before it can reach the Earth's surface

P

pacemaker sinoatrial or SA node; an area of cells within the heart that controls its electrical activity

Pap test cancer screening procedure in which cells removed from the cervix are examined

paracervical anesthetic anesthetic injected into tissues surrounding the cervical opening

paraphilia a preference for unusual sexual practices

particulate phase portion of tobacco smoke composed of small suspended particles

particulate pollutants class of air pollutants composed of small solid particles and liquid droplets

partner abuse violence committed against a domestic partner

parturition childbirth

passionate love state of extreme absorption in another; tenderness, elation, anxiety, sexual desire, and ecstasy

passive smoking inhalation of air that is heavily contaminated with tobacco smoke

passively acquired immunity temporary immunity achieved by providing antibodies to a person exposed to a particular pathogen

pathogen disease-causing agent

peak stage stage of an infectious disease at which symptoms are most fully expressed; acute stage

pedophilia sexual contact with children as a source of sexual excitement

pelvic inflammatory disease (PID) acute or chronic infections of the peritoneum or lining of the abdominopelvic cavity; associated with a variety of symptoms and a potential cause of sterility; generalized infection of the pelvic cavity that results from the spread of an infection through a woman's reproductive structures

periodic abstinence birth control methods that rely on a couple's avoidance of intercourse during the ovulatory phase of a woman's menstrual cycle; also called *fertility awareness* or *natural family planning*

periodontal disease destruction of soft tissue and bone that surround the teeth

peripheral artery disease (PAD) damage resulting from restricted blood flow to the extremities, especially the legs and feet

peritonitis inflammation of the peritoneum or lining of the abdominopelvic cavity

pesticide agent used to destroy pests

phenylpropanolamine (PPA) active chemical compound found in most over-the-counter diet products

physical dependence need to continue using a drug to maintain normal body function and to avoid withdrawal illness; also called *addiction*

pituitary gland "master gland" of the endocrine system; the wide variety of hormones produced by the pituitary are sent to structures throughout the body

placebo pills pills that contain no active ingredients

placenta structure through which nutrients, metabolic wastes, and drugs (including alcohol) pass from the bloodstream of the mother into the bloodstream of the developing fetus

plateau stage second stage of the sexual response pattern; a leveling off of arousal immediately before orgasm

platelet adhesiveness tendency of platelets to clump together, thus enhancing speed at which the blood clots

platonic close association between two people that does not include a sexual relationship

podiatrists specialists who treat a variety of ailments of the feet

polychlorinated biphenyls (PCBs) class of chlorinated organic compounds similar to the herbicide DDT

polyunsaturated fats fats composed of compounds in which multiple hydrogen-bonding positions remain open; these fats are liquids at room temperature; derived from a variety of vegetable sources

positive caloric balance caloric intake greater than caloric expenditure

postpartum period of time after the birth of a baby during which the uterus returns to its prepregnancy size

potentiated effect phenomenon whereby the use of one drug intensifies the effect of a second drug

preferred provider organization a group of physicians who market their professional services to an insurance company at predetermined fees

primary care physician the physician who sees a patient on a regular basis, rather than a specialist who sees the patient only for a specific condition or procedure

problem drinking alcohol use pattern in which a drinker's behavior creates personal difficulties or difficulties for other people

procreation reproduction

prodromal stage stage of an infectious disease process in which only general symptoms appear

professional nurses registered nurses who hold a bachelor's degree in nursing from a college or university

progesterone ovarian hormone that continues the development of the uterine wall that was initiated by estrogen

progressive resistance exercises muscular strength training exercises that use traditional barbells and dumbbells with fixed resistances

proof twice the percentage of alcohol by volume in a beverage; 100 proof alcohol is 50% alcohol

prostaglandin inhibitors drugs that block the production of prostaglandins, thus eliminating the hormonal stimulation of smooth muscles

prostaglandins chemical substances that stimulate smooth muscle contractions

prosthodontics dental specialty that focuses on the construction and fitting of artificial appliances to replace missing teeth

proteins compounds composed of chains of amino acids; primary components of muscle and connective tissue

protooncogenes normal genes that hold the potential of becoming cancer-causing oncogenes

psychoactive drug any substance capable of altering one's feelings, moods, or perceptions

psychological dependence need to consume a drug for emotional reasons; also called *habituation*

psychosocial sexuality masculine and feminine aspects of sexuality

psychosomatic disorders physical illnesses of the body generated by the effects of stress

puberty achievement of reproductive ability

pulmonary pertaining to the lungs and breathing

pulmonary emphysema irreversible disease process in which the alveoli are destroyed

purging use of vomiting or laxatives to remove undigested food from the body

putrefaction decomposition of organic matter

Q

quackery marketing of unreliable and ineffective services, products, or information under the guise of curing disease or improving health

R

radiation sickness illness characterized by fatigue, nausea, weight loss, fever, bleeding from mouth and gums, hair loss, and immune deficiencies, resulting from overexposure to ionizing radiation

radon gas a naturally occurring radioactive gas produced by the decay of uranium

range of motion distance through which a joint can be moved; measured in degrees

rape an act of violence against another person wherein that person is forced to engage in sexual activities

recovery stage stage of an infectious disease at which the body's immune system has overcome the infectious agent and recovery is underway; convalescence stage

recycling ability to convert disposable items into reusable materials

reflexology massage applied to specific areas of the feet to treat illness and disease in other areas of the body

refractory phase that portion of the male's resolution stage during which sexual arousal cannot occur

refractory errors incorrect patterns of light wave transmission through the structures of the eye

regulatory genes genes within the cell that control cellular replication or doubling

rehabilitation return of function to a previous level

relaxation response physiological state of opposition to the fight-or-flight response of the general adaptation syndrome

relaxation training the use of various techniques to produce a state of relaxation

remediation development of alternative forms of function to replace those which had been lost or were poorly developed

resolution stage fourth stage of the sexual response pattern; the return of the body to a preexcitement state

retinal hemorrhage uncontrolled bleeding from arteries within the eye's retina

rheumatic heart disease chronic damage to the heart (especially heart valves) resulting from a streptococcal infection within the heart; a complication associated with rheumatic fever

rheumatoid arthritis the result of autoimmune deterioration of the joints

rigor mortis rigidity of the body that occurs after death

role of health mission of health within a person's life cycle

rubella German (or 3-day) measles

rubeola red or common measles

S

sadism sexual excitement achieved while inflicting injury or humiliation on another person

sadomasochism combination of sadism and masochism into one sexual activity

salt sensitive descriptive of people whose bodies overreact to the presence of sodium by retaining fluid and thus increasing blood pressure

satiety state in which there is no longer a desire to eat; fullness

satiety value food's ability to satisfy feelings of hunger

saturated fats fats made up of compounds in which no further hydrogen bonding can occur; these are fats in solid form at room temperature; primarily animal fats

sclerotic changes thickening or hardening of tissues

screenings relatively superficial evaluations designed to identify deviations from normal

secondary bacterial infection bacterial infection that develops as a consequence of a primary infection

sediments fine particles of soil that are washed into a body of water, become suspended, and eventually settle to the bottom

self-actualization highest level of personality development; self-actualized people recognize their roles in life and use personal strengths to the fullest

self-care movement trend toward individuals taking increased responsibility for prevention or management of certain health conditions

self-esteem the quality of feeling good about yourself and your abilities

self-limiting capable of not progressing beyond a specific point; self-correcting

semen secretion containing sperm and nutrients discharged from the male urethra at ejaculation

sensory modalities vision, hearing, taste, touch, and smell; pathways for stimuli to register within the body

serum lipid analysis analysis of fat substances in the bloodstream; includes cholesterol and triglyceride measurements

set point genetically programmed range of body weight

sex flush reddish skin response that results from increasing sexual arousal

sex reassignment operation surgical procedure designed to remove the external genitalia and replace them with genitalia appropriate to the opposite gender

sexual fantasies fantasies with sexual themes; sexual daydreams or imaginary events

sexual harassment unwanted attention of a sexual nature that creates embarrassment or stress

sexual victimization sexual abuse of children, family members, or subordinates by a person in a position of power

sexuality the quality of being sexual; can

be viewed from many biological and psychosocial perspectives

sexually transmitted diseases (STDs) infectious diseases that are spread primarily through intimate sexual contact

shaft body of the penis

shingles viral infection affecting the nerve endings of the skin

shock profound collapse of many vital body functions; evident during acute alcohol intoxication and other serious health emergencies

sidestream smoke the smoke that comes from the burning end of a cigarette, pipe, or cigar

singlehood the state of not being married

six dimensions of health important areas of health in which specific strengths or limitations will be found: physical, emotional, social, intellectual, spiritual, and occupational

skinfold measurement measurement to determine the thickness of the fat layer that lies immediately beneath the skin

sliding scale method of payment by which patient fees are scaled according to income levels

smegma cellular discharge that can accumulate beneath the clitoral hood and the foreskin of an uncircumcised penis

smog air pollution composed of a combination of smoke, photochemical compounds, and fog

smokeless tobacco tobacco products (chewing tobacco and snuff) that are chewed or sucked rather than smoked

snuff finely shredded smokeless tobacco; used for dipping

spermatogenesis process of sperm production

spermicides chemicals capable of killing sperm

stalking a crime involving an assailant's planned efforts to pursue an intended victim

starch complex carbohydrate; a polysaccharide; a compound of long-chain glucose units

static stretching the slow lengthening of a muscle group to an extended level of stretch followed by holding the extended position for a recommended time period

sterilization generally permanent birth control techniques that surgically disrupt the normal passage of ova or sperm

stewardship acceptance of responsibility for the wise use and protection of the Earth's natural resources

stillborn baby that is dead at the time of birth

stimulants psychoactive drugs that stimulate the function of the central nervous system

stress physiological and psychological state of imbalance caused by the body's response to an unanticipated, disruptive, or stimulating event

stress test examination and analysis of heart-lung function while the body is undergoing physical exercise; generally accomplished when the client walks or runs on a treadmill device while being monitored by a cardiograph

stressors factors or events, real or imagined, that elicit a state of stress

subcutaneous fat fat layer immediately beneath the skin

sudden cardiac death immediate death resulting from a sudden change in the rhythm of the heart

surrogate parenting one of several arrangements in which a woman becomes pregnant and gives birth for an infertile couple

sustainable environment an environment capable of supporting habitation; made possible by the efforts of individuals, organizations, and all levels of government

sympto-thermal method method of periodic abstinence that combines the basal body temperature method and the cervical mucus method

synapse location at which an electrical impulse from one neuron is transmitted to an adjacent neuron

synergistic drug effect heightened, exaggerated effect produced by the concurrent use of two or more drugs

synesthesia perceptual process in which a stimulus produces a response from a different sensory modality

systolic pressure blood pressure against blood vessel walls when the heart contracts

------------------------- T -------------------------

tar particulate phase of tobacco smoke with nicotine and water removed

target heart rate (THR) number of times per minute that the heart must contract to produce a training effect

technical nurses registered nurses (RNs) who hold diplomas or associate degrees from schools of nursing or university nursing programs

teratogenic capable of producing birth defects

testes male reproductive structures that produce sperm and the gonadal hormone testosterone

testosterone male sex hormone that stimulates tissue development

thorax the chest; portion of the torso above the diaphragm and within the rib cage

titration determining a particular level of a drug within the body

tolerance an acquired reaction to a drug; continued intake of the same dose has diminished results

total person holistic view of the person, incorporating the dynamic interplay of physical, emotional, social, intellectual, spiritual, and occupational factors

toxic shock syndrome potentially fatal condition resulting from the proliferation of certain bacteria in the vagina, whose toxins enter the blood circulation

trace elements minerals whose presence in the body occurs in very small amounts; micronutrient elements

training effect significant positive effect that exercise has on the heart, lungs, and blood vessels

transcenders self-actualized people who have achieved a quality of being ordinarily associated with higher levels of spiritual growth

transcervical balloon tuboplasty the use of inflatable balloon catheters to open blocked fallopian tubes; a procedure used for some women with fertility problems

transient ischemic attack (TIA) temporary spasm of a cerebral artery that produces symptoms similar to those of a minor stroke; often a forewarning of a true cerebrovascular accident

transition the third and last phase of the first stage of labor; full dilation of the cervix

transsexualism the profound rejection of the gender to which the individual has been born

transvestism recurrent, persistent cross-dressing as a source of sexual excitement

trimester three-month period of time; human pregnancies encompass three trimesters

tropical oils oils extracted from coconut, palm, and palm kernel that contain much higher levels of saturated fat then other vegetable oils

tubal ligation sterilization procedure in which the fallopian tubes are cut and the ends tied back or cauterized

tumescence state of being swollen or enlarged

tumor mass of cells; may be cancerous (malignant) or noncancerous (benign)

type I alcoholism inherited predisposition supported by environmental factors favoring alcoholism

type II alcoholism male-limited alcoholism; an inherited form of alcoholism passed from father to son

------------------------- U -------------------------

unbalanced diet diet lacking adequate representation from each of the five food groups

underweight condition in which body weight is below desirable weight

unintentional injuries injuries that occur

without anyone's intending that harm be done

urethra   passageway through which urine leaves the urinary bladder

urethritis   infection of the urethra

V

vacuum aspiration   abortion procedure in which the cervix is dilated and vacuum pressure is used to remove the uterine contents

vaginal contraceptive film (VCF)   spermicide-containing film that clings to the cervical opening

variant   different from the statistical average

vas deferens   (pl. vasa deferentia) passageway through which sperm move from the epididymis to the ejaculatory duct

vascular system   body's blood vessels; arteries, arterioles, capillaries, venules, and veins

vasectomy   surgical procedure in which the vasa deferentia are cut to prevent the passage of sperm from the testicles; the most common form of male sterilization

vasocongestion   retention of blood within a particular tissue

vegan vegetarian diet   vegetarian diet that excludes the use of all animal products, including eggs and dairy products

very low-density lipoprotein (VLDL)   the type of lipoprotein that transports cholesterol and other lipid material from the liver into the bloodstream

vicariously formed stimuli   erotic stimuli that originate in one's imagination

virulent   capable of causing disease

vitamins   organic compounds that facilitate the action of enzymes

voyeurism   watching others undressing or engaging in sexual activities

vulval tissues   tissues surrounding the vaginal opening

W

warm-up   physical and mental preparation for exercise

wellness   a broadly based process used to achieve a highly developed level of health

will   legal document that describes how a person wishes his or her estate to be disposed of after death

withdrawal illness   uncomfortable, perhaps toxic response of the body as it attempts to maintain homeostasis in the absence of a drug; also called *abstinence syndrome*

work   movement of mass over distance

Y

yeast   single-cell plant responsible for the fermentation of plant products

young adult years   segment of the life cycle from ages 18 to 22; a transitional period between adolescence and adulthood

yo-yo syndrome   The repeated weight loss, followed by weight gain, experienced by many dieters

Z

zero tolerance laws   laws that severely restrict the right to drive for underage drinkers who have been convicted of driving under the influence of *any* alcohol

zoophilia   sexual contact with animals as a preferred source of sexual excitement; bestiality

EXAM PREP
Chapter 1   Shaping Your Health

MULTIPLE CHOICE

1. What health strategy involves following specific eating plans or exercise programs?
   A. Health screenings
   B. Education activities
   C. Behavior changes
   D. Regimentation

2. Why is it necessary to formulate an initial adult identity?
   A. So you can answer the question, "Who am I?"
   B. To have a productive and satisfying life
   C. It will help you move through other stages of development
   D. All of the above

3. Which developmental task involves using your own resources to follow a particular path?
   A. Forming an initial adult identity
   B. Assuming responsibility
   C. Establishing independence
   D. Developing social skills

4. Which of the following statements is *false?*
   A. The deeper the emotional relationships a person has, the better.
   B. Maintaining and improving your health is an important responsibility.
   C. The need to interact socially will at times negatively influence your health.
   D. Development of social skills can enhance your independence from your family.

5. What is *generativity?*
   A. The process of generating wealth and status in midlife
   B. The process of repaying society for its past support
   C. The negative attitude one generation holds for another
   D. None of the above

6. Which of the following are tasks for the elderly period of life?
   A. Accepting the physical decline of aging
   B. Maintaining high levels of physical function
   C. Establishing a sense of integrity
   D. All of the above

7. Which of the following is *not* a dimension of health?
   A. Transitional dimension of health
   B. Emotional dimension of health
   C. Holistic dimension of health
   D. Both A and C

8. Which dimension of health do some professionals believe to be the "core of wellness"?
   A. Emotional
   B. Spiritual
   C. Social
   D. Intellectual

9. Why is the occupational dimension of health important?
   A. Because you won't be happy unless you make a lot of money after graduation.
   B. Because both external and internal rewards from work affect your happiness.
   C. Because when people feel good about their work, they are more likely to live a healthier lifestyle.
   D. Both B and C

10. Which of the following is a strategy for changing your behavior?
    A. Make a personal contract to accomplish your goals.
    B. Go it alone; it is better not to involve family or friends.
    C. Don't reward yourself until you get to the final outcome.
    D. Don't let any obstacles occur or you will fail.

CRITICAL THINKING

1. What is health?

2. What is meant by the term *wellness?*

3. How does *empowerment* affect overall health and well-being?

4. Which dimensions of your health would you like to improve, and why?

5. How do you plan to successfully complete your developmental tasks?

Chapter 2   Achieving Emotional Maturity

MULTIPLE CHOICE

1. Emotionally well people:
   A. Experience the full range of human emotions, but are not overcome by them.
   B. Are only concerned with their own well-being.
   C. Set goals that are far and above what they can realistically accomplish.
   D. Trust only those who have proven their worth.

2. What factors shape self-esteem?
   A. Warm and supportive physical contact
   B. Religious indoctrination leading to guilt
   C. Failure to be successful in early undertakings
   D. All of the above

3. What three traits show a person's *hardiness?*
   A. Success, direction, and ability
   B. Commitment, control, and challenge
   C. Commitment, self-control, and self-esteem
   D. None of the above

4. Which of the following statements most accurately describes adults in midlife?
   A. Most experience a period of yearning for their youth called *midlife crisis.*
   B. Most experience a multitude of problems that fill them with melancholy and despair.
   C. Most have less to think about than they did when they were younger.
   D. Most see themselves as being in the prime of life.

5. Which of the following factors affects the quality of life of older adults?
   A. Sexual intimacy
   B. Marital status
   C. Economic status
   D. All of the above

6. What type of depression may occur after the death of a spouse or some other period of difficulty?
   A. Primary depression
   B. Reactive depression
   C. Chemically induced depression
   D. None of the above

7. Which is the most mature form of conflict resolution?
   A. Dialogue
   B. Submission
   C. Persuasion
   D. Aggression

8. What is the first step toward taking a proactive approach to life?
   A. Undertaking new experiences
   B. Taking risks
   C. Accepting mental pictures
   D. None of the above

9. Which of the following are motivational needs defined by Maslow?
   A. Physiological needs
   B. Economic needs
   C. Sexual needs
   D. Material needs

10. Which of the following statements describes creative individuals?
    A. They are intuitive and open to new experiences.
    B. They are less interested in detail than in meaning and implications.
    C. They are flexible.
    D. All of the above

CRITICAL THINKING

1. What is meant by a "normal range of emotions"?

2. What are some ways to overcome feelings of loneliness and shyness?

3. What are the warning signs of suicide, and how should they be treated?

4. What is the four-step process that allows one to control the outcomes of experiences and learn about one's emotional resources?

5. How do faith and spirituality affect emotional well-being?

Chapter 3   Managing Stress

MULTIPLE CHOICE

1. An event that produces stress is called a:
   A. Response
   B. Stressor
   C. Type B
   D. None of the above
2. Positive stress is called:
   A. Eustress
   B. Distress
   C. Type R stress
   D. None of the above
3. Which of the following is *not* a stage in Selye's general adaptation syndrome model?
   A. Alarm reaction stage
   B. Relaxation stage
   C. Resistance stage
   D. Exhaustion stage
4. Which part of the body is responsible for the interconnection between the nervous system and the endocrine system?
   A. Hypothalamus
   B. Pituitary gland
   C. Adrenal gland
   D. None of the above
5. When the body perceives stress, a number of responses are brought about by the epinephrine (adrenaline) and corticoids released. Which of the following is an expected response?
   A. Decreased cardiac and pulmonary function
   B. Increased digestive activity
   C. Decreased fat use
   D. Altered immune system response
6. PMR, or progressive muscular relaxation, is:
   A. A procedure of alternately contracting and relaxing muscle groups.

   B. A correct way of breathing, by relaxing the diaphragm.
   C. An Eastern relaxation technique that employs the use of a mantra.
   D. A form of self-hypnosis that costs between $250 to $400 to learn.
7. Which of the following diseases have some origin in unresolved stress?
   A. Irritable bowel syndrome
   B. Allergies
   C. Asthma
   D. All of the above
8. Which of the following personality traits fosters high levels of stress?
   A. Self-confidence and practicality
   B. Anger and cynicism
   C. Both A and B
   D. Neither A nor B
9. Stress is best described as:
   A. Something completely beyond your control.
   B. The leading cause of cynicism.
   C. A physical and emotional response to change.
   D. A realistic and positive outlook on life.
10. What three areas of the body prepare the body to respond to stressors?
    A. Circulatory system, lymphatic system, and brain
    B. Brain, nervous system, and endocrine system
    C. Brain, muscular tissue, and nervous system
    D. Heart, lungs, and brain

CRITICAL THINKING

1. What is stress? Give an example of a stressful situation and how the person might feel.

2. Can stress be positive? Give an example.

3. What physiological reactions occur in the body because of stress?

4. How can repeated stress, if not dealt with properly, affect long-term health?

5. What are some healthy ways to deal with stress? Which would you choose to adopt, and why?

Chapter 4   Becoming Physically Fit

MULTIPLE CHOICE

1. Which of the following is *not* a benefit of physical fitness?
   A. The person can engage in various tasks and leisure activities.
   B. Body systems function efficiently to resist disease.
   C. Body systems are healthy enough to respond to emergency (threatening) situations.
   D. All of the above are benefits.

2. Which of the following areas of physical fitness do exercise physiologists say is most important?
   A. Muscular strength
   B. Muscular endurance
   C. Cardiorespiratory endurance
   D. Flexibility

3. Anaerobic, or oxygen-deprived, energy production:
   A. Is the result of low-intensity activity.
   B. Is the result of short-duration activities that quickly cause muscle fatigue.
   C. Is the result of activities such as walking, distance jogging, and bicycle touring.
   D. None of the above

4. Which of the following types of training exercises are based on the *overload principle?*
   A. Isometric exercises
   B. Progressive resistance exercises
   C. Isokinetic exercises
   D. All of the above

5. Of the following statements, which accurately describes flexibility?
   A. It is relatively the same throughout your body.
   B. Not every joint in your body is equally flexible.
   C. Nothing alters the flexibility of a particular joint.
   D. Gender and age do not affect flexibility.

6. Which of the following statements is true about aging?
   A. Aging is predictable and the same for every person.

   B. The greatest change is in areas of the simplest function.
   C. Change often occurs suddenly and without warning.
   D. Two people of the same age may experience deterioration of different body systems.

7. The American College of Sports Medicine recommends five significant areas to consider for achievement of cardiorespiratory fitness. Which of these is *not* one of the areas?
   A. Mode of activity
   B. Frequency of training
   C. Intensity of training
   D. Popularity of activity

8. What is target heart rate (THR)?
   A. An intensity level of between 60% and 90% of maximum heart rate
   B. An intensity level of between 70% and 100% of maximum heart rate
   C. The maximum number of times your heart should contract each minute to give your respiratory system a work overload
   D. The rate at which you become so fatigued that you must stop exercising

9. What are the three basic parts of a good training session?
   A. Running, weightlifting, stretching
   B. Warm-up, workout, cooldown
   C. Warm-up, stretching, cooldown
   D. Mental warm-up, socialize, workout

10. Which of these is an abnormal sign to be aware of, during or after exercise?
    A. A delay of over 1 hour in your body's return to a fully relaxed, comfortable state after exercise
    B. Difficulty sleeping
    C. Noticeable breathing difficulties or chest pains
    D. All of the above

CRITICAL THINKING

1. What are the components of a well-designed fitness program for older adults?

2. How serious is low back pain, and what should a person do to alleviate or prevent it?

3. Explain what steps you would take to develop a cardiorespiratory fitness program, taking into account all five areas recommended by the American College of Sports Medicine.

4. Describe some of the newest trends in physical activity (such as rollerblading, water exercise, or "street jam"). Which most appeals to you, and why?

5. Why is steroid use dangerous?

Chapter 5   Understanding Nutrition and Your Diet

MULTIPLE CHOICE

1. What three nutrients provide the body with calories?
   A. Sugar, amino acids, and supplements
   B. Carbohydrates, fats, and proteins
   C. Tropical oils, food additives, and carbohydrates
   D. None of the above

2. Which of the following statements accurately describes carbohydrates?
   A. They occur in two forms only, depending on the number of proteins that make up the molecule.
   B. About 20% of our calories comes from carbohydrates.
   C. Carbohydrates are combinations of sugar units, or saccharides.
   D. Each gram of carbohydrate contains 400 calories.

3. Which of the following statements is *false*?
   A. Fats are important nutrients in our diets.
   B. Fats make it impossible for our bodies to absorb vitamins A, D, E, and K.
   C. Fat insulates our bodies, helping us retain heat.
   D. Most of the fat we eat is "hidden" in food.

4. What are vitamins?
   A. Inorganic materials necessary for tissue repair and disease prevention
   B. Pills that can be taken each morning to give the body energy all day
   C. Organic compounds that are required in small amounts for normal growth, reproduction, and maintenance of health
   D. Nutrients that provide more than half our body weight

5. Which of the following nutrients could the body not live without for over a week?
   A. Minerals
   B. Fiber
   C. Vitamins
   D. Water

6. Which of the following is a recommendation based on the USDA Food Guide Pyramid?
   A. Adults should eat two to four servings from the fruit group each day.
   B. Three to five servings from the vegetable group each day are recommended for an adult.
   C. Adults should consume two to three servings from the milk, yogurt, and cheese group each day.
   D. All of the above

7. What are phytochemicals?
   A. Physiologically active components that function as antioxidants and may deactivate carcinogens
   B. The additives used in foods that preserve freshness or enhance flavor, color, or texture
   C. The chemicals used to enrich breads and cereals
   D. None of the above

8. What kind of vegetarian eats milk products but not eggs?
   A. Ovolactovegetarian
   B. Macrobiotic vegetarian
   C. Lactovegetarian
   D. Vegan vegetarian

9. What factors may influence nutritional changes as a person ages?
   A. Changes to the structure and function of the body resulting from age
   B. The progressive lowering of the body's basal metabolism
   C. Both A and B
   D. Neither A nor B

10. Which of the following is a suggested step toward increasing the availability of food?
    A. Increase the yield of land under cultivation.
    B. Increase the amount of land under cultivation.
    C. Use water more efficiently for the production of food.
    D. All of the above

CRITICAL THINKING

1. Based on your personal assessment of your current diet, are you getting all the nutrients you need? In which areas do you need to improve?

2. What role does cholesterol play in the diet?

3. Explain the difference between *water-soluble* and *fat-soluble* vitamins and the characteristics of each.

4. Would you consider becoming a vegetarian? Why or why not?

5. What is *nutrient density?* Why is it important to consider this concept when making food choices?

Chapter 6 Maintaining a Healthy Weight

MULTIPLE CHOICE

1. Which weight measurement technique precisely measures relative amounts of fat and lean body mass by comparing underwater weight with out-of-water weight?
   A. Skinfold measurements
   B. Body mass index (BMI)
   C. Electrical impedance
   D. Hydrostatic weighing

2. Which may be the simplest method of determining a person's amount of body fat?
   A. Appearance
   B. Height-weight tables
   C. Body mass index (BMI)
   D. Waist-to-hip ratio

3. What influences obesity?
   A. Environment
   B. Genetics
   C. Both environment and genetics
   D. None of the above

4. Which area(s) within the hypothalamus tell the body when it should begin and end food consumption?
   A. Feeding and satiety centers
   B. Central nervous system (CNS)
   C. Thyroid and pituitary glands
   D. None of the above

5. Which of the following statements describes "brown fat"?
   A. It is located in small amounts in the upper back between the shoulder blades.
   B. There is a renewed interest in the study of it.
   C. It burns calories as heat without generating energy units that are stored in fat cells.
   D. All of the above

6. Which of Sheldon's three body types is characterized by a tall, slender build?
   A. Ectomorph
   B. Mesomorph
   C. Endomorph
   D. None of the above

7. What is hypercellular obesity?
   A. The increase of fat cells later in life as a result of being overfed in infancy or substantially gaining weight in childhood or adolescence
   B. When fat cells increase in size as a result of long-term positive caloric balance in adulthood
   C. Excessive fat around the waist, which can contribute to the onset of diabetes mellitus
   D. None of the above

8. What would most experts cite as the most important reason for the widespread problem of obesity?
   A. Family dietary practices
   B. Endocrine influence
   C. Infant feeding patterns
   D. None of the above

9. What is basal metabolic rate (BMR)?
   A. The rate of caloric intake to caloric output
   B. The minimum amount of energy the body requires to carry on all vital functions
   C. The rate of a food's thermic output
   D. None of the above

10. Which weight management technique involves the use of pharmaceuticals?
    A. Balanced diets supported by portion control
    B. Fad diets
    C. Hunger/satiety-influencing products
    D. Self-help weight reduction programs

CRITICAL THINKING

1. What factors influence your body image and self-concept?

2. What steps might you take to successfully control your weight throughout your lifetime?

3. Why is dieting alone not a good technique for achieving and maintaining weight loss?

4. What are reasons someone might develop anorexia nervosa or bulimia? How should a person be treated for the disorders?

5. What does it mean to exercise or eat compulsively?

Chapter 7   Choosing a Drug-Free Lifestyle

MULTIPLE CHOICE

1. Which of these is an aspect of addictive behavior?
   A. Exposure
   B. Compulsion
   C. Loss of control
   D. All of the above

2. What kind of drugs alter the user's feelings, behaviors, or moods?
   A. Medicines
   B. Over-the-counter drugs
   C. Psychoactive drugs
   D. Steroids

3. Which type of dependence creates *full* withdrawal symptoms when the drug use is stopped?
   A. Psychological
   B. Physical
   C. Cross-tolerant
   D. None of the above

4. What are neurotransmitters?
   A. Chemical messengers that transmit electrical impulses
   B. Organic messengers that transmit the chemicals in drugs directly to the brain
   C. Hallucinogenic drugs that are currently popular with college students
   D. None of the above

5. How do drugs "work"?
   A. By blocking the production of a neurotransmitter
   B. By forcing the continued release of a neurotransmitter
   C. Either A or B
   D. Neither A nor B

6. Which type of psychoactive drug *excites* the activity of the central nervous system (CNS)?
   A. Inhalants
   B. Hallucinogens
   C. Narcotics
   D. None of the above

7. What is "crack"?
   A. Powdered cocaine that is alkalized in benzene or ether and smoked through a waterpipe
   B. A small, rocklike crystalline material made from cocaine hydrochloride and baking soda
   C. A white powder that is snorted in "lines" through a rolled dollar bill or tube
   D. A pure form of methamphetamine that looks like rock candy

8. Which type of psychoactive drug *slows down* the function of the central nervous system (CNS)?
   A. Inhalants
   B. Hallucinogens
   C. Cannabis
   D. Depressants

9. What is THC?
   A. A hallucinogen derived from the peyote cactus plant
   B. A drug popular in the 1960s
   C. The active ingredient in marijuana
   D. A new "designer" drug

10. Which drugs are among the most dependence-producing?
    A. Inhalants
    B. Hallucinogens
    C. Depressants
    D. Narcotics

CRITICAL THINKING

1. What is the difference between drug *misuse* and drug *abuse?*

2. How has cocaine use affected poor urban areas?

3. What are possible long-term effects of marijuana use?

4. What is a synergistic effect, and why is it dangerous?

5. What do you think about the legalization of drugs and about drug testing?

Chapter 8   Taking Control of Alcohol Use

MULTIPLE CHOICE

1. What is *binge drinking?*
   A. The practice of drinking and then purging
   B. A harmless activity popular among college students
   C. The practice of consuming five drinks in a row, at least once during the previous 2-week period
   D. The practice of consuming two drinks in a row, at least once a day

2. What is the alcohol content of a bottle of 140-proof gin?
   A. 140% of the fluid in the bottle
   B. 70% of the fluid in the bottle
   C. 14% of the fluid in the bottle
   D. 1.4% of the fluid in the bottle

3. What type of drug is alcohol?
   A. Stimulant
   B. Hallucinogen
   C. Depressant
   D. Narcotic

4. What should be done with people who become unconscious resulting from alcohol consumption?
   A. They should be given a cold shower to wake them up.
   B. They should be made to drink coffee.
   C. They should be taken to bed and left undisturbed for several hours.
   D. They should be put on their side and monitored frequently.

5. Which of the following leading causes of accidental death has connections to alcohol use?
   A. Motor vehicle collisions
   B. Falls
   C. Drownings
   D. All of the above

6. Which of the following is a good guideline to follow for responsibly hosting a party?
   A. Make alcohol the primary entertainment, especially with a keg or other popular way to serve alcohol.
   B. Ridicule those who are too afraid to drink.
   C. If friends say they are just fine to drive home even though they have been drinking, let them go.
   D. None of the above

7. Which alcohol awareness group promotes responsible party hosting among university students?
   A. AA
   B. MADD
   C. BACCHUS
   D. SADD

8. What is the main difference between problem drinking and alcoholism?
   A. Problem drinkers stay away from hard liquor.
   B. Alcoholics usually don't engage in binge drinking.
   C. Alcoholism involves a physical addiction to alcohol.
   D. Problem drinking is easier to detect.

9. Which support group appeals to the children of alcoholics?
   A. Al-Anon
   B. AA
   C. Alateen
   D. MADD

10. Which new drug, approved by the FDA in 1995, is being used to treat alcoholism?
    A. Naltrexone
    B. Antabuse
    C. Heroin
    D. Maltodextrine

CRITICAL THINKING

1. Why do people drink alcohol?

2. What physiological differences in women make them more susceptible to the effects of alcohol?

3. What are the possible effects of drinking alcohol while pregnant?

4. What role does alcohol use play in violent crime, family violence, and suicide?

5. Explain *denial, enabling,* and *codependence* as they occur with alcoholism.

Chapter 9   Rejecting Tobacco Use

MULTIPLE CHOICE

1. Which factor most affects a person's decision to smoke?
   A. Gender
   B. Age
   C. Education
   D. Race

2. What are psychosocial factors of tobacco dependence?
   A. Manipulation
   B. Advertising
   C. Modeling
   D. Both A and C

3. What consumer group is the FDA focusing its education efforts on to discourage increased tobacco use?
   A. Women
   B. African-American men who attend predominately black universities
   C. Teens
   D. Older adults who began smoking before health risks were known

4. Which phase of tobacco use includes nicotine, water, and a variety of powerful chemical compounds known collectively as *tar*?
   A. Active phase
   B. Particulate phase
   C. Gaseous phase
   D. Nicotine phase

5. What signals the beginning of lung cancer?
   A. Changes in the basal cell layer resulting from constant irritation by accumulating tar in the airways
   B. An inability to breathe normally
   C. A "smoker's cough"
   D. Mucus swept up to the throat by cilia, where it is swallowed and removed through the digestive system

6. What is COLD?
   A. Chronic obstructive lung disease
   B. A chronic disease in which air flow in and out of the lungs becomes progressively limited
   C. A disease state made up of chronic bronchitis and pulmonary emphysema
   D. All of the above

7. Which of the following statements is *false?*
   A. It is strongly recommended that women who smoke not use oral contraceptives.
   B. Chewing tobacco and snuff generate blood levels of nicotine in amounts equivalent to those seen in cigarette smokers.
   C. Contrary to some claims, second-hand smoke is not a serious health threat.
   D. Children of parents who smoke are twice as likely to develop bronchitis or pneumonia during the first year of life.

8. Which of the following statements is *true?*
   A. Chewing tobacco is a safe alternative to smoking.
   B. Sidestream smoke makes up only 15% of our exposure to involuntary smoking.
   C. Spouses of smokers may have a 30% greater risk of lung cancer.
   D. The only effective way to quit smoking is to go "cold turkey."

9. Which is more effective as a means of quitting smoking?
   A. Nicotine-containing chewing gum
   B. Transdermal patch
   C. Neither A nor B work
   D. Both A and B are equally effective

10. What is the main debate concerning smoking today?
    A. The validity of health warnings
    B. The rights of the nonsmoker vs. the rights of the smoker
    C. The rights of young adults to buy cigarettes
    D. None of the above

CRITICAL THINKING

1. What advertising tactics do tobacco companies use to offset the potential decline in sales from reports of health risks?

2. In what ways is tobacco addictive?

3. How does smoking adversely affect health?

4. Why should a pregnant or breastfeeding woman refrain from smoking?

5. Do you think smoking should continue to be banned from public places? Why or why not?

Chapter 10   Reducing Your Risk of Cardiovascular Disease

MULTIPLE CHOICE

1. Why has the rate of death caused by cardiovascular disease declined?
   A. Changing American lifestyles
   B. Medical advances in diagnosis and treatment
   C. A breakthrough new drug
   D. Both A and B
2. What is the nation's number one "killer"?
   A. AIDS
   B. Lung disease
   C. Cancer
   D. Cardiovascular disease
3. Which of the following is a function of the blood?
   A. Regulation of water content of body cells and fluids
   B. Transportation of nutrients, oxygen, wastes, and hormones
   C. Buffering to help maintain appropriate pH balance
   D. All of the above
4. What are three cardiovascular risk factors that cannot be changed?
   A. Age, gender, body composition
   B. Heredity, weight, glandular production
   C. Age, heredity, and metabolism
   D. None of the above
5. What is a risk factor that can be changed?
   A. Cigarette/tobacco use
   B. Physical inactivity
   C. High blood pressure
   D. All of the above
6. Which disease predisposes people to developing heart disease?
   A. Cancer
   B. Epilepsy
   C. Diabetes
   D. Multiple sclerosis
7. Which form of cardiovascular disease involves damage to the vessels that supply blood to the heart muscle?
   A. Hypertension
   B. Stroke
   C. Coronary heart disease
   D. Congenital heart disease
8. What is cholesterol?
   A. The oil used to fry food
   B. A soft, fatlike material manufactured by the body
   C. A material necessary for reproduction of blood
   D. None of the above
9. What is hypertension?
   A. A consistently elevated blood pressure
   B. Stress on arterial walls resulting from plaque build-up
   C. The tendency for blood to clot
   D. Abnormally low blood pressure
10. What is the name of the cardiovascular disease that begins as a streptococcal infection of the throat?
    A. Peripheral artery disease
    B. Rheumatic heart disease
    C. Phlebitis
    D. Congestive heart failure

CRITICAL THINKING

1. What components make up the cardiovascular system? How does the system work?

2. Do you exhibit any risk factors for cardiovascular disease? What steps can you take to change them, if they can be changed?

3. What is the difference between HDLs and LDLs?

4. How can hypertension be prevented?

5. What are the different causes of stroke?

Chapter 11   Living with Cancer and Chronic Conditions

MULTIPLE CHOICE

1. What happens to cells that leads to cancer?
   A. Their normal behavior ceases.
   B. They become severely dysfunctional.
   C. Neither A nor B
   D. Both A and B

2. What are protooncogenes?
   A. Genes that repair damaged cells
   B. Genes that suppress the immune system
   C. Genes that have the potential to become cancerous
   D. Abnormal genes

3. What is the Human Genome Project?
   A. The testing of new cancer-fighting drugs
   B. A scientific study of genes
   C. A secret military project that exposed World War II troops to carcinogens
   D. The study of cancer-producing viruses

4. Which type of cancer is found in cells of the blood and blood-forming tissues?
   A. Lymphoma
   B. Neuroblastoma
   C. Carcinoma
   D. Leukemia

5. Which is the most common site of the body to develop cancer in women?
   A. Breast
   B. Uterus
   C. Lung
   D. Skin

6. Which test greatly improves the chances of preventing cervical cancer?

   A. Mammography
   B. MRI
   C. Pap test
   D. Biopsy

7. Which type of cancer is referred to as the "silent" cancer because of its vague symptoms?
   A. Ovarian
   B. Prostate
   C. Vaginal
   D. Lung

8. Which traditional method of cancer treatment has had many successful advances in recent years?
   A. Surgery
   B. Chiropractic manipulation
   C. Chemotherapy
   D. Radiation

9. Which chronic disease most often appears in early adulthood and continues intermittently for the next 20 to 25 years?
   A. Diabetes mellitus
   B. Lupus
   C. Multiple sclerosis
   D. Asthma

10. Which type of asthma is caused by stress or as a consequence of frequent respiratory tract infections?
    A. Extrinsic
    B. Intrinsic
    C. EIA
    D. Childhood-onset asthma

CRITICAL THINKING

1. What social and environmental factors contribute to the onset of cancer?

2. What steps can women take to prevent cancer or to detect the early stages of cancer?

3. What steps can men take to prevent cancer or to detect the early stages of cancer?

4. What are the seven warning signs of cancer?

5. What are the differences and similarities between insulin-dependent and non–insulin-dependent diabetes?

Chapter 12   Preventing Infectious Diseases

MULTIPLE CHOICE

1. What is a pathogen?
   A. A disease-causing agent
   B. A virus, bacterium, or fungus
   C. Neither A nor B
   D. Both A and B
2. What is the function of a reservoir in the chain of infection?
   A. To cause disease
   B. To offer a favorable environment in which an infectious agent can thrive
   C. To act as a portal of exit
   D. To transmit the agent from person to person
3. Which term describes insects, animals, or birds that carry diseases from human to human?
   A. Vectors
   B. Pathogens
   C. Reservoirs
   D. Agents
4. During which of the following stages of infection is the infected person *most* contagious?
   A. Prodromal stage
   B. Clinical stage
   C. Decline stage
   D. Incubation stage
5. Which type of immunity is the result of vaccination or immunization?
   A. Naturally acquired immunity
   B. Artificially acquired immunity
   C. Passively acquired immunity
   D. None of the above
6. Which viral infection has mental fatigue and depression as side effects?
   A. Influenza
   B. Common cold
   C. Mononucleosis
   D. Pneumonia
7. What is chronic fatigue syndrome (CFS)?
   A. A mononucleosis-like condition most commonly seen in women in their thirties and forties
   B. A condition that may be linked to neurally mediated hypotension
   C. A condition that may be a psychological disorder
   D. All of the above
8. How is Lyme disease transmitted?
   A. Through droplet spread
   B. Through fecal-oral spread
   C. Through the deer tick nymph
   D. Through inhalation
9. Which sexually transmitted disease occurs as blisterlike lesions on the genitals or lips?
   A. Herpes simplex
   B. Gonorrhea
   C. Syphilis
   D. Human papillomavirus
10. Of the following STDs, which has no cure?
    A. Vaginal infections
    B. Cystitis and urethritis
    C. Herpes simplex
    D. Gonorrhea

CRITICAL THINKING

1. What are the two main components to the body's protective defense? How do they work?

2. Why do the elderly and people with additional health complications need to take extra precaution to avoid contracting influenza?

3. Why should people pay close attention to their immunization history, especially college students?

4. What precautions should women take when using tampons to avoid toxic shock syndrome?

5. How is AIDS transmitted, and what precautions can be taken to avoid contracting it?

Chapter 13   Understanding Sexuality

MULTIPLE CHOICE

1. Which basis for biological sexuality refers to the growing embryo's development of gonads?
   A. Genetic
   B. Gonadal
   C. Structural
   D. None of the above

2. At which age are typical children able to correctly identify their gender?
   A. 4 years
   B. 2 years
   C. 18 months
   D. 6 months

3. What part of the testis produces sperm?
   A. Seminiferous tubules
   B. Scrotum
   C. Epididymis
   D. Interstitial cells

4. Which is the most sensitive part of the female body?
   A. Mons pubis
   B. Vagina
   C. Clitoris
   D. Prepuce

5. During which phase of the menstrual cycle does ovulation occur?
   A. Menstrual
   B. Proliferative
   C. Secretory
   D. None of the above

6. Which phase of the sexual response pattern prevents men from having multiple orgasms?
   A. Excitement
   B. Plateau
   C. Orgasmic
   D. Refractory

7. Which of the following statements is not true about celibacy?
   A. Celibate people may have intimate relationships without sex.
   B. It is defined as the self-imposed avoidance of sexual contact.
   C. Psychological complications often result from a celibate lifestyle.
   D. All are true.

8. Which type of oral-genital stimulation involves kissing and licking the vulva of the female?
   A. Foreplay
   B. Fellatio
   C. Cunnilingus
   D. None of the above

9. Which type of love is enduring and capable of sustaining long-term mutual growth?
   A. Infatuation
   B. Passionate love
   C. Companionate love
   D. Devotional love

10. Which of the following statements is not true of cohabitation?
    A. It is an alternative to marriage.
    B. It can sometimes exist between people sharing a platonic relationship.
    C. Approximately half of all cohabiting couples will disband.
    D. Couples who cohabit are more likely to get married than those in a more traditional dating relationship.

CRITICAL THINKING

1. How do biological and psychosocial factors contribute to the complex expression of our sexuality?

2. How has a blending of feminine and masculine qualities benefitted society?

3. Why might the "withdrawal" method of contraception not work?

4. What changes, both physiological and psychological, might menopause create in a woman's life?

5. What effect does the aging process have on the sexual response pattern?

Chapter 14   Managing Your Fertility

MULTIPLE CHOICE

1. Which form of birth control *does not* prevent STDs?
   A. Withdrawal
   B. Calendar method
   C. IUD
   D. All of the above

2. Which two forms of birth control, when used together, provide a high degree of contraceptive protection *and* disease control?
   A. IUD and spermicides
   B. Spermicides and condoms
   C. Calendar method and spermicides
   D. Oral contraceptive and spermicides

3. Which of the following statements is *not* true of oral contraceptives?
   A. The use of antibiotics lowers their contraceptive effectiveness.
   B. They regulate a woman's menstrual cycle.
   C. The user may experience more frequent vaginal infections, weight gain, mild headaches, and mild depression.
   D. They are useful in the prevention of STDs.

4. What are "minipills"?
   A. Smaller versions of the regular oral contraceptive that can be swallowed more easily
   B. The placebo pills taken between cycles
   C. Oral contraceptives that contain no estrogen— only low-dose progesterone
   D. Less expensive versions of the pill that are slightly less effective

5. What is Depo-Provera?
   A. An injectable contraceptive
   B. A subdermal implant contraceptive
   C. A type of diaphragm
   D. A brand of oral contraceptive

6. Which type of abortion is performed in the earliest stages of the first trimester?

A. Menstrual extraction
B. Dilation and curettage
C. Dilation and evacuation
D. Hypertonic saline procedure

7. What is RU-486?
   A. The "morning after" pill
   B. The process of using prostaglandin to influence muscle contractions that expel uterine contents
   C. A hypertonic saline solution
   D. A drug that blocks the action of progesterone, thus producing an early abortion

8. What is the first thing a parent should do on arriving home?
   A. Collapse in front of the television.
   B. Hug or hold his or her young children for at least a few minutes.
   C. Begin making dinner.
   D. Encourage children to do their chores.

9. Which of the following is an obstacle to pregnancy?
   A. 200 to 500 million sperm cells are deposited in each ejaculation.
   B. Sperm cells are capable of moving quickly.
   C. The acidic level of the vagina is destructive to sperm.
   D. Once inside the fallopian tubes, sperm can live for days.

10. Which type of artificial fertilization involves transferring fertilized ova from a laboratory dish into the fallopian tubes?
    A. In vitro fertilization and embryo transfer (IVF-ET)
    B. Gamete intrafallopian transfer (GIFT)
    C. Zygote intrafallopian transfer (ZIFT)
    D. Surrogate parenting

CRITICAL THINKING

1. What factors should you consider when choosing a method of birth control?

2. Which of the available methods of birth control would you be most likely to use, if you needed to?

3. What are the guidelines set forth under *Roe v. Wade*, the landmark 1973 Supreme Court case?

4. What serious questions need to be considered before deciding to have children?

5. Describe the birth process from beginning to end.

Chapter 15   Making Consumer and Health Care Choices

MULTIPLE CHOICE

1. Which of the following statements is *false?*
   A. The accuracy of health information from friends and family members may be questionable.
   B. The mass media routinely supply public service messages that give valuable health-related information.
   C. Never trust the labels and directions on prescription medication; it is usually misleading and intended to make you buy more of the product.
   D. Folk wisdom is on occasion supported by scientific evidence.

2. Which health resource has the most effective way of distributing information to the public by mail?
   A. On-line computer services
   B. Voluntary health agencies
   C. Government agencies
   D. Qualified health educators

3. What is the difference between allopathy and osteopathy?
   A. Osteopaths engage in quackery.
   B. Allopathic physicians are board-certified; osteopaths are not.
   C. Osteopaths perceive themselves as being more holistic.
   D. Only osteopaths function as primary care physicians.

4. Which type of health care professional provides services relating to understanding behavior patterns or perceptions but does not dispense drugs?
   A. Dentist
   B. Psychiatrist
   C. Podiatrist
   D. Psychologist

5. What does an optician do?
   A. Specializes in vision problems due to refractory errors
   B. Provides prescriptions for eyewear products
   C. Grinds lenses according to a precise prescription
   D. Specializes in vision care with a base in general medicine

6. What type of nursing position is helping to provide communities with additional primary care providers?
   A. Nurse practitioner
   B. Registered nurse
   C. Licensed practical nurse
   D. Technical nurse

7. The established amount that the insuree must pay before the insurer reimburses for services is:
   A. Fixed indemnity
   B. Coinsurance
   C. Deductible
   D. Exclusion

8. What are Medicare and Medicaid?
   A. Preferred provider organizations (PPOs)
   B. Independent practice associations (IPAs)
   C. Health maintenance organizations (HMOs)
   D. Forms of governmental insurance

9. Which is the most frequently prescribed drug in the United States?
   A. Prozac (for depression)
   B. Vasotec (for high blood pressure)
   C. Mevacor (for high cholesterol)
   D. Zantac (for ulcers)

10. Which of the following is a sign of quackery?
    A. Makes promises of quick, dramatic, painless, or drugless treatment
    B. Claims a product provides treatment for multiple illnesses
    C. States that the treatment is secret or not yet available in this country
    D. All of the above

CRITICAL THINKING

1. What are some pros and cons of obtaining health information from mass media?

2. What are some sources of health information available to you?

3. What are some alternative health care practices? Would you be willing to try them?

4. How can self-care benefit both individuals and the health care industry as a whole?

5. What are the advantages and disadvantages of HMOs?

Chapter 16   Protecting Your Safety

MULTIPLE CHOICE

1. Which form of violence received national attention because of the deaths in 1994 of Nicole Brown Simpson and Ronald Goldman?
   A. Child abuse
   B. Carjacking
   C. Domestic violence
   D. Elder abuse

2. Who is most often a victim of partner abuse?
   A. Prostitutes
   B. Teenage girls
   C. Spouses or former spouses of the assailant
   D. Men

3. Which form of child abuse occurs most frequently?
   A. Neglect
   B. Physical
   C. Psychological
   D. Sexual

4. What may be the "single greatest crime problem in America today"?
   A. Youth violence
   B. Hate crimes
   C. Bank robberies
   D. Organized crime

5. Aside from the physical harm of rape, what other effects may occur?
   A. Posttraumatic stress syndrome
   B. Guilt
   C. Emotional damage resulting from "broken trust"
   D. All of the above

6. Which of the following constitutes sexual harassment?
   A. Excessive pressure for dates

   B. Sexually explicit humor
   C. Unwanted physical contact
   D. All of the above

7. Which of the following can help increase safety around your home?
   A. Make sure your name is spelled correctly in the phone book.
   B. Try to live in apartments on the first floor.
   C. Require repair people to show valid identification.
   D. Leave windows unlocked in case you need to escape in a hurry.

8. Over half of all murders result from:
   A. Random crime
   B. Domestic abuse
   C. Arguments between acquaintances or relatives
   D. None of the above

9. Which of the following profiles is a most likely candidate for death by motor vehicle accident?
   A. Male, 55–65 years of age, driving in rainy conditions on a weekend afternoon
   B. Female, 35–45 years of age, driving on a freeway with the noise of children playing in the back seat
   C. Female, 65–75 years of age, driving in rush-hour traffic
   D. Male, 15–25 years of age, driving on a two-lane rural road on a Saturday night

10. Which of the following resources will help improve your safety on campus?
    A. University-approved escorts
    B. Campus security departments
    C. Campus counseling center
    D. All of the above

CRITICAL THINKING

1. What factors may have contributed to a drop in U.S. homicide rates?

2. How should suspected child abuse be properly handled?

3. What is rape? What is acquaintance rape? What is date rape?

4. How can you increase your personal safety?

5. What steps can you take to protect children and the elderly?

Chapter 17 Controlling Environmental Influences

MULTIPLE CHOICE

1. Each year, the population of the world grows by:
   A. 90 million people
   B. 90,000 people
   C. 90%
   D. 90 billion people

2. What is the leading source of air pollution?
   A. Kuwait oil fires
   B. Chemical production plants
   C. Internal combustion engines
   D. Coal-fired power plants

3. What has caused the greenhouse effect?
   A. A progressive increase in carbon dioxide in the atmosphere
   B. A hole in the ozone layer
   C. A slight warming of the Earth's surface
   D. All of the above

4. What substances produce acid rain when they combine with moisture in the atmosphere?
   A. Coal and hydrogen
   B. Hydrocarbons and particulate matter
   C. Chlorofluorocarbons
   D. Nitrogen and sulfur

5. Which type of pollution disproportionately affects children of low-income families?
   A. Radon gas
   B. Lead
   C. Subsidence inversion
   D. Radiation inversion

6. What is eutrophication?
   A. A biological imbalance that causes fish to die in great numbers from lack of oxygen
   B. The overabundance of aquatic plants that results when water is rich in nitrates and phosphates
   C. Both A and B
   D. Neither A nor B

7. Which of the following is the name of a hydrocarbon found in the water supply that has been linked to cancer?
   A. Chlorine
   B. PCB
   C. DDT
   D. EPA

8. Which of the following sources of water pollution comes from power plants?
   A. Oil spills
   B. Thermal pollution
   C. Sediments
   D. None of the above

9. Which type of solid waste disposal is discouraged or illegal in many urban areas?
   A. Ocean dumping
   B. Incineration
   C. Sanitary landfill
   D. Open dumping

10. Which of the following devices generates electro-magnetic fields?
    A. Water bed heater
    B. Electric razor
    C. Cellular phone
    D. All of the above

CRITICAL THINKING

1. How do different types of air pollution adversely affect us?

2. Why are metals, such as mercury, arsenic, and copper, particularly dangerous when they pollute our water supply?

3. What factors have kept recycling from being fully adopted in many areas?

4. What are some concerns related to nuclear energy?

5. What steps can you take to improve your environment and reduce your exposure to harmful environmental pollutants?

Chapter 18   Accepting Dying and Death

MULTIPLE CHOICE

1. Which of the following is a criterion by which death may be determined?
   A. Lack of heartbeat and breathing
   B. Lack of central nervous system function
   C. Presence of rigor mortis
   D. All of the above

2. Which type of euthanasia is illegal in the United States?
   A. Direct euthanasia
   B. Indirect euthanasia
   C. Both A and B
   D. Neither A nor B

3. What does the physician's order "DNR" stand for?
   A. Death not recorded
   B. Do not resuscitate
   C. Do not release
   D. Do not recognize

4. Which psychological stage for dying people serves as the earliest temporary defense mechanism?
   A. Denial
   B. Anger
   C. Bargaining
   D. None of the above

5. Which of the following describes the appropriate way to act toward someone who is dying?
   A. Refrain from crying so as not to upset them
   B. Remain optimistic even when there is no hope for recovery
   C. Try to be genuine and honest
   D. Try to distract the person from talking about death

6. Adults coping with the death of a child should:
   A. Have another child and name that child after the deceased.
   B. Move to a different home for a change of environment.
   C. Give themselves time and space to grieve.
   D. All of the above

7. Which of the following is *not* a normal, healthy expression of grief over the loss of a loved one?
   A. Physical discomfort
   B. Sense of numbness
   C. Guilt
   D. Extreme hostility

8. How long do periods of grief usually last?
   A. A few weeks
   B. 2 to 5 years
   C. A few months to a year
   D. 10 years or more

9. What is a wake?
   A. An established time for friends and family to share emotions and experiences about the deceased
   B. A formaldehyde-based fluid used to replace blood components during embalming
   C. A container for ashes from cremation
   D. None of the above

10. Which of the following is the word for a notice of death printed in a newspaper?
    A. Eulogy
    B. Epitaph
    C. Obituary notice
    D. None of the above

CRITICAL THINKING

1. What are living wills and durable power of attorney documents? Why would it be prudent to have these documents?

2. How do the emotional stages of dying described by Elisabeth Kübler-Ross affect those close to the dying person?

3. Describe what might occur during an out-of-body experience.

4. How does a hospice differ from a traditional hospital with respect to care of the terminally ill?

5. In what ways do death rituals aid people in dealing with death?

ANSWERS

Chapter 1
1. C; 2. D; 3. C; 4. A; 5. B; 6. D; 7. D;
8. B; 9. D; 10. A

Chapter 2
1. A; 2. D; 3. B; 4. D; 5. D; 6. B; 7. A;
8. D-Constructing mental pictures is the answer;
9. A; 10. D

Chapter 3
1. B; 2. A; 3. B; 4. A; 5. D; 6. A; 7. D;
8. B; 9. C; 10. B

Chapter 4
1. D; 2. C; 3. B; 4. D; 5. B; 6. D; 7. D;
8. A; 9. B; 10. D

Chapter 5
1. B; 2. C; 3. B; 4. C; 5. D; 6. D; 7. A;
8. C; 9. C; 10. D

Chapter 6
1. D; 2. A; 3. C; 4. A; 5. D; 6. A; 7. A;
8. D-Inactivity is the answer; 9. B; 10. C

Chapter 7
1. D; 2. C; 3. B; 4. A; 5. C; 6. D-Stimulants
is the answer; 7. B; 8. D; 9. C; 10. D

Chapter 8
1. C; 2. B; 3. C; 4. D; 5. D; 6. D; 7. C;
8. C; 9. C; 10. A

Chapter 9
1. C; 2. D; 3. C; 4. B; 5. A; 6. D; 7. C;
8. C; 9. A; 10. B

Chapter 10
1. D; 2. D; 3. D; 4. D-Age, gender, and heredity
is the answer; 5. D; 6. C; 7. C; 8. B; 9. A;
10. B

Chapter 11
1. D; 2. C; 3. B; 4. D; 5. C; 6. C; 7. A;
8. C; 9. C; 10. B

Chapter 12
1. C; 2. B; 3. A; 4. B; 5. B; 6. C; 7. D;
8. C; 9. A; 10. C

Chapter 13
1. B; 2. C; 3. A; 4. C; 5. B; 6. D; 7. C;
8. C; 9. C; 10. D

Chapter 14
1. D; 2. B; 3. D; 4. C; 5. A; 6. A; 7. D;
8. B; 9. C; 10. C

Chapter 15
1. C; 2. C; 3. C; 4. D; 5. C; 6. A; 7. C;
8. D; 9. D; 10. D

Chapter 16
1. C; 2. C; 3. A; 4. A; 5. D; 6. D; 7. C;
8. C; 9. D; 10. D

Chapter 17
1. A; 2. C; 3. A; 4. D; 5. B; 6. B; 7. B;
8. B; 9. D; 10. D

Chapter 18
1. D; 2. A; 3. B; 4. A; 5. C; 6. C; 7. D;
8. C; 9. A; 10. C

Credits

Chapter 1: p. 2 (Star Box), Source: Guyton R, et al: College students and national health objectives for the year 2000: a summary report, *Journal of American College Health* July 1989, 38:9-14; **p. 2 (Table 1-1),** From National Center for Health Statistics: *Monthly Vital Statistics Report* 44:1, July 20, 1995, pp. 17-18, Hyattsville, MD, United States Public Health Service, for the 12-month period ending December 1994; **p. 4 (Star Box),** Source: *Healthy People 2000: Midcourse Review and 1995 Revisions,* Department of Health and Human Services, Washington, DC, 1996.

Chapter 2: p. 26, From Study Guide and Personal Explorations for *Psychology applied to modern life: adjustment in the 80s,* by Wayne Weiten. Copyright © 1983 by Wadsworth, Inc. Reprinted by permission of Brooks/Cole Publishing, Pacific Grove, CA 93950; **p. 29 (Star Box),** From Depression is a sign of illness, not a sign of weakness, *Ball State University Campus Update* Dec 12, 1988, p. 1; **p. 31 (Star Box),** From Blumenthal SJ: Suicide: a guide to risk factors: assessment and treatment of suicidal patients, *Medical Clinics of North America* 72:937-971, 1988; **p. 36 (Figure 2-2),** "HIERARCHY OF NEEDS" from MOTIVATION AND PERSONALITY, 3RD ED. by ABRAHAM H. MASLOW. Revised by Robert Frager, James Fadiman, Cynthia McReynolds, and Ruth Cox. Copyright 1954, © 1987, Harper and Row, Publishers, Inc. Copyright © 1970 by Abraham H. Maslow. Reprinted by permission of HarperCollins Publishers, Inc.

Chapter 3: p. 45, Modified from Holmes TH and Rahe RH: The social adjustment rating scale, *Journal of Psychosomatic Research* 11:213-218, 1967; **p. 46,** Modified from an inventory developed by Rosellen Bohlen, University of Scranton; **p. 61,** *Dilbert* © 1996, United Feature Syndicate.

Chapter 4: p. 67 (Health Action Guide), Source: Dr. Steven Blair, Director of Epidemiology at the Aerobics Institute, Dallas, and author of *Living with exercise,* American Health Publishing Co., 1991; **pp. 69, 77 (Star Boxes),** From Prentice WE: *Fitness for college and life,* ed 4, St Louis, 1994, Mosby; **pp. 74-75,** Data from the National Fitness Foundation; **p. 84,** Copyright 1987, *USA Today,* excerpted with permission, art by Donald O'Connor; **pp. 85-86 (Star Boxes),** Copyright 1986, *USA Today,* excerpted with permission, art by Donald O'Connor.

Chapter 5: pp. 95-96, From *Nutrition for a healthy life,* courtesy of Marcy Leeds; **p. 98 (Figure 5-1),** Adapted from Procter & Gamble, 1989; **pp. 100-106, 109 (Tables 5-1, 5-2, 5-3, 5-4, 5-6),** From Wardlaw G, Insel P: *Perspectives in nutrition,* ed 3, St Louis, 1996, Mosby; **pp. 106-108 (Table 5-5),** Modified from Food and Nutrition Board, National Research Council: *Recommended dietary allowances,* ed 10, Washington, DC, 1989, National Academy of Sciences; **p. 108 (Figure 5-2),** US Department of Agriculture/US Department of Health and Human Services, August, 1992; **pp. 112-113 (Star Box),** Modified from Hegarty V: *Decisions in nutrition,* St Louis, 1988, Mosby; 132-133; **pp. 115-116 (Figure 5-3, A-B),** Source: Food and Drug Administration, and Wardlaw G, Insel P: *Perspectives in nutrition,* ed 3, St Louis, 1996, Mosby; **pp. 117 (Health Action Guide) 118 (Table 5-7),** US Department of Health and Human Services, Pub-

lic Health Service: *The Surgeon General's report on nutrition and health,* Washington, DC, 1988, US Government Printing Office; **p. 110,** Data on four food groups from Guthrie H: *Introductory nutrition,* ed 7, St Louis, 1989, Mosby; **p. 117 (Star Box),** From *Nutrition and your health: dietary guidelines for Americans,* ed 4, 1995, USDA, Home & Garden Bulletin no. 232; **p. 119 (Health Action Guide),** © 1986, American Diabetic Association. HEALTH FOOD CHOICES, used with permission; **p. 120 (Figure 5-5),** National Dairy Council, Rosemont, IL.

Chapter 6: p. 128 (Star Box), C. Everett Koop Foundation, American Diabetes Association; **p. 129 (Table 6-1),** Reprinted with permission of Metropolitan Life Insurance Company; **p. 130 (Table 6-2),** US Department of Agriculture; **p. 131 (Figure 6-1),** Modified from George A. Bray; **p. 137 (Table 6-4),** Based on data from Bannister EW, Brown SR: The relative energy requirements of physical activity. In HB Falls, editor: *Exercise Physiology,* New York, 1968, Academic Press Inc; Howley ET, Glover ME: The caloric costs of running and walking a mile for men and women, *Medicine and Science in Sports* 6:235, 1974; and Passmore R, Durnin JVGA: Human energy expenditure, *Physiological Reviews* 35:801, 1955; **p. 140,** Modified from Foreyt J, Goodrick GK: *Living without dieting,* Houston: Harrison Publishing; **p. 141 (Health Action Guide),** © 1987, *USA Today,* excerpted with permission; **pp. 142-143 (Table 6-5),** Adapted from Guthrie H: *Introductory nutrition,* ed 7, St Louis, 1989, Mosby, pp. 226-227.

Chapter 7: p. 155 (Figure 7-1), Source: National Institute on Drug Abuse, 1990 survey; **p. 158 (Star Box),** Source: Interagency Drug Alcohol Council: Why people use drugs, Ft Wayne, IN, The Council; **p. 161 (Table 7-1),** Modified from Muncie Star © 1987. Reprinted with permission; **p. 162 (Table 7-2),** Sources: C Lecos: The latest caffeine scoreboard, *FDA Consumer,* March 1984, p. 14; Measuring your life with coffee spoons, *Tufts University Diet and Nutrition Letter,* April 1984, pp. 3-6; and Expert Panel on Food Safety and Nutrition, Institute of Food Technologists: Evaluation of caffeine safety, from the Institute of Food Technologists, 221 N. LaSalle Street, Chicago, IL 60601, 1986; **p. 163 (Figure 7-2),** Source: American Management Association Survey.

Chapter 8: p. 182 (Table 8-1), US Department of Health and Human Services: Alcohol and health: fourth special report to the US Congress, Washington, DC, 1981, DHS Pub No ADM 81-1080; **p. 183 (Figures 8-1 and 8-2),** Source: Presley CA, Melman, PW: *Alcohol and drugs on American college campuses: a report to college presidents,* June 1992, US Department of Education, Drug Prevention in Higher Education Program, (FIPSE Grant), Southern Illinois University Student Health Program Wellness Center; **p. 184 (Table 8-2),** US Department of Transportation, National Highway Safety Administration: Adapted from Alcohol and the impaired driver (AMA); **p. 187 (Figure 8-3),** From Wardlaw G: *Perspectives in nutrition,* ed 3, St Louis 1996, Mosby; **p. 191 (Health Action Guide),** Modified from brochure of the Indiana Alcohol Countermeasure Program; **p. 196 (Star Box),** Modified from Woititz JG: *Adult children of alcoholics,* Pompano Beach, FL, 1983, Health Communications,

Inc. In Pinger R, Payne W, Hahn D, Hahn E: *Drugs: issues for today,* St Louis, 1991, Mosby.

Chapter 10: pp. 229 (Figure 10-1), 230 (Star Box), 244 (Health Action Guide), 1995 Heart and Stroke Facts, American Heart Association; **p. 238 (Health Action Guide),** Reproduced with permission, © 1988, American Heart Association: Heart Facts; **p. 240 (Figure 10-4),** 1990 Heart Facts, art by Donald O'Connor; **p. 232,** From Howard E: *Health Risks,* Tucson, 1986, Body Press; **p. 239 (Table 10-1),** Report of the Expert Panel on Detection, Evaluation and Treatment of High Blood Cholesterol in Adults, US Department of Health and Human Services (DHS: NIH Pub No 89-2925), 1989, Washington, DC, US Government Printing Office.

Chapter 11: p. 252 (Figure 11-1), National Cancer Institute: *Horizons of cancer research,* NIH Pub No 89-3011, © 1989; **pp. 253 (Figure 11-2), 254, 258, 260, 265 (Health Action Guides), 263 (Star Box),** Reprinted with permission of the American Cancer Society, Inc; **pp. 256-257,** Modified from American Cancer Society, Inc.; **p. 262 (Health Action Guide),** American Academy of Dermatology; **p. 266 (Table 11-2),** From Hasler CM: *Nutri-News,* St Louis, 1995, Mosby; **p. 271 (Health Action Guide),** courtesy of Allergy and Asthma Network, Mothers of Asthmatics, Inc.

Chapter 12: p. 284, Sources: Centers for Disease Control and Prevention and American Academy of Pediatrics; **p. 288 (Table 12-3),** courtesy of the National Institute of Allergy and Infectious Diseases; **p. 298,** Centers for Disease Control and Prevention, Atlanta.

Chapter 13: p. 331, Modified from *USA Today;* **p. 334 (Health Action Guide),** Adapted from Haas K, Haas A: *Understanding sexuality,* ed 3, St Louis, 1993, Mosby; **p. 335,** Quiz from *The joy of being single,* by Janice Harayda, copyright © 1986 by Janice Harayda, used by permission of Doubleday, a division of Bantam Doubleday, Dell Publishing Group, Inc.

Chapter 14: pp. 346-347 (Table 14-1), Modified from Lisken L, et al: Youth in the 1980s: social and health concerns, Population Reports, Series M, No 9, Population Information Program, Johns Hopkins University, November-December 1985; **p. 348,** From Haas K, Haas A: *Understanding sexuality,* ed 3, St Louis, 1993, Mosby.

Chapter 15: p. 381 (Figure 15-1), First Databank, The Hearst Corporation; **p. 384 (Health Action Guide),** Source: Pell AR: *Making the Most of Medicare,* DCI Publishing, 1990, in *in-synch,* Erie, PA, Spring, 1994, Erie Insurance Group; **p. 389 (Figure 15-2),** Source: SAMSHA News, Vol I, #4, p. 3.

Chapter 16: p. 407 (Figure 16-1), courtesy of the National Committee to Prevent Child Abuse, Chicago, IL; **p. 413 (Health Action Guide),** From the American College Health Association; **p. 416 (Health Action Guide),** Adapted from Pynoos J, Cohen E: *Creative ideas for a safe and livable home,* Washington, DC, American Association of Retired Persons, 1992; and Van Tassel D: *Home, safe home,* St Louis, 1996, GenCare Health Systems.

Chapter 17: pp. 424-425, Modified from *Being green: some tips on how to help the earth*, Scripps Howard News Service; **p. 425 (Figure 17-1)**, Source: UN Population Fund; **p. 426 (Figure 17-2)**, World Resources, 1988-1989; **p. 429 (Table 17-1)**, Source: Water Pollution Control Federation; **p. 437 (Star Box)**, From McGrath M, Dadd DL: *Nontoxic, Natural, and Earthwise*, Los Angeles, 1990, Jeremy P. Tarcher; **p. 440**, logos courtesy of The Wilderness Society, USDA, Forest Service, and Sierra Club; Greenpeace logo courtesy of Greenpeace USA, a nonprofit, environmental organization, 1436 U Street, NW, Washington, DC 10009; Cousteau Society logo used with permission of the Cousteau Society, © 1990, a non-profit, membership-supported organization, dedicated to the protection and improvement of the quality of life for present and future generations.

Chapter 18: **p. 451 (Star Box)**, Reprinted with permission of Concern for Dying, formerly Concern for Dying/Society for the Right to Die, 250 W 57th Street, New York, NY 10107; **p. 460 (Figure 18-1)**, The National Kidney Foundation Uniform Donor Card is reprinted with permission from the National Kidney Foundation, Inc. Copyright 1970, 1991, New York, NY.

Inside back cover: (Ovolactovegetarian food pyramid) Data from Wardlaw GM, Insel PW: *Perspectives in nutrition*, ed 3, St Louis, 1996, Mosby.

Photo Credits

Chapter 1: **pp. 6, 19**, Stewart Halperin; **p. 7**, Ed Self/Photographic Services, Ball State University.

Chapter 2: **pp. 34, 41**, Stewart Halperin.

Chapter 3: **pp. 43, 47**, Stewart Halperin; **pp. 48, 54**, Ed Self/Photographic Services, Ball State University.

Chapter 4: **pp. 68, 82**, Ed Self/Photographic Services, Ball State University; **pp. 71, 74-75, 77, 91**, Stewart Halperin.

Chapter 5: **pp. 92, 94, 125**, Stewart Halperin; **p. 97**, NutraSweet, Monsanto Corp.; **p. 113**, Ed Self/Photographic Services, Ball State University.

Chapter 6: **p. 132**, Linsley Photographics; **p. 136**, Stewart Halperin; **pp. 138, 139**, CLG Photographics.

Chapter 7: **pp. 163, 175**, Stewart Halperin; **p. 167**, From Drug Enforcement Administration: Drugs of abuse, US Department of Justice; **p. 170**, Charles Gupton/The Stock Market; **p. 172**, courtesy of Partnership for a Drug Free America.

Chapter 8: **p. 180**, Stewart Halperin; **p. 184**, From G. Heilman Brewing Company, Inc., LaCrosse, Wisconsin; **p. 188**, George Steinmetz; **p. 195**, Bob Daemmrich/Stock Boston.

Chapter 9: **pp. 203, 207, 215, 219**, Stewart Halperin; **p. 206**, Ed Self/Photographic Services, Ball State University; **p. 213**, Courtesy of American Cancer Society.

Chapter 10: **p. 235**, Richard Hirneisen/The Stock Shop.

Chapter 11: **p. 259**, Stewart Halperin; **pp. 261, 262**, From Thibodeau G, Patton K: *Anatomy & physiology*, ed 3, St Louis, 1996, Mosby; **p. 262**, From Habif TP: *Clinical dermatology*, ed 3, St Louis, 1996, Mosby; **pp. 264, 270**, CLG Photographics.

Chapter 12: **p. 290**, courtesy of Dr. Farrar: *Slide atlas of infectious diseases, 2/e*; **p. 294**, courtesy of Beth and William Kenk; **pp. 300, 301**, Centers for Disease Control and Prevention.

Chapter 13: **p. 330**, CLG Photographics.

Chapter 14: **p. 349**, Courtesy of Ortho Pharmaceutical Corp.; **p. 350**, Courtesy of Apothocus, Inc.; **pp. 351 (left), 355**, Stewart Halperin; **pp. 351 (right), 353 (top)**, Laura J. Edwards; **p. 353 (bottom)**, Courtesy of the Alza Corporation; **p. 353 (left)**, Linsley Photographics; **p. 357**, Courtesy of Wyeth-Ayerst Laboratories; **p. 363**, Photo Researchers; **p. 365**, Science Photo Library/Photo Researchers.

Chapter 16: **pp. 406, 412**, CLG Photographics.

Chapter 17: **p. 431**, Norbert Wu; **p. 433**, Greig Granna/Stock Boston.

Chapter 18: **p. 450**, The Gamma Liaison Network; **p. 454**, CLG Photographics.

Index

Page numbers in italics indicate illustrations; *t* indicates tables.

Index

I-11

Health Reference Guide

EMOTIONAL HEALTH

National Institute of Mental Health
Public Inquiries Branch
5600 Fishers Lane
Room 15C-05
Rockville, MD 20857
(301) 443-4513
www.nimh.nih.gov

National Mental Health Association
1021 Prince Street
Alexandria, VA 22314
(800) 969-6642
(703) 684-7722
(416) 484-7750 (Canada)
www.worldcorp.com/dc-online/nmha

Recovery, Inc.
Association of Nervous and Former
Mental Patients
802 N. Dearborn
Chicago, IL 60610
(312) 337-5661

FITNESS AND NUTRITION

**National Eating Disorders
Organization (NEDO)**
6655 S. Yale Ave.
Tulsa, OK 74136
(918) 481-4044

**President's Council on Physical
Fitness and Sports**
701 Pennsylvania Ave., N.W.
Suite 250
Washington, D.C. 20004
(202) 272-3430

**TOPS Club, Inc. (Take Off Pounds
Sensibly)**
P.O. Box 07360
Milwaukee, WI 53207
(414) 482-4620
www.tops.org

Weight Watchers International, Inc.
(516) 390-1400

SUBSTANCE ABUSE

**Al-Anon Family Group
Headquarters, Inc.**
P.O. Box 862
Midtown Station
New York, NY 10018-0862
(800) 344-2666 (USA)
(800) 245-4656 (New York)
(800) 443-4525 (Canada)

Alcohol and Drug Referral Line
(800) ALCOHOL

Alcoholics Anonymous
P.O. Box 459
Grand Central Station
New York, NY 10163
(212) 870-3400
(416) 487-5591 (Canada)
www.alcoholics.anonymous.org

Scripps Memorial Hospital
McDonald Center
9904 Genesee Avenue
La Jolla, CA 92037
(619) 626-4300

**Mothers Against Drunk Driving
(MADD)**
(214) 744-6233
(800) 438-6233 (24-hour hotline for
victims only)

National Cocaine Hotline
P.O. Box 100
Summit, NJ 07902
(800) COCAINE

**National Council on Alcoholism and
Drug Dependence Hope Line**
(800) 622-2255

Remove Intoxicated Drivers (RID)
(518) 372-0034

**Students Against Driving Drunk
(SADD)**
(508) 481-3568

CONDITIONS AND DISEASES

AIDS Information Hotline
(800) 342-AIDS
(800) 344-7432 (Spanish)
(800) 243-7889 (TDD)
(416) 972-6281 (Canada)

**Centers for Disease Control National
AIDS Clearinghouse**
(800) 458-5231
www.cdcnac.aspensys.com:86

American Cancer Society
1599 Clifton Road, N.E.
Atlanta, GA 30329
(800) 227-2345
(416) 961-7223 (Canada)
www.cancer.org

American Diabetes Association
(800) 232-3472
(703) 549-1500 (Virginia)
(416) 362-4440 (Canada)

American Heart Association
(800) 242-8721
(514) 482-3407 (Canada)
www.amhrt.org

American Kidney Fund
(800) 638-8299
(800) 492-8361 (Maryland)
(301) 881-3052
www.arbon.com\kidney

American Lung Association
(800) LUNG-USA
(613) 747-6776 (Canada)
www.lungusa.org
info@lungusa.org

American Red Cross
(202) 737-8300

**Asthma & Allergy Foundation of
America**
(800) 7-ASTHMA
(202) 265-0265
(416) 244-9312 (Canada)

NCI Cancer Information Service
(800) 4-CANCER
(800) 638-6070 (Alaska)
(808) 524-1234
(202) 636-5700 (Washington, D.C.)
(416) 961-7223 (Canada)
www.nci.nih.gov

Center for Sickle Cell Disease
(202) 806-7930

**Centers for Disease Control and
Prevention**
1600 Clifton Road, N.E.
Atlanta, GA 30333
(404) 639-3286

CDC National STD Hotline
(800) 227-8922

American Social Health Association
(for information about STDs)
(919) 361-8400
www.sunsite.unc.edu/asha

Juvenile Diabetes Foundation
International Hotline
(800) 223-1138
(212) 889-7575 (New York)
(800) 668-0274 (Canada)
(416) 889-4171 (Canada)

Leukemia Society of America, Inc.
(800) 955-4LSA
www.leukemia.org

Lungline Information Service
(800) 222-LUNG
www.njc.org

**March of Dimes Birth Defects
Foundation**
(914) 428-7100
www.modimes.org

Medic Alert Foundation
(800) 344-3226

National Association for Sickle Cell Disease
(800) 421-8453

National Headache Foundation
(800) 843-2256
(312) 878-7715
(800) 663-3557 (Canada)
(416) 920-4916 (Canada)

PMS Access
(800) 222-4PMS

Y-ME National Breast Cancer Organization
(800) 221-2141
www.y-me.org

SEXUALITY, THE FAMILY, AND FERTILITY CONTROL

Child Help USA/Child Abuse Hotline
(800) 422-4453
(705) 526-5647 (Canada)

National Childwatch
4065 Page Ave.
P.O. Box 1368
Jackson, MI 49204
(800) 222-1464

National Abortion Federation
Consumer Hotline
(800) 772-9100
(202) 546-9060

National Center for Missing & Exploited Children
2101 Wilson Blvd.
Suite 550
Arlington, VA 22201
(800) 843-5678
(703) 235-3900
(800) 826-7653 (hearing impaired line)

National Committee to Prevent Child Abuse
(800) 55NCPCA
(312) 663-3520

National Runaway Switchboard
(800) 621-4000
(312) 880-9860

SIDS Alliance (Sudden Infant Death Syndrome)
(800) 221-SIDS
(410) 964-8000 (Maryland)
(416) 488-3260 (Canada)

Parents Anonymous
(for abusive parents)
(909) 621-6184
hn3831@handsmet.org

Parents Without Partners, Inc.
International Headquarters
401 N. Michigan Ave.
Chicago, IL 60611-4267
(800) 637-7974

Planned Parenthood Federation of America
810 7th Avenue
New York, NY 10019
(800) 829-7732
(613) 238-4474 (Canada)
www.ppfa.org/ppfa

Runaway Hotline
(800) 231-6946
(800) 392-3352 (Texas)

Women Against Rape
P.O. Box 02084
Columbus, OH 43202
(614) 221-4447 (crisis phone)
(614) 291-9751 (business office)

Rape Education and Prevention Center
408 Ohio Union
1739 High Street
Columbus, OH 43210
(614) 292-0479
repp@life1.saa.ohio-state.edu

Rape Abuse Shelter Hotline
(800) 548-2480 (Missouri)
NOTE: Check local yellow pages for a rape crisis listing in your area. There is no national hotline number; any of the above three numbers can refer you state-by-state to a local rape crisis center.

National Domestic Violence Hotline
(800) 799-SAFE

CONSUMER AND ENVIRONMENTAL SAFETY

DOT Auto Safety Hotline
(800) 424-9393
(202) 366-0123 (Washington, D.C.)
www.nhtsa.dot.gov

U.S. Consumer Product Safety Commission Hotline
Washington, D.C.
(800) 638-CPSC
(613) 238-2533 (Canada)

Energy Conservation
(800) 428-2525
www.erecbbs.nciinc.com

Environmental Protection Agency (EPA)
PM 211-B
401 M Street, S.W.
Washington, D.C. 20460
(202) 260-2080 (Public Information Center)
(202) 260-7751
www.epa.gov

U.S. Department of Transportation
National Highway Traffic Safety Administration
Office of Public and Consumer Affairs
400 7th Street, S.W.
Room 5232
Washington, D.C. 20590
(202) 366-9550

THE MATURING ADULT

Alzheimer's Association
919 N. Michigan Ave.
Suite 1000
Chicago, IL 60611
(800) 272-3900
(312) 335-8700
(312) 335-8882 TDD
(416) 925-3552 (Canada)
www.alz.org/
develop@alz.org

American Association of Retired Persons (AARP)
601 E. Street, N.W.
Washington, D.C. 20049
(800) 424-3410
(202) 434-2277
(613) 728-9347 (Canada)
www.aarp.org

Arthritis Consulting Services
(800) 327-3027
(416) 967-1414 (Canada)
www.newreach.net/acs
arthritis@juno.com

Choice in Dying
(800) 989-WILL
(212) 366-5540
www.choices.org

Living Bank
(800) 528-2971

Medic Alert Foundation
(800) 344-3226
(209) 668-3333
(800) 668-1507 (Canada)
(416) 696-0267 (Canada)

United Network for Organ Sharing
(800) 24-DONOR (Organ Donor Information Line)
(613) 727-1380 (Canada)
NOTE: Check your local directory for additional information on poison control, suicide prevention, Social Security, and for additional Canadian resources.